Health Care of Women

HEALTH CARE OF WOMEN

Leonide L. Martin, R.N., M.S.
Family Nurse Practitioner
Lecturer, Department of Nursing
Sonoma State College
Rohnert Park, California

J. B. LIPPINCOTT COMPANY
Philadelphia
New York   San Jose   Toronto

Distributed in Great Britain by
Blackwell Scientific Publications
London   Oxford   Edinburgh

ISBN 0-397-54219-4

Library of Congress Catalog Card Number 78-15633

Printed in the United States of America
2   4   6   8   9   7   5   3   1

Library of Congress Cataloging in Publication Data

Martin, Leonide L
  Health care of women.

  Includes index.
    1. Gynecologic nursing.   2. Obstetrical nursing.
I. Title.
RG105.M34   610.73′678   78-15633
ISBN 0-397-54219-4

Preface

As nursing roles evolve, additional responsibilities and functions fall within the scope of professional practice. With the expansion of nursing practice, there are many opportunities for nurses to respond creatively to women's health care needs. In assuming major responsibility for the management of normal pregnancy and postpartum, nurses can incorporate education on childbearing and provide support for exploration of family concerns and problems. Contraception can be provided with respect for individual choices and life styles, and with dangers as well as benefits honestly discussed. With full information, women and their partners can make better choices in terms of their values and priorities. Common health problems of women can be given the attention they deserve, and a thorough assessment combined with careful attention to emotional and informational needs enables the nurse to provide a high level of comprehensive care. Serious illnesses can be responded to with consideration of the entire range of human needs when the nurse, physician, and other professionals collaborate as a team in the management of complex problems.

This work is undertaken to create a new kind of text for nurses, not bound by old concepts about appropriate content and organization. It is a response to recent developments in nursing and health care, and to the evolution of ideas. Women do not separate childbearing and gynecological problems from other aspects of their lives, and they need practitioners who will respond to many types of concerns with deep understanding of the experience of being female. Nurses no longer wish to separate physiological and psychosocial aspects of patients' needs for health care, and are seeking greater authority to participate directly in all aspects of care. This book will encompass the common health needs and problems of women seen in primary ambulatory care, and will approach these from the viewpoint of the practitioner.

There are several features of this book which make it especially useful to the nurse in ambulatory settings. The general approach in presenting material follows the pattern encountered by the practitioner in actually providing care. The patient does not present with an established diagnosis, but with a complex of symptoms or concerns. The practitioner must then reason from these data, gathering more information through the process of history-taking, physical examination, and diagnostic testing. The complete data base is then combined to arrive at the diagnosis or assessment of the patient's problem, and a plan for treatment formulated, implemented, and evaluated. The chapters in the book are organized around such symptom complexes or patient concerns, and information unfolded in the logical sequence of the care process.

Greater depth in history-taking and physical assessment pertinent to the particular problem than found in most nursing texts is included, to provide a knowledge base congruent with the practitioner's increased responsibilities for patient care. The many details of clinical management, and specifics of decision-making in each stage of the care process, are emphasized because these are the crux of clinical judgment. A foundation is provded for the practitioner to assume a high level of responsibility and to deliver complete patient care in the areas of developmental concerns, preventive health needs, and common illnesses of women in primary care settings.

Knowledge of physical assessment skills, the ability to perform a complete physical examination, familiarity with systematic history-taking, and a basic nursing background are assumed. The book is primarily intended for nurses assuming expanded responsibilities in the management of patient care. It will be most useful to practicing nurses who are responsible for the care of women, and for educational programs which prepare them. This material will also be helpful as an adjunct to basic texts, particularly as baccalaureate nursing programs are moving toward greater inclusion of physical diagnosis and nursing management in the curricula.

It is recognized that not all possible health needs of women are included, for these extend into many areas of highly specialized knowledge, but all endeavors must have their limits. Although this work focuses primarily upon women, men and children constitute an important part of most women's lives and thus must be included in consideration of certain problems. However, their needs and concerns will not receive the extensive consideration given to women's problems.

Leonide L. Martin, R.N., M.S.

Acknowledgments

A simple and heartfelt thanks to Avner Perry, Ph.D., for his belief in the importance of this effort and collaboration in creating the life space necessary to carry it out. His multitalented assistance in researching the literature, reviewing content, suggesting manuscript revisions, photography and preparation of illustrations, and general encouragement was invaluable.

I am also indebted to Len Hughes Andrus, M.D., Chairman of the Department of Family Practice at the University of California, Davis, School of Medicine for his assistance in reviewing the manuscript for accuracy, currency and applicability in the overlapping areas of patient care management shared by nursing and medicine.

Without the enthusiastic support of Mr. David T. Miller, Managing Editor of the Nursing Department, J. B. Lippincott Company, this work would not have been launched. His continuing interest and assistance made possible the transition from concept to reality.

Contents

Introduction

Women want more from health care than the system is presently providing them. Quantitavely, women need greater access to care, particularly comprehensive and ongoing primary care. Qualitatively, women desire health care which is more sensitive to the experience of being a woman in contemporary society. Increasingly, women are expecting to receive honest and complete information from health providers, to be a central part of decision-making which affects their bodies and lives, and to be treated with respect as adults fully capable of understanding their health problems and responsible for their own destinies.

Much of what is included in women's care concerns the exercise or control of normal physiological processes. Pregnancy and childbirth are natural conditions, though relatively infrequent during a lifetime, and not pathological events. The changes and difficulties associated with the menstrual cycle, including menopause, frequently prompt women to seek medical care. Although disease may be present, more typically the woman's symptoms are related to physiological variations or dysfunctions. Contraception involves the woman's control of her own body, and reflects her desire to decide on its uses. Concerns related to sexuality also involve a natural human function. For many of these conditions, the treatment indicated is counseling, education, support, and assistance rather than highly technical, expensive procedures. Woman want to play a decisive part in decisions related to these conditions, and do not want them inappropriately labeled as illness.

The provider's response to women's needs in both health maintenance and the treatment of illness must take into account recent social and attitudinal changes related to women's roles. Shrinkage of the proportion of a woman's lifetime which is monopolized by childbearing and raising children is having a profound effect upon family patterns. Having fewer children, with her last child often born by the mid-20s, today's woman finds herself in her late 30s with mothering no longer an all-consuming use of her energies. Technological advances have freed her from hours of household chores, so homemaking no longer provides her a full-time occupation. Her lifespan has lengthened and her state of health has improved, so at age 35 to 40 she is healthy and vigorous, looking ahead to another 20 to 25 productive years in which mothering and homemaking cannot utilize all of her time and energy.

Changes in values among a significant number of people also helped to expand the options open to women. It was once necessary for a woman to make a choice between family and career; now women increasingly combine these spheres of life as men have always been privileged to do. Many types of work previously closed off to women are opening gradually. Federal statutes support equal treatment of women workers, and although change is slow, there is a mechanism to challenge discrimination and unfair employment practices which often served to discourage women from pursuing certain occupational commitments. Antidiscrimination laws also are having significant impact on educational institutions, forcing a gradual change in the social bias toward male privilege perpetuated through values taught in primary and secondary schools, and culminating in the admissions practices and sex-linked career choices fostered by colleges.

Growing numbers of women no longer accept traditional definitions of female identity and women's roles. They seek a more individualized definition of self that offers a wide range for expression of their unique characteristics, whether "masculine" or "feminine" in traditional terms. The common qualities shared by women and men are felt to far outweigh their sex-related differences. Social roles providing each sex with a wider range of behaviors are seen as promoting human potential. Such women expect more choices of life style to be open to them: they may marry or not, have children or not, pursue any career suited to their individual talents and interests, have access to high level decision-making positions, and enjoy economic and social rights on an equal footing with men.

Between the traditional "feminine" woman whose identity is established in the wife-mother role and the radical "feminist" woman who would erase all sex-linked distinctions and completely restructure family and social patterns, there are all shades of variation. Women seeking health care represent the entire spectrum, and the provider must be open to responding at many levels to the patient's needs. Awareness of women's history and the continuous process of social change enables providers to develop flexibility and understanding in their approach to their female patients.

The push to change health care is part of this larger evolution toward more equitable distribution of rights and recognition of human potential. Changes are reflected in the achievements of the civil rights movement, the women's movement, and the rise of consumer rights which have occurred over the last two decades. Conflict is developing between professionals and their clients in many fields, including nursing, medicine, law, teaching, city planning and others. Professionals no longer can exercise sole province over their bodies of knowledge and practice standards. Clients want consideration of personal needs, individualized attention, and a greater voice in decisions of vital importance to themselves.

Women's health problems and needs have, in recent time, been handled largely by a specialty of males (about 95 percent of all gynecologists are men[1]). History reveals that this was not always so, however; the fields of maternity and women's problems had been primarily the domain of female midwives and healers until the late nineteenth century. Then the male physicians took over, incorporating women's care into the general format of medical practice. The revival of the women's movement in the early 1970s brought increasing dissatisfaction with health care in general and gynecologists in particular. Women often feel forced into the socially approved feminine role of passive submission to the male physician's authority. Dependency is commonly enforced by the withholding or selective sharing of information and plans, and the intimation that the patient is incapable of making appropriate decisions about treatment. The woman also may feel vulnerable to humiliation through a depersonalized access to her most intimate thoughts and body parts, or through judgments or decisions made about her reflecting personal bias or social values. The fear of personal suffering also may be present, as an unsympathetic physician could cause the woman greater pain in examinations, unnecessary suffering in childbirth, or greater risks of complications during gynecological procedures. Anger and resentment toward the physician, nurse or other health provider is often the result of such experiences, accompanied by the demand for alternative types of health care.

The nurse is in a particularly favorable position to bring about many of the changes women desire in their health care. As an occupational group consisting mainly of women, nurses have a built-in propensity to understand and respond empathetically to women's concerns. Men in nursing also have an advantage in responding sensitively to women's health needs, through their close association with many women and the socialization process of the profession. Professional norms and values internalized through nursing education emphasize the patient as an individual and promote practice which considers the person's unique needs, relation to the family and community, psychological and social factors as well as physical, and concentrate much of nursing care on the meaning and impact of illness rather than the illness itself. Nursing also emphasizes education about health and maintenance of well-being as a major function of the profession. The teaching and counseling aspects of nursing, and the involvement of patient, family and community in the planning and treatment of illness, are areas of professional focus which distinguish nursing from medicine and other health professions.

Nurses can continue this humanistic approach to patient care, but with an additional dimension previously not well developed in nursing practice: the responsibility for the full range of care for an appropriate patient population. With the knowledge base and necessary skills to assess physical as well as

---

[1]Nelson, Alix, "Sexual Bias in Medicine," *The New York Times Book Review*, August 28, 1977, p. 13. A review of *Women's Health Care: The Hidden Malpractice*, by Gena Corea, William Morrow & Co., New York; and *Doctors Wanted: No Women Need Apply*, by Mary Roth Walsh, Yale University Press, New Haven.

psychosocial problems at a sophisticated level, nurse practitioners and other nurses are able to fill a new position in the health care delivery structure. They have become primary providers, with direct patient access, individual or shared practices, and can assume complete responsibility for patient care within the boundaries of their expertise. By merging nursing and medical knowledge, a quality of care can be offered which is not achievable by either profession alone.

The major purpose of this book is to bring together information needed by nurses, information which usually must be sought in a variety of texts, clinical references, periodicals, and pamphlets, or is common but largely unwritten practice knowledge. In recognizing that people do not separate their health needs into physical and emotional realms, an effort is made to bridge both physiological and psychological components of care. The emphasis of the content is on primary care in the ambulatory setting. Increasingly, the health system is shifting focus from inpatient hospital care after disease is established or critical to community-based care which identifies disease in earlier, more treatable stages or seeks to prevent illness and maintain health. Primary care encompasses the initial contact for care, continuous care over time to people in various states of health and illness, and the responsibility and coordination for the entire spectrum of care including maintenance and promotion of health, management of illness, restoration of health or rehabilitation, and a system of referral for more specialized services.[2] Nursing functions and responsibilities are expanding rapidly in the primary care field. The care of patients in ambulatory settings within their communities holds promise for nursing to have major impact on improving our nation's health.

[2]Nursing's Role in the Delivery of Primary Care—A Position Paper. Western Council on Higher Education for Nursing, Boulder, Colorado, October, 1976, p. 1.

1

Health Maintenance
for Women

The goal of health care is to restore and maintain the highest possible level of health for the individual. Because our health care system is far from perfect, people enter at various points along a continuum from elective screening, when completely asymptomatic, to emergency life-sustaining measures, when critically ill. A significant proportion of the efforts and resources in the health care field is directed toward correction or alleviation of disease and injury once these have occurred. Relatively little is allotted to the early detection of disease before symptoms are produced, and even less to a determination of future risk or prevention. There are many complex reasons why we really have a "disease care system" rather than a health care system, including professional values, social attitudes, and economic forces. However, evidence mounts that there is a growing emphasis on the prevention of disease and the maintenance of health, rather than just the management of illness.

Far-reaching changes are needed in our health (illness) care system, in order to reduce its escalating costs, inefficiency, lack of continuity, maldistribution of resources, and its numerous gaps in responding to the public's needs for care. The role of nurse practitioner has emerged as one response to this demand for change, with the hope that services would be made more widely available and that the care would include a greater concern for the prevention of disease and the promotion of health. In considering expectations of the health care system, what medicine can provide in the treatment of illness, where responsibility for various components of social and individual health needs lies, and what people are seeking when they enter the health system, it is evident that confusion and conflict in goals, purposes, and intent are rampant.

In the past, individuals had to accept the full responsibility for most, if not all, of their own care during illnesses. Family, experienced friends, and clergy were the main sources of help when illness struck. Even if physicians or nurses were available, the science of medicine was primitive and could offer little more than could the ministrations of concerned others. Gradually, technology and research enabled medicine to provide more definitive treatment for certain types of illnesses. Society as a whole became involved in the control of sanitary conditions and epidemics, then increasingly in environmental and occupational hazards and in subsidizing the health system. As medicine and society took over the management of more and more health problems, folk knowledge about how to care for illness at home was slowly lost. People now turn to the health system for every type of problem from the common cold, boils, and diarrhea to emotional crises, obesity, and alcoholism. The health system, however, concentrates on the type of illness to which therapy can be applied effectively, such as removing the cause of the illness through eradication of microorganisms by drugs; repairing damage by setting fractures

1

and suturing lacerations; or replacing or correcting malfunctioning parts, for example, insulin for diabetics, antihypertensive drugs, prosthetics, and surgery for diseased organs. And it is creaking under present demand.

It is time to return the knowledge of health care measures to the people. When people understand their bodies, their normal physiological functioning and adaptive responses, when they know how to treat and alleviate minor symptoms and how to recognize truly serious problems, they are able to use the health system appropriately.

Many minor ills and common human miseries cannot be more effectively treated by prescriptions provided by the health care system than by home remedies. It is thus an unnecessary cost to patients and a drain on the health system to attempt treatment of these problems through the system. And many of the diseases with real organic pathology are caused by habits and practices of living, the control of which rests entirely within the choice and will of the individual. Health care providers cannot assume responsibility for the conduct of their clients' lives, nor should patients give over the responsibility for their health to the providers. But, in order to accept and carry out their responsibility for their own health maintenance, people must have knowledge. Sharing knowledge about health and illness is one of the basic requirements of health maintenance.

The nurse practitioner is in a key position to provide health maintenance. Emphasis on primary care and health maintenance was integral to the development of the nurse practitioner's role. By tradition the nurse is concerned about the whole patient, in both health and illness, and nurses have always tried to help patients and their families cope with health problems and with the impact of illness. It is a logical extension of this orientation for the nurse practitioner to assist people to recognize health risks and to take action to prevent illness. With direct access to patients in a way not possible before, with credibility because of pathophysiological knowledge, with real authority and decision-making power in the health system, the nurse practitioner brings expertise from both nursing and medicine to the patient encounter. A knowledge of the natural history and management of disease is combined with knowledge of teaching, counseling, and interpersonal dynamics. With a philosophy of pro-

vider accountability and patient responsibility and a commitment to both health teaching and disease management, the nurse practitioner has the opportunity as well as the background to act as a strong advocate for health maintenance.

DEFINITION OF HEALTH

The meaning of health and illness is determined culturally, with varying definitions of abnormality as well as expected behaviors when one is sick. A universal definition is thus elusive. Within the United States the meaning of health and illness is different according to, for example, social class, ethnic subculture, age, and personal beliefs. However, there is usually some picture of wholeness or soundness of body and mind implicit in the concept of health. In 1947 the World Health Organization defined health as "a state of complete physical, emotional, and social well-being, and not merely the absence of disease or infirmity."[1] An unattainable ideal seems implied in this definition, for occasional dysfunction and some degree of disability are inevitable components of life, at least as it is attainable today. This definition also raises the question whether a person is diseased at any point short of the epitome of physiological functioning and the zenith of mental health. Obviously, few of us achieve these heights, particularly for any length of time.

The social environment must also be taken into account, because detrimental social or occupational factors can cause both physical and psychological illness. All body systems may be functioning normally, but distorted behavior may place the person at variance with the social structure, leading to types of "dis-ease" such as delinquency, violence, child abuse, addiction, neurosis, and psychosis. Organic disease frequently occurs in people living in unfavorable environments. The poor are known to have a higher incidence of illness, and certain occupations are associated with particular diseases due to a high risk of injury or exposure to carcinogens. A life style with excessive stress is increasingly implicated in several diseases, including cardiovascular and endocrine disease.

Health, then, can be conceptualized as freedom from disease, dysfunction, and disability insofar as these interfere with a person's functioning effectively in a particular environment. It is a state of ecological balance between a person's internal and external environment:

> Health is a state of feeling well in body, mind, and spirit, together with a sense of reserve power; based upon normal functioning of the tissues, a practical understanding of the principles of healthy living, a harmonious adjustment to the environment (physical and psychological); it is a means to a richer life.[2]

Instead of perceiving health as a static or perfect state, we must review it as a dynamic ever-changing process, in which the person has the opportunity to grow, develop, and improve. Individual potential can be maximized by maintaining a purposeful direction and harmony with the functional environment. The healthy person does not exist passively in the environment, but constantly appraises possibilities, weighs choices, plans and takes action to create change; in short, creatively attains comfort and satisfaction—the concept of "high-level wellness."[3] People are part of ecological systems, open, active, ever evolving, and interacting in totality with their environment. Harmony, wholeness, social integration, and affectional ties must be balanced with challenge, stimulation, conflict, and the drive for self-determination.

CONCEPTS OF HEALTH MAINTENANCE

In its broadest sense, health maintenance includes all activities to prevent illness or minimize its effects, and to promote well-being. Within this scope are public education, individual teaching, preventive health measures, improvement of the level of wellness, reduction of disability and distress, screening for early diagnosis and treatment, and prediction of risks for the avoidance of disease or the reduction of death or disability. The overall goal of health maintenance is to help people live healthier and more satisfying lives, both physically and emotionally.

Society practices health maintenance through its public health agencies by informing the public about current dangers, such as new strains of flu, rabies outbreaks, or measles epidemics. Preventive care may also be provided through public immunization programs for flu and measles and by local drives to promote special rabies vaccination clinics for dogs and cats. One of the mainstays of preventive care is immunization against childhood illness, which is widely practiced in both private and public health care institutions. The teaching and counseling aspect of health maintenance is very important and encompasses both information about healthy living patterns and education about special diseases such as cancer, heart disease, and diabetes. Balanced nutrition is a growing public and professional concern, as the relation of foodstuffs to a myriad of diseases is gradually deciphered. Dietary management is central in the prevention and control of such diseases as diabetes, hyperlipoproteinemia, obesity (which is associated with hypertension, low back pain and other musculoskeletal problems, and diabetes), gout, anemia, and allergies. The relation of the American diet—rich in saturated fats and refined sugar and low in roughage and fiber—to such diseases as hypertension, myocardial infarction, atherosclerosis, diabetes, colonic and rectal cancer, breast cancer, and other chronic degenerative diseases is under considerable scrutiny.

Environmental dangers and occupational hazards are being increasingly identified and linked to specific diseases. The relation of smoking to the incidence of lung cancer and heart attack is well documented. Chronic obstructive pulmonary disease in the forms of chronic bronchitis and emphysema, often closely connected to smoking, causes considerable morbidity and decreases the quality and comfort of life in those afflicted. Workers in asbestos plants have a greatly increased risk of asbestosis, lung cancer, mesothelioma and other cancers. The carcinogenic properties of radiation, policyclic hydrocarbons, metabolites of some dyes, nitrosamines, excessive ethyl alcohol, vinyl chloride, ultraviolet light, silica, herpesvirus type II, and many other chemicals and industrial fumes place industrial workers and other persons exposed to these agents at increased risk of developing various types of cancer. Health maintenance in many of these instances depends upon government regulations and industrial standards, augmented by the efforts of individuals through unions and other organizations to demand conditions of safety for workers and for the public. Health providers are responsible for educating patients and disseminating information about environmental hazards, for important follow-up, and for advising against future exposure.

As factors which indicate a high or low incidence of a certain disease are identified, it is the health provider's obligation to keep up-to-date. This new information is then used for the patient's benefit through appropriate screening and risk appraisal procedures. Through this process, the annual Pap smear and the monthly breast self-examination have become common, widely used screening procedures to detect cervical and breast cancer in women at early stages when cure is most likely. Certain characteristics of a woman's past history and family history have been found to be predictive of an increased or decreased risk of these two diseases (see Chapter 13, Breast Masses and Chapter 14, Abnormal Pap Smears), and the provider can use this information to identify risk and to educate the patient about future risk and risk reduction.

Helping the patient to gain greater knowledge about the self and the body during each phase of development is a step toward high-level wellness. Worry and concern over different, but normal, body sensations and feelings, changes which accompany various life stages, and unhealthy practices due to misinformation or ignorance can be minimized or prevented through patient education. Dangerous habits can be avoided or stopped. Positive behaviors to promote health, such as good nutrition, adequate exercise, weight control, and a balance between stimulation and rest, can be encouraged.

Prevention and Prediction

Preventive maintenance is a well-established concept in a technological society for complex, expensive machinery such as computers, airplanes, and automobiles. Periodic servicing to maintain efficient function and to prevent deterioration of these machines is as standard as major repairs during breakdowns. For people, this concept is not nearly as widely accepted, despite the common knowledge that many diseases can be prevented or minimized by early intervention. However, in many large industries and the military, periodic health maintenance examinations for executives and key personnel are standard practice. These programs have demonstrated a significantly decreased disability and a continued productivity of management personnel.[4]

Medical literature has contained articles advocating periodic health examinations for over 100 years, and in 1922, the American Medical Association adopted a resolution recommending such examinations. They are of demonstrated effectiveness in the detection of disease, case finding, health surveillance, and disease monitoring. In a long-term study of the value of multiphasic health check-ups on adults done by Kaiser-Permanente, these check-ups were associated with significantly lower death rates from potentially postponable causes for adults age 35 to 54 and were cost-effective for middle-aged men as measured by their decreased disability and increased earning capacity. Health maintenance organizations (HMOs) have utilized periodic health examinations as a mode of entry into the health care system. These examinations enable the providers to identify their patients' health and sick care needs, to initiate additional diagnostic studies and treatment, and to offer referral services. These organizations call upon the appropriate professional resources to meet the patients' needs rather than having the patients arrange for the services they think are needed.[5]

Under the umbrella of health maintenance, many different approaches are included whose goals may range from screening for the early detection of specific diseases to the development of a comprehensive patient profile which predicts individual risks of contracting certain diseases in the future. Some of the different methods are discussed below.

SCREENING   is directed at an apparently well population in order to identify unrecognized disease or the risk of disease through the use of tests, examinations, or other procedures which can be rapidly applied. Screening differentiates people who probably have a disease from those who probably do not, but screening tests and procedures are not meant to be diagnostic. People with positive or suspicious findings are referred to physicians or other providers for diagnosis and treatment. Pap smears, blood pressure, tonometry, stool guiuac, and blood tests for sickle cell trait are all common screening tests and procedures.

MULTIPHASIC TESTING   is the application of a combination of screening tests to large groups of people, and it is often combined with a physical examination for the "multiphasic check-up." A self-administered history, the battery of tests, and a physical examination are analyzed, and follow-up care is provided, including any special procedures needed to establish a final diagnosis and indicate a line of treatment. Prepaid and enrollment health care plans, such as Kaiser-Permanente and HMOs, often use multiphasic testing.

DIAGNOSTIC EVALUATION is frequently an outcome of screening, or it may be directed toward patients who present with problems. The objective here is to diagnose the problem underlying the abnormal screening test or the patient's symptoms and to seek a resolution of this problem.

A PERIODIC HEALTH EXAMINATION usually includes a complete history, a physical examination, and selected laboratory tests. Generally it is part of a personal or organization-sponsored preventive health maintenance program which seeks to establish a medical data base, detect disease at an early stage, and provide health education and counseling. It is called periodic because it is done at regular intervals, usually yearly. The "annual check-up" is another term for a periodic health examination. In these examinations, the extent of the evaluation varies considerably.[6,7]

PREDICTIVE HEALTH CARE is directed toward the identification of the future risk of disease or disability and the establishment of prognostic characteristics for the development of such illnesses. It also includes recommendations of methods for reducing individual risk. This anticipatory approach is also called "prospective medicine." The identification of profiles which find people at risk for certain types of cancer, heart disease, or diabetes is one approach to predictive health care. The most comprehensive approach is the Health Hazard Appraisal approach developed at Methodist Hospital of Indiana. The objective of this approach is to identify specific risks of death and disease by comparing data from the history, physical examination, and selected laboratory tests of patients with charts showing the leading causes of death by age, sex, and race. The goal is to predict risks before the onset of diseases (or in the early asymptomatic stages) so the provider can use health counseling and teaching to change patients' habits and behaviors, with the

hope of preventing or minimizing disease. Early treatment can also be instituted, thus preventing some of the serious consequences of disease.[8]

While the concept of health maintenance is widely embraced, the state of the art is in the beginning stages of development. Accurate and specific predictive factors are often hard to identify, and there are many diseases for which no good treatment exists, even if they are diagnosed early. Caution in promoting the benefits of periodic health examinations or of screening has been advised in order to avoid making implicit promises which cannot be kept. For example, a negative screening test may be taken to indicate that all is well and that the patient need not worry about the condition for which he or she is being screened. While this is generally true for a negative Pap smear (given the natural history of cervical carcinoma, the chances are excellent that a woman with a negative Pap smear need not worry for several months or years), it is certainly not true for a normal electrocardiogram (the classic case being the man who is admitted to the coronary care unit with a myocardial infarction one month after a normal ECG).

The effects on the patient and his or her family of detecting an incurable disease early, the changes in life style and self-concept which may result when a diagnostic label is applied, and the worry and expense in following up false positive screening tests must all be considered. Another concern is the allotment of limited health care resources to evaluating the "worried well" which might be better applied to the treatment of the symptomatic sick. Suggestions for meeting these considerations include using efficient screening tools for certain populations with known risks and improving the sensitivity and specificity of history taking, physical examinations, and laboratory tests. The following criteria have been developed to justify screening for a given disease:

1. The disease must have a significant effect on the quality or length of life.
2. Acceptable methods of treatment must be available.
3. The disease must have an asymptomatic period during which detection and treatment reduce morbidity or mortality.
4. Treatment in the asymptomatic phase must yield a therapeutic result superior to

that obtained by delaying treatment until symptoms appear.

5. Tests must be available at reasonable cost to detect the condition in the asymptomatic period.
6. The incidence of the condition must be sufficient to justify the cost of screening.[9]

These rigorous criteria have been applied to current screening practices, an action which has led to specific recommendations for 36 selected diseases and a longitudinal screening program for asymptomatic adults. Some of the results of this study are startling (see pp. 24-28), because some commonly used screening techniques, for instance x-ray examination of the chest for lung cancer and urine or blood tests for diabetes in the asymptomatic adult, fail to meet all the criteria and are therefore not recommended. Other criteria suggested for screening tests are that compliance following early diagnosis must be enough to alter the natural history of the disease, that long-term beneficial effects must outweigh long-term detrimental effects, that benefits to a community at large must withstand scientific scrutiny, and that screening procedures must be integrated into a system of care which provides treatment and follow-up.[10,11]

Health Maintenance in Daily Practice

The health provider may place special emphasis on health maintenance by incorporating it into the care provided to patients in day-to-day practice. There are many ways, both formal and informal, to include various aspects of education, risk prediction, prevention, and screening. The care of women in particular lends itself to health maintenance because of the frequent contacts between women and the health system relating to the control or exercise of reproductive functions. In general women use the health system more frequently than do men, and it is more culturally acceptable for women to seek help for physical or emotional problems. They also have contact when they bring their children in for care, and these encounters are profitable opportunities both to learn how to maintain the child's health and to discuss parenting or personal concerns.

Many examples come to mind, in the primary care of women, of opportunities for providing health maintenance, and specific approaches will be discussed in more detail later.

Briefly, health providers have the opportunity, when providing information about contraception to do a considerable amount of teaching and counseling about normal physiology, sexual concerns, common side effects and their management, prevention of vaginitis and urinary tract infections, and principles of choice and self-determination. In treating vaginitis and urinary tract infections explanations of the cause and methods of prevention should be part of routine care. Prenatal care offers an ongoing opportunity for important health teaching to prevent complications during pregnancy, to prepare women for a satisfying experience in labor, to facilitate the transition to parenthood and the inclusion of the new child into the family, and to learn the skills and attitudes necessary for successful infant care. Preventive care for the fetus includes the mother's family history of abnormality, a seriological test for syphilis (VDRL), blood type and Rh factor, antibody titers if Rh negative, rubella testing, evaluation of nutritional state and supplementation when needed, and monitoring of the mother throughout pregnancy for signs of infections, preeclampsia, and diabetes. Other preventive measures include avoidance of exposure to x-rays, the administration of live virus vaccines, or the use of drugs during pregnancy.

The visit for a Pap smear is a good time to teach breast self-examination and to discuss with the woman factors which place her at increased or decreased risk for cervical and breast cancer. In at risk groups, venereal disease screening can also be done. Every visit provides information about blood pressure, and, as women progress toward middle age, they can be counseled on the increasing risk of hypertension and cardiovascular disease and on ways to prevent these. Menstrual problems are frequent reasons for seeking care, and informing women about the danger signs and the increasing risk with age of endometrial and ovarian carcinoma should be part of the plan of care.

Virtually every patient encounter can be utilized for health maintenance. Whether teaching how to use a medication properly and recognize its side effects or engaging in a thorough work-up and health hazard appraisal, the nurse practitioner has a special mandate to encourage and promote health-maintaining behaviors. The opportunity is ever-present; a consciousness of the need for it and a determination to include health maintenance should enable the nurse practitioner to be a pacesetter in this critical aspect of primary care.

HEALTH MAINTENANCE NEEDS OF WOMEN
Health Needs and Illnesses at Various Life Stages

ADOLESCENCE. The most common problems presented by adolescent girls in seeking health care include vaginitis, dysmenorrhea, irregular menstrual cycle, contraception, contraceptive failure, pregnancy, and venereal disease. Drawing from these problems, the health maintenance needs of adolescents include sex education to assist the girl to understand and accept herself and to develop a positive feminine identity. By helping girls anticipate body changes, understand sexual drives, demystify menstruation and view it as a healthy normal body function, a considerable amount of sexually related morbidity could be prevented. Attitudes exert considerable influence upon the response to menstruation. Knowledge of physiology and a sense of self-worth could help to prevent unplanned pregnancy and venereal disease. Choice, considered decision making, and readiness could encourage more satisfying early sexual experiences and decrease orgasmic dysfunction. Contraceptive knowledge allows choice and control over girls' bodies and lives and helps to prevent unwanted pregnancy. Girls also need to understand vaginal physiology and methods of preventing vaginitis.

Pap smears are indicated once the adolescent girl has become sexually active. Discussing with girls the correlation between early sexual activity and multiple sexual partners with cervical carcinoma is part of health maintenance. The rising incidence of vaginal herpes and its dangers during pregnancy and in relation to cervical carcinoma can also be included. Because of the increased incidence of vaginal and cervical adenocarcinoma in girls whose mothers were given diethylstilbestrol (DES) during pregnancy, it is important to ask adolescents if their mothers took hormones while carrying them. Screening for DES should be carried out whenever the response is positive.

Health maintenance for adolescents should ideally include education and counseling about drug abuse, alcohol abuse, and smoking. While the dangers of drug use, including death and disability, are usually readily apparent to the teenager, smoking and alcohol may not appear as so great a threat because their effects are often not seen until later adulthood. Presenting some mortality statistics about cirrhosis, lung cancer, and arteriosclerotic heart disease may impress young girls with the significant health risks caused by long-term heavy use of tobacco and alcohol. Morbidity from chronic lung disease, hypertension and other cardiovascular diseases, and alcoholism can also be shown to reduce the quality of life and the person's functional capacity. However, working with adolescents requires great patience and interpersonal skill; in the flush of youthful vigor it is hard to imagine later disability, and many barriers are raised against adults' laying their "heavy trips" about the future on the young.

Examining the leading causes of death among teenagers provides additional guidelines for health maintenance (Table 1-1).

Automobile safety and driver education are an obvious priority in preventing the greatest cause of death in the 10 to 19 age group. While the government and the education system have a more broadly based responsibility in this area, health providers can contribute by counseling individual patients about seat belt use, alcohol, drugs, and medications. Among potentially preventable causes, suicide figures prominently in white females. Health maintenance includes the detection of depression or a family history of suicide and the initiation of family or individual psychotherapy for girls found to be depressed. Chronic rheumatic heart disease affects black teenagers and should be screened by history of rheumatic fever, signs or symptoms, and presence of heart murmur. Pneumonia is a leading cause of death in both races, and factors placing a person at increased risk include previous episodes of bacterial pneumonia, heavy alcohol use, emphysema, and smoking over one-half pack of cigarettes per day. High risk teenagers can be identified and counseled on ways to reduce their risk, particularly regarding smoking and alcohol, and to seek treatment early for respiratory infections. Among black females, socioeconomic conditions and the lack of health resources no doubt contribute to the deaths from anemias and complications of pregnancies and abortions.

Table 1-1
Ten-Year Deaths per 100,000 Population

White Female, Age 10-14				Black Female, Age 10-14		
Rank	*Cause*	*Number*	*Percentage*	*Rank*	*Cause*	*Number*	*Percentage*
1	Motor vehicle accidents	158	36.7	1	Motor vehicle accidents	91	13.7
2	Leukemia	17	3.9	2	Homicide	84	12.7
3	Suicide	17	3.9	3	Complications of pregnancy and abortions	26	3.9
4	Pneumonia	14	3.2	4	Drowning accidents	26	3.9
5	Homicide	13	3.0	5	Poisonings	22	3.3
6	Drowning accidents	11	2.5	6	Pneumonia	21	3.2
7	Congenital circulatory defects	10	2.3	7	Suicide	18	2.7
8	Poisonings	9	2.0	8	Accidents due to fire	16	2.4
9	Vascular lesions of the central nervous system	9	2.0	9	Anemias	15	2.3
10	Malignant neoplasms of the brain	8	1.8	10	Congenital circulatory defects	14	2.1
White Female, Age 15-19				Black Female, Age 15-19		
1	Motor vehicle accidents	222	37.0	1	Homicide	198	17.2
2	Suicide	47	7.8	2	Motor vehicle accidents	147	12.8
3	Homicide	25	4.1	3	Complications of pregnancy and abortions	53	4.6
4	Pneumonia	16	2.6	4	Poisonings	49	4.2
5	Vascular lesions of the central nervous system	15	2.5	5	Suicide	49	4.2
6	Poisonings	15	2.5	6	Pneumonia	32	2.8
7	Leukemia	14	2.3	7	Vascular lesions of the central nervous system	28	2.4
8	Congenital circulatory defects	10	1.6	8	Anemias	25	2.2
9	Malignant neoplasms of the brain	8	1.3	9	Rheumatic heart disease	15	1.3
10	Complications of pregnancy and abortion	8	1.3	10	Nephritis and nephrosis	15	1.3

Material in this and the following five tables based upon Geller-Steele probability figures, in L. C. robbins and J. H. Hall, *How to Practice Prospective Medicine* (Methodist Hospital of Indiana, 1970), pp. 27-50, 76-100. Tables updated in 1971, personal communication from Gregory Steele. First ten causes of death are included.

These conditions reinforce the importance of screening populations at risk and societal obligations to combat poverty and maldistribution of health care. Increasing awareness of child abuse has led to programs to help abusive parents. Still, homicide due to parental or other violence remains a leading cause of death.

YOUNG TO MID-ADULTHOOD. Women in the 20s through the 40s seek health care frequently for the treatment of vaginitis or urinary tract infections, menstrual problems, pregnancy and its complications, sexual problems, depression, anemia, obesity, neoplasia of the breast, cervix, or uterus, diabetes, and hypertension. Health maintenance for women during these years most commonly includes regular Pap smears, breast examinations and teaching breast self-examination. Taking the time to do a short, focused history to identify the risk factors for cervical and breast cancer would greatly increase screening effectiveness. Women found to have high risk characteristics could then receive Pap smears and breast examinations more frequently, with mammography if appropriate. Contraception-related morbidity becomes a concern for this age group, particularly due to complications from oral contraceptives and IUD use over time. Reassessing contraceptive methods periodically, discussing alternatives and problems, and keeping the women well informed about new data as they appear are part of health maintenance activities. Education about the prevention of vaginitis, urinary tract infections, and venereal disease are also included.

Menstrual concerns and problems constitute a sizeable portion of women's care during these years. The opportunity is often present to educate women about menstrual functioning and to encourage the acceptance of their bodies and physiology. Women at high risk for uterine cancer can be identified and informed, and all women can be taught the danger signs of unexplained irregular vaginal bleeding. Good prenatal care is itself a preventive procedure aimed at maintaining the health of both the mother and the fetus. As discussed previously, many facets of personal and family health can be promoted while providing prenatal, intrapartal, and postpartal care. Sexual and interpersonal problems often surface in young to mid-adulthood, as do depression and anxiety. Early accurate diagnosis, referral, and treatment are important for attaining positive outcomes. Nutritional counseling plays an important part in the prevention of anemia, obesity, and diabetes as well as in their treatment. Prompt treatment of these problems reduces morbidity and promotes higher levels of health.

Mortality tables show that motor vehicle accidents remain among the top ten causes of death. Suicide, homicide, and pneumonia continue to take their toll. Chronic rheumatic heart disease drops below the tenth cause of death, due to the widespread practice of culturing sore throats in children for beta-hemolytic streptococcus and of pursuing treatment and follow-up vigorously. The death rates from complications of pregnancy and abortion in the early 20s emphasize the need for widely available prenatal and abortion services (Table 1-2).

Among white women in the 25 to 29 age group, breast and cervical cancer have entered the list of top ten killers—testimony to the importance of keeping these diseases in mind,

even for younger women. Black women have significantly higher total mortality figures, even in these young adult ages, and the greater incidence of arteriosclerotic and hypertensive heart disease at this early stage is probably related to the excessive stresses placed upon black women in contemporary society. Cirrhosis also makes its appearance—a mute testimony to the hopelessness and despair drowned in alcohol.

After age 30, breast cancer becomes the third cause of death among white women, with cervical cancer not far behind. Arteriosclerotic heart disease rises rapidly during these years to attain second place toward the end of the 30s. Lung cancer enters the top ten causes of death in both races. Among black females, arteriosclerotic heart disease and hypertensive heart disease remain leading causes of death throughout this decade. Because of this rapid ascendance, it is important for nurse practitioners to know the factors which place women at increased risk of heart disease: hypertension, elevated serum cholesterol, diabetes, sedentary habits with little exercise, family history of arteriosclerotic heart disease, smoking more than one-half pack of cigarettes per day, and overweight greater than 15 to 20 percent (Table 1-3). Prevention consists of counseling women to change those factors which they can control (weight, exercise, smoking, diet) and treating hypertension to maintain blood pressure within normal limits.

These same factors, with the exception of weight are predictive of vascular lesions of the central nervous system. Central nervous system infarcts and hemorrhages are leading causes of death throughout life. Diabetes, while itself not often listed as the cause of death, is involved in many other causes such as arteriosclerotic heart disease and vascular lesions of the central nervous system. Adult onset diabetes might well be a preventable disease, if the American eating pattern of infrequent heavy meals and the intake of large amounts of concentrated and refined sugars did not exert a continuing stress upon pancreatic function. Certainly it is controllable, but not primarily with medication; therapy is largely under the patient's control and involves weight reduction and a carbohydrate-restricted diet. The extent of the alcohol abuse problem in this country is borne out by statistics on cirrhosis as a leading cause of death. In both black and white

Table 1-2
Ten-Year Deaths per 100,000 Population

White Female, Age 20-24				Back Female, Age 20-24			
Rank	Cause	Number	Percentage	Rank	Cause	Number	Percentage
1	Motor vehicle accidents	169	25.2	1	Homicide	276	17.1
2	Suicide	73	10.9	2	Motor vehicle accidents	158	9.8
3	Homicide	33	4.9	3	Vascular lesions of the central nervous system	64	3.9
4	Vascular lesions of the central nervous system	22	3.3	4	Suicide	61	3.8
5	Pneumonia	18	2.6	5	Poisonings	57	3.5
6	Poisonings	15	2.2	6	Complications of pregnancy and abortions	54	3.3
7	Leukemia	14	2.1	7	Pneumonia	41	2.5
8	Complications of pregnancy and abortions	13	1.9	8	Cirrhosis	41	2.5
9	Hodgkin's disease	11	1.6	9	Arteriosclerotic heart disease	33	2.0
10	Malignant neoplasms of the brain	10	1.5	10	Anemias	30	1.8
White Female, Age 25-29				Black Female, Age 25-29			
1	Motor vehicle accidents	127	15.3	1	Homicide	294	12.8
2	Suicide	88	10.6	2	Motor vehicle accidents	150	6.5
3	Vascular lesions of the central nervous system	37	4.4	3	Vascular lesions of the central nervous system	138	6.0
4	Homicide	35	4.2	4	Cirrhosis	124	5.4
5	Malignant neoplasms of the breast	34	4.0	5	Arteriosclerotic heart disease	96	4.2
6	Pneumonia	22	2.6	6	Pneumonia	63	2.7
7	Arteriosclerotic heart disease	21	2.5	7	Suicide	60	2.6
8	Diabetes mellitus	18	2.1	8	Malignant neoplasms of the breast	58	2.5
9	Malignant neoplasms of the cervix	17	2.0	9	Poisonings	50	2.2
10	Leukemia	17	2.0	10	Hypertensive heart disease	49	2.1
11*	Cirrhosis	17	2.0	11*	Complications of pregnancy and abortions	49	2.1

*Included because of identical numbers.

women, cirrhosis is among the top ten killers from the ages of 30 to 60, and alcohol consumption is directly related to risk. Women who drink to mild excess have twice the risk of dying of cirrhosis that the average moderate and occasional social drinker does; those who drink heavily to definite excess are at five times greater risk than average; and twelve times as many frank alcoholics as average

drinkers die of cirrhosis. Nondrinkers are at one-tenth the average population risk, and if drinking is stopped before symptoms appear, the risk may be reduced to two-tenths of average.

Cardiovascular disease, breast and cervical cancer, and cirrhosis remain leading killers as women traverse the fifth decade of life. White women still commit suicide and die in motor

Table 1-3
Ten-Year Deaths per 100,000 Population

	White Females, Age 30-34				Black Female, Age 30-34		
Rank	*Cause*	*Number*	*Percentage*	*Rank*	*Cause*	*Number*	*Percentage*
1	Motor vehicle accidents	114	9.5	1	Homicide	296	8.5
2	Suicide	109	9.1	2	Vascular lesions of the central nervous system	274	7.8
3	Malignant neoplasms of the breast	88	7.4	3	Arteriosclerotic heart disease	260	7.5
4	Vascular lesions of the central nervous system	68	5.7	4	Cirrhosis	247	7.1
5	Arteriosclerotic heart disease	59	4.9	5	Motor vehicle accidents	152	4.4
6	Cirrhosis	47	3.9	6	Malignant neoplasms of the breast	120	3.4
7	Malignant neoplasms of the cervix	35	2.9	7	Pneumonia	101	2.9
8	Homicide	35	2.9	8	Malignant neoplasms of the cervix	100	2.9
9	Pneumonia	29	2.4	9	Hypertensive heart disease	95	2.7
10	Diabetes mellitus	25	2.1	10	Nephritis and nephrosis	64	1.8
	White Female, Age 35-39				Black Female, Age 35-39		
1	Malignant neoplasms of the breast	191	10.1	1	Arteriosclerotic heart disease	588	11.9
2	Arteriosclerotic heart disease	152	8.0	2	Vascular lesions of the central nervous system	421	8.5
3	Suicide	130	6.9	3	Cirrhosis	365	7.4
4	Motor vehicle accidents	119	6.3	4	Homicide	277	5.6
5	Vascular lesions of the central nervous system	115	6.1	5	Malignant neoplasms of the breast	215	4.3
6	Cirrhosis	104	5.5	6	Malignant neoplasms of the cervix	169	3.4
7	Malignant neoplasms of the lung	57	3.0	7	Motor vehicle accidents	154	3.1
8	Malignant neoplasms of the cervix	57	3.0	8	Hypertensive heart disease	149	3.0
9	Malignant neoplasms of the intestines and the rectum	48	2.5	9	Pneumonia	142	2.6
10	Malignant neoplasms of the ovary	45	2.4	10	Malignant neoplasms of the lung	89	1.8

vehicle accidents, and cancer of the intestines, rectum, and the ovary becomes more significant. Black women continue to die of pneumonia, homicide, and motor vehicle accidents. Lung cancer progressively increases in both groups (Table 1-4).

The toll of cardiovascular disease increases during the fifth decade, especially during the last half. Among black women age 45 to 49 it causes over 30 percent of all deaths, and in white women over 20 percent. Stress, smoking, obesity, lack of exercise, a diet high in saturated fat, familial predisposition, and neglect of diabetes are reaping their bitter fruit as the numbers in mortality tables tell the story. Cancer of the intestines and rectum gains a prominent place, and the nurse practitioner needs to know the predictive factors: the pres-

Table 1-4
Ten-Year Deaths per 100,000 Population

	White Female, Age 40-44				Black Female, Age 40-44		
Rank	Cause	Number	Percentage	Rank	Cause	Number	Percentage
1	Arteriosclerotic heart disease	338	11.4	1	Arteriosclerotic heart disease	1082	15.9
2	Malignant neoplasms of the breast	335	11.3	2	Vascular lesions of the central nervous system	665	9.7
3	Vascular lesions of the central nervous system	186	6.2	3	Cirrhosis	430	6.3
4	Cirrhosis	175	5.9	4	Malignant neoplasms of the breast	367	5.3
5	Suicide	138	4.6	5	Homicide	230	3.3
6	Malignant neoplasms of the lung	125	4.2	6	Malignant neoplasms of the cervix	221	3.2
7	Motor vehicle accidents	121	4.1	7	Hypertensive heart disease	212	3.1
8	Malignant neoplasms of the ovary	101	3.4	8	Pneumonia	178	2.6
9	Malignant neoplasms of the intestines and the rectum	88	2.9	9	Malignant neoplasms of the lung	159	2.3
10	Malignant neoplasms of the cervix	84	2.8	10	Motor vehicle accidents	155	2.2
	White Female, Age 45-49				Black Female, Age 45-49		
1	Arteriosclerotic heart disease	684	15.3	1	Arteriosclerotic heart disease	1923	20.0
2	Malignant neoplasms of the breast	497	11.1	2	Vascular lesions of the central nervous system	1052	10.9
3	Vascular lesions of the central nervous system	290	6.5	3	Malignant neoplasms of the breast	528	5.5
4	Cirrhosis	235	5.2	4	Cirrhosis	424	4.4
5	Malignant neoplasms of the lung	219	4.9	5	Hypertensive heart disease	275	2.8
6	Malignant neoplasms of the ovary	163	3.6	6	Malignant neoplasms of the cervix	263	2.7
7	Malignant neoplasms of the intestines and the rectum	161	3.6	7	Malignant neoplasms of the lung	259	2.7
8	Suicide	142	3.2	8	Pneumonia	214	2.2
9	Motor vehicle accidents	127	2.8	9	Malignant neoplasms of the intestines and the rectum	194	2.0
10	Malignant neoplasms of the cervix	104	2.3	10	Homicide	168	1.7

ence of polyps, undiagnosed rectal bleeding, a history of ulcerative colitis, and a diet low in roughage and fiber. The most sensitive, inexpensive, and simple screening test for intestinal and rectal cancer is the stool guiuac test, which should be done regularly on women after the late 20s. Malignant neoplasms cause over 25 percent of all deaths among white women, and over 12 percent among black women, during late 40s.

LATE ADULTHOOD. Women in the late adult years, approximately the 50s to mid-60s, seek care for menopausal related concerns, which usually begin in the mid-40s, mid-50s. Health maintenance for women should include preparation for menopause and counseling and support during the process. As the reproductive years end, menstrual irregularities become more common and pose a potentially greater danger. Contraception is a thorny issue; risks associated with oral contraceptives and IUDs are increasing at a time when conception becomes less likely, but, as the exact moment of infertility cannot be clearly identified, the risk of pregnancy remains present, and the physical and emotional complications of "change of life" pregnancies pose significant problems. After menopause, women and health providers are faced with the controversy of estrogen use and must weigh the pros and cons for each individual (see Chapter 8, Menopause). Prompt diagnosis of abnormal bleeding in peri- and postmenopausal women is essential, and patient education is an important part of the effective diagnosis and treatment of cervical and uterine cancer.

Pap smears continue to be routine health maintenance activities, as do breast examinations. Problems of pelvic relaxation become more common as vaginal tone decreases; many such problems can be managed with Kegal's exercises and weight control rather than with surgery. Many of the problems of the middle years continue, including obesity, hypertension, diabetes, anemia, and depression. Cardiovascular disease and cancers remain the leading killers among older adults. Lung cancer is not as prominent a killer of women as it is of men. Predictive factors are based on smoking habits, with nonsmokers having six-tenths the average population risk; those smoking one-half pack per day have one and three-tenths times the average risk, one pack per day two times, and two packs per day three times the average risk of dying of lung cancer. About one-third of the lung cancers in women are diagnosed under the age of 55, and other factors which contribute to an increased risk are a family history of cancer of the lung, colon, or larynx, exposure to airborne carcinogens (chromates, asbestos, arsenic, uranium, polonium), alcoholism, recurrent pneumonia, and chronic obstructive pulmonary disease. Rheumatic heart disease begins to take its toll among white women. Kidney diseases, uterine cancer, and diseases of the arteries appear as significant causes of death among black women (Table 1-5).

ADVANCED YEARS. Women in the years spanning the mid-60s to the mid-70s present problems related to atrophic vaginitis, pelvic relaxation, osteoporosis, and various chronic illnesses including malignancies and cardiovascular conditions. Ability to care for the self and functional capacity vary widely, and families must face the question of whether to provide home care or institutional care for aging parents. Many health problems which are not in themselves life-threatening decrease the quality of life, such as the limitations of activity due to arthritis, back, spine, and hip problems, visual impairment, respiratory conditions, hearing impairment, and mental deterioration. Loss, grief, loneliness, and the prospect of facing death confront the elderly person, for living sufficiently long in itself brings inevitable loss of people, places, and values. Health providers are becoming more aware of the dynamics of death and dying and are slowly assuming a more active role in helping patients and families prepare for and cope with this final human dilemma.

Health maintenance can have an enormous payoff in the advanced years if it is carefully attended to during all the preceding years. Caring for the body, mind, and spirit, developing healthy habits and avoiding undue stress, whether physical or emotional, and identifying and dealing with health problems before significant damage is done can all contribute to an old age in which vigor, zest for life, and ability to function are preserved. The burden of this responsibility is upon the individual, for ultimately most choices are the person's to make, but society, with its unequal treatment of citizens, the health system, with its often misplaced priorities and many shortcomings, and the provider, with the obligation to seek the best level of health for patients within her or his practice, all share in this responsibility.

Pneumonia has been rising again as a cause of death among both black and white women. This no doubt reflects a decreased resistance, secondary to debilitation, poor nutrition, and chronic illness. Many nursing home deaths are due to pneumonia, and probably many would be preventable if principles of health maintenance were applied. Cardiovascular disease continues to be the leading cause of death among the elderly; it is responsible for over 50 percent of the deaths among women over 65. Cancers of the breast, cervix, uterus, intestines and rectum, and stomach cause approximately

Table 1-5
Ten-Year Deaths per 100,000 Population

	White Female, Age 50-54				Black Female, Age 50-54		
Rank	Cause	Number	Percentage	Rank	Cause	Number	Percentage
1	Arteriosclerotic heart disease	1344	20.2	1	Arteriosclerotic heart disease	3030	23.5
2	Malignant neoplasms of the breast	656	9.8	2	Vascular lesions of the central nervous system	1430	11.1
3	Vascular lesions of the central nervous system	443	6.6	3	Malignant neoplasms of the breast	621	4.8
4	Malignant neoplasms of the lung	313	4.7	4	Hypertensive heart disease	374	2.9
5	Cirrhosis	279	4.2	5	Cirrhosis	366	2.8
6	Malignant neoplasms of the intestines and the rectum	276	4.1	6	Malignant neoplasms of the lung	327	2.5
7	Malignant neoplasms of the ovary	214	3.2	7	Malignant neoplasms of the intestines and the rectum	319	2.4
8	Motor vehicle accidents	139	2.1	8	Malignant neoplasms of the cervix	291	2.2
9	Rheumatic heart disease	137	2.0	9	Pneumonia	258	2.0
10	Suicide	135	2.0	10	Nephritis and nephrosis	183	1.4
	White Female, Age 55-59				Black Female, Age 55-59		
1	Arteriosclerotic heart disease	2615	26.1	1	Arteriosclerotic heart disease	5056	26.8
2	Malignant neoplasms of the breast	765	7.6	2	Vascular lesions of the central nervous system	2343	12.4
3	Vascular lesions of the central nervous system	751	7.5	3	Malignant neoplasms of the breast	684	3.6
4	Malignant neoplasms of the intestines and the rectum	425	4.2	4	Hypertensive heart disease	515	2.7
5	Malignant neoplasms of the lung	381	3.8	5	Malignant neoplasms of the intestines and the rectum	465	2.4
6	Cirrhosis	286	2.8	6	Malignant neoplasms of the cervix	370	1.9
7	Malignant neoplasms of the ovary	274	2.7	7	Malignant neoplasms of the lung	349	1.8
8	Rheumatic heart disease	198	1.9	8	Pneumonia	344	1.8
9	Pneumonia	154	1.5	9	Cirrhosis	305	1.6
10	Motor vehicle accidents	150	1.5	10	Diseases of the arteries	277	1.4
	White Female, Age 60-64				Black Female, Age 60-64		
1	Arteriosclerotic heart disease	4746	31.4	1	Arteriosclerotic heart disease	8365	29.6
2	Vascular lesions of the central nervous system	1354	8.9	2	Vascular lesions of the central nervous system	3969	14.1
3	Malignant neoplasms of the breast	823	5.4	3	Hypertensive heart disease	718	2.5
4	Malignant neoplasms of the intestines and the rectum	614	4.0	4	Malignant neoplasms of the breast	706	2.5

Table 1-5 (continued)

	White Female, Age 60-64				Black Female, Age 60-64		
Rank	Cause	Number	Percentage	Rank	Cause	Number	Percentage
5	Malignant neoplasms of the lung	423	2.8	5	Malignant neoplasms of the intestines and the rectum	696	2.4
6	Malignant neoplasms of the ovary	326	2.1	6	Diseases of the arteries	488	1.7
7	Cirrhosis	260	1.7	7	Pneumonia	467	1.6
8	Diseases of the arteries	258	1.7	8	Malignant neoplasms of the cervix	460	1.6
9	Rheumatic heart disease	254	1.6	9	Malignant neoplasms of the lung	397	1.4
10	Pneumonia	236	1.5	10	Malignant neoplasms of the uterus	312	1.1

9 percent of the deaths among white women and 8 percent among black women. An increased risk of cancer of the stomach is associated with a positive family history, hypochlorhydria, pernicious anemia, and a diet with large amounts of smoked fish and soy sauce. Positive stool guiuacs for occult blood raise this diagnostic possibility and may also suggest cancer of the colon or rectum.[12] Accidental falls are the tenth leading cause of death among white women age 70 to 74, pointing to the need for home safety measures and patient education for prevention. Pap smears and breast examinations remain part of health maintenance, and stool guiuacs should be done yearly. Proctosigmoidoscopy is often recommended every 5 years after age 40, but particularly in the advancing years (Table 1-6).

APPROACHES TO HEALTH MAINTENANCE

The ideal toward which the health provider can strive is to put some health maintenance into each patient visit. Even in a 15-minute visit for a viral upper respiratory infection, health maintenance can be carried out by educating the patient about ways to stay healthy and avoid these infections, or ways to manage such minor illnesses at home. Every practice could benefit from the use of some method to organize and give direction to health maintenance activities such as a preventive or screening flow sheet, patient education check list, or a formal health appraisal. Many different approaches are possible and can be tailored to the population served and to the style of the practice. Three approaches to health maintenance will be described here which can be used as designed or as models which the practitioner can modify to develop a unique method.

Preventive or Screening Flow Sheets

The purpose of flow sheets is to pull out essential or critical information in the management of patient problems over time and to arrange these in a clear, orderly manner for the rapid review of data. Usually flow sheets are used for complex, chronic problems which need regular monitoring via several physical, laboratory, or treatment programs. Diabetic flow sheets generally include such data as weight, blood pressure, blood sugar, urine sugar and acetone, skin condition, medication dosage, and diet. Hypertension flow sheets cover weight, blood pressure and pulse rate, chest auscultation, cardiac sounds, edema of extremities, symptoms (chest pain, dyspnea, palpitations, headaches, and so on), laboratory tests such as serum potassium and electrolytes, x-ray examinations of the chest, ECGs, medication dosage, and diet. The principle of arranging key information vertically on one sheet to facilitate rapid scanning has also been adapted to health maintenance.

Flow sheets for health maintenance are usually arranged by age and are directed toward screening tests and procedures which allow early detection of disease. General measures which provide information about overall health

Table 1-6
Ten-Year Deaths per 100,000 Population

	White Female, Age 65-69				Black Female, Age 65-69		
Rank	*Cause*	*Number*	*Percentage*	*Rank*	*Cause*	*Number*	*Percentage*
1	Arteriosclerotic heart disease	8504	35.3	1	Arteriosclerotic heart disease	13393	30.7
2	Vascular lesions of the central nervous system	2667	11.1	2	Vascular lesions of the central nervous system	6417	14.7
3	Malignant neoplasms of the intestines and the rectum	884	3.6	3	Malignant neoplasms of the intestines and the rectum	1060	2.4
4	Malignant neoplasms of the breast	871	3.6	4	Hypertensive heart disease	963	2.2
5	Diseases of the arteries	533	2.2	5	Diseases of the arteries	962	2.2
6	Malignant neoplasms of the lung	445	1.8	6	Malignant neoplasms of the breast	811	1.8
7	Pneumonia	425	1.7	7	Pneumonia	744	1.7
8	Malignant neoplasms of the ovary	338	1.4	8	Malignant neoplasms of the cervix	501	1.1
9	Rheumatic heart disease	288	1.2	9	Malignant neoplasms of the lung	496	1.1
10	Hypertensive heart disease	257	1.0	10	Malignant neoplasms of the stomach	402	0.9

	White Female, Age 70-74				Black Female, Age 70-74		
1	Arteriosclerotic heart disease	14231	36.5	1	Arteriosclerotic heart disease	16204	31.4
2	Vascular lesions of the central nervous system	5123	13.1	2	Vascular lesions of the central nervous system	7912	15.3
3	Malignant neoplasms of the intestines and the rectum	1180	3.0	3	Diseases of the arteries	1342	2.6
4	Diseases of the arteries	1061	2.7	4	Malignant neoplasms of the intestines and the rectum	1179	2.3
5	Malignant neoplasms of the breast	936	2.4	5	Hypertensive heart disease	1035	2.0
6	Pneumonia	798	2.0	6	Pneumonia	967	1.8
7	Hypertensive heart disease	479	1.2	7	Malignant neoplasms of the breast	811	1.5
8	Malignant neoplasms of the lung	446	1.1	8	Malignant neoplasms of the stomach	475	0.9
9	Malignant neoplasms of the ovary	348	0.9	9	Malignant neoplasms of the lung	461	0.9
10	Accidents due to falls	305	0.8	10	Malignant neoplasms of the cervix	430	0.8

status, such as weight and health history questionnaires, may also be recommended. The tests or procedures included are those which can identify common correctable problems such as anemia, bacteriuria or syphilis; chronic controllable conditions such as diabetes and hypertension; and the more frequent cancers for which there are reasonable screening tests such as the Pap smear for cervical cancer, breast examination for cancer of the breast, and rectal examination with stool guiuac for occult blood for cancer of the colon and rectum. Immunizations and purified protein derivative (PPD) testing for tuberculosis are part of preventive care and may be included in flow sheets.

One example of preventive flow sheets is from Rochester, New York, courtesy of Dr. Stephen Stowe. The sheet is arranged by age and by screening test or procedure. When a test or procedure is indicated, the box beneath the age at which it is to be done is left blank so that the date of the screening can be entered. At ages when a particular screening test or procedure is not recommended the box is darkened. Figures 1-1 and 1-2 show these preventive flow sheets for ages 12 to 30 and 45 to 65. Sheets are available for ages 0 to 65+. Unless indicated by symbols for gender, screening is to be done for both men and women.

Health Hazard Appraisal

The Health Hazard Appraisal is a formalized approach to health maintenance. It is described in the booklet *How to Practice Prospective Medicine* by Lewis C. Robbins, M.D. and Jack H. Hall, M.D. of the Methodist Hospital of Indiana. The goal of the Appraisal is to provide a format for continuous comprehensive care based upon the identification of specific risks of death and disease for men and women of various ages. Tables showing the leading causes of death and associated risk factors by age, sex, and race are utilized to predict risks of disease during a 10-year period. The prediction of risks before the onset of diseases (or in the early asymptomatic stages) allows the practitioner to use health counseling, education, and prompt treatment to avert illness or disability. It is envisioned that the Health Hazard Appraisal will be used in practices providing primary, ongoing care.

Utilizing data from insurance companies, major medical prognostic studies and prognostic reviews in the literature, teaching cases at several university medical schools, and other special studies related to particular diseases, risk factors are identified for the leading causes of death. These are combined with population statistics so that numbers, percentages, and a decimal weighting system can be assigned to average risks. Any given individual's risks, as determined by that person's prognostic characteristics, can be compared to the population average. A person can then be found to have an average, decreased, or increased risk of dying from a given cause.

For example, the leading cause of death among black females age 40 to 44 is arteriosclerotic heart disease, and the predictive factors include blood pressure, cholesterol, diabetes, exercise, family history of arteriosclerotic heart disease, smoking, and weight. Depending upon an individual's characteristics in these areas, she may be at an increased or decreased risk of dying of arteriosclerotic heart disease over the succeeding 10 years when compared to the population average. To convey this risk to the patient, the Health Hazard Appraisal relies upon numbers and percentages. In this category, the population average is 1082 deaths per 100,000 over the succeeding 10 years. If the patient, a 43-year-old black women, has a blood pressure of 150/94, a cholesterol level of 225 (N 180–300), is not diabetic, is sedentary, has no family history of arteriosclerotic heart disease, smokes one pack of cigarettes per day, and is 50 percent overweight, her overall or composite risk of dying of arteriosclerotic heart disease is three times the average risk. Thus she has 3571 chances per 100,000 of dying over the next 10 years, instead of the 1082 chances per 100,000 that the average person in her age-sex-race category faces (Figure 1-3, pp. 20-21).

To use the Health Hazard Appraisal, certain data must be obtained from the person so that individual prognostic characteristics can be identified. These data are quite specific for each cause of death and are readily attainable from a self-administered history, a physical examination, and selected laboratory tests. Historic data are summarized on the Personal Risk Registry Form (Figure 1-4, p. 22). Physical examination and laboratory data are taken from any comprehensive physical write-up and from lab slips. Specific data are then entered on the Health Hazard Appraisal Form which is designed for the person's age-sex-race group. The person's prognostic characteristics are compared with the risk for the average population, and, by using the Health Hazard Appraisal manual, a composite risk factor for the individual is determined. From this, her chances of dying are calculated for each cause of death, as well as her total risk of dying. The total risk of dying is used to determine her "appraisal age." If she has few risk factors and her total risk of dying is below the population average, then her appraisal age will be less than her actual age. However, if she has many risk factors and a higher than average total risk of

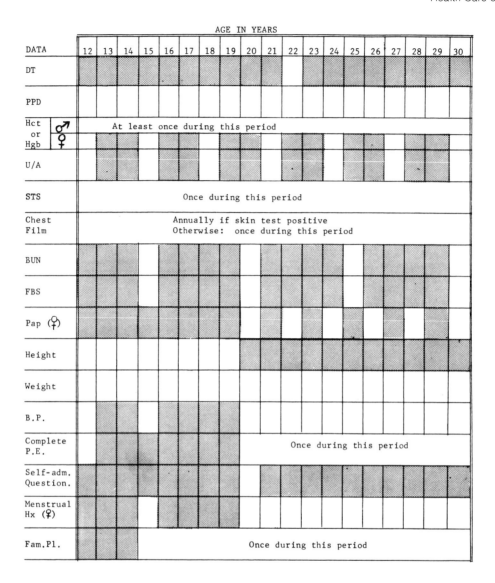

Figure 1-1. Preventive flow sheet, ages 12-30. Family Practice Center, Community Hospital, Santa Rosa, California.

dying, a woman's appraisal age will be more than her actual age. Another way to view this is that her characteristics place her in an age group with higher mortality statistics. Or more simply stated, "The condition of your body makes you older than your chronological age."

All is not hopeless, however, for those at increased risk. The Health Hazard Appraisal includes suggestions for ways to reduce risks and has methods for calculating how much any one therapy will reduce the risks and improve the chances of survival. Therapies may include changes in personal habits, health practices, diet, and medication. In the case of the 43-year-old black woman, recommended therapies include diet or drugs to reduce blood pressure, a regular exercise program, no smoking, and a diet to reduce weight. If the woman's blood pressure were reduced to normal, she exercised moderately, stopped smoking, and reduced to average weight for her height and bone structure, she could reduce her risk to 80 percent of the average. Thus she would have 887 chances out of 100,000 of dying from arteriosclerotic heart disease in the next ten years, instead of her original 3571. By following recommended

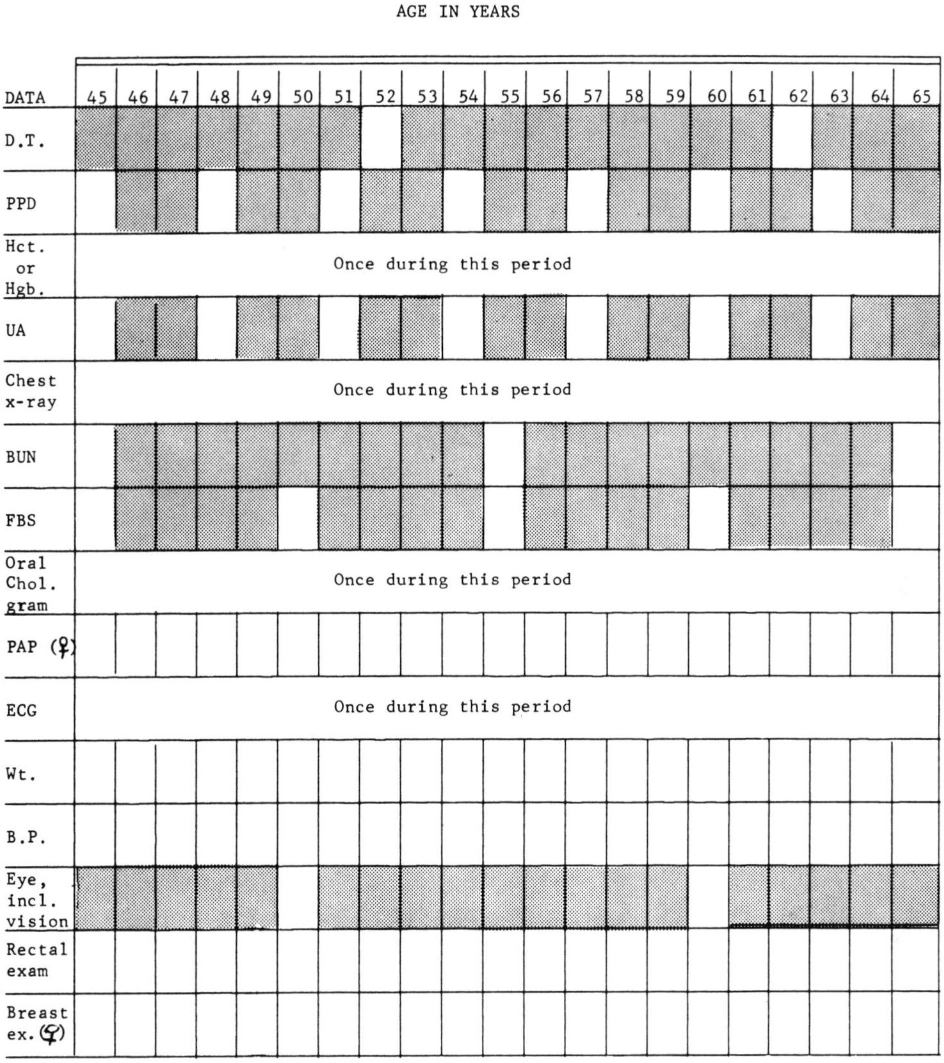

AGE IN YEARS

DATA	45	46	47	48	49	50	51	52	53	54	55	56	57	58	59	60	61	62	63	64	65
D.T.																					
PPD																					
Hct. or Hgb.						Once during this period															
UA																					
Chest x-ray						Once during this period															
BUN																					
FBS																					
Oral Chol. gram						Once during this period															
PAP (♀)																					
ECG						Once during this period															
Wt.																					
B.P.																					
Eye, incl. vision																					
Rectal exam																					
Breast ex. (♀)																					

Figure 1-2. Preventive flow sheet, ages 45-65. Family Practice Center, Community Hospital, Santa Rosa, California.

therapies, this woman can increase her survival advantage by 27 percent. Likewise, by improving her health and reducing risks in the other categories on the Health Hazard Appraisal, she can attain a "compliance age" which is lower than her "appraisal age." This represents years of life that she can theoretically gain if she follows recommendations to improve her state of health (see Figure 1-3).

The Health Hazard Appraisal is a statistical tool in the practice of prospective health care. It is a concrete way to show patients the health risks they face and the increased chances for survival if they take action to reduce their risk factors. As a numbers game, the Health Hazard Appraisal can be very effective in reaching pa-

tients who are at risk but relatively asymptomatic, who know that smoking and overeating saturated fats increase their chances of heart disease and cancer, but who have never had the opportunity to play the odds with actual numbers. Seeing their risk double or triple, stated as deaths per 100,000 or diagrammed in a bar graph with certain bars extending way beyond the average is most impressive (Figure 1-5, p. 23). In certain populations, the Health Hazard Appraisal is an excellent motivator for change in behavior and greatly increases the patient's

HEALTH HAZARD APPRAISAL CHART

Quality control: Evaluate performance of a predetermined goal.

Goal: "Get this patient safely through the next ten years."

Name __A. B.__   Patient No. _____   Birthdate _____

Street _____   State _____   Zip _____   Race, Sex, Age __BF 43__

City _____   Date __SEPT. 19 77__

BF 40-44   AVERAGE TO INDIVIDUAL RISK

POPULATION AVERAGE 10 YEAR DEATHS PER 100,000		INDIVIDUAL PROGNOSIS — RISK APPRAISAL				PROGNOSIS AFTER INTERVENTION — RISK REAPPRAISAL*				SURVIVAL ADVANTAGE	
Disease/Injury	Average Risk	Prognostic Characteristics	Risk Factor	Composite Risk Factor	Present Risk	Prognostic Characteristics	Risk Factor	Composite Risk Factor	New Risk	Amount Reduction	Per Cent Reduction
From Manual	From Manual	Listed in Manual Physician Select	From Manual x / +	See Instructions	(2) x (5)	After Physician's Prescription	From Manual x / +	See Instructions	(2) x (9)	(6) - (10)	**
(1)	(2)	(3)	(4)	(5)	(6)	(7)	(8)	(9)	(10)	(11)	(12)
1. ARTERIOSCLEROTIC HEART DISEASE	1082	BLOOD PRESSURE 15%4	1.3	3.3	3,571	DIET/DRUGS TO REDUCE BP	.8	.82	887	2,684	27%
		CHOLESTEROL 225	1				1				
		EXERCISE Sed.	1.4			REGULAR EXERCISE PROGRAM	.9				
		FAMILY HISTORY No	1				1				
		SMOKING 1 pk.	2.1			STOP SMOKING	1.1				
		WEIGHT 50% over	1.5			REDUCE TO AVERAGE WT.	1				
2. VASCULAR LESIONS OF CNS	665	BLOOD PRESSURE 15%4	1.3	1.8	1,197	DIET/DRUGS TO REDUCE BP	.8	.8	632	565	5.6%
		CHOLESTEROL 225	1				1				
		DIABETIC No	1				1				
		SMOKING 1 pk.	1.5			STOP SMOKING	1				
3. CIRRHOSIS	430	ALCOHOL Mod.	1	1	430		1	1	430	0	0
4. MALIGNANT NEOPLASMS OF THE BREAST	367	FAMILY Hx. No	1	1	367		1	.5	184	183	1.8%
		MONTHLY SELF-EXAM No	1			DO MONTHLY SELF-EXAM AND HAVE ANNUAL MD PALPATION	.5				
		ANNUAL MD EXAM No	1								
5. HOMICIDE	230	ARREST RECORD No	1	1	230		1	1	230	0	0
		WEAPONS No	1								
6. MALIGNANT NEOPLASMS OF THE CERVIX	221	PAP SMEAR 1 in 5yr	.7	.7	155	ANNUAL PAP SMEAR	.1	.1	22	133	1.3%
		ECON. & SOCIAL STATUS									
		ONSET OF INTERCOURSE									
7. HYPERTENSIVE HEART DISEASE	212	BLOOD PRESSURE 15%4	1.3	1.8	382	DIET/DRUGS TO REDUCE BP	1	1	212	170	1.6%
		WEIGHT 50% over	1.5			REDUCE TO AVERAGE WT.	1				
8. PNEUMONIA	178	ALCOHOL Mod.	1	1.2	214		1	1	178	36	.3%
		BACT. PNEUMONIA No	1				1				
		EMPHYSEMA No	1				1				
		SMOKING	1.2			STOP SMOKING	1				

Figure 1-3. Health Hazard Appraisal chart. C. E. Robbins and G. Steele, Methodist Hospital of Indiana, and Ken Bubb, CommonHealth Club, Santa Rosa, California.

	AVERAGE TO INDIVIDUAL RISK — INDIVIDUAL PROGNOSIS RISK APPRAISAL					RISK REDUCTION FOR INDIVIDUAL — PROGNOSIS AFTER INTERVENTION RISK REAPPRAISAL				SURVIVAL ADVANTAGE	
POPULATION AVERAGE 10 YEAR DEATHS PER 100,000 Disease/Injury *From Manual* (1)	Average Risk *From Manual* (2)	Prognostic Characteristics *Listed in Manual Physician Select* (3)	Risk Factor *From Manual* x + (4)	Composite Risk Factor *See Instructions* (5)	Present Risk (2) x (5) (6)	Prognostic Characteristics *After Physician's Prescription* (7)	Risk Factor *From Manual* x + (8)	Composite Risk Factor *See Instructions* (9)	New Risk (2) x (9) (10)	Amount Reduction (6) - (10) (11)	Per Cent Reduction (12)
9. MALIGNANT NEOPLASMS OF THE LUNG	159	SMOKING 1 pk.	2.0	3.0	495	STOP SMOKING 1.6	1.6	2.6	413	82	.8%
10. MOTOR VEHICLE ACCIDENTS	155	ALCOHOL Mod. 1, MILEAGE 10,000 1, SEAT BELTS 50% .9, DRUGS & MEDS. 1	.9		140	USE SEAT BELTS 100% .8	.8	.8	124	16	.15%
11. MALIGNANT NEOPLASMS OF INTESTINE & RECTUM	106	POLYP No 1, RECTAL BLEEDING No 1, ULCERATIVE COLITIS No 1, PROCTOSIGMOIDOSCOPY No 1	1	1	106	HAVE PERIODIC PROCTO. .3	.3	.3	32	74	.7%
12. NEPHRITIS & NEPHROSIS	95	1	1	1	95		1	1	95	0	0
13. MALIGNANT NEOPLASMS OF THE OVARY	87	1	1	1	87		1	1	87	0	0
14. RHEUMATIC HEART DISEASE	86	MURMUR No 1, RHEUMATIC FEVER No 1, SIGNS OR SYMPTOMS No .1	.1	.1	9	.1	.1	.1	9	0	0
15. ALCOHOLISM	76	ALCOHOL Mod. 1	1	1	76		1	1	76	0	0
Other Causes	2650										
Total	6799				10,204				6,261	40	

Health Appraisal Age __46__ Compliance Age __40__ Appraiser __COMMON HEALTH, SANTA ROSA, CALIF.__ (SIGNATURE)

Physician ____ (SIGNATURE)

*Reappraise on assumption that physician's prescription is complied with. Columns (7) through (10) same as columns (3) through (6) except where the physician's prescription changed prognostic characteristics.

**Divide figures in column (11) by total of column (6).

L. C. ROBBINS, M.D. ● N. B. GESNER, M.C.A. ● 1604 N. CAPITOL AVENUE ● INDIANAPOLIS, IND. 46202

Form CH-969

PERSONAL RISK REGISTRY   Date: _____

NAME: _____ AGE: ____ SEX: ____ RACE: ___
(PLEASE ANSWER EVERY QUESTION. IF YOU ARE UNCERTAIN OF THE ANSWER, CHECK *NO*)

PERSONAL HISTORY AND HEALTH HABITS
YES   NO
____ ____ History of bacterial pneumonia. (serious pneumonia, probably hospitalized for treatment, treated with antibiotic
____ ____ Do you have diabetes?
____ ____ Emphysema?
____ ____ Frequent, severe depression. (have considered seeking professional help)
____ ____ Rectal polyps (elongated growths inside lower bowel; *not* hemorrhoids).
____ ____ Undiagnosed (don't know the cause of) rectal bleeding.
____ ____ Ulcerative colitis, When? _____.
____ ____ Arrest record for violence or threat of violence.
____ ____ Weapon carried on person.
____ ____ Rheumatic fever (did you undergo chemoprophylaxis for this—drug treatment?) _____
____ ____ Hypochlorhydria (lack of acid in the stomach). (If uncertain about this, answer *no*.) How long? _____
____ ____ Signs or symptoms of rheumatic heart disease.
____ ____ Have you had a proctosigmoidoscopy (rectal exam with a tube or proctoscope)? When? _____

FAMILY HISTORY
YES   NO
____ ____ Did either of your parents die of heart attack? If yes, age at death. _____
____ ____ Did either parent, a brother or sister have diabetes?
____ ____ Has there been a suicide in your family? (If yes, what was your relationship to that person? _____)

Do you currently smoke?   How much per
YES NO   day?
____ ____Cigarettes   _____
____ ____Cigars   _____
____ ____Pipe   _____

Did you smoke but have stopped?   How much per   Date Quit?
YES NO   day?
____ ____Cigarettes   _____   _____
____ ____Cigars   _____   _____
____ ____Pipe   _____   _____

How many drinks of alcohol do you have *each week*? (includes beer, wine, liquor). _____

How many miles do you travel (as driver and/or passenger) in an automobile each year? _____ (The average
person travels 10,000 miles annually in an automobile. Try to estimate mileage.)
What percentage of the time do you use a seat belt? _____%.

Last chest x-ray: Date _____ Result (Circle one):   Positive (some TB activity indicated past/present.)
                                                          Negative (no indication of any TB activity)

Exercise (Check one)
_____a) Sedentary—under 5 flights of stairs or half mile walking daily and no comparable activity.
_____b) Some—between 5 and 15 flights of stairs or 0.5 to 1.5 miles walking daily or comparable activity.
_____c) Moderate—programmed exercise 4 times per week which activity equals 1.5 to 2 miles walking or 15 to
              20 flights of stairs daily or comparable activity.
_____d) Vigorous—greater than moderate.

FEMALE PATIENTS ONLY
YES   NO
____ ____ Have you had breast cancer?
____ ____ Did your mother or sister have breast cancer?
____ ____ Do you examine your own breasts for lumps and other problems? How often? _____
____ ____ Do you have a yearly breast exam by your physician?
____ ____ Have you had a mammography (breast x-ray)? When? _____
____ ____ Do you have undiagnosed (don't know the cause of) bleeding from the vagina?
____ ____ Have you had a hysterectomy?

How many Pap smears have you had within the last five years? _____
If the results were anything other than negative, please explain. _____

CURRENT TEST RESULTS (to be filled in by CommonHealth Club staff).

Blood Pressure: _____

THE HEALTH HAZARD APPRAISAL ATTEMPTS TO POINT OUT THOSE AREAS IN WHICH PREVENTIVE ACTION WILL BE EFFECT
THE RESEARCH TO ESTABLISH RISK FACTORS FOR SPECIAL CONDITIONS (such as asthma, ulcers, allergies, major operati
etc.) HAS NOT YET BEEN DONE. AS A RESULT, WE ARE UNABLE TO INFORM YOU AT THIS TIME AS TO THE IMPACT OF S
SPECIAL CONDITIONS ON YOUR OVERALL RISK OR OF THE APPROPRIATE PREVENTIVE MEASURES.

PROSPECTIVE MEDICINE — PERSONAL RISK CHART

RISK FACTOR — AS COMPARED TO OTHERS OF THE SAME AGE, SEX, RACE

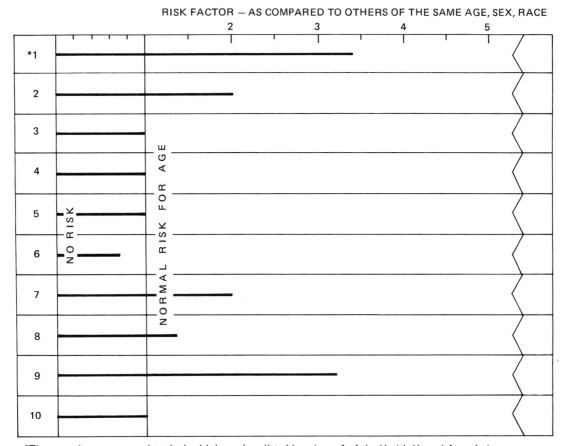

*These numbers correspond to the health hazards as listed in column 1 of the Health Hazard Appraisal Chart.

NAME ___A.B.___   DATE ___SEPT. 1977___

Age _____ 43
Appraisal Age _____ 46
Compliance Age _____ 40

Figure 1-5. Health Hazard Appraisal personal risk chart. CommonHealth Club, Santa Rosa, California.

awareness and sense of responsibility for maintaining her or his own health.[13] The overall goal in using the Health Hazard Appraisal is to "get the patient safely through the next 10 years" through practicing prospective care which is

1. comprehensive in its concern for the individual's total risk
2. continuous in its search for new risks
3. initiated before disease and injury, beginning with a quantitative estimate of the patient's own risks and a program for their reduction.[14]

Figure 1-4. Personal risk registry. CommonHealth Club, Santa Rosa, California.

Periodic Screening Recommendations

While no one argues about the importance of prevention and early recognition of disease, the practical question to be answered is, what health examinations or tests should be done, at what intervals, on which asymptomatic patients? In a series of articles which assembled and condensed data on periodic screening, recommendations were made for selective screening and longitudinal risk factor analysis for 36 diseases. Paul S. Frame and Stephen J. Carlson, in "A Critical Review of Periodic Health

Screening Using Specific Screening Criteria" in the *Journal of Family Practice*, also developed a periodic screening flow sheet for asymptomatic adults.[15] The criteria for acceptable screening tests or procedures are listed on page 28.

Diseases examined critically which are of importance in the health care of women will be discussed below. Findings and recommendations include the following:

SMOKING. While not a disease, smoking is a significant health hazard associated with considerable mortality from several diseases. Cessation of smoking decreases mortality. Generally, the more cigarettes smoked daily the greater the risk: the death rate for those who smoke 10 cigarettes per day is 40 percent higher than that for nonsmokers, an increase to 40 cigarettes per day creates a death rate 120 percent higher than for nonsmokers. In women ages 45 to 74, death rates from cerebrovascular disease are 38 to 111 percent higher in smokers. Smokers with bronchopulmonary disease are more symptomatic and have mortality ratios ranging from 4.6, for up to 9 cigarettes per day, to 18.2 for 40 or more, compared to nonsmokers. Lung cancer statistics are even more impressive, with a mortality ratio of 7.0 for up to 9 cigarettes and 33.8 for 40 or more cigarettes per day. Duration of smoking, and the amount of inhalation also influence lung cancer death rates.

Smoking is usually easy to diagnose by history. It is a widespread habit with 60 percent of the men and 36 percent of the women in this country smoking by age 25; the incidence of smoking increases up to about age 40, after which it drops, and by age 65, 20 percent of the men and 4 percent of the women smoke. It is well documented that the discontinuation of smoking substantially reduces morbidity and mortality from cardiovascular disease, chronic obstructive pulmonary disease, and lung cancer. For screening, a smoking history should be taken initially and repeated at ages 30 and 40.

HYPERTENSION. Fifteen percent of the adult population has a blood pressure greater than 140/90, and another 15 percent is borderline. By age 60, 35 percent of all women and 30 percent of all men are hypertensive. It tends to be a familial problem and is more common in blacks than in whites. Diagnosis is quick, reliable, and simple using the sphygomomanometer. There is a long asymptomatic stage, but often serious consequences, which include coronary artery disease, cerebrovascular disease, and renal failure, eventually occur. These diseases are related to the degree and duration of hypertension. Medication is a reasonably effective treatment. Hypertension meets all criteria for screening; thus all adults should have blood pressure checks every two years.

ISCHEMIC HEART DISEASE (arteriosclerotic heart disease). Death rates from arteriosclerotic heart disease increase steadily with age, and men are affected three times as often as women. However, it is a leading cause of death among women, especially after age 40. While the exact nature of the presymptomatic phase is not known, it is thought that the atherosclerotic process can start very early in life, especially if risk factors are present. The disease may present as myocardial infarction, angina, incidental diagnosis in the asymptomatic person or even sudden death. Once disease is manifest, the person's risk of dying from it within five years is increased five times. Risk factors for the development of arteriosclerotic heart disease include hypertension, hyperlipidemia, smoking, diabetes, obesity, sedentary life style, psychosocial tension, and hyperuricemia.

The only specific treatment for ischemic heart disease in its earlier stages is the identification and elimination of risk factors in order to prevent and possibly reverse atherosclerosis formation. The standard approaches to diagnosing the disease using physical examinations, x-ray examinations of the chest, and ECGs are unreliable and generally detect only advanced cases. The ECG is not recommended as a routine screening device because finding an abnormality does not lead to any different treatment, and, because the test is not very sensitive, a normal result may lead to a false reassurance. The recommended screening procedure is to identify risk factors by blood pressure check every 2 years, cholesterol every 4 years, history of smoking every 10 years, and check for obesity every 4 to 6 years.

RHEUMATIC HEART DISEASE. The prevalence of rheumatic heart disease is decreasing in the United States, particularly among the younger population. Primary rheumatic heart disease is a disease of children with new cases unusual after the age of 25. About 10 percent of the children with rheumatic fever will develop rheumatic heart disease; those with the disease are susceptible to bacterial endocarditis throughout life. Complications can usually be controlled with antibiotic therapy, but, if the disease goes unrecognized, the asymptomatic adult is at an increased risk of suffering a recurrence of rheumatic fever and endocarditis. A single screen of adults is recommended when first seen or at age 21 by complete cardiovascular history and physical examination. An ECG does not improve screening; a positive history and presence of a murmur are the significant factors.

STROKE. Cerebrovascular disease is most common in people over 55, and is often a sudden catastrophic event. However, about one-third of these patients have transient ischemic attacks with subsequent recovery. Risk factors include hypertension, elevated serum lipids, and diabetes. Although the presence of carotid bruits or other signs of cardiovascular insufficiency raise the suspicion of a potential stroke, there is no good way of predicting it in advance of any symptoms. The only treatment in the asymptomatic stages is the reduction of risk factors. The recommended screening is a blood pressure check every 2 years and a cholesterol check every 4 years.

TUBERCULOSIS. This is still a common disease with significant morbidity and is often asymptomatic. People with a positive PPD have a 5 percent chance of developing tuberculosis and are a high risk group. Pharmaceutical treatment will effectively arrest or cure the disease. The PPD is 90 percent sensitive but does not distinguish between active and latent disease; it is a good screening test but diagnosis is made by x-ray examination of the chest. Positive yield by x-ray examination in mass screening is so low (0 to 3 per 1000) that it is no longer recommended for this purpose. Screening by PPD or other tuberculin testing is recommended initially and then every 10 years. High risk populations should be screened more frequently.

LUNG CANCER. The incidence of lung cancer shows a recent upward trend with a strong relation to age; for men age 40 it is 10 per 100,000 and age 65 it is 150 per 100,000; for women age 45 it is 4 per 100,000 and age 65 to 70 it is 20 per 100,000. Risk factors are male gender, increasing age, cigarette smoking, asbestosis, and other lung conditions. Lung cancer is a rapidly growing neoplasm with a short asymptomatic period and a rapidly fatal course. Ninety percent of new cancers are symptomatic before changes are evident on x-ray examination, early radiologic signs are subtle and easily missed, and one-third of the lesions are incurable before they are evident on x-ray examination. The latent period between the onset of signs and incurability is probably less than 6 months, and even x-ray screening every 6 months only increases the 5-year survival by 5 to 8 percent. No screening is recommended because with present techniques, attempts at early diagnosis do not significantly decrease mortality.

DIABETES. Maturity onset diabetes increases from 650 per 100,000 for the ages 25 to 44 to 2,700 per 100,000 for the ages 45 to 64. Onset is usually insidious over a period of years, and there is a considerable amount of morbidity and mortality, with vascular, infectious, ocular and neurologic complications. The major risk factors are heredity and obesity; 80 percent of new adult onset diabetics are overweight. Chemical diabetes, manifest by an abnormal glucose tolerance test in an asymptomatic person, lasts weeks to years before the disease becomes overt. Diagnosis is readily established by a glucose tolerance test or a 2-hour postprandial blood sugar test. A fasting blood sugar or urine sugar test is an adequate screen for overt diabetes. While treatment can control acidosis and hypoglycemia, there is controversy over whether complications (vascular, ocular, neural, renal) can be arrested or minimized. There is little evidence that treatment in the asymptomatic stage affects long-term morbidity better than withholding treatment until symptoms appear. The major treatment for chemical diabetes is weight reduction, which would not apply to people of normal weight. Therefore, screening is not recommended for asymptomatic adults. It would be indicated as part of a work-up for obesity and in patients with a positive family history of diabetes.

CIRRHOSIS AND ALCOHOLISM. Alcoholism develops slowly over many years, primarily affects the 30 to 50 age group, with men having a 6:1 ratio to women. Incidence is reported at 4,200 per 100,000. There are significant complications including liver, gastrointestinal, cardiac, and neural damage as well as psychological, financial, and social disruption of patient and family. Cirrhosis is a leading cause of death in middle-aged and older people, and about 90 percent of people with cirrhosis are alcoholics. Diagnosis of alcoholism is made by history; cirrhosis can be detected by abnormal liver function tests (SGOT, SGPT, alkaline phosphatase). There is no specific treatment for cirrhosis except cessation of drinking. Treatment of alcoholism consists of achieving abstinence from drinking, and a variety of therapies are utilized. Screening for cirrhosis is not recommended as there is no treatment; alcoholism should be screened by questioning people between the ages 30 and 60 every 5 to 10 years about their drinking habits.

OBESITY. Among Americans, 20 percent of the men and 30 percent of the women are obese, that is, at least 20 percent over ideal body weight. The incidence of obesity rises gradually with age. Onset is gradual, and people 20 to 30 percent above ideal weight have increased risk of death from all causes by 50 percent, cardiovascular and renal disease by 50 percent, diabetes by 283 percent, cirrhosis by 150 percent, and gallbladder and biliary tract disease by 52 percent. The most important risk factor is a family history of obesity. Treatment is weight loss, which depends upon patient motivation, and overall success rates are poor. Achievement of a sustained weight reduction does decrease the death risks from the above causes. Diagnosis is simple and treatment can be quite effective in reducing morbidity and mortality. Screening is recommended for all adults using height and weight measurements for comparison with a table of ideal weights every 4 years.

CANCER OF THE COLON AND RECTUM. Carcinoma of the colon and rectum has an overall incidence of 45 per 100,000, occurs equally in both sexes, and is 95 percent a disease of people over 45 with the median age at diagnosis being 60 to 67 years. Risk factors include ulcerative colitis, familial polyposis, villous adenomas, and increasing age to the seventh decade. Adenomatous polyps are thought to have very little malignant potential. Most colorectal cancers occur in the distal 25 cm. of the bowel, and 81 percent of the people who have rectal cancer have bloody stools. There are several possible screening tests. The barium enema is expensive, a poor detector of rectal lesions, but 90 percent accurate in diagnosing cancer of the colon. The digital rectal examination only detects 15 percent of existing tumors, but is easy to do and has few complications. Proctosigmoidoscopy is expensive and uncomfortable, can cause perforations, is accurate in detecting colorectal cancer, but its effectiveness decreases markedly with repeated examination. Testing stools for occult blood has a low number of false negatives and few false positives if the patient follows a meat-free high-residue diet during specimen collection. The method is cheap, causes no discomfort, and can detect cancers from a large area of the bowel. Recommendations are that all patients over 40 have stools tested for occult blood (stool guiuac) every 2 years until age 50, and yearly thereafter. A single sigmoidoscopy on all patients at age 55 is also recommended. Early detection and treatment of colorectal cancer clearly improves the prognosis.

BACTERIURIA. The prevalence of bacteriuria among women is 6,000 per 100,000, and risk factors include frequent sexual intercourse and pelvic relaxation. Most women with bacteriuria have a history of urinary tract infection, and while associated with intravenous pyelogram (IVP) changes and elevated blood urea nitrogen (BUN) and blood pressure, bacteriuria may be an effect rather than a cause. Chronic nephritis cannot be related to bacteriuria, and there are no good data to indicate a relationship to kidney scarring. Diagnosis is by urine culture and is simple and relatively inexpensive. Although antibiotic treatment will eradicate bacteria from the urine, after 1 year only 55 percent will still have sterile urine, and 36 percent will have spontaneously developed sterile urine even though untreated. The long-range benefit from treatment and the amount of morbidity due to renal damage is controversial. Screening asymptomatic persons for bacteriuria is not recommended.

VENEREAL DISEASE. Primary and secondary syphilis have an incidence of 11.5 per 100,000 and latent and late syphilis 24.6 per 100,000. Most cases occur in young and middle-aged adults. There are several excellent, reliable, and cheap serologic tests for syphilis available. Seventy-five percent of undetected cases will progress to irreversible tertiary complications with significant morbidity and mortality. It is recommended that all persons aged 20 to 50 be screened by STS every 6 years, and high risk groups more frequently.

Gonorrhea, although common and readily diagnosed by culture and treated by antibiotics, is not recommended for routine screening in asymptomatic persons. In men, this is because most are symptomatic. In women, it is because morbidity is low (75 percent asymptomatic). Women with pelvic inflammatory disease or other complications will present with symptoms, although cases treated late may result in sterility. Given the present technology and social values, it is believed that gonorrhea cannot be eliminated or controlled, and with relatively low morbidity and mortality as well as little advantage to treatment in the asymptomatic stage, routine screening is not indicated. This conclusion is controversial and no doubt many providers will disagree.

CERVICAL CANCER. The Pap smear is well established as an inexpensive, reliable test for cervical cancer, and it is recognized that diagnosis and treatment in early stages is important in decreasing death rates and achieving cures. The disease meets the criteria for effective periodic screening, but an annual Pap smear is probably too frequent. Cancer of the cervix progresses slowly, requiring between 5 and 10 years to progress from dysplasia to invasive carcinoma. The yield of positive smears decreases markedly in women with several previous negative smears. Therefore, recommendations are for all women over 20 to have annual Pap smears for 2 years, then a smear every other year indefinitely. High risk groups (low socioeconomic class, frequent and multiple sexual partners) should be screened more often.

ENDOMETRIAL CANCER. This is primarily a disease of perimenopausal and postmenopausal women. Abnormal bleeding is the presenting symptom in 79 percent of the patients and most endometrial cancer is diagnosed in Stage I. There is currently no good screening test to detect endometrial cancer prior to symptoms. Educating the patient to report any postmenopausal bleeding and menopausal metrorrhagia is the best approach to screening for this disease. Risk factors include diabetes, hypertension, and estrogen stimulation.

BREAST CANCER. After age 25, breast cancer becomes increasingly common, reaching an incidence of 150 to 200 per 100,000 in women aged 45 to 65. The rate of growth is quite variable and treatment in early Stage I has a much better prognosis than later treatment. Ninety percent of breast cancers are detected by self-examination, but there may be a time lag averaging 10 months before treatment is sought. Small breasts are more easily examined than large, pendulous, or fatty breasts. Mammography is useful in identifying about 42 percent of the tumors in women over age 50 which could not be palpated, but palpation is more effective in younger women. Recommendations for screening include 1) detailed instruction in breast self-examination at age 20, repeated every 10 years; 2) encouraging women to do a systematic breast self-examination every month; 3) breast examination by a health provider every 2 years until age 50, then yearly; and 4) annual or biannual mammography done routinely, only in women over 50 with large, fatty breasts.

ANEMIA. About 10 percent of nonpregnant women are anemic, and 85 to 90 percent of these cases are due to iron deficiency. Frequently anemia is asymptomatic, and there is no evidence that asymptomatic anemia is harmful per se, or that treatment then is superior to treatment after symptoms appear. Symptoms and cardiovascular reserve show no correlation with hemoglobin level until values below 7 to 8 Gm. per 100 ml. are reached. The frequency of serious underlying disease is less than 10 percent. Thus, no routine screening for anemia in asymptomatic nonpregnant women is advised.

GLAUCOMA. Chronic open-angle glaucoma has a high incidence, a long asymptomatic course, and a significant degree of morbidity and treatment is probably effective in reducing complications and disability. It is usually a disease of people over age 40, with an overall prevalence of about 360 per 100,000. However, there is no single diagnostic test that is sensitive and specific enough. Tonometry is most often used but has a 50 to 90 percent false positive rate and a 40 to 60 percent false negative rate. Ophthalmoscopy is another method, and

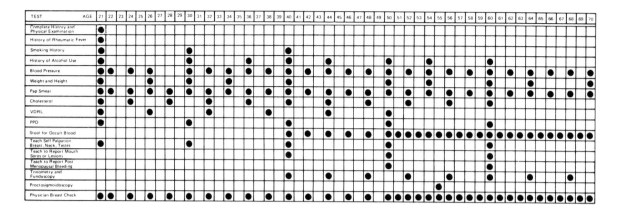

Figure 1-6. Flow sheet for periodic screening for asymptomatic adults. Frame and Carlson, "A Critical Review of Periodic Health Screening Using Specific Screening Criteria." *Journal of Family Practice* 2, 4 (1975): 289.

enlargement of the optic cup greater than one-third the disk diameter suggests glaucoma but is not pathognomonic. Recommendations for screening include tonometry plus ophthalmoscopy every 4 years after age 40. Figure 1-6 summarizes these recommendations for periodic screening in a flow sheet.

In considering these screening recommendations, it must be remembered that they apply only to completely asymptomatic adults. Persons with symptoms or characteristics placing them at increased risk would naturally be screened from a different perspective. In any screening program, patients need to be educated about the importance of prevention, health screening, and risk reduction. The plan for screening must be carefully explained and they must understand that the possibilities of their having specific diseases are being evaluated. Screening is not a guarantee to overall good health. It is but one part in the complex mosaic of seeking high-level wellness and maintaining a state of good health.

NOTES

1. World Health Organization, *Constitution* (WHO Chronicles, Vol. 1, 1947).

2. F. Brockington, *World Health* (London and New York: Churchill Livingstone, 1975), p. 6.

3. C. J. Braden and N. L. Herban, *Community Health: A System Approach* (New York: Appleton-Century-Crofts, 1976), p. 39.

4. M. F. Collen, "Periodic Health Examinations: Why? What? When? How?" *Primary Care* 3,2 (June 1976): 197-204.

5. *Ibid.*

6. R. C. Rock and C. R. Baisden, "Preventive Medicine—Health Screening: Early Detection of Disease." In *Family Practice*, H.F. Conn, et al. (eds.) (Philadelphia: W. B. Saunders, 1973), pp. 82-94.

7. T. L. Delbanco, "The Periodic Examination of the Adult: Waste or Wisdom?" *Primary Care* 3,2 (June 1976): 205-14.

8. L. C. Robbins and J.H. Hall, *How to Practice Prospective Medicine* (Methodist Hospital of Indiana, 1604 W. Capitol, Indianapolis, Indiana 46202, 1970).

9. P. S. Frame and S. J. Carlson, "A Critical Review of Periodic Health Screening Using Specific Screening Criteria," Part 1. *Journal of Family Practice* 2,1 (1975): 29-30.

10. Delbanco, "Periodic Examination of the Adult," pp. 206-7.

11. Rock and Baisden, "Preventive Medicine," pp. 83-84.

12. "Roundtable: Developing Cancer Risk Factor Profiles," and "Charting Determinants of Cancer Risk." *Patient Care* 10,3 (February 1, 1976): 65-84 and 57-61.

13. "The Case for Doing Health Hazard Appraisals." *Patient Care* 8,17 (October 1, 1974): 106-41.

14. Robbins and Hall, *Prospective Medicine*, p. 12.

15. Frame and Carlson, "Periodic Health Screening," Part I, "Selected Diseases of Respiratory, Cardiovascular, and Central Nervous Systems," *Journal of Family Practice* 2,1 (1975): 29-35; Part II, "Selected Endocrine, Metabolic, and Gastrointestinal Diseases," 2,2, pp. 123-9; Part III, "Selected Diseases of the Genitourinary System," 2,3, pp. 189-95; Part IV, "Selected Miscellaneous Diseases," 2,4, pp. 283-9.

2

Sexuality and Affectional Relationships

It is difficult to know the real nature of female sexuality despite the volumes written on it. Until recently, most of these volumes were written by men. The expression of female sexuality is so inseparable from socialization into the "feminine role" that even the premises from which observations are made are biased. The heavy overlay of psychosocial factors has confounded the search for woman's "natural" sexual nature—if a wide range of choices were available for expressing sexual drive, it would be difficult to know which ones women would prefer. The greatly restricted sexuality allowed women under patriarchal systems is our present inheritance, and its moral codes still exert influence. The contemporary blatant commercial use of female sex to sell everything from toothpaste to automobiles and the sharp rise of pornography in magazines and films reflect a swing toward the opposite excess as women break through the restraints of sexual repression.

There are conflicting and contradictory hypotheses regarding the nature of female sexuality, the most ancient and persistent being the "madonna versus whore" in which women are either seen as asexual childbearers (thus good) or as having uncontrolled eroticism (thus bad). Previous concepts of sexuality based upon androcentric thinking grew from observations of the penetration/being penetrated characteristic of sexual dimorphism; since the man penetrated he was the "active" element, and since the women received the penis she was the "passive" element. Interpretations of the meaning of this physiological necessity were bolstered by women's social role. Restricted from taking part in the business of society, conditioned to deference, prepared for a life of service to others, forced to suppress most modes of self-expression, and physically restrained by clothing (long dresses, corsets, and so on) and violence or threats thereof, it is not surprising that women did not seem active in the sexual arena. Psychoanalytic theory spawned concepts of feminine passivity, masochism, narcissism, receptivity, and "mature vaginal sexuality" as opposed to "immature clitoral eroticism." These characteristics reflect sex role rather than sexual behavior. Sexuality in the female that is active, assertive, and self-regulated is much more in keeping with her mammalian descent and maternal function of protecting the young.

Facts about women's sexuality are emerging, although the interpretations and generalizations made from these facts are often questionable. Kinsey and coworkers[1] initiated a new era in sex research through their large-scale study of the practices and experiences of American men and women. One important outcome of this report was the change in attitude toward masturbation, as lay and professional people became aware of its nearly universal occurrence among normal persons. Masters and Johnson[2] again revolutionized thinking about sex when their careful research on physiology documented the same basic process in men and women and, what is more, that in women there was no difference in physiology whether stimulation was entirely clitoral or vaginal. The same principle holds true for men, who experience the same physiological responses whether through masturbation or intercourse. Fisher[3] compiled an impressive array of information about female orgasm and explored how a woman's personality influenced her sexual responsiveness. He urged that results of his research be viewed as tentative because "One of the lessons the writer has learned from his analysis of the previous literature is that generalizations about the nature of sexual responsiveness in women are risky."[4] Hite[5] conducted a nationwide study of female sexuality and asked women to describe in their own words how they experienced their sexuality, including masturbation, orgasm, intercourse, and clitoral stimulation. She also presented a new cultural interpretation of women's sexual expression and problems.

COMPONENTS OF SEXUALITY

The sexuality of the individual can be conceptualized as a complex of emotions, attitudes, preferences, and behaviors which are related to erotic expression. The evidence that sexuality is largely learned as opposed to innate in its expression is extremely strong, although the significance of relations among gonadal hormones, anatomical structures, and sexual behavior is just beginning to be unraveled.[6,7] Among the multiple components of sexuality are the person's chromosomal (genetic) sex, hormonal sex, gonadal sex, morphological sex, gender identity, behavioral sex (sex or gender role and associated beliefs and attitudes), and sexual partner preference. Although there is usually congruence among components, this is not invariably true. Taking the more common case of a person whose genetic, hormonal, gonadal, and morphological sex are congruent, it is believed that the biological equipment provides a frame through which sociocultural definitions of sexuality are expressed. Among humans there are very few sexual behaviors which are unalterable from this biological template, and these include ejaculation of sperm in the male and menstruation, pregnancy and childbirth, and lactation in the female. The much larger sociocultural expression of sexual behavior includes the following key components.

Gender Identity

The sense of being either male or female begins very early. Before the second year of life, personality characteristics have begun to emerge linked to an identification with one sex or the other. In cases of ambiguous external genitalia at birth in which the child was assigned the wrong sex according to its chromosomal complement, it is possible to bring about a change in gender identity during the first 12 to 18 months. With each subsequent month, however, sex reassignment becomes increasingly difficult. By 3½ years of age, the child's core gender identity has been established. This is also the age of establishing conceptual language, the time of settling a gender-differentiated self-concept.[8]

Sex Role

The person's sense of what constitutes appropriate behaviors, attitudes, beliefs, and emotions for a female or male makes up sex role identification. This includes everything a person says and does to indicate to others and the self that she/he is a female or a male. Sex role is the public expression of gender identity, and gender identity is the private and personal experience of sex role. The beliefs a person has about sexuality and the values which coexist with these beliefs are important shapers of sex role behavior. Sex roles are communicated through family interaction, the influence of peers, the channels of communication within a society including all media forms, codes of dress and manners, and the innumerable social structures which encourage and facilitate certain sex-linked behaviors and inhibit or impede others.

Eloquent testimony to the importance of learning and socialization in establishing gender identity and sex role behaviors is illustrated by the case of a sex-reassigned normal male infant after traumatic loss of the penis. At 7 months of age this normal male child was circumcised using electrocautery, but the current was too powerful and the penis ablated flush with the abdominal wall. After months of agonizing and consultation with specialists, the parents implemented a sex reassignment as a girl when the child was 17 months old. This was done with a change of name, clothing and hair style, as well as surgical genital reconstruction. During the 6 years following the initial surgery, close follow-up enabled a tracing of how the newly created girl learned her sexual identity and role. Dress, hair, adornments, neatness, method of urinating, keeping genitals covered, explanation of female reproduction, toys, rehearsal of adult roles in play, quiet instead of rough play, and plans for the child's future life were all used to establish her femininity. Although the child had abundant physical energy, a high level of activity, stubbornness, and was often dominant in her girls' group, she was unquestionably feminine in appearance, attitude, and preferences.[9]

Femininity and masculinity are not absolute conditions and do not necessarily imply opposite behaviors, unless so defined by the culture. There is wide variation in definitions of sex roles, and the criteria for femaleness or maleness often seem arbitrary rather than the result of anatomical or physiological differences. All humans are bisexual to the extent of harboring the impulses, wishes, attitudes, and basic emotional and physiological equipment of the other sex, excluding reproductive anatomy and physiology. It is society's selective development of certain behavioral potentials that produces the difference:

> The members of any society, as participants in its cultural pattern, inevitably perceive some of the dictates of that cultural pattern as eternal verities, and perhaps even as expressions of immutable natural and moral law. The fact is that the canons by which human behavior is regulated are variable to an extraordinary degree, so that the most sacred rules of one society may be the heresies of another.[10]

Sexual Partner Preference

The person's preference for a sexual partner may be the other sex, the same sex, or either sex. The evolution of specific gender group preference for genital sexual involvement is far from understood; it is not even really understood how heterosexual preference develops. That there is no simple and lineal progression involved is amplified by the great variety of partner preference and associated sex role behavior. For example, there is the aggressive, masculine woman whose sex partner choice is a male; the soft, dependent, submissive and very feminine woman whose lover is a lesbian; the effeminate man who exclusively prefers women as sex partners; the effeminate homosexual male; the masculine appearing and behaving homosexual male; and the masculine "butch" lesbian. Recently there has been increased awareness of bisexual capacity in many people who, having all the signs of sex role behavior "appropriate" to their gonadal sex and thus congruent gender identity, find their genital sexual eroticism responsive to either sex. And, there are a rather large number of people who have had homosexual experiences at some point in their lives, but whose basic preference is heterosexual.

Probably factors as diverse as prenatal hormonal environment, the early mother-infant feedback loop, the child's imitation of most valued parent, the family's interstructure and dynamics which could either forestall or foster developing certain identities and behaviors, sociocultural role privileges and restrictions, and society's tolerance of various types of sexual expression are all involved.[11]

THE NEW SEXUAL MYTHS

With the opening up of sexuality in the last two decades, encompassing public discussion, information and behavior changes, many of the old myths growing from a restrictive view of sex have been replaced or discarded. Myths are used to ward off anxiety and hide ignorance by keeping people from thinking. If people can accept something as fact without inquiring into it, questioning and testing its validity, they do not have to consider other possibilities. They can simply act on the basis of what they presume to be true. Sexual myths are particularly helpful in this respect, because sex remains a threatening and uncomfortable area for many people. Some of the old versus new sexual myths are

> Old myth: Women are basically uninterested in sex.
> New myth: Women have become so sexually aggressive that men cannot keep up with them.

There are no definite data to substantiate that male sexual dysfunction is increasing because women are expecting more out of sex. However, the concept of women as passive and uninterested has changed considerably, often swinging to the opposite extreme of insatiable sex drive. The growing awareness that many women have the capacity for multiple orgasms may contribute to unrealistic expectations by the woman and a sense of inadequacy in the man. Rather than seeking her own level of sexual enjoyment the woman measures herself on an exaggerated scale, and the man is involved in a contest of sexual virtuosity.

> Old myth: Masturbation is immature and harmful.
> New myth: Masturbation is more fulfilling sexually than intercourse.

The fear that masturbation causes pimples or insanity has been dispelled, and it is accepted as a widespread and natural sexual practice. Physiological data have revealed that orgasm during masturbation is more intense than during intercourse. Many women, as will be discussed later, are readily orgasmic when masturbating but experience infrequent orgasm during intercourse, or none at all. The solitary nature of masturbation as compared to the relationship and body contact of intercourse makes it less satisfactory for some people. While masturbation may certainly be the sexual activity of choice for some people at certain times, the meaning of sexual fulfillment is individually defined.

> Old myth: Female orgasm is perverse or a rarity.
> New myth: Female orgasm is a glorious life-changing experience.

When women were believed asexual, it was unthinkable that they would have orgasms. Now their orgasmic capacity is not only recognized, but described in superlatives. This often creates unrealistic expectations, such as lights flashing and bells ringing, with disappointment or discouragement when transcendent experiences are not commonly attained. Women need to understand the many natures of female orgasm, its variety of sensations and ranges of intensity. Although becoming orgasmic certainly will make some changes (like enjoying sex more), it is not likely to make immediate, profound changes in a woman's life.

> Old myth: Love is essential to satisfying sex.
> New myth: Love is irrelevant to sex; technique and a sense of fun are everything.

Women particularly have been socialized to believe that love is necessary before sex is permissible, and that the quality of sex depends upon the amount of love. The bitter disillusionment of untold women attests to the falseness of this myth—women who watched love crumble and die because sex was so unsatis-

fying and conflictive. Conversely, men have always known that, not infrequently, great sex occurs with someone for whom they do not feel love, and women have of late been discovering this also. Sex for fun, using the most effective techniques, is promoted by many popular magazines such as *Playboy*, *Penthouse*, and *Cosmopolitan*. At some point most people find, however, a need for caring and attachment in their sexual relations. For many, sex represents a deep bond and primary source of intimacy; thus it is more broadly satisfying in a love relationship. While fun and recreation are positive aspects of sex, and technique certainly needs to be satisfactory to both partners, the integration of sex into our affectional system makes love still an active value.

> Old myth: Vaginal orgasms are superior to clitoral orgasms.
> New myth: Women experience no difference between vaginally induced and clitorally induced orgasms.

Freud's definition of mature female sexuality in terms of capacity for vaginal orgasm, while seeing clitorally induced orgasm as a sign of immaturity or fixation at a more primitive stage of development, branded many women as emotionally sick and fostered a theory of female sexuality which reinforced traditional patriarchal values. These notions have been rejected as physiological research demonstrated that sexual response and changes in genitals and sex organs were identical, as was the mechanism of orgasm, regardless of the source of stimulation. As the myth of the vaginal orgasm was dispelled, and the clitoris recognized as central to arousal and orgasm whether stimulated directly or not, many believed that all orgasms were subjectively experienced in the same way. Women report that they feel a difference between orgasms during intercourse and during masturbation or clitoral stimulation by a partner. The key differences involve the fullness and diffusion of coital orgasm compared to the sharpness and focus of clitorally induced orgasm. These are discussed in greater detail later.

> Old myth: Simultaneous orgasms are the best sexual experience.
> New myth: Sequential orgasms are best.

It is still rather widely believed that simultaneous orgasms are a peak experience and something everyone should strive for, although the popularity of sequential orgasms is growing. There are disadvantages to simultaneous orgasms, as each person may be distracted from her/his sensations by the activity of the other, or the difficulties posed by such exact timing. This is not to say that sequential orgasms are necessarily preferable, though some people enjoy experiencing their partners' climax without distraction. For some people, or at some times, simultaneous orgasm may be more intense and exciting with no disadvantages. This is entirely a matter for the individual and couple, and the pressure of creating a particular goal to strive for only detracts from sexual pleasure and creates anxiety.

> Old myth: Well-adjusted young people are chaste.
> New myth: All contemporary adolescents are promiscuous.

Speculations about the sexual habits of adolescents have usually been exaggerated and distorted, with their promiscuity and wantonness vastly overrated. It is probable that young people begin sexual experimentation and intercourse somewhat earlier than previous generations, to judge by the current younger age at marriage. However, a substantial minority is more conservative and often has not had intercourse before marriage. Adults engage in fantasies about multiple partners, wild sexuality and uninhibited participation in every conceivable sexual act by adolescents which are certainly the exception, not the rule. As stereotypical sex roles blur and change, teenage boys do not have to prove their masculinity by "balling," and girls need not agree to sex because they fear loss of popularity and affection, as other measures of self-worth are developed.

> Old myth: Any woman who is raped probably wanted it.
> New myth: Many women fantasize rape, and therefore must enjoy it.

Rape is a hostile act often associated with brutality. People may be confusing a woman's desire to be "taken by a strong man" when she really does want intercourse with an entirely forced penetration when she has no interest in sex. Part of our sex role socialization includes pretended resistance by the woman, which is overcome by the man's passion. This grows out of denying women's sexual drives and placing them in a submissive position in which it is not proper to express or act on their sexuality.

Part of the sexes' status differential is that men have historically had access to women's bodies whether the women wanted sex or not. Some of this attitude carries over into rape, which the man may feel is somehow his "right" and that the woman's protests are hollow. However, the violence common with rape makes it an exercise of anger or vengeance involving dominance and power, rather than a sexual act. Women find rape a violation of their personal integrity, debasing and dehumanizing. The so-called rape fantasies of women really involve their participation and express their desires, and thus are not truly rape.

> Old myth: Deep, prolonged therapy is necessary to cure sex problems.
> New myth: Sex problems can now be cured by simple tricks or techniques.

With increased public knowledge about sex therapy, what was once viewed as a lifelong insoluble problem is now often seen as readily amenable to cure with mechanical techniques such as "sensate focus" and "pleasuring" and "stop-start technique" or "squeeze technique." The truth lies somewhere in between; specific techniques for sexual problems are often quite effective provided there are no serious interpersonal or attitudinal conflicts involved. Sex therapists need a background in general therapy, because many sex problems are rooted in marital problems, longstanding inhibitions and fears, difficulties with self-concept and self-acceptance, and the many other human dilemmas which create emotional conflicts. The approach used depends upon identifying the source of the sexual problem. Some problems may be improved in a few sessions; others need much longer.

There are many other sexual myths, some of which are presented elsewhere.[12,13] To enjoy full sexual expression, people must question myths and seek answers for themselves. Otherwise, false assumptions about each other or sexuality in general will continue to place barriers between people and hamper understanding.

PHYSIOLOGY OF THE SEXUAL RESPONSE

The clitoral and penile systems in women and men are exact homologues of each other, each part in one having its counterpart in the other. The counterpart may be structurally the same in both, or modified to perform a different function or the same function in a different way. What is striking about the sexual response is its similarities in females and males, rather than its differences. The same two basic physiological responses occur—the primary reaction is widespread vasocongestion, and the secondary reaction is generalized increase in muscle tension or myotonia. The sexual response cycle progresses through identical phases in both sexes with the same or corresponding changes in genital and other organs. There are certain differences in timing and pattern from the excitement to plateau to orgasm to resolution phases in women and men. Orgasm is an intense, extremely pleasurable physical release from the vasocongestion and myotonia built up in response to sexual stimuli. The anatomic structures and physiological responses of both women and men will be covered in this section, so similarities may be appreciated and differences explored.

Female Sexual Anatomy

The external female genitalia are well-known, but the deeper (cryptic) structures have received considerably less attention. The *mons pubis* or *veneris* is the area above the symphysis pubis covered by pubic hair, slightly mounded in shape due to its padding layer of subcutaneous fat. The *labia majora* originate in the mons pubis and terminate in the perineum. These two rounded mounds of tissue form the lateral boundaries of the vulva and are about 7 to 9 cm. long and 2 to 4 cm. wide. These permanent skin folds are homologous to the scrotum of the male. The cleft just below the anterior meeting of the labia is the *anterior commisure*, while their *posterior commisure* is less well defined. The labia majora are well endowed with fatty tissue, hair, sweat glands, blood vessels, lymphatic vessels, and nerves. The *labia minora* are two skin folds lying inside the labia majora, about 5 cm. long, 0.5 to 1 cm. thick, and varying in width from 2 to 3 cm. at the narrowest diameter to 5 to 6 cm. at the widest. The surface has multiple corrigations and no hair. The upper labia minora is continuous with the *prepuce* (clitoral hood) which drapes over the clitoris. Continuing medially the labia line the vaginal opening and end posteriorly in the pudendal frenulum just above the posterior commisure. On their medial aspects beneath the clitoris, they unite to

form the frenulum adjacent to the urethra and vagina, terminating along the hymen. The labial skin is pigmented, the color varying with the state of sexual arousal. Well supplied with blood vessels and nerves, the labia minora distend with sexual arousal and play an important part in the sexual response cycle. The labia minora and vestibule are homologous to the skin of the male urethra and penis.

The area of the *vestibule* is bordered by the labia minora laterally, the posterior commisure and the urethra and clitoris anteriorly. Its inner border is the hymenal ring. The shape and openings of the hymenal membrane vary with sexual experience and parity; after intercourse and pregnancy, the eminences of the hymen are called carunculae myrtiformes. The *external urethral opening* is about 2 to 3 cm. posterior to the clitoris, slightly elevated with depressed areas on the sides, and may be stellate or crescent-shaped. Bilaterally are the openings of the paraurethral (Skene) and periurethral (Aztruc) glands. Just below the vaginal opening, at about 5 and 7 o'clock are the openings of the ducts of the larger vestibular (Bartholin) glands. The blood supply to the vestibule is an extensive capillary plexus. Its innervation is notable for the absence of the usual modalities of touch, although the vestibular portion of the hymenal ring contains an abundance of pain fibers (Figure 2-1).

The *clitoris* consists of four parts: the *glans, shaft, crus,* and *vestibular bulbs.* Its most external portions, the shaft and glans, are located above the vestibule and below the mons, largely hidden under the prepuce in the anterior commisure formed by the fusing of the labia majora. The tiny clitoral shaft with its even tinier glans comprises only one-tenth of the volume of the clitoris in its resting state; this discrepancy is increased during arousal when the cryptic structures may become three times larger. The shaft contains two small erectile cavernous bodies enclosed in a dense fibrous membrane. The length of the shaft is approximately ¼ to ¾ inch, but marked variations exist and substantial normative studies have not been done to establish ranges in size reliably. The glans is on the average 4 to 5 mm. in both transverse and longitudinal measurements, though normal limits encompass transverse diameters from 2 to 3 mm. to 1 cm. The glans is the most sensitive erotogenic area of the body, with its mucous membrane so

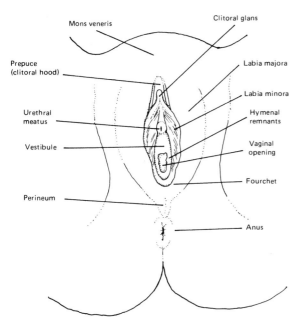

Figure 2-1. External female genitalia.

densely packed with nerve endings that there is hardly room for blood vessels. The entire female sexual cycle can be initiated and maintained to orgasm by light stimulation of the glans of the clitoris alone. At rest, the clitoral shaft is sharply retroflexed posteriorly. As erection occurs, the tip of the clitoris traces an elliptical curve forward, moving through approximately an 180 degree arc. It is retracted and foreshortened as arousal proceeds due to the action of the muscles and cryptic structures of the woman's pudendum.

The clitoral structures divide at the end of the shaft and fan out into the female's lower pelvic area. The two *crura of the clitoris* extend inward bilaterally, following the inferior rami of the pubic symphysis downward. The crura lie below the ischiocavernosus muscles and bodies. The lower portion of the crura becomes tough and tendinous, serving to anchor the clitoris to the inner surface of the ischium. Due to their tendinous nature, the crura play a lesser role in distention during arousal than the vestibular bulbs. The crus of the clitoris is homologous to the corpus cavernosum which becomes the crus of the penis. (See Figures 2-2, 2-3, and 2-4 for homologous female and male sexual anatomy).

The *vestibular bulbs* also divide and descend from the clitoral shaft. They extend outward bilaterally to their position in the anterior portion of the vulva, wrapping about ¾ of the way around the vagina. Each bulb presses closely against the lower third of the vagina just above the level of its opening. The vestibular bulbs are erectile and highly distensible, covered with a mass of coiled blood vessels, conveying blood to and from the bulbs to the clitoral shaft. Called the *commisure of the bulbs*, these vessels also become distended during arousal as part of the total vasocongestion of the area. Located at the bottom of the vestibular bulbs are the greater vestibular glands. The homologous structures in the male are the corpus spongiosum which becomes the bulb of the penis.

The muscles of the female perineum have an important function in sexual arousal and orgasm. The *ischiocavernosus muscles* envelop the clitoral crura in a thin layer of muscle extending from the ischium to the anterior surface of the symphysis at the base of the clitoris. The *bulbocavernosus muscles* envelop the vestibular bulbs and surround the lower third of the vagina. Arising in the midline below the vagina, from the central tendon of the perineum, these muscles ascend around the vagina and terminate in three areas: the fibrous tissue dorsal to the clitoris, the fibrous tissue overlying the crura, and join the ischiocavernosus to form the striated sphincter of the urethra. The *transverse perineal muscles* and *levator ani muscles* converge on the lateral walls of the lower third of the vagina, and unite behind the vaginal opening to form the perineal body. At the lower border of the symphysis pubis, a small triangular fibrous band (suspensory ligament) extends onto the clitoris. The *rectus abdominus muscle* attaches to the suspensory ligament, thus also gaining attachment to the clitoral shaft.

The female pelvic muscles participate in engorgement during sexual arousal, and their contractions on the distended clitoral crura, vestibular bulbs, and circumvaginal venous plexus cause orgasm. Many women are aware that voluntary contractions of perineal muscles can serve to heighten arousal. The three perineal compartments between the urogenital diaphragm and the peritoneum allow extensive room for expansion. This accommodates vaginal expansion during arousal and intercourse, congestion and expansion of bulbs and blood

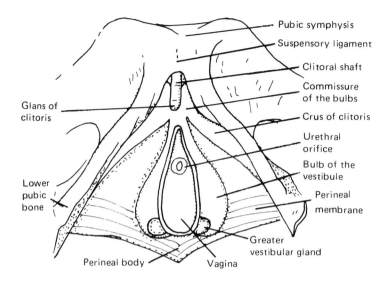

Pubic symphysis
Suspensory ligament
Clitoral shaft
Commissure of the bulbs
Crus of clitoris
Urethral orifice
Bulb of the vestibule
Perineal membrane
Greater vestibular gland

Glans of clitoris
Lower pubic bone
Perineal body
Vagina

Figure 2-2. Dissection of female perineum showing the clitoris, shaft, crus, and vestibular bulbs.

vessels, and the compartments become flattened and virtually obliterated during labor with descent of the fetus through the pelvic canal. The size of the pelvic outlet is considerably wider in females than males to accommodate childbearing. This also contributes to the area available for distention and vasocongestion during sexual arousal.

The *vascularity* of the female pelvis is greater than that of the male. In men, most of the erectile chambers are within the sheath of the cavernous bodies of the penis. Some additional distention is achieved by the pelvic venous plexi around the prostate and rectum. The sheath surrounding the woman's cavernous bodies is not as strong as the man's, allowing greater distention. The area around the bulbs, vagina and uterus is one of the most vascularized in the body, including the large commissure of the bulbs, circumvaginal plexus, and uterine plexus. There is thus more room for expansion in the female pelvis, more structures to expand, and a greater blood supply to accomplish congestion.[14]

Male Sexual Anatomy

Male external genitalia consist of the *penis* with its *shaft* and *glans*, and the *scrotal sacs* containing the *testes* and *epididymis*. The *vas deferens* conveys the sperm to the urethra, where secretions from the *seminal vesicle* and *prostate* join to form the ejaculate. The penis is divided into three long cylinders of erectile tissue surrounded by an elastic sheath, each containing blood vessels and spaces which fill with blood. The two upper cylinders, the *corpora cavernosa*, are responsible for the increased size, especially in width, and rigidity of the erect penis. At the base of the pendulous shaft of the penis, these two cylinders diverge into the *crura*, which become tough tendinous fibers and attach to the pelvic bones. These are homologous to the clitoral crura of the female. The lower cylinder on the underside of the penis is the *corpus spongiosum*, and it terminates on its external end in the *glans* and on its internal end in the *bulb*. The urethra runs through the corpus spongiosum, and is prevented from collapse during erection by tiny struts which hold it patent. The spongy body remains softer during erection, and the glans enlarges to almost twice its usual size, providing a soft protective cushion for the rigid corpora cavernosa. It is highly endowed with nerve endings and is the area of maximal erotic sensation.

The bulb becomes quite rigid and distended during arousal, almost filling the space between the pubic rami. When distended, it lengthens and markedly increases in diameter, pressing downward on the testicles. The bulb of the penis is homologous to the female vestibular bulbs. There is a small groove at the end of the bulb (embryonic groove) which reveals that in early embryonic development there were two bulbs in the male, as in the

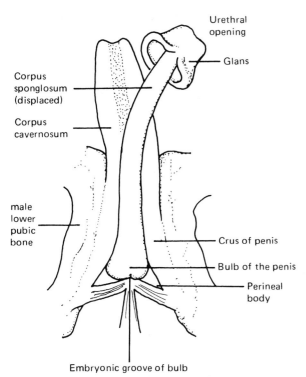

Figure 2-3. Male sexual anatomy.

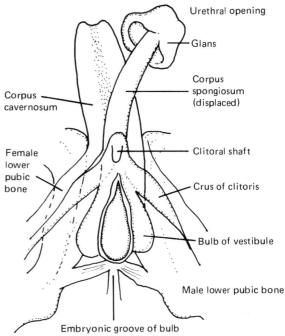

Figure 2-4. Comparison of female and male anatomy.

female, and these later fused to produce the single penile bulb.

There are no muscles which play an important role in the pendulous shaft of the penis, either for erection or ejaculation. Erection occurs by rapid filling of the cavernous bodies against the resistance of their sheaths. In the cryptic portion, however, the bulb and corpora cavernosa become enclosed in a muscular coat. These muscles, with some assistance from practically all other muscles in the area, are responsible for final erection and ejaculation. Contracting in a coordinated, downward rhythm, they compress the cryptic erectile bodies, which compress the urethra and force semen forward with considerable pressure. Blood is also forced out of the distended cavernous spaces, leading to detumescence of the penis. One other structure aids slightly in erection; the suspensory ligament running from the upper margin of the penis toward the symphysis, attaching to the lower abdominal muscles. Its homologue is the suspensory ligament in the female.

The Sexual Response Cycle

The sexual response is an orderly sequence of physiological events which bring about marked changes in the genital organs, both in shape and function, from their resting state. Sexual stimulation, regardless of source, brings about neurological, vascular, muscular, and hormonal reactions which affect almost the entire body. Masters and Johnson, in their pioneering book *Human Sexual Response* (1966)[15] described four successive stages in the response cycle. Characteristic changes occur during each stage involving not only the genitals but also the breasts, skin, muscles, and other pelvic structures. Figures 2-5, 2-6, and 2-7 show the characteristic changes in the genital organs that occur during each stage. A general description of genital changes during the four stages follows.

EXCITEMENT. The onset of erotic feelings begins the excitement stage, producing an immediate and intense vasocongestion and increased muscle tension. In males, excitement is signalled by erection, with scrotal thickening and elevation of the testes also occurring.

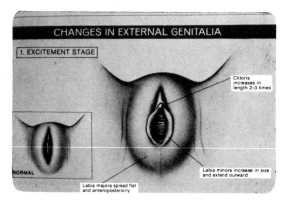
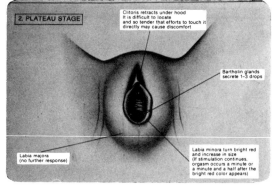
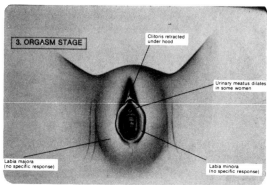
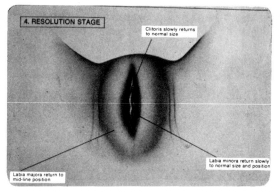

Figure 2-5. Characteristic changes in female external genitalia during the four stages of the sexual response.

In the female, venous dilatation and congestion are quickly followed by passage of fluid from the venous networks into tissue spaces, causing edema. Droplets of clear fluid (transudate) appear within 30 seconds of arousal, which coalesce on the vaginal walls and produce vaginal lubrication. The rapidity and quantity of this transudate indicates that a massive fluid transfer must take place in a few minutes. There is some vasocongestion of the clitoris, which increases slightly in size and may become erect in some women. The uterus enlarges due to vascular engorgement and begins to rise, and the vagina begins to enlarge and balloon in its upper portion.

PLATEAU.   As arousal progresses the plateau stage is reached, occurring just before orgasm. The vasocongestive responses are at a peak in both sexes. In the male, the penis is fully distended and the shaft at its maximum size. The testes are engorged and enlarged, and elevated closely against the perineum. Two or three drops of clear mucoid fluid appear, possibly from Cowper's gland. In the female, a broad "platform" of distended tissues occurs as pelvic congestion and edema reach a peak. Especially involved are the lower third of the vagina, the vestibular bulbs, the labia minora, anterior commissure, and the uterus. The thickened area of congested tissue surrounding the vaginal entrance and its lower third is called the "orgasmic platform." The labia minora reach maximum coloration, the uterus completes its ascent from the pelvic floor, and the upper third of the vagina is widely ballooned. The clitoris arcs upward and retracts under the prepuce and behind the symphysis.

ORGASM.   When the vasocongestive distention reaches a critical point, a reflex stretch mechanism is set off in the muscles surrounding the congested tissues. This causes them to contract vigorously, expelling the blood trapped in the tissues and venous plexi, and creating the sensations of orgasm. The same muscles are involved in both sexes: primarily

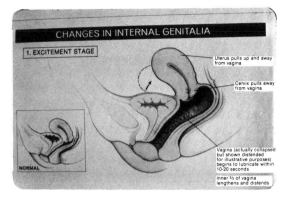
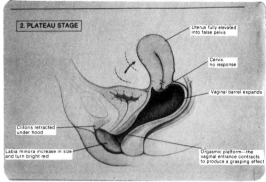
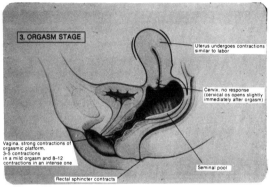
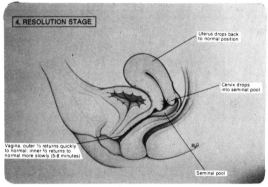

the bulbocavernosi, transverse perineals, external anal sphincter, and rectus abdominus; and to a lesser degree the ischiocavernosi and levator ani. In the male, semen spurts out of the penile urethra at 0.8 second intervals, for 3 to 7 ejaculatory spurts. As muscle contractions around the seminal vesicles and prostate cause emission of the ejaculate into the upper urethra, the man feels the sensation of "ejaculatory inevitability," followed immediately by the propulsive orgasmic contractions. After orgasm, the male usually has a "refractory period" of varying length during which he is not responsive to sexual stimulation. In the female, the muscular contractions producing orgasm also occur at 0.8 second intervals, moving blood from the distended pelvic tissues and veins. Orgasm consists of 8 to 15 contractions, of which the first 5 or 6 are most intense. Many women are capable of restimulation seconds after orgasm, while still distended to plateau levels, to go on to repeated orgasms. It appears women do not have a refractory period, although the capacity for multiple orgasms varies greatly.

Figure 2-6. Characteristic changes in female internal genitalia during the four stages of the sexual response.

RESOLUTION.   In the final stage of the sexual cycle, the changes which occurred in genital and other organs reverse, and the body returns to its resting state. In males, the testes detumesce and descend at once to their usual position suspended away from the body. The penis becomes flaccid more slowly in two stages. It is reduced to half its erect size soon after orgasm, and by 30 minutes has returned to its resting size. In the female the clitoris returns to its normal position 5 to 10 seconds after orgasm, and there is rapid detumescence of the orgasmic platform. The vagina may take 10 to 15 minutes to return to its relaxed state, and the cervical os gapes for about 30 minutes, at which time the uterus has completed its descent into the pelvis placing the cervix in the seminal basin. The labia minora loses its deep coloration in 10 to 15 seconds, with its edema taking longer to resolve.

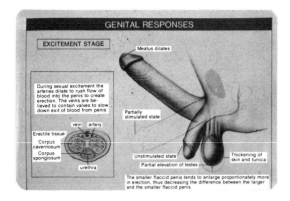

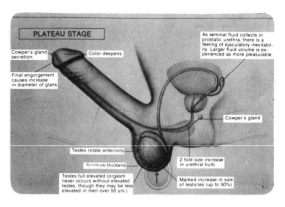

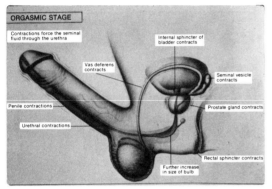

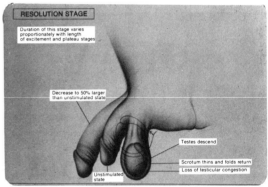

Figure 2-7. Characteristic changes in male internal genitalia during the four stages of the sexual response.

Patterns of Sexual Response

There are wide variations in the patterns of sexual response among different women and in the same woman at different times. The basic anatomical and physiological responses are always the same, appearing sequentially under all conditions of arousal, but variations occur in timing or duration of each phase, intensity of reactions, according to parity and phase of the menstrual cycle, and if the woman has suffered obstetrical damage. Because there is also considerable variation in precise construction of women's sexual anatomy, variations in response often result from these subtle differences, particularly in effectiveness of stimulation methods.

Certain differences occur in the responses of men and women, although the similarities far outweigh the differences. In the excitement phase, men attain an erection very rapidly, within 3 to 5 seconds, as compared to the 30 seconds required for the woman's vaginal transudate to appear. The reason for this is that the woman attains greater generalized vasocongestion and edema to fill the larger structures in her pelvic area, which simply takes longer. Men have three erectile bodies to fill: the two corpora cavernosi and one bulb with its shaft extension, the corpus spongiosum. Women have five erectile bodies: the two corpora cavernosi, the two vestibular bulbs with their anterior commissure extension, and a large circumvaginal plexus into which drain all the veins of the perineum. With all venous plexi and bulbs maximally distended, the total blood volume which the woman must remove during orgasm is considerably greater than that of the man. Because of the greater diameters of the pelvic outlet in women, their muscles are longer in this area. In the male, much of the strength of the orgasmic muscles' contractile force is expended in the first 3 to 4 contractions. This strong, concentrated muscular activity assures deposition of semen deep within the vaginal barrel, resulting in a short and intense orgasm. In the woman, the first few contractions are not as strong and the orgasm is more prolonged, a nice adaptive device to remove the greatest amount of her more widespread vascular congestion. Therefore, as far as effective contractions are concerned, the woman's orgasm generally lasts about twice as long as the man's—the most forceful and pleasurable contractions in the man last about 3 to 4 seconds and in the woman about 5 to 6 seconds.[16]

Women experience basically three types of response patterns, while men experience one basic type. In the male, excitement and plateau phases build continuously to one definitive, usually strong orgasm. The excitement phase can be prolonged by deliberate use of delaying techniques. Once ejaculation begins, the orgasmic contractions continue involuntarily whether or not stimulation is applied. This is in contrast to the female, in which orgasmic contractions will stop at any point if stimulation ceases. Resolution usually occurs rather rapidly in the male, with the refractory period during which restimulation is not possible. The refractory period is much shorter in younger men, who may have another erection in a few minutes.

In the female, one pattern resembles this male pattern, in which excitement and plateau phases build rapidly, with some peaks and dips, to one intense orgasm and rapid resolution. In a second pattern, excitement and plateau phases may be prolonged. There can be one definitive orgasm, a milder and less intense orgasm, or multiple orgasms while rising from and falling into plateau levels of arousal, usually followed by slower resolution. A third pattern involves achieving plateau levels of arousal with minor surges toward the orgasmic level, causing a repeated and prolonged "pleasant or tingly" sensation without definitive orgasm. Resolution is also slower in this pattern.[17]

BIPHASIC NATURE OF SEXUAL RESPONSE. The division of the sexual response into four stages as described by Masters and Johnson allows inclusion and correct placement of the specific physiological responses in sequence on a continuum. Although this is the normal progression, the sexual response does not comprise a single entity, but consists of two distinct and relatively independent components. One component is the genital vasocongestive reaction which produces erection in the male and vaginal lubrication and swelling in the female; the other is the reflex clonic muscular contractions which cause orgasm in both sexes. These two components involve different anatomic structures which are ennervated by different parts of the nervous system. The erectile and congestive component is mediated by the parasympathetic division of the autonomic nervous system, and the muscular contractive (orgasmic) component by the sympathetic division. As a result, sexual problems involving one or the other component present distinctly different clinical syndromes, probably caused by different pathophysiological mechanisms, and responsive to different types of treatment.[18]

The Clitoris and Orgasm

Masters and Johnson have aptly called the clitoris the "transmitter and conductor" of erotic sensation. The clitoris is exquisitely sensitive and highly responsive to all types of stimulation, as long as touch and pressure are not direct enough or hard enough to cause pain. Clitoral erection causes the shaft to retract into the swollen prepuce (clitoral hood) shortly before orgasm. This is accomplished by contraction of the ischiocavernosi muscles (which lengthen in men to allow erection), distention of the crura, and shortening of the suspensory ligament via its attachment to the rectus abdominus. The swelling of the prepuce causes it to envelop the clitoral shaft and glans closely, and the clitoris is pulled up onto the anterior border of the symphysis which increases the pressure against it. Friction applied to the area of the clitoris, whether by the tongue, fingers, a vibrator, or the penis, moves the clitoris back and forth under its prepuce. Although stimulation can be applied more directly to the clitoral glans or shaft in earlier stages of arousal, once into the plateau stage with full retraction of the clitoris, the final stimulation which triggers orgasm is provided to the clitoris by friction against its own hood. This final stimulation of the clitoris leads to maximal distention and the reflex muscular contractions of orgasm.

The "preputial-glandar" mechanism works extremely well as long as there is adequate stimulation. During masturbation, when women can apply exactly the type and amount of stimulation which causes the best response for them, orgasm is frequently attained in 3 to 4 minutes and multiple orgasms are not uncommon. During intercourse, however, orgasm is less reliable and often more difficult to produce. Penile thrusting causes intermittent traction on the woman's labia, which in turn pulls the clitoral hood. This mechanical traction moves the hood against the clitoris and pulls the clitoral shaft downward with insertion, releasing it to return to its more erect position upon withdrawal. Continued friction by this method then leads to orgasm. While this thrusting mechanism works well in some women, it is not generally as effective as manual stimulation of the clitoris. Due to individual variations in anatomy and sexual technique, a significant number of women either never or rarely have orgasm by coitus alone.

EFFECTS OF PREGNANCY AND THE LUTEAL PHASE.   There is an increase of sexual interest in women during the second half of the menstrual cycle, the luteal phase. Although psychogenic factors can mitigate these physiological processes, women during the luteal phase demonstrate greater desire to initiate sex, reach plateau stages of arousal more easily, have a more copious transudate of a slipperier consistency, and achieve orgasms more readily. This facilitation of sexual response is primarily due to the greater baseline of pelvic congestion and edema produced by the progesterone effects of the luteal phase. The extent of pelvic congestion possible, or more easily achieved, is greater when the woman is sexually stimulated at this time. Hormonal effects may also play some role, as the presumed erotic hormone in both men and women (androgen) may be increased at this time, possibly from conversion of progesterone.

Many women have their first orgasm from coitus either during or after their first pregnancy. This increase in orgasmic capacity with pregnancy is probably related to greater vascularity of the entire pelvis induced by pregnancy hormones. The growth of new blood vessels spurred by pregnancy, and persisting to some extent afterwards, and the elaboration of huge amounts of progesterone and androgen during pregnancy are involved. An increased vascular bed allows greater vasocongestion and distention of erectile structures; the hormones have an effect on the responsivity of the clitoral system and the strength of the muscles

producing the orgasmic response. Barring obstetrical damage, subsequent pregnancies will increase the volume capacity of the pelvic venous system and edema which it produces, enhancing the capacity for both sexual tension and premenstrual congestion.[19]

MULTIPLE ORGASMS.   Many women are capable of repeated orgasms if effectively stimulated. Masturbation and manual clitoral stimulation are usually necessary for multiple orgasms, because the male cannot sustain coitus long enough and because clitoral stimulation is more effective. Women may have 5 to 6 full orgasms within a few minutes, although as many as 20 to 50 consecutive orgasms have been reported. The mechanisms for multiple orgasms is inherent in the dynamics of female sexual response. The immediate results of the woman's orgasmic contractions are emptying of the vestibular bulbs and commissure, emptying of the circumvaginal plexi, and relaxation of the ischiocavernosi muscles and suspensory ligament allowing clitoral return. However, with full venous engorgement and edema, the emptied bulbar cavities and plexi refill immediately, and fluid from the tissues moves back into the vascular bed. Thus vasocongestion recurs rapidly after orgasm, and if effective stimulation is continued, the clitoris again retracts and the muscles of the pelvic floor are again distended to the point of reflex orgasmic contractions. Some women use continuous stimulation to go from one orgasm to the next with almost no time lapse, and others prefer to return to the plateau or excitement phase for restimulation to the next orgasm.

The labia majora contribute to capacity for multiple orgasms, for they act as reservoirs of congested vessels and edema which are not emptied during orgasm. Venous return from the labia goes directly to the bulbar and pudendal plexi, aiding in their prompt refilling. The labia are increasingly vascularized with pregnancies, and in multiparous women they become so edematous and engorged during intense sexual arousal that their resolution may take several hours. Continuous labial congestion and edema are central in maintaining sexual tension, and account for the sensation of continued arousal in multiparous women even after one or two orgasms.

As each orgasm is followed by prompt refilling of the venous erectile chambers, with engorgement and edema creating distention and leading to another orgasm, it appears that the female's orgasmic capacity is theoretically insatiable. The more orgasms a woman has, the more she can have, and the stronger they become. Women experiencing multiple orgasms can continue until muscle fatigue sets in, and the pelvic orgasmic muscles are too tired to continue contracting.[20] All women, although potentially having this capacity, do not desire multiple orgasms, may not have found an effective method of stimulation, or do not have the frame of mind conducive to producing them. Although the male is at a physiological disadvantage in respect to multiple orgasms, in our culture men have a much stronger drive to fulfill their orgastic potential.

WOMEN'S EXPERIENCE OF SEX

To understand female sexuality, large numbers of women must be asked numerous questions concerning how they feel, what they like, and what they think of sex. In her book *The Hite Report*,[21] Shere Hite summarizes the results of her nationwide survey of female sexuality, including responses from 3,000 women ages 14 to 78. By structuring her extensive questionnaires to avoid conveying expectations about what was "normal" in sexual practices, Hite enabled respondents to describe all ranges of sexual experiences and feelings. The results speak eloquently to a new way of conceptualizing female sexuality:

> Female sexuality has been seen essentially as a response to male sexuality and intercourse. There has rarely been any acknowledgement that female sexuality might have a complex nature of its own which would be more than just the logical counterpart of (what we think of as) male sexuality.[22]

Women's experience of various sexual practices as reported in this work will be discussed below.

Masturbation

From 65[23] to 80[24] percent of women masturbate and most discover it on their own at a very early age. In many homes, sexual exploration, nudity, and masturbation are prohibited by parents and feelings of guilt and shame are common among women from such families. Although masturbation often continues through the life cycle, there is still cultural proscription against it, creating in many women reluctance and uncomfortable feelings associated with masturbation. More men than women masturbate, approaching 100 percent of men, and the practice seems more culturally acceptable for men. One reason for repression of masturbation in women is that in so doing, they are not fulfilling the socially approved feminine role. In the area of sex, giving pleasure to men and participating in mutual activities is expected. This solitary and noncoitally connected activity threatens established sex roles.

While most women who do masturbate experience intense orgasms and enjoy it physically, they often do not enjoy it psychologically. Many feel lonely and isolated, and use masturbation as a substitute for sex or orgasm with a partner. Masturbation is seen by some women as a learning experience which helps them know their bodies and have better sex with another person. A few women view it as a pure pleasure, important for their sexual satisfaction and a means of independence and self-reliance.

The type of motion used by women during masturbation is a massaging, rubbing, patting or stroking of the clitoral/vulval area with hand or fingers. Some use direct clitoral contact, and others indirect contact; but the touch usually remains soft and light. Motion often becomes faster as excitement progresses, with some increase in pressure. The constancy of pressure and rhythm seems most important in achieving orgasm, usually requiring very rapid agitation similar to a vibrator. While leg position varies among women, in the same women a particular position is generally necessary for orgasm.

Orgasm

Approximately 90 percent of women have experienced orgasm, perhaps 75 percent on a reasonably regular basis.[25] Women clearly find orgasm important, as most would not enjoy sex without it and tolerate only occasional nonorgasmic intercourse. Many women feel left out and cheated when only their partner experiences orgasm, leading to anger and frustration. Women occasionally can derive vicarious satisfaction from the man's orgasm in this situation. There seems to be a great pressure for women to have orgasm during intercourse. This arises from a need to perform well sexually, to make the man feel potent and accomplished in sex, or to meet society's expectations for being a real woman.

Some women have physical signs of orgasm such as pelvic rocking, shuddering, moaning, and rapid breathing. Many do not show discernible signs, however, remaining largely still and quiet. A regular partner would know from subtle signs but new or inexperienced partners might not be able to recognize the woman's orgasm. Sexual arousal is experienced as intense tingling, aching, heat, swelling or pressure focused in the genital area. As peak arousal is reached (plateau) sensations are exploding, overflowing, or like an electric shock. The pelvic and vaginal contractions of orgasm feel like rolling pulses, throbbing waves or spasms, vibrations or pulsations, or waves of heat up through the body. Feelings after orgasm include relaxation, elation, euphoria, peacefulness, or aliveness.

Although capable of restimulation to several orgasms, the vast majority of women desire only one. This probably results from cultural conditioning, making the woman feel guilty, self-conscious, greedy, or unnatural if she wants additional orgasms. Although generally satisfied with one orgasm, women do not return to a sexually insensitive state afterwards. They often feel strong, energetic and alive, or tender and loving. These are similar to the feelings accompanying arousal, and probably represent the woman's continued capacity for restimulation. Women who do prefer several orgasms relate that each subsequent one is stronger, deeper and more satisfying.

Orgasm with the presence of a penis (during intercourse) feels different from orgasm without this (during masturbation or clitoral stimulation by a partner). Coital orgasm is more diffuse and noncoital orgasm more intense. The overall body pleasure and feelings of closeness during intercourse make coital orgasm more satisfying emotionally, richer, deeper and more joyous for some women. Orgasm due to clitoral stimulation without penetration is more intense, focused, and localized. This may be due to less self-consciousness when alone, perfect centering and coordination of stimulation, and easy assumption of the best leg position. Another factor might be less distraction and constriction from the other person's body movement or weight.

Coital orgasm feels more diffuse, covering the entire body, partly because there is a longer buildup period than with masturbation. Some women feel an intense desire for penetration (vaginal ache) just before orgasm which is soothed and diffused with a penis present. While felt as an unpleasant, hollow feeling by certain women, others find this most pleasurable. Occasionally women describe an "emotional orgasm" felt as an intense emotional peak, sometimes with an opening sensation in both vagina and throat, accompanied by strong feelings of yearning, closeness, or exaltation. The intense clitoral feelings and vaginal contractions of orgasm are not present.[26] While this experience can be satisfying emotionally, it does not provide the physical release of actual orgasm.

Intercourse

Significant numbers of women do not experience orgasm regularly as a result of intercourse. Over 70 percent of the women Hite studied could not have an orgasm during intercourse without more direct clitoral stimulation manually at the time of orgasm. Only 30 percent could experience orgasm regularly from intercourse alone. Thus, orgasm as a result of intercourse alone is the exceptional, rather than the usual, experience (Table 2-1).

These figures are corroborated by data from other studies of female sexuality. Fisher found that about 39 percent of the 300 young, married, middle-class women in his 5-year study always or nearly always had orgasm during intercourse. However, only 20 percent of this group said they never required a final push to orgasm from manual clitoral stimulation.[27] Kaplan, using her extensive clinical experience as a sex therapist and psychoanalyst, arrived at the impression that, while about 90 percent of women can achieve orgasm by some means, only half or fewer can reach a climax during coitus without additional clitoral stimulation.[28] The works of both Kinsey and Masters and Johnson recognize that women experience orgasm much more frequently from masturbation or clitoral stimulation than from intercourse. The fact that 50 percent of all women are unable to have orgasm during coitus was corroborated by Romney.[29] The consensus of these studies is that most women do not naturally have orgasm during intercourse from

Table 2-1
Orgasm During Intercourse

Orgasm Regularly from Intercourse Alone	Orgasm Rarely from Intercourse Alone	Orgasm During Intercourse with Simultaneous Manual Clitoral Stimulation	No Orgasm During Interourse
30%	22%	19%	29%

penile thrusting and the traction this produces on the labia and clitoris.

The inability to have orgasm during intercourse is the most common female sexual problem. In large measure, this is a problem of attitudes and ignorance. Cultural definitions of femininity maintain that women should have orgasm with coitus alone and find this maximally satisfying. Ignorance of female sexual physiology leads to intercourse techniques which do not provide adequate stimulation. Long-standing attitudes continue to bind sexual pleasure with reproduction, making coitus the "real" sexual activity and all other types perversions or substitutions. In a sexist tradition, intercourse symbolizes male dominance and gives men direct access to reproductive control. By demanding virginity at marriage and monogamy thereafter, patrilineal descent can be established, property transferred in the male lineage, and maximum population growth encouraged. Power politics and the suppression of women probably underlie some of the difficulties in approaching the problem of coital nonorgasm. With such a large group of women involved, this must be considered a normal variation rather than a sign of pathology.

The Freudian model of female sexuality with its vaginal primacy added the dimension of neuroses when women were nonorgasmic during coitus. However, relations between immature personality structure, poor ego integration, and unconscious conflicts with inability to have orgasm during intercourse have not been demonstrated. As an outgrowth of this model, however, women often feel emotionally abnormal or personally at fault when they do not have orgasm during intercourse. Therapy based on the assumption that normal women should experience orgasm with intercourse alone serves to perpetuate these problems.

Women often must work toward developing specific techniques to achieve orgasm during intercourse. Centering on some type of clitoral contact is a frequent method. The position of woman on top with its freedom of movement allows adjustment of penetration, and the woman can seek her best leg position and control mons area rubbing or pressure. Some women prefer a grinding of the pubic areas together with little thrusting, or frequent penile reentry with small movements at the introitus. The plateau level may be reached with clitoral stimulation and intromission may occur just prior to orgasm, or the woman may experience orgasm clitorally before penetration. Simultaneous clitoral stimulation with the partner's or woman's hand during intercourse is a popular method of achieving coital orgasm.[30]

A significant number of women fake orgasm with intercourse, for a number of complex reasons. If a woman does desire coital orgasm, the key point is that she must take an active role and not passively expect the man to be responsible. She needs to learn what types of stimulation are effective, and how to keep the arousal progressing and trigger the orgasm. Cooperation of her partner must be elicited as necessary. Knowing her body and being responsible for her own pleasure are the essential factors in finding effective approaches to intercourse.

Older Women

There is an increase or peaking of female responsiveness after the late 30s, often continuing through menopause and thereafter. Although decreased vaginal lubrication and atrophic changes can occur after menopause, women who have regular sexual activity continue responsiveness into old age. Both physical and social factors are involved in this later blossoming of women's sexuality, as compared to men's peak responsiveness occurring in the late teens. Cultural influences which diminish the ability of younger women to enjoy their sexuality are probably most important in this delay of full expression of sexual potential.

Unlike men who are given early social sanction to value and enjoy genital sexuality, women are conditioned to undervalue or disown theirs. Social approval for sex after the woman is married cannot undo overnight 20 or more years of conditioning; but, with repeated pleasurable sexual experiences, many women are able to overcome the taboos of youth by their middle years. For women fulfilling the traditional feminine role, the years after age 30 are freer from unrelenting demands of raising babies and toddlers. With more time for herself, the woman can become more conscious of both her sexuality and self-identity. This may enable her to be more assertive in sex and less willing to settle for unsatisfying experiences. Seeing her partner as less susceptible to ego damage due to increased self-confidence often makes her comfortable with discussing improvement of sexual techniques. Better communication may lead to appropriate expression of anger and diminution of marital power struggles often involved in holding back sexual responsiveness.[31]

Physiological changes augment increased sexuality, with enhanced pelvic vascularity after childbirth and reduced circulating estrogen levels, which reduces their check on the sexually stimulating action of androgens. Experience no doubt is important, as women have had more time to learn about their bodies and what practices stimulate them most. Most women in Hite's study reported that their sexual pleasure increased with age. Others, however, felt sex was not important to them any more, or had difficulty finding partners if they were interested in sex. Some older women had extramarital lovers, had begun to relate sexually to women, or enjoyed sex with younger men. Some were disappointed and bitter about their sexual experiences:

> My current sexual life is zero. It has been zero for 21 years... I am 62, and have been married 25 years (in my present marriage). I am married to a typical male boor, selfish and insensitive, also alcoholic, but I stay here because I am aging, I have no skills, and I have cardiac problems.[32]

Not infrequently older women come to rely more on masturbation, because of their partner's decreasing capacity and the lack of socially permissible alternative relationships. Cultural stereotypes are equally destructive for aging men, who suffer decreased self-esteem as erection takes longer to achieve, orgasm is slower and less reliable, the refractory period longer, and sex drive lessened. The cultural emphasis on penile function and coitus prevents men from exploring other ways of expressing their sexuality, which could otherwise be complementary to the older woman's increased sexual desire and capacity.

The "Sexual Revolution"

The changes in sexual behavior and mores apparent since the 1960s are a long-range result of changes affecting the structure of the family and women's role in it. "Sexual freedom," the right of women to have sex without marriage and decreased emphasis on monogamy, is a function of the decreased importance of childbearing to society and of paternity to men. Although many women like these changes because there is more openness about sex, others feel there has not been real freedom for women and men to explore their total sexuality, resulting in another form of exploitation as women are put under pressure to have more of the same kind of sex. Some contend it has merely taken away the woman's right not to have sex, for fear of rejection or being considered "up tight" or abnormal. Most women—still tied to the cultural definition of one (male) model of sex: foreplay, penetration, intercourse, and ejaculation—habitually satisfy men's needs during sex and ignore their own.

The basic value of sex and intercourse for women involves closeness and affection; indeed, sex is almost the only way people can be really physically and emotionally intimate in our society. Most women know how to have orgasms, but do not insist on their satisfaction with male partners, partly out of habit and social conditioning ("women are used to serving men their orgasms"), partly because of fear of losing love ("men give love for sex, women give sex for love"), and partly for economic reasons. A woman who is totally dependent for food and shelter upon the man with whom she has sex, and has no economic alternatives, is subject to obvious economic intimidation. Even women who work have less economic security than men, are pressured to marriage or secondary roles, or are still conditioned to modifying their sexual desire to meet other needs of survival and comfort.

...you cannot decree women to be "sexually free" when they are not economically free; to do so is to put them into a more vulnerable position than ever, and make them into a form of easily available common property.[33]

APPROACH TO SEXUAL PROBLEMS

It is difficult for a woman to admit to her health provider that she is having a sexual problem, although there is an increasing tendency for openness. Many physical symptoms may mask or result from underlying sexual difficulties. Problems involving the genitalia can suggest sexual problems, particularly complaints of increased vaginal discharge, foul-smelling vaginal discharge, or vaginitis when there are no confirmatory physical findings. Pelvic or abdominal pain in the absence of pathology is also suspect. "Organ language" in response to stress, such as backache, headache, chest tightness, throat tightness, and so forth, can be caused by sexual as well as other emotional conflicts. Abnormal vaginal bleeding may also be triggered by stress. Women experiencing dyspareunia or reporting lax vaginal muscles are speaking more directly to sexual problems. Some may say outright that they cannot become sexually excited or cannot have orgasm.

Sexual History

A careful, detailed history using a direct approach and precise terms enables the provider to understand the type of sexual problem and gain data about possible cause. Questions in the history include the following:

What is the specific sexual problem?
When did it begin? Any associated factors?
When does it occur? Associated factors?
Has it always been present, or does it come and go? What brings it on, what makes it go away?
What makes the problem better, what makes it worse?
What have you (and your partner) done about it? Does your partner know about it?
Is the problem about the same, or is it getting worse?
Does it occur with only your regular partner, or other partners also?
(If indicated) How does your partner feel about sex? About this problem?

(If indicated) How do you feel about sex? About this problem?

The history also includes menstrual pattern, pregnancies, gynecological problems and surgery, birth control, illnesses, and operations. To gain information about attitudes toward sexuality, questions may explore how the woman first learned about sex, feelings about menarche, experiences with masturbation, reaction to first intercourse, and beliefs about conditions under which sex is acceptable or types of sexual practices considered appropriate. Other data which may be important are the woman's age, marital status, occupation, religion, number and ages of children, and personal characteristics of her partner. Previous traumatic or unpleasant experiences connected with sex are important.

The quality of the woman's relationship with her partner may also be important to explore, including common interests and activities, sharing confidences, recreation when first together and now, frequency of sex when first together and now, sexual encounters with other people, types of sexual practices, and whether both partners are satisfied with sex.[34]

Physical Examination

Certain findings on physical examination can be indications of sexual problems. Inflammation, lesions or smegma of the clitoris may cause pain or reduce clitoral sensitivity. Varicosities, lesions, inflammation or infection of vulva or vagina are often related to dyspareunia. A narrow perineal body with gaping introitus, and inability of the woman to squeeze down on two examining fingers with vaginal musculature can indicate reasons for failure of response to stimulation with coitus. Involuntary contraction of the vaginal opening when the perineum is approached is classical for vaginismus. Vaginal atrophy can lead to painful intercourse and lessened sexual response.

Cul-de-sac masses caused by a retroverted uterus, prolapsed adnexa, pelvic inflammation, or endometriosis are often associated with pain on deep penetration. Some chronic illnesses may cause decreased sensitivity to stimulation or decreased sexual desire, including diabetes, heart disease, multiple sclerosis, and endocrine disorders. Certain types of surgery are particularly difficult to accept in terms of sexual self-image, such as mastectomy, hysterectomy, ileostomy, colostomy, and sometimes tubal ligation. Chronic illnesses and surgery exert a stronger psychological than physical effect, however, and may serve as a vehicle for expression of psychogenic sexual conflicts rather than be the actual cause.

Medications

Sedatives, narcotics, tranquilizers, alcohol, some antihypertensive and other drugs may decrease sexual drive or function. A partial list includes

narcotics	methantheline bromide
alcohol	propantheline bromide
all sedatives	monoamine oxidase
tranquilizers	inhibitors
tricyclic anti-	amphetamines
depressants	(in excess)
methyldopa	cyproterone acetate
guanethidine	progesterone (some-
phenotolamine	times)
imipramine	nicotine (possibly)
	estrogen (in excess)

COMMON SEXUAL PROBLEMS OF WOMEN

LACK OF AROUSAL. General sexual dysfunction in which the woman does not become aroused by sexual stimuli has been called "frigidity," a derogatory and misleading term. Often women with this problem are warm, affectionate, and caring people who enjoy physical contact. However, they derive little if any erotic pleasure from sexual stimulation. Physiologically, such women have an impairment of the vasocongestive component of the sexual response—there is no or little lubrication, the vagina does not expand, and the orgasmic platform does not form. Or, there may be partial response with light lubrication. Sex may be an ordeal for the woman, who may endure it only to maintain her marriage, or assiduously avoid it.

Female sexual arousal is a visceral reaction of the autonomic nervous system (as is male). The physiological discharge of negative emotions impairs this response. If the woman is in a state of rage or fear while having sex, her visceral outflow is disrupted and reflex genital vasocongestion does not take place. The cause of her emotional state can be present anxieties about whether she will have orgasm, judgmental self-observation, reluctance to express her erotic wishes to her partner, or failure to develop sexual autonomy. Or, its origins may lie in deeper psychological problems, with the result being the same. It is often compounded by having her body used for her partner's pleasure, witnessing his satisfaction, and feeling exploited and dehumanized. She may develop a strong antagonism toward sex, hostility toward her partner, and feelings of self-hatred, depression and hopelessness.[35]

ORGASMIC PROBLEMS. Women with specific orgasmic dysfunction experience erotic feelings with stimulation, develop the vasocongestive response and lubricate normally, enjoy the sensation of penetration, but get "stuck" at or near the plateau phase. They are unable to achieve orgasm, or have great difficulty in doing so. The woman may have never experienced orgasm (primary) or may have previously been orgasmic (secondary). If the problem is absolute, she is unable to achieve either clitorally induced or coital orgasm under any circumstances; if situational, she can reach orgasm under some circumstances but not others. Problems with orgasm are the most common type of female sexual complaints. Especially common are women who experience orgasm readily with masturbation or clitoral stimulation, yet do not experience orgasms from intercourse alone.

The immediate cause of failure to reach orgasm is the involuntary inhibition of the orgasmic reflex. Female orgasm can be conditioned easily and is subject to inhibition, but the woman is usually not aware of the conditioning process. The fear of losing control over feelings and behavior is very prevalent, resulting in the defense mechanism of "holding back" or overcontrol to reduce anxiety. Orgasm may be inhibited because of its acquired symbolic meanings, its intensity frightens the woman, or because unconscious conflicts are evoked by erotic feelings, such as ambivalence about the relationship, fear of abandonment, fear of asserting independence, guilt over sexuality, or hostility toward the partner.[36] The adequacy of stimulation may be a key factor, as intercourse has been seen to provide less effective stimulation than clitoral contact. Women who are not free enough to discuss this with their partners, or to experiment with positions and techniques, may be nonorgasmic simply because of inadequate stimulation.

To insist that women have orgasm with intercourse, and to call them abnormal if they do not, is both fallacious and destructive. Orgasm by masturbation or clitoral stimulation is women's major mode, which needs to be widely accepted and reinforced. Women who for reasons of their own strongly want to have orgasm with intercourse can be counseled to apply their masturbatory techniques, either by themselves or by teaching their partner effective clitoral stimulation. The "no hands" approach to intercourse is unrealistic for the vast majority of women, and grows out of our cultural inhibitions concerning women's sexuality.

VAGINISMUS. This relatively rare sexual disorder is characterized by conditioned spasm of the vaginal introitus whenever entry is attempted. This involuntary response can be brought about by pelvic examination as well as attempts at penile penetration. Women with vaginismus are often sexually responsive and orgasmic on clitoral stimulation. Vaginismus is a frequent finding in unconsummated marriages, often associated with primary impotence of the male. It may not develop until after several unsuccessful attempts at coitus. Occasionally vaginismus develops in women who first experienced severe dyspareunia, which may result from trauma, infection, and inflammation (see below). Guilt about sex and fears of penetration accompanied by fantasies of bodily damage may underlie vaginismus, or the original noxious stimulus may have been physical pain or trauma with vaginal entry.

DYSPAREUNIA. Painful intercourse can be due to physical or psychological factors. Pain on insertion can be caused by an intact hymen or irritated hymenal remnants, vaginitis, Bartholin's gland inflammation or enlargement, scar tissue in the perineum, and loss of elasticity and size of the introitus after menopause. Smegma beneath the prepuce can cause irritation, or there may be clitoral adhesions causing pain on insertion and thrusting. Burning, itching or aching during and after intercourse is often due to inadequate vaginal lubrication, secondary to lack of arousal or atrophic vaginal changes. Pain on deep thrusting may be due to masses in the cul-de-sac, peritoneal irritation, pelvic inflammation, or lacerations of the broad or sacrouterine ligaments following childbirth.

Chronic lower abdominal aching and pain might indicate orgasmic problems, as the woman's massive vasocongestive response is elicited by stimulation, but there is no orgasmic release.[37] The most frequent cause of dyspareunia is lack of adequate vaginal lubrication during sexual arousal, generally due to ineffective stimulation.

Treatment

EDUCATION AND REINFORCEMENT. Ignorance or misinformation often contributes to concern over sexual performance or normality. Myths about frequency of intercourse, type and number of orgasms, masturbation, oral-genital techniques, positions in intercourse, penis size and female satisfaction, sex drive, aging, and so on can prevent people from being comfortable with and enjoying their unique sexuality. Lack of understanding about the erotic significance of the clitoris, varying tempos of sexual arousal, and difference in the woman's sex drive during pregnancy or the menstrual cycle can diminish the couple's pleasure. Fears created by minor unpleasant symptoms may lead to avoidance of sex if the underlying physiology is not understood and the benefit of treatment not sought. In this era of public discussion of sexuality, it may be surprising that ignorance still persists; however, misconceptions and misinterpretations of information are common. Some people simply need reinforcement that their sexual practices are normal.

IMPROVING COMMUNICATION. People find it hard to talk about their sexual feelings, or to accept criticism or suggestions regarding sexual performance. Often miscommunication occurs involving sexual techniques that either "turn off" the woman or fail to turn her on. For many reasons previously discussed, women are reluctant to share with partners their sexual preference, to make demands that could lead to more satisfying sexual experiences, and to be more assertive and take more initiative in sex. Therefore, many women receive inadequate sexual stimulation, decreasing their enjoyment and satisfaction. Encouraging the couple to discuss feelings about sex, sexual preferences, and effective techniques often can be of considerable assistance.

However, many factors may complicate communication. The bed as the battlefield, and sex with a hidden agenda are familiar syndromes to those involved in marital counseling. Perceptions of male and female roles may hamper communication, for example, the cultural idea that the woman is there to serve the man sexually, and that her enjoyment of sex is secondary and her sexual needs do not deserve much attention. Or, a struggle for power and dominance may be raging between the pair, part of the game being to frustrate the other sexually or mete out sex as a reward for compliance. Anger or fear can interfere with the woman's releasing herself to the sexual experience. Usually formal counseling is necessary to deal with problems in the relationship before progress can be made on the sexual problems.

SEX THERAPY.   Often sexual problems can be helped by specific types of sex therapy, which usually include the above approaches. The aim of sex therapy is to facilitate the woman's abandonment to the sexual experience by changing the sexual system in which she functions. This is implemented by creating a nondemanding, relaxed, and sensuous atmosphere which permits the natural unfolding of the sexual response. Open communication between partners about sexual feelings and wishes helps create this atmosphere. Various sensuous and erotic experiences are usually prescribed systematically. The reorientation to sex which occurs with improved communication, permission to experience sensuousness, and learning new and effective techniques can improve sexual satisfaction and resolve problems.

In managing sexual problems the health provider must be guided by her or his individual interest, knowledge and experience. Appropriate selection of cases is also important, with an initial assessment of whether the woman is a reasonably healthy person with a sexual problem, or a person with significant psychopathology for which referral is indicated. The provider must also decide whether the problem lies primarily within the patient herself or within the relationship. If interaction between the sexual partners seems to be the primary reason for the woman's problem, then conjoint therapy is probably necessary and the provider needs to decide whether to handle it alone, to seek a cotherapist, or to refer the couple to a marriage counselor or sex therapist. Conjoint counseling of both sexual partners is important

because the couple's interaction may be causing or perpetuating the sexual problem, the partner's cooperation is often critical to successful treatment, and the partner is inevitably affected when there is a sexual problem, regardless of its origin.

While relief of the symptom is the primary objective of sex therapy, treatment often involves exploring conflicts between the partners, irrational fears and phobias affecting sexuality, inhibitions and previous conditioning, and destructive impulses or defenses operating in the relationship. Improvement of the couple's communication and general relationship is frequently an outcome of the treatment process. While the treatment format varies, common features include prescribed sexual experiences or exercises, office sessions for discussion of reactions to these experiences and provision of information and education, and limitation of the length of therapy to about 2 to 10 weeks. If the problem is not resolved by this time, another treatment method is needed. While the mechanism by which short-term sex therapy exerts its therapeutic influence is not well understood, three factors are believed to contribute to the improvement in sexual functioning produced by the prescribed sexual experiences. 1) The previously destructive sexual system is altered, as sexual interactions are structured so that guilt and fear of failure and rejection are largely eliminated. A favorable milieu is created in which new and more appropriate responses can be acquired. The pleasure and success provided by the exercises gradually extinguish negative associations and replace these with positive ones. The actual experiences of erotic pleasure are more effective than a therapist's verbal reassurances or interpretations. 2) The resolution of sexual conflict is facilitated, as couples are compelled to experience previously avoided feelings and sensations. The sexual exercises often require what are new experiences, such as masturbation or being completely selfish in receiving pleasure. The woman may be unaware that she has avoided these experiences, and bringing them into conscious focus makes the associated guilt and anxiety available for exploration and resolution. 3) Previously unrecognized fears and conflicts in other areas may also surface in the course of sex therapy, including marital problems, ambivalence toward sexuality, and other motivations and feelings. As the usual defenses against awareness of such problems fall, they become available for therapeutic exploration often leading to insight and modification of unrealistic and judgmental attitudes toward sexuality and the marital relationship.[38]

TREATMENT OF LACK OF AROUSAL. The usual treatment sequence for the woman who does not become erotically aroused includes sensate focus exercises (nondemand pleasuring experiences), genital stimulation, and nondemand coitus. Commonly involved in this problem are inadequate stimulation of the woman or her inability to receive or ask for pleasuring. In the first two stages, coitus is prohibited so the woman will be freed from the pressure to produce an orgasm or serve her partner. The sensate focus exercise consists of having the partners gently caress and touch each other's bodies, using hands or lips, and avoiding the genitals and nipples. If the woman performs the caressing first, this may reduce her guilt about being on the receiving side and her fear of not performing. The woman is instructed to concentrate on how it feels to caress her partner, then how she feels being caressed. Each partner is to tell the other what kind of touch pleasures most, and to seek adjustments of pressure, tempo, and location to receive increased pleasure.

The woman may experience sensuous feelings and erotic responses for the first time during these exercises. Additionally, she has the opportunity to assume active responsibility for her own sensual pleasure, and discovers that her partner will not reject her for her assertiveness. The partner must defer his desire for orgasm and willingness to do so expresses his concern and caring. Both partners often are gratified by receiving pleasure and providing pleasure for each other. If responses to sensate focus exercises are positive, the couple can move to the next phase. If responses are negative, or the couple has difficulties carrying out the exercise, exploration of these obstacles is necessary followed by repeat of the experiences.

In the second phase, breasts and genitals are stimulated following body caressing. Light, gentle touch is used by the partner to the nipples, clitoral area and vaginal entrance with the help of a lubricant if necessary. Demanding, orgasm-oriented stimulation must be avoided

and the woman allowed to experience non-pressured, reassuring genital play. If this genital pleasuring is too stimulating and frustrating for the partner, he can be brought to orgasm manually or orally after the woman has been genitally pleasured. The couple is advised to experiment and find the position most comfortable for them in this exercise. If the relationship is without serious conflicts, and the woman does not have complex intrapsychic factors causing her lack of arousal, genital stimulation will produce a sharp increase in her sexual responsiveness.

Intercourse is the next step, conducted under the woman's control with elimination of any pressure to have an orgasm. After the woman reaches a high level of arousal following sensate focus and genital stimulation, she initiates coitus. Generally, the female superior position allows her greater control of thrusting. Beginning with slow, exploratory thrusting, the man remains essentially passive while the woman focuses her attention on physical sensations in the vagina. Contracting her pubococcygeal muscles while she thrusts often increases the woman's sensations. If the man's urge to ejaculate becomes too intense during exploratory thrusting, the partners should separate for several seconds (30 seconds to a minute or so). The man can continue to manually stimulate the woman, and his excitement decreases somewhat. This interruption of intercourse with resumption after the man's excitement decreases may occur several times. If eventually the woman feels like driving for orgasm, she communicates this to her partner. If she does not, after a reasonable time, coitus may be used to bring the man to orgasm.

Relieved of the pressure to produce an orgasm, remaining in control of the sexual experience, and seeking her own erotic pleasure through these prescribed exercises, the woman often deactivates her defenses against the perception of erotic sensations. With increased interest in sex, a relaxed atmosphere, and better communication, the woman often is able to become responsive and orgasmic.[39]

TREATMENT OF PRIMARY ORGASMIC DYSFUNCTION. The primary objective in treating orgasmic dysfunction is to diminish or extinguish the woman's involuntary overcontrol of the orgasmic reflex. The woman who has never had orgasm must learn to recognize the premonitory sensations associated with the orgasmic reflex, and to not shut off these sensations but allow them to proceed to their natural conclusion. Often the woman must be distracted from the inhibitory overcontrol she unconsciously exerts to allow this natural response to occur. Masturbation is generally used to achieve the first several orgasms, because the presence of another person (audience) is strongly inhibitory, and the lengthy time necessary for adequate stimulation to overcome the orgasmic inhibition may be destructive to the couple's relationship if the man was required to provide the stimulation. The treatment format includes use of masturbation, resolution of unconscious fears of orgasm, distraction, muscle contraction, fantasy, and transfer of the orgasm to intercourse.

Instructing the woman to masturbate often evokes anxiety as masturbation may be seen as shameful or dangerous due to childhood teachings. Therapeutic sessions are used to deal with this anxiety, give the woman permission to release the orgasmic discharge, and encourage masturbation under reassuring situations free from fear of interruption or discovery. The woman often can reach a certain level of excitement, but then begins to feel tense and uncomfortable and stops stimulation. She is instructed to stay with these uncomfortable feelings and continue stimulation, often with use of a distractor such as tensing her abdominal and perineal muscles. If orgasm does not ensue, it may be necessary to use a vibrator which provides the strongest, most intense stimulation known. Although highly effective, the vibrator has certain disadvantages, including conditioned reliance on this method with inability to transfer to manual masturbation, and negative feelings about mechanical devices. If the vibrator must be used, after several orgasms the woman is instructed to resort to manual stimulation to finish off orgasm after reaching high levels of excitement with the vibrator, and eventually to use only manual methods.

If the woman experiences great difficulty in having an orgasm, a large amount of support and encouragement is needed from the therapist. She is instructed in how to let go when on the verge of orgasm, how to tense her muscles, breathe, and to use fantasy to distract herself from inhibition. Insight into the variety of fears which underlie orgasmic inhibition may be needed. Some women fear they will die if they have an orgasm, or they equate orgasm with loss of control. Others fear the extent to which becoming orgasmic may change their lives, such as causing preoccupation with sex, promiscuity, or fear of facing anxieties about success. Paradoxically, helping the woman realize that achieving orgasm will not drastically alter her life is often effective in breaking the inhibition. Exploring the symbolism of orgasm in terms of life changes assists this process.

Distraction plays a very important role in treatment of orgasmic dysfunction. The inhibited woman consciously focuses attention on her sexual experience and watches herself for the progression of arousal. She generally stands apart and judges herself, making orgasm virtually impossible even with intense stimulation. Having the woman focus her attention on an erotic fantasy, or on breathing, or contracting vaginal and abdominal muscles, has the effect of "distracting the distractor." Fantasy is excellent for these purposes, as it both distracts the woman from watching herself and provides an additional source of stimulation. Some women may feel guilty about their erotic fantasies, however, requiring the therapist's encouragement and reassurance that these are acceptable and normal. Contraction of the pubococcygeal and circumvaginal muscles, as well as those of the lower abdomen, increases tone of the muscles of orgasm, enhances excitation, and also serves as a distraction.

After successful use of masturbation to achieve orgasm, the partner is involved so the woman can experience orgasm with intercourse. The general approach is to have the partners engage in coitus in their usual way, with no pressure on the woman to achieve orgasm. After the man has ejaculated, he may use the vibrator or his hand to stimulate the woman clitorally for orgasm. She guides him in this technique, and is to guard against again becoming a spectator by focusing completely on her own sensations, using her favorite erotic fantasy, or contracting her muscles to provide distraction.[40]

A high level of success can generally be expected in helping an inorgasmic woman to attain orgasm by the methods described. Many progress to the ability to have orgasm with intercourse. If this presents difficulties, these women can be treated with methods used for women who are orgasmic with masturbation but not during intercourse (see below).

TREATMENT OF COITAL ORGASMIC DYSFUNC-
TION. Significant numbers of women are sexually responsive, become highly aroused with intercourse, are readily orgasmic with masturbation, but cannot have orgasm during intercourse. There remains controversy over whether or not this represents true dysfunction or is a normal variant, but if the woman desires orgasm with intercourse, it is unquestionably a sexual problem. In some cases, the woman's inability to reach orgasm with coitus is associated with a specific orgasmic inhibition, inadequate stimulation techniques, or problems in the couple's relationship. These situations are amenable to treatment and the woman often attains orgasm through coitus. Other women seem to have high orgasmic thresholds and require intense clitoral stimulation for orgasm, which no technique of coitus alone can provide. As millions of women fit in this category, it is unreasonable to consider them sick and, should this be the situation, the couple is counseled that reliance on clitoral stimulation for orgasm is normal and authentic, is not second best or an inferior mode of sexual expression, and has advantages in permitting a rich and fulfilling sexual life for both partners. Myths surrounding vaginal orgasm versus clitoral orgasm, and simultaneous orgasms often must be dispelled.

The strategies for treating coital nonorgasm include identifying and removing intrapsychic and interpersonal blocks as much as possible, attaining high degrees of sexual arousal so the woman is close to orgasm when coitus begins, enhancing her awareness of and pleasure in vaginal sensations, and maximizing clitoral stimulation. Sensate focus and genital pleasuring exercises may be used if the woman seems generally inhibited or the couple's sexual communication needs improvement. The couple engages in foreplay until the woman is highly aroused, at which point penile entry occurs and the man begins thrusting in a slow, teasing manner. After a brief period, he withdraws, waits a short while, then penetrates and begins thrusting again. This stop-start technique is very stimulating and the woman may have orgasm. If not, the man stimulates the woman's clitoris during interruptions in intercourse. Coitus begins again when the woman is highly aroused. When the man is near orgasm, he stops thrusting while the penis remains in the vagina, and he stimulates the clitoris while he regains ejaculatory control. Clitoral stimulation stops just short of orgasm, which may then be evoked by resumed coital thrusting.

The woman uses whatever distraction and heightened arousal techniques are helpful, including fantasy and muscle contraction. As orgasm nears, she can quicken her thrusting motions and sometimes climax this way. However, changing from intense clitoral stimulation to the less intense stimulation of coital thrusting often causes a decrease in excitement, and anxiety often sets in. When this occurs, the woman must communicate to her partner, and the above procedures of interrupted coitus and clitoral stimulation are repeated. Concentrating on vaginal sensations can often assist orgasm, as the woman learns to identify the pleasurable sensations produced by vaginal distention and deep pressure on the circumvaginal muscles. These are distinctly different sensations from those produced by clitoral stimulation and do not usually produce orgasm; it is the rising clitoral sensations which trigger this. However, concentrating on the pleasurable sensations produced by slow movement of the penis inside the vagina, and the contractions of perineal muscles against the erect penis, is occasionally sufficient to cause or lead to orgasm.

Techniques to increase clitoral stimulation are very useful, including coital position and simultaneous manual clitoral stimulation. With the woman on top, she can control thrusting and press her clitoris down on her partner's pubic bone, enhancing clitoral stimulation. Direct clitoral stimulation by the man during intercourse can be accomplished in the female superior or side-to-side position. The woman is stimulated to near orgasm with the man either not thrusting or moving very slowly. When she feels near orgasm, she signals him to stop clitoral stimulation and begin active thrusting. If orgasm does not ensue, thrusting stops and manual stimulation of the clitoris begins again. This may be repeated several times, until eventually the woman reaches orgasm with coital thrusting. Often, after using this technique for several weeks, coital orgasm can be reached with less and less clitoral priming. Variations on this approach include use of a vibrator or self-stimulation.[41]

If these techniques are not successful, the couple can be reassured that there are millions of women who achieve orgasm only with clitoral stimulation. This can be combined with intercourse for orgasm during penetration, or used in whatever combination or sequence the couple desires. Emphasis on the normality of this situation makes it more acceptable to both partners.

TREATMENT OF VAGINISMUS. Pelvic conditions making vaginal entry painful or difficult must be corrected, such as infections, hymenal tags, endometriosis, atrophy, and so forth. If none of these are present, or vaginismus persists after correction, treatment aimed at modifying the conditioned response is undertaken. The method is simple, consisting of use of graduated dilators made of rubber or glass, combined with therapeutic sessions to deal with ignorance, fears, and phobias. Examination of the woman with her partner present provides information about sexual anatomy, and self-examination by the woman in this situation serves to reduce the phobic element and facilitate insertion of the dilator. Irrational fears can be extinguished by repeated evocation of imagery of the feared situation while the woman is deeply relaxed and in a safe, supportive environment.

Beginning with a wire-thin dilator, progressive dilatation occurs over time, eventually with the woman placing her finger in the vagina and then her partner placing his. The woman is instructed to contract and relax her vaginal muscles to gain a sense of voluntary control. At the point at which the larger dilators can be tolerated without discomfort, intercourse can be attempted, with the woman guiding the penis with her hand. As the mechanism of avoidance plays a significant part in vaginismus, the woman is encouraged to tolerate anxiety and stay with her unpleasant feelings as treatment progresses. After initial penetration, the penis is simply held still in the vagina for a period of time. The man proceeds with slow gentle thrusting only at the woman's signal, and withdraws immediately on her request. Coitus with thrusting to orgasm is deferred for some time. The success rate for treatment of vaginismus by these methods is very high, although this is no guarantee that the woman will respond to sexual stimulation and become orgasmic. Other sexual problems may emerge and require treatment; or, the couple may proceed to mutually satisfying sexual experiences with no further therapy.[42]

TREATMENT OF DYSPAREUNIA. Identification and treatment of the physical factors causing dyspareunia often resolve the problem. This may be a temporary situation readily remedied by clearing vaginitis, treating postmenopausal vaginal atrophy, and temporary use of a lubricant during times of relative hormonal depletion, such as during the postpartum period. If no physical problems are identified, and history reveals that lack of adequate lubrication before intercourse is attempted seems to be the problem, a discussion of the couple's sexual techniques and the woman's usual sexual responses is indicated. The provider may decide that general lack of arousal underlies the pain caused by intromission, and undertake treatment methods previously described for this condition. Or, the partner's techniques may be ineffective, with communication difficulties or marital conflicts preventing the woman from discussing this with him. If the woman becomes highly aroused, but does not have orgasm, she may eventually complain of aching pain following intercourse and lasting several hours. Determination must be made of whether she is ever orgasmic, under what circumstances, and appropriate treatment undertaken depending on her type of orgasmic dysfunction.

Women often mask sexual problems in complaints of painful intercourse, as they recognize pain to be readily understandable language to the health provider. Many are hoping there is a physical problem, for which a simple treatment will be prescribed, and some do not want to explore their sexual or interpersonal relationships as probable causes of dyspareunia. Deep pelvic pathology is often difficult to rule out, or findings may be so subtle as not to be recognized by the provider. However, by far the most common cause of dyspareunia is intercourse without adequate vaginal lubrication.[43] A thorough sexual history is essential if the cause underlying this symptom is to be unraveled.

LESBIANISM

There is a growing propensity to consider homosexuality, the desire to be physically intimate with a person of the same sex at some time during one's life, or always, as a natural and normal experience. Homosexuality is "abnormal" only when, by definition, interest in reproductive sex is necessary to be "normal." Obviously, most sex is not engaged in for reproduction, and to call all nonreproductive sex "unnatural" is a very constricted view. Varieties of sexual contact are common among same-sexed animals, and the origins of Western religious proscriptions against homosexuality have more to do with breaking pagan customs and establishing a separate group identity than with morality. Practices necessary for in-group solidarity soon become customs themselves, are translated into morals, and finally institutionalized into law.

In Hite's study of female sexuality, 8 percent of the women questioned said they preferred sex with another woman, and 9 percent identified themselves as bisexual or said they had sexual experiences with both men and women without identifying preference. Kinsey estimated that about 12 to 15 percent of the women interviewed had incidental or more specific homosexual relations at some point during their adult lives. Sexual preferences can change more than once during a lifetime, and with cultural conditioning lessening its inhibition on sexual expression, greater numbers of people will no doubt seek wider ranges of sexual experiences. There may now be an increase in lesbianism and/or bisexuality partly for political reasons, as women dissociate from male dominance and female dependence as a sexual interpersonal mode.

In relating physically to each other, women utilize a wide range of activities with no standard format. The two most striking differences reported by women between homosexual and heterosexual relations are the greater tenderness, higher level of feelings, affection and sensitivity with women, and longer lovemaking with more and stronger orgasms. More overall body sensuality is involved, and sex is less goal-directed than with men. There was often a feeling of equality in the relationship, a sense of understanding and being understood, a closeness between female lovers expressed in the study.[44]

Professional controversy still exists concerning origins or causes of homosexuality, whether it is biological or psychological, and whether it represents sexual pathology or is within the normal range of variation. As pre-

viously discussed we must answer the questions of why and how a person becomes heterosexual before there will be any lucid answers as to why a person becomes homosexual. There are many forces in our society, most also concerned with suppression of women as a group, which violently oppose recognition of homosexuality as a legitimate form of sexual expression. Many of the emotional problems presented by homosexuals to therapists result from cultural taboos and values. Often the goals of treatment are to help the person become more self-accepting, and to resolve conflicts, thus leading toward greater comfort with homosexual relationships.

REDEFINING FEMALE SEXUALITY

There is no need to limit sexuality to the traditional reproductive pattern, especially since this is often unsatisfactory to women. Sex is intimate physical contact for pleasure, and need not have any one particular goal. Women's ideas about change go much deeper than just "having an orgasm too." The entire range of sensuousness needs to be included, with intercourse only one of many types of physical contact. Women would like to be held and caressed by men without it automatically meaning coitus, to have genital contact without it necessarily culminating in penetration, to be free not to have orgasm as the ultimate goal of every sexual encounter, to enjoy their bodies themselves, to love other women, to explore and discover their own sexuality. All kinds of physical intimacy, so important in expressing affection and receiving comfort, and part of our biological heritage as a social species, need to be rediffused throughout our lives, rather than channeled into narrowly defined heterosexual intercourse as is now prevalent. Touching other people in friendship or affection needs to be accepted, and the sharp distinction of sexual touching erased. Physical intimacy, with its highly pleasurable feelings, needs to be a common experience in many parts of our lives.

NOTES

1. A. Kinsey, et al, *Sexual Behavior in the Human Female* (Philadelphia: W. B. Saunders, 1953).
2. W. H. Masters, and V. E. Johnson, *Human Sexual Response* (Boston: Little, Brown, 1966).
3. S. Fisher, *The Female Orgasm.* (New York: Basic Books, 1973).

4. *Ibid.*

5. S. Hite, *The Hite Report* (New York: Macmillan, 1976).

6. R. Green, *Sexual Identity Conflict in Children and Adults* (New York: Basic Books, 1974).

7. J. Money, and A. A. Ehrhardt, *Man & Woman, Boy & Girl* (Baltimore: The Johns Hopkins University Press, 1972).

8. *Ibid.*, p. 176.

9. *Ibid.*, pp. 118-23.

10. *Ibid.*, pp. 125-26.

11. Green, *Sexual Identity*, pp. 297-305.

12. W. Pomeroy, "Sexual Myths of the 1970's." *Medical Aspects of Human Sexuality* 11,1 (January 1977): 62-74.

13. E. Stanley, "Emergence of Strong Sexual Drives in Women Past Thirty." *Medical Aspects of Human Sexuality* 11,6 (June 1977): 18-27.

14. M. J. Sherfey, *The Nature & Evolution of Female Sexuality* (New York: Random House, 1972), pp. 57-66, 146-65.

15. Masters and Johnson, *Human Sexual Response.*

16. Sherfey, *Nature & Evolution of Female Sexuality*, pp. 74-80.

17. Masters and Johnson, *Human Sexual Response*, pp. 134-38, 212-17.

18. H. S. Kaplan, *The New Sex Therapy* (New York: Brunner/Mazel, 1974), pp. 13-14.

19. Sherfey, *Nature & Evolution of Female Sexuality*, pp. 96-101.

20. *Ibid.*, pp. 104-12.

21. Hite, *The Hite Report.*

22. *Ibid.*, p. xi

23. S. L. Romney, et al., eds., *Gynecology & Obstetrics: The Health Care of Women* (New York: McGraw-Hill, Blakiston, 1975), p. 546.

24. Hite, *The Hite Report*, p. 3.

25. Romney, *Gynecology & Obstetrics*, p. 546.

26. Hite, *The Hite Report*, pp. 111-13.

27. Fisher, *Female Orgasm*, p. 193.

28. Kaplan, *New Sex Therapy*, p. 341.

29. Romney, *Gynecology & Obstetrics*, pp. 546-47.

30. Hite, *The Hite Report*, pp. 209-11.

31. Stanley, "Emergence of Strong Sexual Drives."

32. Hite, *The Hite Report*, p. 358.

33. *Ibid.*, p. 305.

34. "Ferreting Out Covert Sex Problems." *Patient Care* 10,4 (February 15, 1976): 45-56.

35. Kaplan, *New Sex Therapy*, pp. 361-65.

36. *Ibid.*, pp. 374-84.

37. J. A. Batts, "Somatic Warning Signs of Sexual Problems in Women." *Medical Aspects of Human Sexuality* 11,5 (May 1977): 89-97.

38. Kaplan, *New Sex Therapy*, pp. 187-220.

39. *Ibid.*, pp. 361-73.

40. *Ibid.*, pp. 384-92.

41. *Ibid.*, pp. 397-411.

42. *Ibid.*, pp. 412-28.

43. Romney, *Gynecology & Obstetrics*, p. 547.

44. Hite, *The Hite Report*, pp. 257-77.

3

Contraception

The control of reproductive functions holds potentially revolutionary impact for the woman-man relationship and for the woman's self-concept. Underlying the idea of birth control are concepts of freedom of choice and individual rights to self-determination—concepts not applied to women until the midtwentieth century. Before control of reproduction was feasible and reliable, Freud's notion that biology is destiny had much truth for women: unless they abstained from sex (and heterosexual or marital relations with all their substrata of social approval) women continually risked becoming pregnant. Once pregnant, numerous social, psychological, and biological processes solidified women into appropriate roles and gave them status within the social structure. Motherhood, with all its demands, unpredictable, nearly inevitable, and more or less continual throughout the major portion of the adult women's life span, was the inescapable lot of most women. It heavily influenced their relation with men, their position in society, and their concept of themselves.

Women and men have from time immemorial tried to control reproduction, but until the development of oral contraceptives and intrauterine devices, the only available methods carried significant risk of pregnancy. Of the more ancient methods, coitus interruptus and the condom made the women dependent upon her male partner. Breast feeding, thought to be a means of preventing pregnancy, made her dependent upon having a nursing child, and was unreliable and only useful for a limited time. Spermicidal creams, jellies, and foams are more effective but are closely connected with the sex act in time and have a relatively high failure rate. The diaphragm, once the leading contraceptive method among the more educated, requires the mastery of insertion techniques, discipline for constant use, and a sense of ease about touching the genitals. Highly effective when used properly, its popularity declined after the introduction of oral contraceptives. Recently, interest in the diaphragm has revived as data accumulate on the dangers of "the pill" and as concern grows about interference with natural functions and body ecology. Sterilization, for both women and men, is steadily gaining favor as an effective and permanent means of contraception among those who have completed their families and those who desire no children. The 1973 U.S. Supreme Court decision making first trimester abortion a matter between the woman and her physician, with certain regulations for later abortions, has made this method of birth control widely available as a backup for contraceptive failure or as a primary intervention in unwanted pregnancies (see Chapter 7, Induced Abortion).

When the goal is to avoid pregnancy, any method of contraception is better than none. Individuals vary in their attitudes toward conception control, their feelings about their bodies and sexuality, their concepts of health and well-being, their ideas about medication or invasive devices, and a myriad of other personal predilections which influence their approach to contraception. The health provider must understand that individual goals are different when patients present seeking contraception. Exploring such goals and the personal characteristics which will affect contraceptive practices are of great value in assisting the patient or couple to find the most suitable method. Even the most effective contraceptive methods have a significant failure rate when not used properly, for use effectiveness is in the patient's control. An open mind on the practitioner's part and a flexible approach which can maximize the values of all types of contraceptive methods will best encourage long-term effective contraceptive use.

MEANINGS OF CONTRACEPTION FOR WOMEN

A woman may desire to limit her fertility for any number of reasons related to personal convenience, economics, social values, and life style. A deeper motivation, often unconscious, may stem from the drive to achieve, to be in control. Part of the quality of being human is creating circumstances to meet our needs, rather than yielding helplessly to every impinging force or event. For the woman, the control of this body function also represents freedom of choice. Not only can unwanted pregnancies be avoided, with relief from the burden of multiple childrearing, but other life experiences can be opened up, other options made possible. It is no accident that the women's liberation movement followed closely upon the widespread use of highly effective contraceptive agents.

Whether it is in order to have more time to devote to mothering and wifehood, to relieve the family of oppressive economic burdens and enhance upward socioeconomic mobility, or to pursue an all-consuming career, women in America today are using birth control at an unprecedented rate. The repercussions of this change for society are already being felt and are manifest in the changing roles of women and changing values related to sexuality and parenthood. While individual contraceptive choices must be viewed apart from concerns for population control, there are parallels between the declining birth rate in the United States and an increasing awareness of the dictates of ecology. For many women, these factors no doubt enter into the desire for fertility control.

Contraceptive use has implications for a woman's concept of her sexual self and her expression of sexuality. Her feelings can be positive or negative, facilitating or inhibiting the sexual experience. For the woman who is comfortable with herself and for whom sex has no hidden agendas, freedom from the fear of pregnancy provided by effective contraception would be likely to enhance sexual enjoyment. For other women, sex is more pleasurable when it is associated with some degree of risk, whether this is the risk of pregnancy or of discovery, or a defiance of authority such as parents or social values. Effective contraception reduces or eliminates the risk, and, thus, for these women takes the excitement out of sex. Closely connected to this attitude is the view of sex as dirty or bad. From this viewpoint, it is permissible to have intercourse, which is "bad," only if the goal is to have children or if there is the possibility that pregnancy, although not directly desired, will result. In this way one can be "punished" for one's wrongdoings; thus, intercourse is made psychologically acceptable and laced with a titillating touch of danger.

When the risk of pregnancy is virtually eliminated by effective contraception, these psychological games are interrupted. The woman clearly makes a commitment to sex for pleasure, without extenuating circumstances. Although the woman may accept this philosophy intellectually, older emotional mores and taboos produce a considerable degree of guilt, which can interfere with sexual enjoyment. Depending upon the type of contraception used, decreased interest or enjoyment of sex can be associated with various mechanical, aesthetic, or hormonal factors. However, attitudes toward sex and sexuality are far more important than real or imagined side effects of contraceptive use.

Contraceptives are not panaceas for unsatisfying sexual relations. Women who expect a great surge in sexuality after beginning contraceptive practices will generally be disappointed. Others may have to face their lack of sexual responsiveness squarely when the fear of pregnancy can no longer serve as an excuse to put off sex or as a rationale for nonorgasm. If the use of contraceptive measures provides an impetus to deal more effectively with sexual dysfunction, it can benefit both partners. Men too find that contraception inhibits sexual pleasure, mechanically as with the condom, or psychologically as described above for women. These attitudes contribute to contraceptive failure rates and to not using birth control. One other significant factor contributing to nonuse, particularly among teenagers, is the need to feel that sex is unplanned and spontaneous. Somehow it is all right if sex just happens but wrong if it is planned and prepared for. This creates the problem of unwanted pregnancies and the need for abortion (see Chapter 7).

For the poor and underprivileged woman, contraception means some relief from want and hardship. Having fewer children means that the family's resources can be less thinly stretched, with more opportunity for each member and less susceptibility to crises for the family. The woman's daily burden can be lightened when a new baby is not a yearly event. Although family-planning clinics have been accused of genocide by some black men, black women have continued to use these clinics to obtain contraception according to their own personal needs.[1] Many Mexican-American, or Chicano women, although predominantly Catholic, use other types of birth control than the Church-approved rhythm method, which has a high failure rate. One report found that 78 percent of young Catholic women in the United States used contraceptive methods not approved by the Church.[2] The motives and concerns of the lower income women concerning contraceptive use are unique and compelling and may present a different perspective on the risk-benefit ratio of the various methods.

Contraceptive choice and its related meanings are highly individual matters, and these differences must be respected by the practitioner. The professional's obligation is to present the range of possibilities to the individual, fairly and without undue bias, so that a fully informed choice can be made.

CONTRACEPTIVE EFFECTIVENESS VERSUS RISK

With any contraceptive method, or with unprotected intercourse, the risk-benefit ratio must be considered by the professional while counseling individuals or couples. Certain mortality and morbidity rates occur with pregnancy as well as with mechanical and chemical contraception. The risks with any method are different for different people, and there are wide possibilities for benefits according to individual needs and perceptions. Often practitioners, nurses, physicians, lay counselors, and others involved in contraceptive counseling have their favorite methods, based on personal preferences and the extent of professional information at their command. It is only human to tend to encourage patients to use the professional's preferred method and to subtly or directly discourage the use of less preferred ones. This may close off the best method for a given individual or couple, possibly leading to contraceptive failure and unwanted pregnancy. Regardless of the professional's convictions about the risk-benefit ratio of various contraceptive methods, the choice is basically the individual's or the couple's to make, and it should be a fully informed choice based on a fair presentation of information on effectiveness and a complete discussion of complications by the professional.

Theoretical and Use Effectiveness

The *theoretical effectiveness* of any contraceptive method is its effectiveness in preventing pregnancy when used under ideal conditions, in which the method is completely understood and always used correctly. If a given method is used under such ideal conditions, any pregnancies which might occur result from *method failure*, the imperfection factor in the nature of the contraceptive method itself. The degree of successful use of a method under ideal conditions is the maximum effectiveness of the method. *Use effectiveness* takes into consideration the contraceptive method's effectiveness in preventing pregnancy under actual conditions of use, in which some people use the method correctly and others use it incorrectly or carelessly. Pregnancies that result from incorrect or careless use of a method are the results of *patient failure*, the human imperfection element. Obviously, use effectiveness figures show a higher percentage of failure rates (i.e., pregnancies) than do the theoretical effectiveness figures. Failure rates are usually expressed in pregnancies per 100 woman years by using the Pearl formula, in which the number of pregnancies per woman years equals 1,300 times the total number of failures per total number of cycles.

Counselors may respond to the question about the effectiveness of various contraceptive methods by quoting theoretical effectiveness rates for their favorite methods and use effectiveness rates for less preferred methods.

This biases the data available to the patient in making a selection of methods. Table 3-1 summarizes the data on theoretical and use effectiveness for the common contraceptive methods. It is apparent from this table that the theoretical effectiveness of every method except coitus interruptus, rhythm, and lactation is excellent, and that there is not as wide a variation in the use effectiveness of oral contraceptives/IUD and condom/diaphragm/foam as might be expected. If couples are properly counseled and given adequate instruction in any of the methods that have a high theoretical effectiveness, no doubt their use effectiveness could be increased. To quote consistently either theoretical or use effectiveness figures for all methods, with adequate instruction, allows the health provider to offer couples an unbiased range of choice in contraceptives.

Risk Factors of Contraceptive Use and Pregnancy

The only completely safe contraceptive for the prevention of death due to pregnancy is total abstinence, and whether this method prevents morbidity is a moot question. Pregnancy carries a greater risk of death than does any common method of birth control, for only late abortion and laparoscopic tubal ligation have higher mortality rates (Table 3-2). When considered from this viewpoint, any contraceptive is safer than no contraceptive, and even rhythm has a substantial risk due to the pregnancies which occur because of rhythm's high failure rate. Mortality is expressed in deaths per 100,000 users per year, and morbidity is expressed in percentage of users.

Often the risk to a particular individual of a given contraceptive method cannot be determined in advance. There are certain characteristics which can be identified by history or physical examination which may contraindicate the use of a given method, such as the pill, IUD, or diaphragm. Even with a completely negative history and physical examination, however, complications do occur. It is the patients' right to know the statistics on complications, so that they may take this information into consideration in deciding upon a contraceptive method. The issue of informed consent is particularly critical in the field of contraception because most methods are initiated at the

Table 3-1
Pregnancies Per First Year of Use per 100 Women: Theoretical and Use Effectiveness

Method	Used Correctly and Consistently	Average U.S. Experience Among 100 Women Wanting No More Children	Theoretical Effectiveness	Use Effectiveness
Abortion	0	0+	0	0
Abstinence	0	?	0	?
Hysterectomy	.0001	.0001	0	.0001
Tubal ligation	.04	.04	0	.04
Vasectomy	.15	.15+	0	.15
Oral contraceptive (combined	.34	4-10	.1	3
Combination pill	—	—	.1	.2
Low dose oral progestin	1-1.5	5-10	1	3
IUD	1-3	5	2	5
Condom	3	10	3	15
Diaphragm with spermicide	3	17	3	13
Foam or jelly alone	3	22	3	20
Coitus interruptus	9	20-25	3	15-23
Rhythm (calendar)	13	21	14	35-40
Douche	?	40	—	35-40
Chance (sexually active)	90	90	80	80

Adapted from R. A. Hatcher, et al, *Contraceptive Technology 1976-1977*, ed. 8 (New York: Halsted Press, Division of John Wiley & Sons, 1976), pp. 25, 100 and S. L. Romney, et al, *Gynecology and Obstetrics: The Health Care of Women* (New York: McGraw-Hill, Blakiston, 1975), p. 552.

Table 3-2
Continuing Pregnancy Rates and Deaths due to Contraceptive Methods or Pregnancies per 100,000 Fertile Women per Year Having Regular Intercourse

Method	Continuing Pregnancies	Death due to Continuing Pregnancies	Deaths due to Birth Control	Total Deaths	Major Morbidity	Minor Morbidity
No Contraception	80,000	16	0	16		
Rhythm	25,000	5	0	5		
Early abortion	0	0	2.6-4	2.6-4	1%	8%
Diaphragm	12,000	2	0	2		
IUD	3,000	1	1	2	1%	40%
Oral contraceptive	500	0	3	3	1%	40%
Laparoscopic tubal ligation	150	0	12-50*	12-50*	.6%	1%
Vasectomy	150	0	0	0	1%	5%

*High mortality rate reflects use of general anesthesia. Adapted from Hatcher, et al, *Contraceptive Technology*, pp. 77, 99 and Romney, et al, *Gynecology and Obstetrics*, p. 551.

request of a healthy patient in the absence of traditional "medical" indications for treatment. Although the potential for serious danger is small, it is tragic when complications occur as a result of contraceptive use. The professional provider is responsible for seeing that the patient has sufficient information about the proposed method and is competent to consent in her or his own behalf.

The question of how much to tell the patient continues to plague professionals, especially regarding side effects and the complications of oral contraceptives and IUDs. Some professionals think that to discuss specific problems, such as headache, has a suggestive effect and may actually create the problem. Although this is true for certain personalities, it is not an adequate reason to avoid discussing major and minor complications. Legally and morally the professional is required to provide adequate information for the patient to make a reasonable decision, and the patient has a right to such information. Practically, a thorough understanding of the method chosen and of its problems leads to more intelligent and effective use. The U.S. Department of Health, Education and Welfare guidelines for informed consent to voluntary sterilization serve as a model for this approach:

Informed consent is the voluntary, knowing assent from the individual on whom any procedure is to be performed or contraceptive provided after she or he has been given

1. a fair explanation of the procedures or proposed method;

2. a description of attendant discomforts and risks, including all major (life-threatening) and all common minor risks;
3. a description of the benefits to be expected;
4. an explanation of alternative methods and effectiveness rates with indication that nothing is 100 percent, and that sterilization is permanent;
5. an offer to answer any questions about procedures or method;
6. an instruction that the individual is free to withdraw consent to the procedure or method at any time prior to the procedure, or to discontinue the method, without affecting future care or loss of benefits;
7. a written consent document detailing the basic elements of informed consent and the information provided. This should be signed by the patient, an auditor-witness of the patient's choice, and by the person obtaining the consent.[3]

The ideal contraceptive is one that is 100 percent safe and 100 percent effective, simple to use and to understand, inexpensive, not intimately connected with the act of intercourse, completely reversible, and able to be widely distributed and made easily available. Although one or the other of the presently available methods may meet some of these criteria, none comes close to fulfilling all of them. Even methods being tested or soon to be released do not satisfy all these criteria. Thus we are left with making personal choices based on our understanding of risk-benefit ratios and the individual meanings of these ratios.

The risks and benefits of the various methods of contraception are discussed in more detail later in this chapter.

CONTRACEPTIVE METHODS: SELECTION, PROCEDURES, AND COUNSELING

The most important objective in assisting individuals or couples in the use of contraceptives is to find a method that *will be used*. The use factor outweighs any consideration of the absolute reliability of a given method. Complete and relative contraindication of a particular method in individual cases must also be given weighty consideration. The outcome should be the selection of a method that the patient understands and is comfortable with, and one that is compatible with the health problems and physical status of the patient.

The History and Physical Examination

Ideally, an interval history should be taken and a screening physical examination should be done on all women seeking contraception. Certain minimal laboratory work is also indicated when the method of choice is the IUD or an oral contraceptive. More historical and physical data are needed for these two methods, and when tubal ligation and the diaphragm are under consideration, than for other nonprescription methods.

HISTORY. Inquire whether there is a history in the immediate family of diabetes, bleeding or clotting problems, heart problems or high blood pressure, migraine headaches or seizure disorders, kidney or liver disease, anemia, tuberculosis, stroke, cancer, or mental problems. This information provides a baseline on diseases the patient may be at risk for and is a cautionary factor when oral contraceptives are being considered. The woman's own past medical history is elicited, covering the above problems in addition to previous hospitalizations, operations, and other major illness. Menstrual and obstetrical history is of particular importance, with any complications or abnormalities carefully noted (see Chapter 4 for details of menstrual history and Chapter 5 for obstetrical history). Previous use of and experience with contraceptives is also included. Allergies and the current use of medications alert the practitioner to potential problems.

Key points in the history include the following:

When did menarche occur, and have menses been irregular or skipped? Late menarche and irregular menses indicate a possible endocrine abnormality, and the woman may be having anovulatory cycles. In this case, oral contraceptives should not be used until her endocrine status has been investigated. Otherwise, permanent anovulation with subsequent infertility could result.

Are menstrual periods heavy with clotting and cramping? The IUD will cause these problems to become worse, and often the oral contraceptive will improve them. However, extremely heavy flow, particularly in the woman over 30, needs investigation before the pill is prescribed. The diaphgram may be a better choice in this situation.

Is there a history of pelvic inflammatory disease? This is a contraindication for the IUD.

Is there a history of severe migraine, cerebral arterial insufficiency, cardiovascular disease, liver disease, severe diabetes, genital or breast cancer, thrombotic problems, high blood pressure, or a family history of stroke? These are contraindications for oral contraceptives.

What type of contraceptive was used before? Was it effective or did a pregnancy occur? Information is gained here about the probability of the successful use of certain contraceptive methods, and some idea is provided about the patient's level of knowledge and understanding of these methods.

What are the most important reasons for contraceptive use? This question helps the health provider assess the presence of realistic or unrealistic expectations on the part of the patient. Misconceptions should be cleared up in discussion, and the patient should be helped to understand the practical benefits of contraception. Goals and priorities can also be identified; if the woman feels strongly that pregnancy must be prevented, a highly effective method is indicated. If delay or spacing of pregnancy is actually the goal and if the woman is quite concerned about any alterations in her body physiology and functions, a method with somewhat greater pregnancy risk but no systemic or local alterations would be more appropriate.

Any positive responses in the history must be fully explored and considered in making decisions about the appropriateness of any particular method.

PHYSICAL EXAMINATION. The extent of the physical performed will depend upon policies and practices in the particular setting, positive responses from the history, and the type of contraceptive method desired. A breast check, pelvic examination, and Pap smear constitute a minimum; at least some health screening should be done when the woman presents this opportunity. A preferred screening physical examination, mainly with the IUD and oral contraceptives in mind, would include the following:

Eyes. Check for signs of glaucoma such as narrow anterior chamber and cupping of discs or increased cup-disc ratio; conditions of veins and arteries, particularly anteriolar narrowing or venous nicking; and condition of retina.

Ear, nose, and throat. This may or may not be done; no specific abnormalities to watch for.

Thyroid. Examine for nodules and diffuse enlargement. Oral contraceptives alter thyroid function tests, although there is no evidence at present that they cause either hypo- or hyperthyroidism. Seek consultation for positive findings.

Chest. Examine lung fields, heart, and great vessels. Any heart murmurs, bruits, or adventitious lung sounds indicate the need for consultation.

Breasts. Any masses, nodules, or discharge from the nipples contraindicates oral contraceptives, at least initially, and calls for consultation. There is some evidence that the pill may be helpful in certain types of benign breast disease, but it is recommended that the pill not be used in cases of suspected or proven breast cancer.

Abdomen. Examine for bruits, masses, and hepatosplenomegaly. Seek consultation for any positive findings.

Skin. Signs of chloasma (mask of pregnancy) or history of this is a relative contraindication for oral contraceptives. Acne may be improved.

Extremities. Varicose veins are a relative contraindication for oral contraceptives. Peripheral pulses which are weak or absent indicate circulatory or arteriosclerotic problems, and further investigation is necessary with avoidance of oral contraceptives until the safety of their use is determined.

Pelvic examination. Significant pelvic relaxation with prolapse, cystocele or rectocele make effective use of the diaphragm impossible. Anatomical anomalies such as a small cervix or short anterior vaginal wall also dictate against this method. An infantile cervix and uterus suggest endocrine problems, and oral contraceptives or an IUD should not be used until this possibility has been ruled out. Pelvic inflammatory disease and extensive cervicitis contraindicate the use of IUDs. Suspicious cervical lesions should be biopsied before any contraceptive method is instituted. Uterine myomata make IUD placement difficult and may be stimulated to increase with the use of oral contraceptives, so foam, a condom, or a diaphragm would be the method of choice. Ovarian or tubal masses should be referred at once for consultation, and no contraceptive given until their nature has been ascertained and the problem treated. Vaginitis is not a contraindication to either the IUD or oral contraceptive, although it may influence the type of pill used and should, of course, be treated. Severe retroversion or anteversion of the uterus contraindicates the IUD.

Weight. Obesity must be viewed as a serious problem when oral contraceptives are desired. Some consider it a contraindication due to the pill's effects on carbohydrate and lipid metabolism. It definitely puts the patient at increased risk for several complications. The obese woman also presents difficulties in fitting a diaphragm and inserting an IUD. It is difficult to find anatomical landmarks and determine the size and position of the uterus. Foam and/or condoms seem to be the contraceptives of choice until weight is lost.

Age. Oral contraceptives carry a greater risk for the very young woman whose endocrine system is immature, and for the woman over 35 who is increasingly susceptible to thromboembolic problems and hypertension.

Blood pressure. Even marginal elevation of the blood pressure contraindicates the use of oral contraceptives. There is a direct relation between the estrogen in the pill and hypertension, and even a certain percentage of normotensive women will develop high blood pressure under the influence of these drugs. When there is already marginal or established hypertension, the risk of serious complication and of a higher blood pressure is increased. Another method of contraception is indicated.

LABORATORY TESTS. A Pap smear should be performed during the pelvic examination, and it is also wise to obtain a culture for gonorrhea in sexually active women. Urinalysis is simple and inexpensive and provides some screening for diabetes, urinary tract infections, and kidney function. A complete blood count rules out anemia or systemic infection in most cases and gives an indication of the condition of the platelets. If there is any question about liver function, liver enzymes should be obtained because impaired liver function is an absolute contraindication to oral contraceptives. A VDRL or other serological test for syphilis would also be a good screening measure.

Abstinence

Among teenage women in the United States, abstinence from sexual intercourse is the most widely used method of birth control. Although on the average, menarche occurs at age 12½, with ovulatory cycles and fertility about 1 to 2 years later, only 14 percent of teenage women are sexually active at age 15 and 46 percent by the age of 19.[4] In some societies, abstinence from sexual intercourse is nearly 100 percent among unmarried males and females, and in certain religious and ethnic groups in the United States premarital abstinence may approach this rate.

Some adults, though probably few, choose a life of abstinence. More go through phases of periodic abstinence, due to separation from or death of a partner. The significance of abstinence for general emotional adjustment is subject to considerable debate, and no doubt the motivation for avoiding sexual intercourse and the associated circumstances play a major role. Although sex is a biological drive, sexual activity may be controlled, delayed, or omitted for long periods of time due to the human's capacity for cortical control of such psychophysiological functions.

Rhythm is a method of periodic abstinence in which sexual intercourse is avoided during the fertile period of the menstrual cycle; it will be discussed in more detail later. Abstinence may be entirely appropriate for a person at a given point in her or his life, or it may represent an expression of intrapersonal or interpersonal conflict. This method is 100 percent effective if used, is always available, and its only risks are the psychological problems or conflicts that underlie it or may be created within the relationship.

Coitus Interruptus (Withdrawal)

One of the most ancient techniques, coitus interruptus is reported to still be the most widely used contraceptive in the world today. In this method, the couple proceeds with intercourse until the male reaches the point of ejaculatory inevitability. He then withdraws his penis from the female's vagina and ejaculates completely away from her genitals. The advantages of this method are that it is always available, costs nothing, and requires no chemicals or devices. There are no medical risks, although there can be psychological and interpersonal adverse effects. Under conditions of ideal use, the couple develops a technique in which both partners derive full satisfaction. However, the actual ability of couples to achieve such ideal circumstances is open to question.

There are many disadvantages to coitus interruptus. It requires great self-control and experience on the part of the man, who must be acutely aware of his sexual response pattern. There is a time lag of about 3 to 5 seconds from the awareness of ejaculatory inevitability to actual ejaculation. At this peak of sexual excitement, rational thought is difficult, and there is a cerebral clouding which is part of the pleasure of orgasm. For the man to anticipate ejaculation accurately under these circumstances, a truly unusual level of awareness and will power is required. Even if the man can accomplish this, there is an inherent source of error in coitus interruptus because a small amount of preliminary ejaculatory fluid often escapes without his knowledge. This fluid, from the prostate and Cowper's glands, ranges from a few drops to 1 cc. in amount and often contains motile sperm. Multiple sex acts over a short period of time increase the possibility of sperms being present in the preejaculatory fluid.

Both the man and the woman are placed under considerable stress when this method is used. The man must carefully control his sexual experience, creating an unnatural situation in which he must withdraw at the time of impending orgasm rather than achieve a deeper penetration, as he strongly desires. The woman must trust the man's intentions and judgment, and her pleasure in intercourse is diminished or blocked by the inevitable worry about his ability to use withdrawal and by the shock of suddenly interrupted contact at a time when she is highly excited or preorgasmic. The couple's sense of closeness is often lost.

Coitus interruptus is one of the more ineffective contraceptive methods, with a failure rate of 15 pregnancies per 100 woman years in constant users and 20 to 25 pregnancies per 100 woman years in actual users. It also contributes to "sexual morbidity" in that many of its users in America are teenagers beginning their sexual experiences. Surrounded by circumstances contributing to haste, fear, and guilt, coitus interruptus sets into motion patterns which can lead to premature ejaculation in the male and orgasmic dysfunction in the female. It is truly a primitive and male-oriented method; it is probably a satisfactory method for both partners in only a small minority of cases.

Methods Other than Penile-Vaginal Intercourse

Some couples have developed techniques of sexual stimulation in which penile-vaginal contact is completely avoided. These techniques include mutual manual masturbation, oral-genital contact, or the use of stimulating devices. While these techniques are more commonly only a part of a couple's sexual repertory, among some couples, for certain periods of time, they may constitute the total of sexual activity. Such methods are very effective provided ejaculation takes place completely removed from the vaginal introitus. Deposition of seminal fluid on the upper thighs or labia puts the sperm in position for ascent into the vagina and can cause pregnancy. Used well and by mutual desire, the couple can achieve complete sexual satisfaction from such methods. However, it is likely that few couples use such methods as a means of contraception.

The Condom

A sheath worn over the penis has been used for decorative purposes, to prevent infection, and as a contraceptive since ancient times. Present-day condoms are made of rubber or processed collagenous tissue (lamb caecum), and are thin sheaths which fit over the erect penis to contain the ejaculate, acting as a mechanical barrier to prevent the sperm from entering the vagina (See Figure 3-1). Condoms are available in only one size and may be plain or colored; some are lubricated, and some have a small pouch at the tip to collect the ejaculate. The advantages of the condom include its availability without a prescription, its ease of use and the simplicity of a method which can readily be understood, absence of side effects except occasional sensitivity of the man or woman to the rubber used, and its ability to prevent the transmission of infections. The two major disadvantages most often expressed by condom users are decreased sensation in the man, and the need to interrupt foreplay to put the condom on. Although the use of thinner condoms (lambskin) can increase sensation, there is also the increased danger of the condom's tearing. The couple's approach to foreplay could include the woman's putting the condom on the man, or dexterity could be developed by the man so that this interruption would hardly be noticed.

The condom is a quite effective contraceptive if used properly. In constant users, who use the condom with every act of intercourse and exactly as directed, the failure rate is 3 pregnancies per 100 woman years. In actual use, however, the failure rate is 15 to 20 pregnancies per 100 woman years. Effectiveness is increased if the condom is used in conjunction with a spermicidal foam or jelly. The key points in effective condom use are to use it *every time* and *properly*. Instructions for the use of condoms must be explicit with the following points stressed: A condom should be used only once and should not be more than 2 years old. It must have been protected from heat, which causes deterioration. The condom must be put on before there is any contact between the penis and the external genitals or the vagina because of the seepage of preejaculatory fluid. There should be about one-half inch of empty space at the tip, not filled with air, or a nipple tip condom should be used so that there is room for the ejaculate. This precaution reduces the likelihood of tearing or the overflow of seminal fluid. Lubricated condoms or good vaginal lubrication also reduces the risk of tears. If additional lubricant is needed, use a water soluble one such as K-Y jelly or Lubrifax rather than a petroleum-based one such as Vasoline, which causes the rubber to deteriorate. After ejaculation, hold on to the condom rim while withdrawing the still partly erect penis. This is to prevent the overflow of seminal fluid and its leakage into the vagina. Care should be taken to avoid spilling any semen onto the woman's external genitals. For every act of intercourse, a new condom should be used. If the condom tears or comes off in

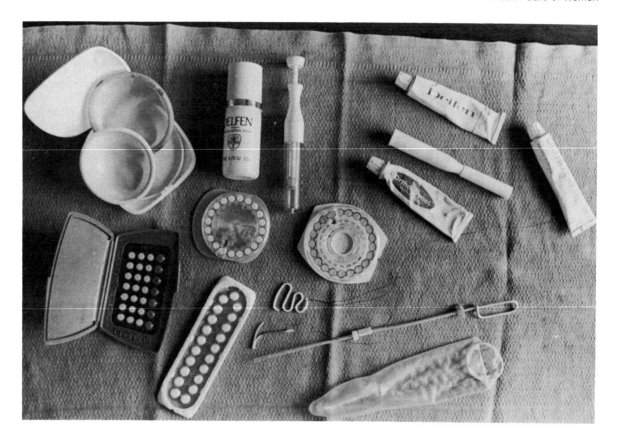

Figure 3-1. Common methods of contraception.

the vagina, contraceptive foam or jelly should be inserted at once.

Vaginal Foam, Jelly or Cream

Spermicidal preparations are inserted into the vagina shortly before intercourse and act as a chemical barrier at the cervical os (Figure 3-1). The aerosol foams expand immediately to cover all of the vaginal folds and then seem to disappear, leaving a long-lasting invisible coating. Cream spreads more evenly then jelly, while jelly offers greater lubrication. Cream and jelly take longer to spread over the vaginal surface than foam—at least several minutes. When these preparations mix with semen after ejaculation, they release an immobilizing spermicide, thus inhibiting the movement of the sperm through the cervical os into the uterus. Because semen and spermicidal chemicals neutralize each other, a separate application is needed for each act of intercourse, no matter how close together they might be.

The advantages of spermicidal preparations include their availability without a prescription, relatively simple method of use, and absence of side effects except for an occasional sensitivity of the woman or man to the chemicals. They are particularly useful interim methods, offering protection until a more effective contraceptive can be started. Postpartum, spermicides are recommended until the 6-week check up. They are also very useful for the 2 weeks to a month following the institution of oral contraceptives or the insertion of an IUD, before these methods should be relied upon alone. When the woman desires to go off the pill for a few cycles or is between IUDs, spermicides are often the method of choice. Used with the condom or diaphragm, their effectiveness is substantially increased. The disadvantages of these preparations include the close association of spermicides with the sex act, for they must be inserted at least a few minutes before penetration and no longer than 30 minutes should elapse between insertion and intercourse. Otherwise, the activity of the spermicide decreases. Some couples find these preparations aesthetically unpleasant, causing too much lubrication, feeling unpleasant to the touch, tasting bad, or creating oral anesthesia.

The major disadvantage, however, is the low use effectiveness of spermicides when used alone. Similar to the condom, among constant users who use spermicides properly and every time, the failure rate of this method is 3 pregnancies per 100 woman years. In actual use, this is 22 pregnancies per 100 woman years. To be effective, spermicides must be used *every time* and *properly*. In counseling, the following instructions should be given: use an inserter following the manufacturer's instructions for filling and place it as far back in the vagina as possible, then back the inserter out slightly before pushing the plunger. This places the spermicide close to the cervix (Figure 3-2). Put in two full applicators for additional protection. Be sure to insert the spermicide before penile contact with the external labia or vagina. Wait several minutes but not more than 30 minutes between application and intercourse. For each additional sex act, use two more applications. Do not douche for several hours following the use of a spermicide.

Some spermicidal preparations (Lorophyn, Koromex) contain an organic mercuric compound, phenylmercuric acetate. Although this substance does not cross the cell wall, there is a chance of absorption should the woman have a vaginal or cervical laceration. Many brands are available which do not contain mercuric compounds.

The Diaphragm

The diaphragm is a dome-shaped rubber cup with a circular metal spring, ranging in size from 55 to 100 mm. in diameter (See Figure 3-1). It is used with spermicidal cream or jelly placed within the dome and around the ring, and it is inserted into the vagina to cover the cervix and part of the anterior vaginal wall (Figure 3-3). The main purpose of the diaphragm is to hold the spermicidal agent in place over the cervix. It has been shown that the diaphragm moves about during intercourse, although when it is properly positioned neither partner can feel it. Diaphragms have been in use since the end of the nineteenth century and have been quite effective in limiting pregnancies for three generations.

The key factor in the effective use of the dia-

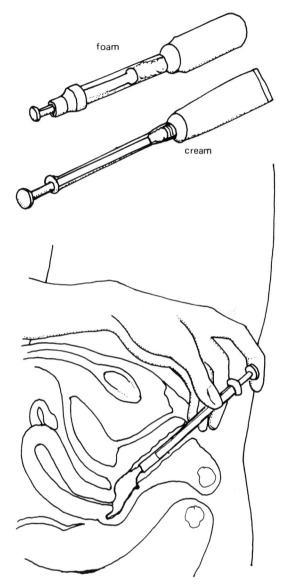

Figure 3-2. Insertion of spermicidal foam or cream near the cervix.

phragm is the motivation of the woman. A responsible, determined woman, without inhibitions about touching her genitals, one who seeks a safe contraceptive which does not interfere with body functions, can do very well with the diaphragm. There is presently a reawakening of interest in this method on the part of professionals and women, particularly among those who are more aware of the complications of oral contraceptives and IUDs. It is also frequently the method of choice for

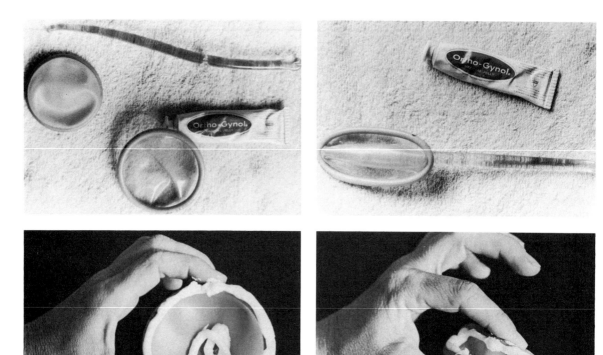

Figure 3-3. (Top, left to right) Diaphragms, spermicidal jelly, and inserter. Diaphragm in position on inserter. (Bottom, left to right) Diaphragm with spermicidal cream applied. Diaphragm compressed ready for manual insertion.

women for whom the pill or IUD is contraindicated. When fitted and used properly, the diaphragm has a failure rate of 3 pregnancies per 100 woman years; and among all users the failure rate is 20 to 25 pregnancies per 100 woman years.

The advantages of the diaphragm include its safety and lack of side effects, except for an occasional sensitivity to the rubber or spermacides used, its good track record when used conscientiously by well-motivated women, its relative separation from the sex act (it can be inserted up to 2 hours before), its unobtrusiveness (it leaves considerably less cream or jelly in the vagina than a spermicide alone), and the control it gives the woman over contraceptive use. The disadvantages can be many or few, depending upon the woman's attitudes toward her sexuality and the diaphragm's inconvenience. It is a prescription method and requires that the woman be fitted by a professional. The woman must learn the techniques of insertion and removal and must clean and store the diaphragm properly between use. Some women find that trying to anticipate sex and inserting the diaphragm early leads to a lot of trouble for nothing in many instances. If they wait, foreplay must be interrupted for insertion. Some dislike touching the cream or jelly, or touching their genitals (an inserter may obviate this difficulty). Refitting a diaphragm is necessary following pregnancy or if there is a substantial weight loss or gain. The diaphragm must be checked periodically for tears and holes, and douching is usually done after removal.

Diaphragm failures are almost always related to one of the following factors: not using it consistently, using a modified rhythm method in which the diaphragm is only used during the estimated midcycle fertile period, cutting the time of use too closely, improper fitting or placement so that the spermicide is not held in position over the cervix, and insufficient spermicide or failing to add extra spermicide for subsequent ejaculations. To be effective, diaphragms have to be *properly fitted*, *properly used*, and *used each time*.

FITTING FOR A DIAPHRAGM.   There are two types of diaphragms in current use, the flat or coil spring in which the entire ring is flexible and which is flat in side view when compressed for insertion, and the alflex or arc spring in which the ring bends only at a certain place and forms an arc when compressed. The coil spring diaphragm is better for nulliparous women with good vaginal tone and can be used with an inserter. The arc spring was designed for ease of manual insertion and cannot be used with an inserter, and some believe it is better with moderate degrees of pelvic relaxation.

Fitting rings are used by the nurse practitioner to determine the correct diaphragm size (Figure 3-4). Most nulliparous women take a 65 to 75 mm. rim size, and multiparas usually take the 75 to 90 mm. sizes. It is a good practice to begin with a 75 mm. rim size and go up or down as needed. With the woman in the lithotomy position, and after examination for anatomical defects which would preclude the use of the diaphragm, a lubricated fitting ring is inserted by the health provider. After tucking the ring behind the symphysis, the provider checks the position of the cervix in relation to the edges of the ring. The cervix should be within the ring, without too much space beyond the posterior rim in the posterior fornix, and without too much space between the anterior rim and the symphysis. The anterior rim should not protrude onto the lower border of the symphysis, and the ring should not move downward or protrude out more when the woman strains. The largest sized diaphragm ring which fits easily behind the symphysis and does not create any sensations for the woman when it is in place is the correct size. Distention of the lateral walls of the vagina is not important unless it causes sensations.

When the proper size has been determined, the woman is instructed how to insert and remove the diaphragm herself. If manual insertion is used, she pinches the rim together in the middle, spreads the labia with the other hand, and inserts the diaphragm down and back in the vagina as far as it can go (Figure 3-5). This can be done lying down, squatting, or

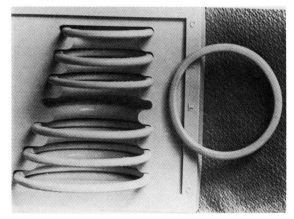

Figure 3-4.   Diaphragm fitting rings.

standing with one leg propped on something. Once the diaphragm is in the vagina, she tucks the anterior rim up behind the pubic bone and feels the cervix inside the fitting ring to be certain that the placement is right. To remove it, the woman hooks one finger under the anterior rim and pulls. It usually will come out quite easily. The health provider should have the woman insert and remove the diaphragm (or fitting ring) while standing by to encourage her and to answer her questions. After the woman has inserted the ring, the provider should also check its position. The woman should practice until she has accomplished several correct insertions and removals before she leaves the examining room. If an inserter is used, the woman should practice positioning the ring or diaphragm on the inserter, stretching it out between the two nobs on one end of the inserter. The inserter is curved to fit the vagina. Assuming the same positions as for manual insertion,

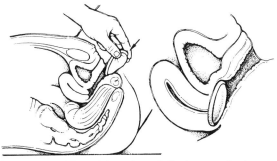

Figure 3-5.   Manual insertion of diaphragm; diaphragm in proper position.

the woman spreads the labia and places the diaphragm on the inserter as far as it will go back into the vagina. She then twists the inserter about one-half rotation, which dislodges the diaphragm from the nobs. She withdraws the inserter, and with one or two fingers tucks the anterior rim up behind the pubic bone. She then checks for position in relation to the cervix. The diaphragm is removed in the way described above.

INSTRUCTIONS FOR USING THE DIAPHRAGM. The diaphragm can be inserted, with spermicidal cream or jelly applied, up to 2 hours before intercourse. About 1 teaspoon of spermicide is placed in the dome, and some is also spread around the rim. Always check the position of the diaphragm by feeling the cervix through the rubber dome. The cervix feels firm and smooth, about the consistency of the tip of the nose. If more than 2 hours elapse between insertion and sex, an extra application of spermicide must be used. Each time intercourse is performed after the diaphragm is in place, spermicide must be inserted. Do not remove the diaphragm to do this, for it should not be disturbed once it is in place. It must be left in place for 6 to 8 hours after the last intercourse for the spermicide to act completely. After removing the diaphragm, wash it with mild soap and water, dry it, and dust it with cornstarch. Keep it in its container until the next use. Many women like to douche after removing the diaphragm because they feel fresher, but this is not required. Before using, or periodically, hold the diaphragm up to the light and inspect carefully for tears or holes. Diaphragms usually last 2 to 3 years.

CONTRAINDICATIONS. Complete uterine prolapse, significant pelvic relaxation, severe cystocele, vesicovaginal or rectovaginal fistula, and severe retroversion or anteversion of the uterus are contraindications to the use of the diaphragm.

Rhythm

Rhythm involves periodic abstinence during the fertile phase of the woman's menstrual cycle. It is a method with many risk factors and requires particular attitudes and convictions on the part of both partners. Some couples choose rhythm for religious reasons (it is the only officially approved method for Roman Catholics) and others because they perceive it as the only truly "natural" method. Lengthy preparation, intelligence, self-control and high motivation are all necessary to practice rhythm effectively. Even then, there is a significant method failure rate.

The concept of rhythm is simple—abstinence during the unsafe phase—but the practice is complicated. Ovulation precedes the next menstrual period by 14 ± 2 days, so it is possible to estimate the time of ovulation by determining the length of menstrual cycles and calculating for variations. Other factors that must be taken into consideration are the ability of sperm to fertilize for about 2 days after ejaculation (though this can be as long as 5 to 7 days), and the capacity of the ovum to become fertilized on the day of ovulation and for 1 day afterwards. Theoretically there is a 4-day period which is unsafe if the moment of ovulation can be exactly determined; of course, this is not possible so the actual time of abstinence, depending upon the amount of variation in cycle length, can be from 7 to 14 days out of each cycle.

CALENDAR METHOD. The woman must keep a record of her menstrual cycles for about 1 year. If her cycle is always 28 days, ovulation occurs between days 12 and 16 ($28 \pm 14 = 2$). She must allow 2 days before this for survival of the sperm, and 1 day at the end for survival of the ovum. Thus the fertile or unsafe period for a regular 28-day cycle would be from day 10 to day 17. If there is any variation in cycle length, however, even greater abstinence is involved. The woman must take her shortest cycle and subtract 18 days to find the start of the fertile period, and then subtract 11 days from her longest cycle to determine the end of the fertile period. If her cycles ranged from 26 to 32 days, 26 = 18, or day 8, would be the start of the fertile period, and 32 − 11, or day 21, would be the end. This means abstinence for 14 days, day 8 to day 21, of each cycle no matter how short or long. Such abstinence may or may not present a problem to the couple. However, other unpredictable variables further complicate the picture. The sperm may survive up to 7 days, or the woman may have an unusually early or late ovulation, or an anovulatory cycle. After an episode of anovulatory bleeding, ovulation can occur at any time, even during bleeding. This can account for conception during a menstrual period which was actually an episode of anovulatory bleeding. Actually, no part of the menstrual cycle can be considered 100 percent safe.

BASAL BODY TEMPERATURE METHOD (BBT). The use effectiveness of rhythm can be increased by the BBT method, which attempts to identify more accurately the time of ovulation. Just before ovulation the woman's basal body temperature, or lowest waking temperature, drops slightly and then rises after ovulation. A rise of 0.5 to 1 degree following a drop, usually within 24 to 72 hours, which is sustained for 3 days indicates that ovulation has occurred. After 3 consecutive days of elevation, the safe period has begun. To calculate the time of ovulation, again records must be kept for 3 to 4 months on a BBT chart (Figure 3-6). Special thermometers are available, and a woman's temperature should be taken before getting out of bed in the morning. When the range of ovulation time has been determined, abstinence should begin 5 days before the shortest time and 3 days after the longest time. Temperature elevation can be caused by infections, tension, irregular sleeping habits, electric blankets, and other factors. Longer sperm survival and unexpected early or late ovulation are also hazards.

CERVICAL MUCUS METHOD. Many women have changes in cervical secretions prior to ovulation and can use these changes to calculate their fertile period. There is an increased quantity of cervical mucus which becomes egg-white or clear and stringy. Due to low saline content and high estrogen level, a drop of this mucus can be stretched into a thin strand of 6 cm. or more (spinnbarkeit). At other times before and after the ovulatory phase, cervical secretions are thick, viscous, and more yellowish. Women who experience such changes in mucus, and not all do, can avoid intercourse once the changes are noticed, and until the mucus becomes thick again. Vaginal infections and other factors influence the appearance of vaginal discharge. If the woman can also identify mittelschmerz and preovulatory heaviness or swelling, this can help identify ovulation.

All rhythm methods are more effective if intercourse is avoided through the entire preovulatory period. In constant users, failure rates as low as 15 pregnancies per 100 woman years have been reported. In actual use, the rates are 25 to 40 pregnancies per 100 woman years. In addition to the risks of mortality and morbidity associated with pregnancy, rhythm users run the danger of fertilizing an "overripe" egg. Structural changes occur in the ovum after about 48 hours, and fertilization of these eggs is associated with an increased incidence of early embryonic death, fetal development abnormalities, and chromosomal defects. This hazard is related to conception which does not occur at time of ovulation, and many rhythm method failures fall into this category.[5]

Oral Contraceptives

The pill has been widely available since 1960, and is presently used by some 80 to 100 million women throughout the world and by 10 to 15 million women in the United States. These millions of women regularly swallow a pill a day, or 20 or more pills a month, for a single purpose—to prevent pregnancy. Oral contraceptives are among the most widely used medications in the world, among the most extensively studied, and yet among the most casually taken and supervised in actual practice. Without question, oral contraceptives are one of the most effective methods when used properly and are completely disassociated from intercourse. They require no manipulation or genital contact, are simple to take, and unobtrusive. To be effective, however, they must be taken religiously and thus require the woman to develop a habit of pill taking. And, evidence is steadily accumulating about their widespread effects on the physiology of the body, complex endocrine alterations, long-term side effects, and significant dangers to life and health.

The theoretical effectiveness of combined pills approaches 100 percent and is reported at a failure rate of 0.1 pregnancies per 100 woman years. Other figures include 0.34 for combined pills in the Royal College of General Practitioners report entitled *Oral Contraceptives and Health*[6], and 2.5 for minipills containing progestin only.[7] Occasionally a woman who has taken her pills properly does become pregnant. Use effectiveness is considerably less for the pill, however, when pregnancies resulting from forgetting or skipping pills and discontinuation without using another contraceptive method are taken into account. Only 40 to 75 percent of all women starting pills will continue them for 1 year. Although accurate use

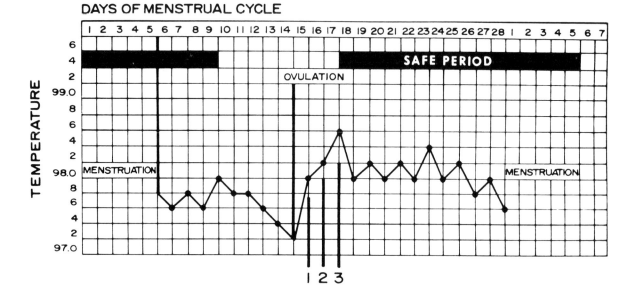

DAYS OF MENSTRUAL CYCLE

Figure 3-6. Basal body temperature chart.

effectiveness is difficult to evaluate, the actual failure rate of pills is in the range of 5 to 10 pregnancies per 100 woman years.[8]

MECHANISMS OF ACTION. There are four means by which oral contraceptives prevent pregnancy, including prevention of ovulation, alteration of tubal transport, changes in the endometrium, and alterations in cervical mucus. Most combination pills have a consistent antiovulatory effect by suppressing the midcycle luteinizing hormone peak and depressing follicle-stimulating hormone. This suppression of gonadotropins is probably mediated via the hypothalamus rather than directly on the pituitary (see Chapter 4 for a discussion of menstrual physiology). Lower doses of estrogen (20 to 50 mcg.) and progestin alone will not always prevent ovulation. Estrogen accelerates the tubal transport of the zygote, while progestins given prior to fertilization seem to slow transport. High doses of estrogen after ovulation cause an alteration in the normal secretory development of the endometrium, producing areas of marked edema alternating with areas of dense cellularity. Reduction in carbonic anhydrase which might cause a decrease in pH also occurs, and these changes make implantation or survival of the zygote impossible. Progestins, either alone or in combinations, cause

a regression of the proliferative endometrium and a rapid progression through the progestational phase, ending with an exhausted, atrophic endometrium. Estrogens have a favorable effect on cervical mucus and capacitate sperm by releasing it from the effects of the seminal fluid. Progestins, however, produce a scanty, cellular mucus of increased viscosity which is resistant to sperm penetration and does not permit the capacitation process to occur.

SYSTEMIC EFFECTS. Originally it was believed that the pill affected only ovulation and fertility. Now it is recognized that these powerful synthetic hormones affect multiple body systems and create many metabolic and endocrine changes. The pill's effects are "profound and protean" and "they probably work because they *have* so many effects."[9] The following is a brief description of certain known physiological alterations:

Ovaries. Under the influence of oral contraceptives, the ovaries appear atretic and inactive. There is some early follicular development, but this is arrested at diameters of less than 1 cm. and then atrophy occurs. The membrane covering the ovaries is white and thickened.

Thyroid. Estrogen causes an increase in thyroxin-binding globulin, leading to an increase in protein bound iodine (PBI) and T4 and a decrease in T3 uptake. The functional state of the thyroid seems unchanged, however, since the basal metabolic rate, I131, cholesterol, and free thyroxin levels are normal. Response to thyroid-stimulating hormone is maintained, and there is no evidence that oral contraceptives cause hypo- or hyperthyroidism. The abnormal tests return to normal 2 to 4 months after discontinuing the pills.

Skin. Chloasma, the discoloration of the skin on the forehead and cheeks and around the mouth, occurs in about 29 percent of oral contraceptive users. Unlike the chloasma of pregnancy, that caused by the pill does not go away entirely after stopping the pill. Women with chloasma of pregnancy or prolonged exposure to sunlight are more likely to develop this problem on the pill. Estrogen causes a decrease in sebaceous gland activity, which may improve acne in women taking estrogen-dominant pills. Some women taking androgenic preparations have an increase in acne. Photodermatitis and erythema nodosum or multiforma have occasionally occurred.

Weight. A 3 to 5-lb. weight gain has been reported in 40 to 50 percent of pill users, usually worse in the first 3 months of use and less after 12 months. One metabolic balance study reported a consistent increase in lean body mass, without a gain in total body weight, and a positive nitrogen balance, indicating an accumulation of body protein. Certain estrogenic preparations cause sodium retention (estradiol), and progestins also lead to this condition with long-term use. Mild sodium and water retention is a common effect of many combination pills.

Carbohydrate metabolism. Women taking oral contraceptives show a threefold increase in human growth hormone (HGH) and a compensatory increase in insulin due to HGH's antiinsulin effect. This relative hyperinsulinism allows them to maintain a normal glucose tolerance test (GTT), although blood sugar levels are also increased by the pill. Fasting blood sugar is elevated in 10 to 25 percent of the women on the pill, and in addition some 20 percent have an abnormal GTT. These patients with abnormal values have some degree of impaired beta-cell functioning. Obesity or a history suggestive of diabetes places the woman at greater risk for abnormalities in carbohydrate metabolism. Studies on short-term pill users show a reversal of all changes after withdrawal of the medication, but the long-term effects are not known.

Lipids. There is an increase in plasma triglyceride and phospholipid levels among pill users which is a dose-dependent estrogen effect. The mechanism is unclear but may be related to increased hepatic production. The long-term effects of this lipid increase are not known, but it may be associated with acute vascular accidents, cardiovascular disease, and circulatory disorders.[10]

Hypertension. Increases in systolic and diastolic blood pressure occur in 15 to 18 percent of women taking the pill, often as early as 1 to 3 weeks after starting the medication. Although the exact mechanism is not known, renin, renin substrate, angiotensin I, and angiotensinase have all been found to be elevated in hypertensive women taking the pill. It is possible that the direct action of estrogen on the juxtaglomerular cells causes a blunting of the normal feedback control. After discontinuation of the pill, blood pressure usually returns to premedication levels within 1 to 3 months. Oral contraceptive users are up to six times more likely to develop hypertension than nonusers.[11] The pill can also produce vascular intimal proliferation within the pulmonary arterial branches, leading to severe pulmonary hypertension and cor pulmonale.[12]

Thromboembolic effects. Women taking oral contraceptives have an increased risk of clotting disorders, with danger of death or disability. Probably several factors are involved in the pill's thrombogenic potential, including the production of vascular lesions, venous stasis, and alterations in the blood. Pill users were found to have more rapid fibrin formation and increased clot firmness, which was not related to dose, estrogen-progestin type, or duration of exposure.[13] Blood changes are thought to begin within a few days of pill use and to disappear 2 months after discontinuation. Estrogen is implicated in clotting problems and causes increases in certain blood factors (VII, IX, X) associated with coagulation, and it also increases the platelet count. There is also a change in electrophoretic mobility of platelets with long-term oral contraceptive use.[14] Women with type O blood may be less susceptible to thromboembolism; one study found the risk three times greater in women with blood types A, B, or AB.[15] The presence of varicosities and other circulatory disorders increase the risk of thromboembolism.

The risk of death from thromboembolic disease due to the pill is 7 to 8 times greater in users than in nonusers. One out of about 2,000 women on oral contraceptives is hospitalized each year for clotting problems; one in 66,000 pill-takers under 35 and one in 25,000 over 35 dies each year from thromboembolic disorders. Among nonusers of the pill, one woman in 500,000 dies annually from clotting disorders. In examining such risks, deaths due to pregnancy must be considered to balance the use of oral contraceptives against other methods with lower effectiveness rates (Table 3-3).

Thromboembolic disorders due to pill use may take the form of thrombophlebitis and deep vein thrombosis, pulmonary embolism, retinal vein thrombosis, cerebral thrombosis, and possibly coronary thrombosis. Dosage has been shown to be important in the development of deep vein thrombosis, with an incidence of 81 per 100,000 among women taking less than 50 mcg. estrogen, and 112 per 100,000 among women taking more than 50 mcg. estrogen.[16]

Effects of cigarette smoking. There is a greatly multiplied risk of fatal heart attack among women over age 30 who smoke and take oral contraceptives, as compared to younger women or those over 30 who do not smoke and who use the pill. While other risk factors (high cholesterol, hypertension) are also associated with greater danger of myocardial infarction, smoking is the most important risk factor. The myocardial death rate caused by pill use is 17 times higher among women who smoke than those who do not, during the age span of 30 to 44. Women without risk factors can continue pill use with relative safety during these years, but those who smoke are in significantly increased danger after age 30.[17]

Cancer. The relationship of oral contraceptives to cancer is problematic and most likely will not be determined for another decade or so. It is well known that the pill causes benign polypoid hyperplasia of the cervix, but there is no evidence that this condition progresses to malignancy. One study found slightly more carcinoma in situ of the cervix in pill users than in diaphragm users, but the pill-using sample came from a population already at risk for cervical carcinoma due to other factors (race, age of first intercourse, number of sexual partners, early and multiple pregnancy, herpes infections).[18] Endometrial adenocarcinoma, though infrequent, has been reported in women on combined oral contraceptive therapy[19] and

in women taking sequential oral contraceptives.[20] There is a distinct relationship between prolonged, unopposed estrogen stimulation and endometrial hyperplasia and adenocarcinoma. Progestins and progesterone generally exert an antitumor effect, but the in vivo effects of synthetic progestins and estrogens used in oral contraceptives are open to question.

To date, no causal relationship has been documented between oral contraceptives and breast cancer in women, although breast cancers have been induced in at least five different species of animals using the same synthetic hormones. Certain types of breast cancer are estrogen dependent and grow more rapidly during hyperestrogen states, such as pregnancy. Because oral contraceptives also create a hyperestrogenic state, there is concern that they might encourage the development of or nourish breast cancer. However, case-controlled studies suggest neither unusually high nor low breast cancer rates among pill users. Long-term pill use is causally related to a low risk of benign fibrocystic breast disease and fibroadenoma.[21] Due to the long latency period of breast cancer, its relationship to oral contraceptive use must still be considered undetermined.

Liver. Studies indicate that an alteration in liver function is caused by oral contraceptives, and that this alteration is apparently related to estrogen rather than progestin, is dose-related, and readily reversible when the medicine is stopped. Bromsulphalein (BSP) retention, transaminase, SGOT, and alkaline phosphatase levels are elevated slightly, and excretory function may be minimally reduced. These effects are thought to be related to an altered hepatic cell permeability and not to hepatotoxicity. The pill has recently been shown to cause liver adenomas, which are related to prolonged use and the type of estrogen. The relative risk increased significantly after 5 years of pill use, and 93 percent of liver adnomas were associated with mestranol but only 7 percent with ethinyl estradiol. Surgery was required to remove the tumors, and all women were doing well 6 months to 11 years later.[22]

Breasts and lactation. About 10 percent of the women on the pill report either an increase or a decrease in breast size with oral contraceptive use, and when a high dose estrogen dominant preparation is used, the incidence of increased size is 20 percent. There may be in-

Table 3-3
Estimates of Risk of Death from Pulmonary Embolism or Cerebral Thrombosis in Users and Nonusers of Oral Contraceptives Compared with Risk of Death from Certain Other Causes

	Age (years)	
	20 to 34	35 to 44
Estimated annual death rate per 100,000 healthy married nonpregnant women from pulmonary or cerebral thromboembolism		
Users of oral contraceptives	1.5	3.9
Nonusers of oral contraceptives	0.2	0.5
Annual death rates per 100,000 female population from		
Cancer	13.7	70.1
Motor accidents	4.9	3.9
All causes	60.1	170.5
Death rates per 100,000 pregnancies from		
Complications of pregnancy	7.5	13.8
Abortion	5.6	10.4
Complications of delivery	7.1	26.5
Complications of puerperium		
phlebitis, thrombosis and embolism	1.3	2.3
Other complications	1.3	4.6
All risks of pregnancy, delivery and puerperium	*22.8*	*57.6*

Swartz and Henriques, "Choosing Methods for Family Planning," *American Family Physician* 13, 4 (April 1976): 140.

creased breast sensitivity, depending upon the preparation, which is usually more pronounced in the early months of use. Low dose pills do not prevent lactation postpartally, but they do cause a significant decrease in milk supply. Small amounts of the exogenous hormones in oral contraceptives are excreted in the milk during lactation. Breast cancer was discussed above.

Gallbladder. There is a suggested relationship between oral contraceptive use and an increased incidence of surgically proven gallbladder disease. Women who developed gallstones tended to become symptomatic early in their pill use, but there may also be a lower long-term risk of gallbladder disease in women on the pill than in women not on the pill.[23]

Corneal edema. Some women develop a mild swelling of the cornea, an estrogen effect due to fluid retention. This may make contact lenses fail to fit properly, necessitating a change in size and shape. Corneal edema is usually worse in the first 3 months of pill use, after which it may improve.

Genetic effects. There is no definitive evidence of an increase in major or minor abnormalities of the fetus among women who used oral contraceptives prior to conception, or that estrogens or progestins cause chromosomal changes in vitro. An increased number of early spontaneous abortions has been linked to the pill, however, and an increased incidence of triploidy among abortuses of women who became pregnant within 6 months of discontinuing oral contraceptives has been reported.[24]

Postpill amenorrhea. Most women resume their normal cycle within a few months of stopping the pill, and their pregnancy rate 3 to 6 months posttherapy is the same as that of women who are nonusers of oral contraceptives. A few women, however, develop true secondary amenorrhea due to the suppressive effect of oral contraceptives on the secretion of gonadotropin. This effect is related more to pretreatment irregularity or anovulatory cycles than to the length of pill use. Patients with a poorly functioning pituitary-ovarian axis are at an increased risk for postpill amenorrhea and possible sterility.

Urinary tract. An increased incidence of urinary tract infections has been noted in users of oral contraceptives. This is probably related to ureteral dilatation and asymptomatic bacteriuria. An increase in vaginitis due to Candida and Trichomonas vaginalis has also been reported.

Depression. The effects of oral contraceptives on depression, libido, and sexual enjoyment are subject to some controversy. It is certainly possible that these steroid hormones with such widespread effects could alter physiology enough to affect sexual functioning and mental state. Many other factors could be involved besides pill taking, however, making accurate assessment difficult. Mood, and sexual interest and enjoyment apparently may change in either direction. There seems to be a fairly widespread belief that the pill causes depression, and if depression is an important clinical concern, a trial discontinuation of oral contraceptives is indicated.

Other effects. Gastrointestinal effects include nausea, with occasional vomiting, which is caused by the estrogen in the pill acting on the vomiting center in the brain. This is a common problem during the first few months of use, then usually the condition improves. Lower dose estrogens cause fewer gastrointestinal problems. Breakthrough bleeding (spotting between periods) occurs when the hormone levels cannot maintain the endometrium. If this happens early in the cycle, it is due to estrogen deficiency, if late to progestin deficiency. Frequently there is a decrease in the length and amount of menstrual flow (actually withdrawal bleeding), or a period may be skipped entirely, due to progestational effects on the endometrium. A decrease in dysmenorrhea and premenstrual symptoms is associated with anovulation and a decreased production of natural progesterone. Women taking oral contraceptives have less iron deficiency anemia than nonusers and fewer ovarian cysts. Table 3-4 lists the side effects and complications of oral contraceptives in a time framework. Figure 3-7 shows the rates of occurrence of certain conditions among those who do and those who have never used the pill and the presumed beneficial and adverse effects of oral contraceptive use.

APPROACH TO MANAGEMENT. Prescribing an oral contraceptive means giving a woman for long-term use a potent medication which has widespread multiple effects on body systems. It should not be undertaken lightly or without adequate pretherapy evaluation. Principles of fully informed consent to treatment should be

followed, and careful follow-up planned. Contraindications to pill use include the following:

Absolute
Thromboembolic disorders (or history of)
Cerebrovascular accident (or history of)
Impaired liver function
Malignancy of breast or reproductive system
Pregnancy

Strong Relative Contraindications
Migraine headaches
Hypertension
Less than 4 weeks postpartum
Prediabetes, diabetes, or strong family history
Gallbladder disease, postcholecystectomy
History of cholestasis during pregnancy
Acute phase of mononucleosis
Sickle cell disease
Undiagnosed abnormal vaginal bleeding

Other Relative Contraindications
Varicose veins
Asthma
Cardiac or renal disease
Chloasma
Uterine fibromyomata
Epilepsy
Depression
Menstrual irregularity or late menarche
Lactation

Selecting the right pill. The health provider has a plethora of pills to choose from in starting a patient on oral contraceptives (Table 3-5). The two forms of estrogen used, ethinyl estradiol and mestranol, are similar in estrogenic potency and contraceptive effectiveness, although ethinyl estradiol is thought to be somewhat more potent. Presently five progestogens are used, and all are 19-nortestosterone derivatives. Their biological properties vary, such as their progestational potency, masculinizing (androgenic) potential, conversion to estrogen, antiestrogenic properties, and anabolic effects (Table 3-6). When different combinations of these synthetic hormones are made into oral contraceptives, it is useful to think of them on a scale from estrogen-dominant to balanced to progestogen-dominant. This helps in selecting an appropriate pill or in changing pills due to certain side effects. Individual women differ in the amount of estrogen and progesterone needed to achieve a balance, and a given oral contraceptive when combined with their own physiology may exceed or fail to meet natural hormone requirements (Table 3-7, p. 80).

Table 3-4
Side Effects and Complications of Oral Contraceptives in a Time Framework

Worse in First 3 Months	Over Time: Steady–Constant	Worse Over Time	Worse Post-Discontinuation
1. Nausea + dizziness (estrogen excess)	1. Headaches during 3 weeks pills are being taken (estrogen excess)	1. Headaches during week pill are not taken (progestin excess)	1. Infertility, amenorrhea; hypothalamic and endometrial suppression**
2. Thrombophlebitis (venous) Leg veins (estrogen excess) *Pulmonary emboli Pelvic veins *Retinal vein thrombosis	2. Arterial thromboembolic events (estrogen excess), blurred vision, *Stroke	2. Weight gain (anabolic progestational)— androgenic effect	2. One form of acne (progesterone excess)
3. Cyclic weight gain edema (fluid retention) (estrogen excess)	3. Anxiety, fatigue, depression (may be due to estrogen excess producing fluid retention, estrogen deficiency or to progestin excess)	3. Candida vaginitis (progestin excess or estrogen deficiency)	3. Hair loss — alopecia (progestin excess)
4. Breast fullness, tenderness (estrogen excess effect on ductal and fatty tissue; progestin excess effect on all alveolar tissue)	4. Thyroid function studies Elevated PBI Depressed T3 resin uptake	4. Periodic missed menses while on oral contraceptives (estrogen deficiency possibly secondary to progestin dominance)	
5. Breakthrough bleeding (early due to estrogen deficiency; late due to progesterone deficiency)	5. Susceptibility to amenorrhea postpill discontinuation (combined effect of progestins + estrogens on hypothalamus, pituitary and also on endometrium)	5. *Chloasma (estrogen excess)	
6. Elevated serum lipid levels even to the extent of pancreatitis	6. Change in cervical secretions - mucorrhea (estrogen excess)	6. *Myocardial infarction	
7. Abnormal glucose tolerance test (estrogen & progestational effect)	7. Decrease in libido (estrogen deficiency or progesterone excess)	7. Spider angiomata (estrogen excess)	
8. Contact lenses fail to fit (estrogen effect via fluid retention)	8. Autophonia, chronic dilatation of eustachian tubes rather than cyclic opening and closing.	8. Growth of myoma (estrogen excess)	
9. Abdominal cramping (estrogen effect via fluid retention)	9. Acne (androgen excess)	9. *Predisposition to gallbladder disease (estrogen or progestin excess)	
10. Suppression of lactation (estrogen excess)		10. Hirsutism (progestin excess)	
11. Pregnancy (failure to understand correct use of oral contraceptives)		11. Decreased menstrual flow (estrogen deficiency)	
		12. Small uterus, pelvic relaxation, cystocele, rectocele, atrophic vaginitis (estrogen deficiency)	
		13. Cystic breast changes (estrogen excess)	
		14. Photodermatitis - sunlight sensitivity with hypopigmentation (estrogen excess)	
		15. One form of hair loss — alopecia (progestin excess)	
		16. Hypertension (?) (progestin or estrogen excess or possibly either)	

*May be irreversible.
**To avoid this complication in many patients, advise women desiring to become pregnant to d/c pills 3-6 mos. prior to desired pregnancy. Hatcher, et al, *Contraceptive Technology*, pp. 52-53.

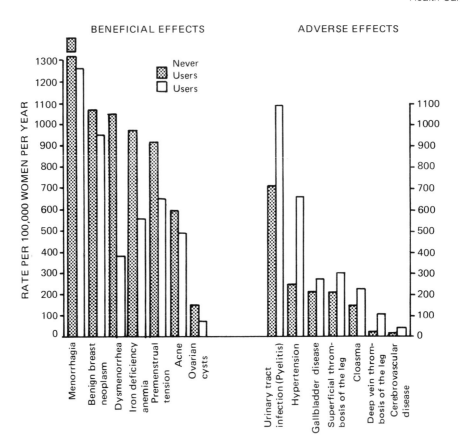

BENEFICIAL EFFECTS   ADVERSE EFFECTS

Figure 3-7. Comparison of the incidence of various conditions in current users and never users of oral contraceptives, Royal College of General Practitioners, 1968–1971. (Rates per 100,000 women)

NOTE: This chart depicts the rates of occurrence of selected conditions in Britain per 100,000 oral contraceptive users and per 100,000 women who have never used oral contraceptives standardized for age, parity, social class, and cigarette consumption. The conditions on the right occur more frequently among oral contraceptive users, that is they can be considered adverse effects of pill use. The conditions on the left occur less frequently among oral contraceptive users, that is, pills have a protective effect against these conditions. The seriousness of these disorders, of course, varies greatly; cerebrovascular disease, although rare, is potentially life threatening and iron deficiency anemia is a cause of continuing morbidity whereas skin disorders are relatively minor.

History or physical findings suggestive of an obvious estrogen or progesterone deficiency or excess can assist in selecting a preparation which might rectify this imbalance. Practically, it is best to begin with a pill having 50 mcg. of estrogen or less in order to minimize thromboembolic risks. Ortho-Novum 1/50 and Norinyl 1/50, which are identical pharmaceutically, are used in many family-planning programs as the initial contraceptive. Use of 20 or 30 mcg. estrogen pills is associated with high rates of breakthrough bleeding, or spotting, which makes these preparations less acceptable to women. Over 90 percent of women can be given pills with 50 mcg. estrogen or less, so the move to 80 or more mcg. should be carefully considered.

If any side effects are reported, evaluate whether these are due to estrogen excess or deficiency, progestin excess or deficiency, or androgen excess (Table 3-8). Encourage the patient to stay for 2 to 3 cycles on her initially chosen pill, because many minor side effects improve after this. For early or late spotting, switch to Ovral, Norlestrin 2.5 or Demulen, or to a higher estrogen pill such as Ortho 1/80 or Norinyl 1/80. For nausea, low estrogen (0 to 50 mcg.) is helpful, as this dosage is for weight

Table 3-5
Most Currently Available Combination and
Microdose Progestin Oral Contraceptives

Product/ Manufacturer	Type	Estrogen	Progestin
Enovid-E/Searle	Comb	100 mcg. mestranol	2.5 mg. norethynordiel
Ortho-Novum/Ortho	Comb	100 mcg. mestranol	2 mg. norethindrone
Norinyl/Syntex	Comb	100 mcg. mestranol	2 mg. norethindrone
Ovulen/Searle	Comb	100 mcg. mestranol	1 mg. ethynodiol diacetae
Ortho-Novum 1+80	Comb	80 mcg. mestranol	1 mg. norethindrone
Norinyl 1+80 Syntex	Comb	80 mcg. mestranol	1 mg. norethindrone
Norlestrin/Parke-Davis	Comb	50 mcg. ethinyl estradiol	2.5 mg. norethindrone acetate
Norinyl 1+50/Syntex	Comb	50 mcg. mestranol	1 mg. norethindrone
Ortho-Novum 1+50 Ortho	Comb	50 mcg. mestranol	1 mg. norethindrone
Norlestrin/Parke-Davis	Comb	50 mcg. ethinyl estradiol	1 mg. norethindrone acetate
Ovral/Wyeth	Comb	50 mcg. ethinyl estradiol	0.5 mg. norgestrel
Demulen/Searle	Comb	50 mcg. ethinyl estradiol	1 mg. ethynodiol diacetate
Zorane 1+50/Lederle	Comb	50 mcg. ethinyl estradiol	1 mg. norethindrone acetate
Brevicon/Syntex	Comb	35 mcg. ethinyl estradiol	0.5 mg. norethindrone
Loestrin 1.5+30 Parke- Davis	Comb	30 mcg. ethinyl estradiol	1.5 mg. norethindrone acetate
Zorane 1.5+30 Lederle	Comb	30 mcg. ethinyl estradiol	1.5 mg. norethindrone acetate
Lo-Ovral/Wyeth	Comb	30 mcg. ethinyl estradiol	0.3 mg. norgestrel
Loestrin 1+20 Parke- Davis	Comb	20 mcg. ethinyl estradiol	1 mg. norethindrone acetate
Zorane 1+20/Lederle	Comb	20 mcg. ethinyl estradiol	1 mg. norethindrone acetate
Micronor/Ortho	Prog		0.35 mg. norethindrone
Nor-Q.D./Syntex	Prog		0.35 mg. norethindrone
Ovrette/Wyeth	Prog		0.075 mg. norgestrel

Table 3-6
Relative Biological Effects of Progestogens in Common Use

	Estrogenic	Antiestrogenic	Androgenic	Progestational
Norethynodrel ENOVID ENOVID-E	++	−	−	±
Norethindrone NORINYL ORTHO-NOVUM	−	+	+	+
Norethindrone acetate NORLESTRIN	−	++	+	+
Ethynodiol diacetate OVULEN DEMULEN	+	++	+	++
Norgestrel OVRAL	−	+++	+	++++

Table 3-7
Hypothetical Spectrum of Estrogen-Progestogen Dominance in Certain Oral Contraceptives

	Most Estrogen Dominant	Progestogen Only
Combined	Enovid-E Enovid 10 Enovid 5 Ovulen Norinyl 2 mg. Ortho-Novum 2 mg. Demulen Norinyl 1/80 Ortho-Novum 1/80 Norlestrin 1 mg. Norinyl 1 mg. Ortho-Novum 1 mg. Ovral Norlestrin 2.5 mg. Ortho-Novum 10 mg. Loestrin	
Mini (Progestogen only)		Nor-Q-D Micronor

Romney, et al, *Gynecology and Obstetrics*, pp. 555 and 557.

Table 3-8
Pill Side Effects: Hormone Etiology

Estrogen Excess	Progestin Excess	Androgen Excess	Estrogen Deficiency	Progestin Deficiency

Nausea, dizziness
Edema and leg
  cramps
Leukorrhea
Increase in
  leiomyoma size
Chloasma
Uterine cramps
Irritability
Increase female fat
  disposition
Cervical exotrophia
Contact lenses
  don't fit
Telangiectasia
Vascular type
  headache
Hypertension(?)
Lactation
  suppression
Headaches while
  taking pills
Cystic breast
  changes
Breast tenderness
  with fluid
  retention
Thrombophlebitis
	Increased appetite
	  and weight gain
	Tiredness and
	  fatigue
	Depression
	Decrease in
	  libido
	Oily scalp, acne
	Loss of hair
	Cholestatic
	  jaundice
	Decreased length
	  of menstrual flow
	Hypertension (?)
	Headaches
	  between pill
	  packages
	Candida vaginitis
	  cervicitis
	Increase in breast
	  size (alveolar
	  tissue)
	Breast tenderness
	  without fluid
	  retention
		Increased appetite
		Hirsutism
		Acne
		Oily skin, rash
		Increased libido
		Cholestatic
		  jaundice
			Irritability,
			  nervousness
			Hot flushes
			Uterine prolapse
			Early and midcycle
			  spotting
			Decreased amount
			  of menstrual flow
			No withdrawal
			  bleeding
			Decreased libido
				Late breakthrough
				  bleeding
				Heavy menstrual
				  flow and clots
				Delayed onset of
				  menses following
				  last pill

Hatcher, et al, *Contraceptive Technology 1976-1977*, p. 51.

gain due to fluid retention. If weight gain is due to increased appetite, use a low progestin pill. For oily scalp or acne, use a low progestin, low androgen pill such as Demulen, Norinyl 1/50, or Ortho 1/50. Ovral may make acne worse. It may be necessary to use Enovid-E if acne continues to be a problem. Depression may be due to fluid retention or to too little estrogen or progestin and is difficult to manage.

Most women use combination pills, and generally a preparation can be found from among the many available which is compatible with individual needs. Sequential pills were banned by the Food and Drug Administration because studies suggested an increased risk of endometrial cancer. These types of pills were previously used for one of four potential advantages: high estrogen effect, low progestational effects, low androgenic effect, or reduced suppression of the hypothalamic-pituitary-ovarian axis. Sequentials provided a higher dose of estrogen alone for 14 to 15 days, and then a progestin was added for the final week or so of the cycle. Their effectiveness rate was lower and complication rate higher than the rates for combination pills. Minipills provide small doses of progestins only and were designed to avoid the complications associated with estrogen. They are less effective than combination pills but in the same range as IUDs. It is not known if minipills contribute to an increased risk of thromboembolic disease, but they do improve the following estrogen-related problems: headache, chloasma, hypertension, breast tenderness, premenstrual depression, and weight gain. They also have less effect on lactation. The main side effect of the minipill is irregular menses. There is increased amenorrhea, spotting, and irregularity of flow which causes concern in some women and may preclude its use. Low dose combination pills such as Loestrin 1/20, Zorane 1/20, Lo-Ovral, and Brevicon have from 20 to 35 mcg. estrogen and can minimize estrogen-associated side effects, but their high rates of breakthrough bleeding and spotting have so far discouraged their widespread use.

Patient education and instruction. Details on how to take the pill, the side effects and symptoms of serious dangers, and follow-up should be discussed. Instructions on taking the pill generally include the following:

1. Start your first pack on the fifth day of your next menstrual period (or after your baby is 1 month old if postpartum). Take one pill a day until the pack is finished. If you have the 21-day pills, stop for 1 week then begin the next pack on the same day of the week you started the first one. You'll always begin each pack on the same day of the week. If you have the 28-day pills, begin the next pack as soon as you finish all the pills. The 28-day pills have 1 week of inert (sometimes with iron added) pills to keep up the habit of taking the pill daily.

2. Use a second method of birth control (such as foam and condom) for the first month you take the pill. Since the pill may not fully protect you for that first month, using another method is generally a good idea.

3. Take your pill at about the same time every day because this keeps a constant blood level of drug and protects you better. In the morning on awakening, at bedtime, or at mealtime are convenient times. Associating the pill with a regular daily activity makes it easier to remember.

4. If you miss *one* pill, take it as soon as you remember, and take today's pill at the regular time. It is unlikely that you would get pregnant. If you miss *two* pills, take both pills as soon as you remember, and two pills the next day. You may have some spotting, and should use another contraceptive for the rest of that pack. If you miss *three or more* pills, stop that pack and use another method at once. You will probably spot or bleed. Start a new pack a week after you stopped the last one, even if you are bleeding. Use another method of birth control all the time you are off the pills and for the first 2 weeks of the new pack.

5. If you *miss one or more pills and skip a period*, you may be pregnant and should see a health provider. If you *miss no pills and skip a period*, it is unlikely that you are pregnant. This happens commonly to women taking pills, and you should begin your next pack at the regularly scheduled time. If you *miss two periods*, even if taking pills regularly, you should be checked for pregnancy.

6. If you want to discontinue taking pills, stop at the end of a pack to avoid irregular bleeding. Be sure to use another method of birth control right away if you want to avoid pregnancy.

A discussion of the side effects includes all the minor ones which usually improve after several cycles on the pill. About 40 percent of pill users have some type of side effects, either minor or major. The woman or couple should be given time to ask questions or voice concerns, and these should be responded to fully. Instructions related to side effects and dangers include the following:

1. If you are concerned about any minor symptom, call for information or make an appointment. If you have spotting for 2 or more cycles, you should be evaluated. If any symptoms persist for more than 3 cycles, they should be evaluated in a return visit.
2. Clotting problems are the most serious complications, and although the incidence of serious trouble is very low, you should be alert to these signs of danger: severe chest pain or shortness of breath might mean a blood clot in the lungs or a heart attack; severe headaches might mean stroke or hypertension; blurred vision, lights flashing before the eyes, or blindness might mean stroke or hypertension; and severe pain in the calf or thigh might mean a blood clot in the legs. Also, severe abdominal pain could mean gallbladder problems. If any of these happen, you must be seen right away.
3. Birth control pills have effects on many systems of the body, and although most of these seem reversible after the pills are stopped, we still do not know for certain whether there will be long-term effects. Although you have no contraindications to taking the pill, you must weigh its hazards against its benefits for you in making your decision.
4. (In the case of relative contraindications) You know that there is a certain risk for you in taking the pill related to (whatever the characteristic is). We have discussed the possible dangers, and you must weigh these against the benefits of the pill for you in making your decision.

Follow-up. Usually a 3-month supply of pills is given on the first visit, and a follow-up appointment scheduled so that the woman may be evaluated after 2 cycles on the pill. If she is doing well and there are no significant side effects, a prescription for that particular pill is given for 6 months to 1 year. Follow-up visits, either every 6 months or annually are continued for as long as the woman takes oral contraceptives. If she has any problems, she is instructed to call for an appointment sooner. On return visits for refills of oral contraceptive medicines, the following procedures are recommended

1. Weight, blood pressure, and urinalysis each visit; Pap smear, hematocrit, gonorrhea culture and serological test for syphilis yearly.
2. Question the patient specifically about headaches, blurred vision, leg pain, chest pain, abdominal pain, bleeding or spotting, and any other symptom she brings up.
3. Review how she is taking the pills to be sure it is correct. Ask if she is satisfied with this method, and offer to discuss alternatives. Review the symptoms of serious complications and what to do about them.

The incidence of complications from oral contraceptives increases with age and in some cases with duration of use. There is a trend toward conservatism which recommends going off the pills periodically to allow the body to reestablish normal gonadotropic functioning. This probably means being off the pills 2 to 3 months per year, and another contraceptive method is needed during that time. Women in the age range of 35 to 40 are well advised to use a method other than the pill, because there is a striking increase in the incidence of myocardial infarctions in women over 40 on the pill.

Other Hormonal Methods

LONG-ACTING PROGESTERONE INJECTION. Medroxyprogesterone acetate (Depo-Provera) is given in 150 mg. doses every 3 months. This method of contraception has a pregnancy rate comparable to the rate for oral contraceptives. The principal side effects are irregular bleeding and amenorrhea, with the same contraindications as combined orals, although it is not known whether there is an increased thromboembolic risk with progestins alone. Because there is the possibility of delayed fertility for as long as 3 years after stopping injections, this method is not recommended for women who want further pregnancies.

SILASTIC IMPLANTS AND DEVICES. Subdermal Silastic capsules containing progestins which provide reversible long-term contraception are being tested. Also there is a Silastic device which is designed to be placed in the endocervical canal and a Silastic vaginal pessary, or ring, placed in the vaginal vault each month postmenses and left in place for 21 days. The

Silicone rubber, impregnated with progestins, provides a continuous release of hormone at a constant rate for up to 3 to 5 years. Effectiveness is dose-related and lower than for combination pills, and the major side effects are irregular bleeding and amenorrhea.

ONCE-A-MONTH PILL. A combined oral contraceptive using quinestrol, a long-acting estrogen stored in body fat and gradually released, and quingestanol acetate, a potent progestin, is taken every 4 weeks regardless of bleeding pattern. The pregnancy rate is reported at 2 to 4 per 100 woman years, with side effects and contraindications similar to conventional combined orals. Withdrawal bleeding usually occurs 6 to 14 days after taking the drug, with nausea in 20 percent and amenorrhea in 5 percent of the cycles.

MORNING-AFTER PILL. Postcoital contraception, or interception, can be accomplished by large doses of estrogen given within 72 hours of unprotected intercourse at midcycle. Accelerated tubal transport and endometrial changes are the mechanisms of action, and nausea and vomiting are the principal side effects. To be effective, the dosage must be high (50 mg. diethylstilbestrol, 3 to 5 mg. ethinyl estradiol, or 25 mg. conjugated estrogen daily for 5 to 6 days), treatment must be started within 72 hours of intercourse, and treatment must continue for 5 to 6 days. If the treatment is adequate, the failure rate is 0.4 pregnancies per 100 woman years. Contraindications include those related to higher estrogen in oral contraceptives, and the possibility of thromboembolic complications does exist. Diethylstilbestrol (DES) can cause vaginal tumors in the daughters of women taking the drug during early pregnancy, and has possible teratogenic effects on the fetus. Thus, abortion is recommended if DES treatment fails. This method of postcoital contraception is quite effective as an emergency measure but should not be used regularly or frequently.

Intrauterine Devices (IUD)

These are small devices made of inert plastic which are placed into the uterus, exerting their contraceptive effect through local action. Usually they are impregnated with radiopaque barium for localization, and newer types also have copper or progesterone added. Many different types of IUDs have been developed and then discontinued due to complications, and new ones tried. The major advantage of the IUD is that once it is in place, its contraceptive effect continues without further effort, motivation, or equipment. The woman does not need to be involved, although checking the IUD string to be sure the device is in place is recommended. For some women, who have trouble remembering to use a method or who find it difficult to follow necessary procedures, the IUD is an excellent choice. The local action of the IUD is appealing to some who consider it safer than the pill because of its lack of systemic effects. The theoretical effectiveness of IUDs is 1 to 3 pregnancies per 100 woman years, while the actual effectiveness is in the range of 5 to 10 pregnancies. About 80 percent of the women with IUDs continue the method after 1 year, the main reasons for discontinuation being expulsions and complications (Table 3-9). Disadvantages of this method of contraception include the necessity for skilled professional insertion of the device, the discomfort associated with insertion, the possibility of expulsions or conception with the IUD in place, an increased menstrual flow and cramping, and the danger of infection. Although mortality is low (1.5 per 100,000 users per year) death occurs in rare instances, usually due to severe pelvic infection. The newer copper and progesterone devices need to be replaced every 1 to 2 years.

MECHANISMS OF ACTION. The precise mechanisms of action of the IUD are not known, but an inflammatory and immune reaction seems to be involved. A local inflammatory effect on the endometrium has been postulated, with the attraction of macrophages to the surface of the IUD. This may cause phagocytosis of spermatozoa or lysis of the blastocyst. The endometrium may also be rendered unfavorable for implantation, or there may be mechanical dislodging after implantation. These possible mechanisms are of significance to couples opposed to abortion. Increased immunoglobulin G and M levels in women with IUDs support the thesis of an immunologic antifertility mechanism.[25]

The addition of copper to the IUD improves its effectiveness, as copper interferes with the migration of sperm and with implantation, probably by disrupting enzymes. Copper may

Table 3-9
IUD Effectiveness and Acceptance per 100 Users During the First Year

	Lippes Loop D	Saf-T-Coil	Copper T	Copper 7		Progesterone T	
				Parous	Nulliparous	Parous	Nulliparous
Pregnancy	1.7	2.8	1.8	0.97	0.99	1.9	2.5
Expulsion	5.1	11.9	5.6	4.77	6.44	3.1	7.5
Medical removal	10.1	8.0	7.3	7.37	10.67	12.3	16.4
Continuation rate	80.1	80.0	83.2	83.5	77.5	79.1	70.9

Romney, et al, *Gynecology and Obstetrics*, Table 32-9, p. 566. Package inserts for Copper 7 provided by Searle and for Progesterone T by Alza Corp.

inhibit carbonic anhydrase and alkaline phosphatase activity, and it may interfere with estrogen uptake by the uterine mucosa or with cellular uptake of DNA in the endometrium. Very small amounts of the copper are absorbed systemically, but most of it is lost vaginally in cervical mucus and menstrual discharge. The IUD does not interfere with ovulation and the normal female cyclicity of gonadotrophic hormones.

SIDE EFFECTS AND COMPLICATIONS. Increased menstrual bleeding, dysmenorrhea, and intermenstrual spotting are the most common side effects of IUDs. These problems are more common the first 1 to 3 months after insertion, although increased flow may persist. Up to 20 percent of women using IUDs will require IUD removal because of these symptoms. Increased blood loss may lead to anemia, and some practitioners routinely provide iron supplements. Expulsion rates vary according to the device used and the skill of the health provider, but generally they are about 6 to 20 percent. Most expulsions occur shortly after insertion or during a menstrual period. Partial expulsions may be felt by the woman, associated with cramping, dyspareunia, or by feeling the plastic tip of the device at the cervical os. In these cases, the device must be removed.

Uterine perforation is a potentially serious complication and is usually due to practitioner error. Carefully determining the position of the uterus and using a gentle technique during IUD insertion can prevent most perforations. Less frequently, the IUD can migrate through the uterine wall or fallopian tubes after insertion. Perforation should be suspected when the IUD string has disappeared and the woman has not noticed expulsion. The uterus can be sounded to detect the presence of the IUD, or

an x-ray examination can be done. Open devices usually do not cause intestinal obstruction, but they can create local inflammation and abscess formation in the abdominal cavity. They should be removed, usually by laparoscopy, but occasionally laparotomy is necessary.

Infection is the leading danger of IUDs and the major cause of the mortality associated with their use. There is evidence that all endometrial cavities are contaminated by IUD insertion, even with a sterile technique, but the uterus actively combats organisms introduced into it and is sterile within 1 month. Pelvic infections occurring shortly after insertion are probably due to the IUD; those occurring later are more likely to be coincidental. The incidence of gonorrheal pelvic inflammatory disease is thought to be the same in women with IUDs as in the population at large, but occasionally the presence of an IUD can lead to a fulminating gonorrheal infection. Many other severe pelvic infections are due to other organisms, with a typical progression from foul-smelling leukorrhea, metrorrhagia, and menorrhagia to frank endometritis and then pelvic peritonitis. There is an increased incidence of endometritis with time in symptomatic women with IUDs in place, and some chronic endometritis associated with IUDs.[26] In most cases removal of the IUD is indicated if infection develops.

Pregnancy occurring with an IUD in place also presents the danger of serious infection and septic abortion. The Dalkon shield was removed from the market because it was associated with several deaths due to septic abortions in the second trimester. Its polyfilamented string had a wicklike effect, providing access for bacteria to the uterine cavity. If the woman wants the pregnancy terminated, the IUD can be removed either before or during the abortion procedure. If she wants to continue the pregnancy, the IUD should be removed because of the danger of infection. There is a 25 to 30 percent chance of spontaneous abortion following the removal of an IUD. Problems of infection and sepsis if pregnancy occurs can happen with any type of IUD, and women should be informed of this potentially serious risk.

APPROACH TO MANAGEMENT. Gynecological history and pelvic findings are important in determining suitability of an IUD for the individual. A woman with very heavy menses and significant cramping or with uterine abnormalities, marked anteflexion or retroflexion, or a uterine cavity that sounds to less than 6 cm. is not a good candidate. Contraindications to IUD insertion include

Absolute

Active pelvic infection
Recent or chronic PID
Postpartum endometritis
Septic abortion
Pregnancy
Endometrial hyperplasia or carcinoma
Abnormalities of the uterine cavity (bicornate
    uterus, myomata, polyps, and so on)

Relative

Acute cervicitis
History of ectopic pregnancy
Valvular heart disease
Cervical stenosis
Endemetriosis
Dysmenorrhea
Abnormal uterine bleeding
Anemia
Small uterus (less than 6 cm.)
Marked anteflexion or retroflexion

Types of IUDs. In choosing an IUD, the most important factor is the practitioner's familiarity with and competence in inserting the particular type. Other factors to consider are the size and shape of the device and the parity of the patient. The Lippes loop comes in four sizes (A to D), is easy to insert and remove, and has stood the test of time. The Saf-T-Coil is a modification of this device, inserted much like the loop, which comes in two sizes, the small one designed for the nulliparous woman. The Copper 7 is small, has the smallest diameter inserter, and has been found to be well tolerated by nulliparas. It has a thin copper wire coiled around its vertical limb which releases a constant amount of copper. While most of the copper is still present after 2 to 3 years in place, there is a question of its availability for contraceptive action after 2 years. A layer of calcium has been found on the surface of copper 7 IUDs which have been in place for 18 to 36 months. Also, an increased pregnancy rate occurs among women during the third year of continuation with the same device.[27] The FDA has approved the Copper 7 for 3 years of continuous use. The Copper T is similar but slightly larger. The Progesterone T (Progestasert) has a reservoir of progesterone in its vertical stem which is released continuously for 1 year, after which it must be replaced. Each type of IUD is packaged with its own inserter and instructions. While the smaller devices are more easily inserted, they also are more readily expelled. Most devices are acceptable for a uterine depth of 6 to 9 cm.; if above 10 cm., another method of contraception should be considered. The Copper 7 and Copper T are reported to cause fewer cramping and heavy menstrual flow problems.

Insertion technique. Insertion differs slightly, depending upon type of IUD and inserter, but instructions generally include the following:

1. Explain the insertion technique in advance and during the procedure to help the woman to relax and understand what is happening.
2. Do a careful speculum and bimanual examination to rule out pregnancy, pelvic infection, and uterine abnormalities, and determine size and position of uterus. Obtain Pap smear and gonorrhea culture, other vaginal smears as indicated.
3. Under sterile technique (for which a second sterile speculum may be used), cleanse the cervix three to four times with antiseptic solution. Grasp the anterior lip of the cervix (some grasp the posterior lip with retroflexion) with a tenaculum 1 to 2 cm. from the os. This usually causes pain or cramping of varying severity. Bend the uterine sound to approximate the angle of curvature of the uterus as determined by bimanual examination. Use gentle traction on the cervix with the tenaculum and insert the uterine sound gradually, steadily and gently through the os. There is often a slight resistance as the sound enters the os, then it slips through without much force needed. If the sound

cannot pass through the cervix, check the position of the tenaculum which may have been closed in such a way as to occlude the endocervical canal. Reposition it if necessary. Do not force the sound, seek consultation for possible dilatation if it does not pass readily through the cervix. Pass the sound into the uterus slowly and gently until resistance is felt, when the end of the sound bumps against the upper fundus. Place a Q-tip at the cervix parallel to the sound, and remove both together (this permits more accurate measurement of depth of fundus).

4. Load the IUD into the inserter barrel, keeping in mind that these devices cannot remain inside the inserter for more than 1 to 2 minutes or the plastic will lose its "memory" and the device will not straighten out or coil into proper shape within the uterus. Follow directions for individual types of inserters for loading.

5. There are two basic techniques of insertion: a) In the push-in method the preset cervical stop on the inserter is left in place and sounding is used to be sure the uterine cavity is large enough (6 cm. or more). Using gentle traction with the tenaculum, and bending the IUD inserter to approximate the uterine angle if this is appropriate, introduce the loaded inserter through the cervix as with the sound until the cervical stop touches the cervix. Be certain that the IUD will be positioned in the proper anteroposterior plane of the uterus. Push the plunger steadily and gently to deposit the IUD in the uterine cavity. Withdraw the inserter, gently pull down the string until resistance is felt, then clip the string leaving 2 inches from the os. (Figure 3-8) b) In the inserter withdrawal method the cervical stop is moved and set at the depth to which the uterus was sounded. Use traction with the tenaculum. Bend the inserter if this is appropriate, and introduce the loaded inserter through the os as during sounding. When the cervical stop reaches the cervix, the end of the inserter should be touching the top of the fundus. Holding the plunger steady, back the inserter downward to deposit the IUD. Withdraw the inserter and clip the string 2 inches from the os (Figure 3-8).

6. Swab the cervix to remove blood, check to be sure that the IUD tip cannot be seen at the cervical os. If it is protruding, remove the IUD and proceed with a new one.

Many practitioners prefer to insert IUDs during or shortly after menses because the cervix is slightly softer and dilated at that time. It also minimizes the risk of pregnancy at the time of insertion, and the slight bleeding caused by insertion will not be noticed. However, it is not essential that IUDs be inserted during menses, particularly the smaller types. Pain and faintness immediately after insertion are not uncommon and usually disappear in a few minutes. Allow the woman to remain flat on the examining table until she feels steady. Occasionally a paracervical block may be necessary to provide local anesthesia. If cramping persists, pain medication for a few days may be given. Rarely, a vagal reaction may cause bradycardia.

Patient education. The following information and instructions should accompany IUD insertion:

1. Spotting and cramping following insertion are normal and will gradually diminish. Irregular spotting may occur for the first 2 to 3 months. Menstrual periods will usually be heavier and longer.
2. The IUD string should be checked to be sure that the IUD is in place. Expulsion is most likely just after insertion and during menses. Feel the string frequently during the first several months, then after each period. If you cannot feel the string, come in to be examined.
3. Use another method of birth control the first 2 months for better protection against pregnancy. Keep another method in reserve in case of the expulsion of the IUD.
4. The Copper 7 and Copper T must be replaced in 2 or 3 years, and the Progesterone T in one year. Other IUDs may stay in place longer if you have no problems.
5. If you develop a fever, pelvic pain and cramping, and unusual bleeding you should be checked right away. These may be signs of infection which can be life-threatening, and treatment should be started at once.
6. If you miss a period or suspect pregnancy, you should be checked. If pregnant, the IUD must be removed because of the danger of infection. Options for abortion or continuing pregnancy will be discussed.
7. Your IUD should be checked at least yearly, and you should have a Pap smear and breast examination yearly.

Follow-up and IUD removal. A recheck in 3 months is a good idea if visits are not a hardship for the woman. Yearly examinations are necessary for Pap smear and breast examination and a gonorrhea culture is recommended.

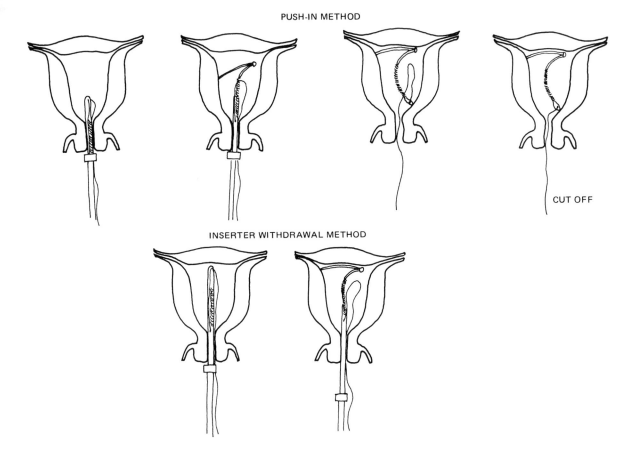

Figure 3-8. Techniques of IUD insertion.

Women with IUDs bleed heavily, so hematocrit is indicated to rule out anemia. Removal of an IUD is usually easier and less painful than insertion, and it is facilitated during menses. The technique for removal is the following:

1. Grasp the string with a sponge forceps close to the cervical os. Apply gentle, steady traction and remove the IUD slowly. There is usually some initial resistance, then the IUD comes out readily.
2. If the IUD does not come out easily, sound the uterus, for this might dilate the internal cervical os. Leave the sound in for 30 seconds and then rotate it 90 degrees slowly. Apply gentle traction again on the string, and the IUD should come out. If it still resists, or if the strings break off, dilatation is necessary with the use of a hook or narrow forceps. A paracervical block may be required, in which case consultation should be sought.

Sterilization

Permanent methods of contraception are be-coming increasingly popular in the United States and are presently the most commonly used method of fertility control among married couples over 30 years of age. [28] There are now about 7 million sterilized adults; approximately 14 percent of these are women and 11 percent are men. Admittedly low estimates report that 25 percent of all white married couples and 47 percent of couples married 10 to 24 years have been sterilized.[29] (Figure 3-9). Sterilization is used not only by men and women who have completed their families, but with growing frequency by couples who desire no children or by single persons. There are no laws or formulas which dictate who may have a sterilization, and its availability depends upon community attitudes, medical standards, and the skill of the individual physician. At the same time that the popularity of sterilization is increasing, so are requests for reversals. The success of reversing the procedure with sub-

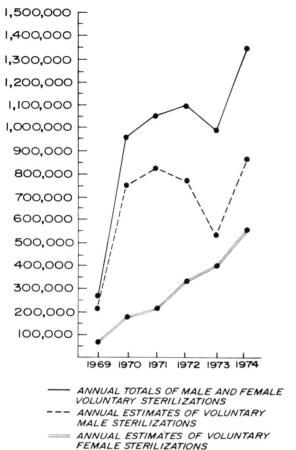

1,500,000
1,400,000
1,300,000
1,200,000
1,100,000
1,000,000
900,000
800,000
700,000
600,000
500,000
400,000
300,000
200,000
100,000

1969 1970 1971 1972 1973 1974

—— ANNUAL TOTALS OF MALE AND FEMALE
      VOLUNTARY STERILIZATIONS
--- ANNUAL ESTIMATES OF VOLUNTARY
      MALE STERILIZATIONS
=== ANNUAL ESTIMATES OF VOLUNTARY
      FEMALE STERILIZATIONS

Figure 3-9. Sterilization of men and women between 1969 and 1974. Hatcher, et al., *Contraceptive Technology 1976-1977*, p. 94.

sequent pregnancy is low, and although reversible techniques are under investigation, presently sterilization must be considered permanent.

COUNSELING FOR STERILIZATION. The maturity, understanding, motivation, and adjustment of couples and individuals seeking sterilization are most important in their later satisfaction with this method. Common concerns involve the pain associated with the procedure, the effects of sterilization on physiology, complications, and repercussions on sexual performance. These problems will be discussed individually under male and female sterilization procedures. Counseling deals with these concerns and provides accurate information, as well as allowing couples to explore their feelings about ending reproductive func-

tioning. Ideally, both partners should agree about sterilization. If there is conflict, sterilization may be performed on the partner so desiring, but this must be an individual decision. Young men and women in their early 20s may seek permanent contraception, and the soundness of this decision should be explored in counseling. If motives are healthy and the individuals well adjusted, sterilization for either man or woman will not adversely affect sexual functioning, physiology, or self-concept.[30]

FEMALE STERILIZATION. There are many abdominal and vaginal procedures available, including postpartal laparotomy with various techniques to transect or interrupt the fallopian tube, interval laparoscopy with tubal coagulation and/or transsection, and culpotomy or culdoscopy using the vaginal approach. Failure rates are very low, .01 to .4 percent, but there are complications associated with the procedure and with anesthesia. Hospitalization is usually required for 1 to 3 days, and immediate access to facilities for major abdominal surgery is essential.

The postpartal laparotomy is done 1 to 3 days after delivery, under general anesthesia, and usually with a small subumbilical incision. The tubes are isolated and may be crushed, ligated, imbedded in surrounding tissue after resection, or clipped or plugged in the newer potentially reversible techniques. The interval mini-laparotomy uses a suprapubic incision with similar techniques for interrupting tubal patency, also requiring about 2 days of hospitalization. Laparoscopic sterilization may be done at any time, and although general anesthesia is usually given, a local is possible in carefully selected cases. A one-incision (in umbilicus) or two-incision (umbilicus and at pubic hairline) approach can be used; incisions are about 1 inch long. The abdomen is distended with carbon dioxide, the laparoscope introduced through its trocar via the umbilical incision, and the fallopian tube visualized. A grasping instrument is introduced either through the same laparoscope or through the second incision, the isthmic portion of the tube grasped, and the tube is coagulated with electric current and may be transsected. This is repeated on the other side, through the same incision(s).

The incidence of complications is low, but the complications can be serious when they occur. Complications include coagulation burns on the bowels, bowel perforations, infection, hemorrhage, and adverse anesthesia effects. The procedures are relatively expensive, require a skilled operator, and emergency back-up facilities. Most women who undergo sterilization are satisfied with the results, but a small number, probably in the range of 10 to 15 percent, regret termination of fertility or are dissatisfied for numerous reasons. Some women find their sexual interest or sense of worth adversely affected when the possibility of pregnancy is removed; others attribute certain gynecological problems such as dysmenorrhea, menorrhagia, premenstrual syndrome, and irregularity to the procedure. Theoretically, tubal interruption should have no effect on hormonal cycles and menstrual patterns. However, it is possible that interference with vascular and lymphatic drainage in the pelvic region, particularly with coagulation, could produce increased pelvic congestion premenstrually, with pain and cramping with the onset of menses. The possibility of hysterectomy some years later due to severe dysmenorrhea cannot be ruled out, and probably does occur in a small number of cases. Salpingoplasty, the surgical reconstruction of the fallopian tubes, results in an overall pregnancy rate of 15 percent; about three-fourths of these result in live births, and 10 percent are tubal pregnancies.

MALE STERILIZATION. Vasectomy, the interruption of sperm transport by severing the vas deferens, is the single most popular method of permanent contraception and one of the three male-oriented techniques available. The procedure is simple, has no mortality rate and a low rate of complications, is relatively inexpensive, can be done under local anesthesia, and does not require hospitalization or absence from work. In an outpatient minor surgery room, a 2 to 3 cm. incision is made over the vas deferens on each side of the scrotum, under local anesthesia. The vas is isolated, occluded by severence with ligation of the ends, coagulation of the lumen, burying the cut ends, or by using clips, silicone plugs or polyethylene tubing with a stopcock for potentially reversible procedures. Absorbable sutures are used to close the skin, and after a brief recovery period, the patient is instructed to apply ice should pain or swelling occur, use a scrotal support for

about 1 week, and then he is able to walk out and go home. It generally takes 4 to 6 weeks to clear sperm from the vas beyond the point of occlusion and the prostate, depending upon sexual activity. Six to 36 ejaculations are often required, so the couple is advised to use another method of birth control and to bring in sperm samples 2 to 3 times for a sperm count. There must be at least two consecutive sperm-free samples before the man may be considered sterile. Rechecks at 6 and 12 months are recommended to be sure that fertility has not been restored by recanalization.

Complications include bleeding and hematoma, infection, sperm granulomas, recanalization, immune responses, and psychological factors. There are no known harmful physiological effects, and hormone production and testicular function are not affected. The vas proximal to the ligation becomes dilated with sperm and macrophages. Occasionally the absorption of antigens from the sperm results in the development of antibodies against sperm, a factor which could reduce fertility if later there were a successful reconstruction of the vas. Psychological factors prevent many men from accepting vasectomy, for they fear reduction of potency or masculinity. After the procedure, most men have intercourse or masturbate during the first 1 to 2 weeks; and there is a trend toward increased sexual activity during the first year postvasectomy. This might indicate some increased need to prove or reinforce sexuality, or it might simply reflect a new-found freedom from the fear of paternity. The great majority of men are satisfied with vasectomy, encourage their friends to consider it when no more children are desired, and find their sexual performance much the same as before. They note that erection, ejaculation, the amount and consistency of seminal fluid, and sexual interest remain unchanged. About 1.5 percent experience decreased sexual pleasure or are dissatisfied with vasectomy.

Vasovasostomy, reanastomosis of the vas deferens, is usually anatomically successful with about 40 to 90 percent of men having sperm present in postoperative ejaculates. The incidence of paternity after reanastomosis is much lower, however, being reported between 5 to 30 percent. The interference with the transport of sperm along the vas, as well as antibody production, probably account for this difference.

The search for reversible methods continues, focusing on removable plastic devices or clips. Alternate methods of occlusion of the tubes or vas are also being explored to produce permanent sterility, such as silver nitrate, quinacrine, silicone polymers, and surgical adhesives. There is some current research into hormonal methods for men, including suppression of sperm production and interference with seminal fluid biochemistry, but numerous problems involving side effects, long-term effects, and reversibility must be solved before these methods will be available.

NOTES

1. W. A. Darity and C. B. Turner, "Attitudes toward Family Planning: A Comparison between Northern and Southern Black Americans." *Advances in Planned Parenthood* 8 (1973):13.
2. C. F. Westoff and L. Bumpass, "The Revolution in Birth Control Practice of U.S. Roman Catholics." *Science* 179. (January 5, 1973):41-44.
3. Adapted from HEW guidelines for informal consent to voluntary sterilization, included in R. A. Hatcher, et al., *Contraceptive Technology 1976-1977*, ed. 8 (New York: Halsted Press, Division of John Wiley & Sons, 1976), pp. 131-132.
4. J. F. Kantner and M. Zelnik, "Sexual Experience of Young Unmarried Women in the United States." *Family Planning Perspectives* 4,4 (October 1972): 9.
5. S. L. Romney, et al., *Gynecology and Obstetrics: The Health Care of Women* (New York: McGraw-Hill, Blakiston, 1975), p. 573.
6. *Oral Contraceptives and Health: Report of the Royal College of General Practitioners* (London: Pitman Medical, 1974).
7. Hatcher, et al., *Contraceptive Technology 1976-1977*, p. 57.
8. *Ibid.* p.41.
9. B. Seaman, *The Doctors' Case Against the Pill* (New York: Peter H. Wyden, 1969), p. 24.
10. M. Stern, et al., "Cardiovascular Risk and Use of Estrogens or Estrogen-Progestogen Combinations." *JAMA* 234, 8 (February 23, 1976): 811-15.
11. S. Ramcharan, F. A. Pellegrin, and E. Hoag, "The Occurrence and Course of Hypertensive Disease in Users and Nonusers of Oral Contraceptive Drugs." In *Oral Contraceptives and High Blood Pressure*, M. H. Fregly and M. S. Fregly, eds. (Gainsville, Fla.: The Dolphin Press, 1974), pp. 1-16.
12. R. E. Kleiger, et al., "Pulmonary Hypertension in Patients Using Oral Contraceptives." *Chest* 69, 2 (February 1976): 143-47.
13. I. R. Fisch and S. H. Freedman, "Oral Contraceptives, ABO Blood Groups, and In Vitro Fibrin Formation." *Obstetrics and Gynecology* 46, 4 (October 1975): 473-79.
14. Romney, et al., *Gynecology and Obstetrics*, p. 562.
15. H. Jick, et al., "Venous Thromboembolic Disease and ABO Blood Type: A Cooperative Study." *The Lancet* (March 8, 1969): 539-42.
16. *Oral Contraceptives and Health: An Interim Report for the Oral Contraceptive Study of the Royal College of General Practitioners* (New York: Pittman Publishing, 1975).
17. "Digest: Cigarettes Plus Pill: Deadly for Women 30 and Over." *Family Planning Perspectives* 9, 1 (January/February 1977): 36.
18. M.R. Melamed, et al., "Prevalence Rates of Uterine Cervical Carcinoma-in-situ for Women Using the Diaphragm or Oral Contraceptive Steroids." *British Medical Journal* 3 (1969): 195.
19. E. R. Novak and J. D. Woodruff, *Gynecologic and Obstetric Pathology* (Philadelphia: W.B. Saunders, 1974).
20. H. W. Kelley, et al., "Adenocarcinoma of the Endometrium in Women Taking Sequential Oral Contraceptives." *Obstetrics and Gynecology* 47, 2 (February 1976): 200-02.
21. H. Ory, et al., "Oral Contraceptives and Reduced Risk of Benign Breast Diseases. *New England Journal of Medicine* 294, 8 (February 19, 1976): 419-22.
22. H. A. Edmondson, B. Henderson, and B. Benton, "Liver-Cell Adenomas Associated with Use of Oral Contraceptives." *New England Journal of Medicine* 294, 9 (February 26, 1976): 470-72.
23. E.B. Connell, "Contraception." *Primary Care* 2,3 (September 1975): 513-39.
24. D. H. Carr, "Chromosome Studies in Selected Spontaneous Abortions. I. Conception after Oral Contraception." *Canadian Medical Association Journal* 103 (1970): 343.
25. D. W. Gump, et al., "Intrauterine Contraceptive Device and Increased Serum Immunoglobulin Levels." *Obstetrics and Gynecology* 41,2 (February 1973): 259-64.
26. Romney, *Gynecology and Obstetrics*, p. 569.
27. J. Newton, at al., "Continuous Intrauterine Copper Contraception for 3 Years: Comparison of Replacement at 2 Years with Continuation of Use." *British Medical Journal* 1 (1977): 197-199.
28. H. S. Presser and L. L. Bumpass, "The Acceptability of Contraceptive Sterilization Among U.S. Couples: 1970." *Family Planning Perspectives* 4, 4 (1972): 18.
29 C. F. Westoff and E. F. Jones, "Contraception and Sterilization in the United States, 1965-1975." *Family Planning Perspectives* 9, 4 (July/August 1977): 153-157.
30. L. Lader, *Foolproof Birth Control: Male and Female Sterilization* (Boston: Beacon Press, 1972), pp. 101-29, 142-83.

4

Menstrual Problems

Bleeding problems constitute the largest group of gynecological difficulties seen in practice. Most women will experience some type of unusual uterine bleeding during their 30 to 35 years of menstruating, and many will seek the aid of a health professional to resolve the problem. Absence of menses (amenorrhea) and painful menses (dysmenorrhea) are also common problems which motivate women to seek health care. While pathology may be the basis of a number of such problems, physiological variations are often an underlying cause for the common functional menstrual problems, and emotional factors play a major role in altering menstrual functioning.

MEANINGS OF MENSTRUATION

Menstruation and childbearing are the only two somatic processes which are exclusive to the female; all of her other body processes are shared in common with the male. These two physiological phenomena have been invested with enormous social significance and thus have a marked psychological overlay which cannot be readily separated from somatic functions. Rites of passage have been associated with menarche in many cultures and used to signify the transition from the status of child to that of adult (reproductive) member of society and the assumption of whatever was deemed the proper role of women. Unfortunately, menarche often had negative associations, related primarily to the low status of woman and the myths of danger surrounding her menstrual functions. Men have been horrified and mystified by menstruation, and

primitive cultures have viewed it as a source of dark power for women and a threat to men. Taboos surrounded menstruating women—they were not to be touched by men and were often physically isolated in separate menstrual huts. Following cessation of menses, cleansing rituals were often performed before women were allowed back into society. The bases of menstrual myths and taboos are thought to lie in three general areas: 1) Men's castration fears were aroused as genital bleeding would symbolize the loss of the male's external and vulnerable genitals. If women were conceptualized as inferior because they had somehow been punished by deprivation of external (male) genitals, their monthly bleeding would be a regular and threatening reminder of that danger. 2) Menses allowed the displacement of a deep-seated guilt associated with the male's aggressive impulses. Some mythologies hold that the man's guilt over the murder of a powerful opponent (the primal father, a relative, or a god), is assuaged by visiting upon his most prized possession (the beautiful woman) a monthly curse of suffering, during which she is inaccessible to him. 3) Menses were used as a guard against incest and its resultant social chaos. Women were thought to have heightened sexuality during menses and to need strict controls to curb their incestuous desires. Also part of menstrual taboos is man's projection of his hatred and fear of the powerful father upon the woman.[1]

Negative Associations

Whatever the primal origins of menstrual taboos, their practical effects have created in

91

women negative feelings about their cyclical physiology and limited their power within the social order. If this frequent and repetitive experience is viewed with disgust, repulsion, and rejection, all of its manifestations become prime targets for psychosomatic complaints. If the status of women is low and the female role is sharply restricted in its possibilities for expression, obvious manifestations of femininity, such as cyclic bleeding, are greeted with remorse, depression, or anger. Menstruation in Western culture is just coming out of a stage of secrecy during which women avoided talking about it among themselves and shielded all evidence of it from external view. Euphemisms for menstruation are a form of avoidance which give ample evidence of its negative connotations: "the curse," being "unwell," "riding the rag," "having a period, "a visit from a friend," "falling off the roof," "having the monthlies," or "flying the flag."

Although attitudes are changing as women gain a sense of self-awareness and increased worth, many women still look upon menstruation with distaste. For many it is associated with pain and premenstrual discomfort; the bleeding is thought of as messy and a nuisance, the odors are perceived as unpleasant, or women may even consider themselves unclean or indecent. The practice of avoiding sex during the menses is still widespread, although most people realize that nothing terrible (such as male loss of potency) will happen. The cosmetics industry capitalizes on these attitudes with such products as feminine hygiene sprays and deodorized tampons. Their message is that all signs of menses can be successfully hidden.

Positive Associations

A growing number of women are thinking of menses positively. As one of the two solely female somatic functions, menses are viewed as an affirmation of femininity and a symbol of femaleness. There is a pleasure in the regular normal body function which attests to the physical health and reliability of the body. Even in a time of widely used contraceptives with high rates of effectiveness, menses is a reassuring sign when the avoidance of pregnancy is desired. Some women tune in to the rhythms of their psychobiology, aware of subtle changes in mood and altered sensitivities. It is seen as an adventure in inner awareness.

Menarche is anticipated with excitement by many girls, for it symbolizes profound changes in self-concept and relations with other people. Girls watch for signs of pubertal development in themselves and their friends, regarding those who begin menses earliest with envy. They seek information about menses and pregnancy from any available source and talk avidly among themselves about womanly functions. Each sign of puberty is greeted as attestment to normal growth, and pride is taken in external bodily changes. The onset of the first menses no doubt causes mixed feelings; there is happiness that the girl has arrived at womanhood, is sexually normal, and is moving toward adult status, but also misgivings about her new responsibilities, changing relations with boys and adults, possible restrictions on activities, and her ambiguous identity as a woman in a changing society.

The implications of the female cyclic hormone pattern are enormous. For fully half of her life, the woman's physical and psychological condition will be influenced by the waxing and waning of estrogen and progesterone. This closeness to physiology, this periodic reminder of essential sexuality, this regular feedback of normality or difficulties in body function are not part of the life experience of men. All of these set women apart, in ways that have previously been filled with negative associations largely related to their status and power within society but which now are embraced as testimony to the human's closeness to the natural world, as signs of strength, harmony and, integration.

Effects of Attitudes and Knowledge

How a woman feels about her major physiological difference, menstrual cyclicity, depends on a complex interaction of internalized values, perceptions of societal and important people's attitudes, the extent of her knowledge and understanding of somatic processes, and the actual physiology of her body. Negative attitudes predispose the woman to experience her menstrual cycles in an unpleasant way. Minor discomforts may be magnified and inconveniences resented. The menses can become a focus for a myriad of psychosomatic complaints: headache, backache, cramps, bloating, irritability, weight gain. All of these may be very real physical symptoms which occur premenstrually and during menstrual flow, but the attitudes of the woman determine whether or not she regards them as incapacitating and abnormal. An example of this power of the psyche over the soma is the difference between perceptions of the minor discomforts of pregnancy and those of menstruation. Pregnancy is surrounded by positive societal values and provides many rewards for the woman; thus, she may tolerate physical discomforts with little complaint or even perceive some, such as the baby's kicking, as pleasurable. Menses, however, with its long history of negative associations is devalued and, thus, its sensations are more likely to be perceived as painful. The woman often seeks removal of these sensations, which in another context might be gladly tolerated or even thought pleasurable.

Women have used menses manipulatively as an excuse for a variety of purposes, ranging from not doing schoolwork to avoiding sex or social obligations. Menstrual discomfort is a readily accepted excuse in most segments of society. It is a leading cause for absence from work or school among women in the menstrual years. This is not to say that menstrual discomfort is purely imaginary, for the symptoms are real and physiologically based. However, psychic processes strongly influence how these symptoms are perceived and responded to and in what form they are expressed behaviorally.

This secondary gain from menstrual discomfort is detrimental to the woman intrapsychically and interpersonally. Such negative feedback cannot but diminish her self-concept and sense of worth as a woman (even her most feminine bodily function is a source of suffering), as do disparaging responses by those involved in her life, although they participate in the social ritual of pseudo-acceptance (how could a woman assume a position of great authority, such as president of the United States, when she is at the mercy of body functions which incapacitate her several days out of the month?).

THE HEALTH PROVIDER'S EDUCATIONAL ROLE

Changing attitudes toward menstruation are gradually being brought about through a variety of influences. Not the least of these is the women's movement which reinforces the value of being female and encourages women to aspire to the full development of their own personalities and personal interests. Feminist and humanist values are infiltrating medical and nursing education, contributing to health providers who view menses in a positive light and who communicate this to their patients. The growing ability of women to gain status and power in society without denying their femininity is a potent force in shaping young women's feelings about female physiology.

Health providers can assist this process by filling in educational gaps for their patients. Counseling premenstrual girls in normal anatomy and physiology, helping them and their parents to understand developing sexuality, dispelling myths and misinformation by providing the correct facts, and conveying an attitude of positive acceptance are all ways to achieve this goal. When dealing with menstrual problems, explaining the mechanisms involved (prevention of menstrual problems, if any, and rationales for management) help the patient to view menstruation in a reasonable context devoid of mysticism.

Primarily, the health provider can convey a respect for female body functions. Helping a woman to understand her body and view its process positively is a major contribution to the woman and to society as a whole.

MENSTRUAL PHYSIOLOGY

The structures involved in cyclic menstrual functions are the uterus and cervix, the vagina, fallopian tubes, ovaries, and the pituitary and hypothalamus glands (Figure 4-1). Estrogen is the major hormone active in female development, and a finely tuned periodicity of estrogen and progesterone secretion regulates the menstrual cycle. The uterus is a pear-shaped, hollow, muscular organ with two sections—the corpus and the cervix. The sizes of these sections change at different times in life, with the cervix relatively larger during infancy, childhood, and postmenopause (Figure 4-2). The nulliparous uterus is about 7 to 9 cm. in length, 6 to 7 cm. in width, and the anteroposterior diameter is 4 cm. After childbirth, the uterus becomes larger, and there is a considerable variation among women in uterine size. The myometrium is composed of involuntary muscle, connective tissue, blood vessels, lymphatics, and nerves derived from the sympathetic nervous system. The endometrium is the mucous

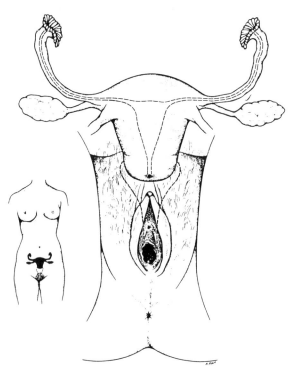

Figure 4-1. Anatomy of the vagina, uterus, tubes, and ovaries.

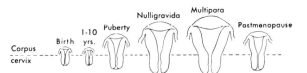

Figure 4-2. Changes in relative size of the cervix and corpus of the uterus. D. W. Beacham and W. D. Beacham, *Synopsis of Gynecology*, ed. 8 (St. Louis: Mosby, 1972), p. 14.

membrane lining the surface of the cavity of the uterus which undergoes morphologic and physiologic changes during the menstrual cycle. It is divided into two layers, the basal and superficial endometrium. The basal layer is contiguous with the myometrium and remains intact during menstruation, beginning reepithelization of its surface as bleeding ceases. The superficial layer is derived from structural elements in the basal layer—arterioles and venules growing from the basal layer under estrogen stimulus with proliferation of glands and stroma. The stroma consists of endometrial stromal cells, blood vessels, and intercellular connective tissue. The glands have columnar cells which produce glycogen and glycoproteins. There is a reticular fiber system present throughout the basilar and superficial layers.

These groups of cells create a velvety soft endometrium which is highly responsive to ovarian hormones. The endometrium is a tissue which has a greater variation in its structure and growth within a short time than any other tissue in the body. It is covered by a superficial columnar epithelium and richly sup-

plied with blood vessels, which also undergo characteristic changes during the menstrual cycle.

The cavity of the uterine corpus communicates with the peritoneum through the lumina of the fallopian tubes superiorly, and with the vagina through the cylindrically shaped cervix below. The cervix is composed of large amounts of connective tissue in proportion to muscle; thus, it is firmer and much less contractile than the uterus. There are no distinct sphincter muscles in the cervix. The endocervical canal traverses the length of the cervix, with an internal and external os, and is lined with columnar epithelium. Glands within the cervix secrete mucus which responds to ovarian hormone stimulation, with differences in viscosity and crystal formation. The outer surface of the cervix is lined with squamous epithelium similar to that of the vagina. Cyclic changes of the cervix and the vagina are discussed in more detail later (See Chapters 9 and 14).

The almond-shaped ovaries are located on either side of the uterus, near the outer end of the fallopian tubes, projecting from the posterior wall of the broad ligament. The average dimensions of the ovary are about 3.5 to 5 cm. in length, 2.5 cm. in width, and 1.5 cm. in thickness, although there is great variation among individuals, and the same woman may have two ovaries of different size. The ovary contains microscopic ova, about 400,000 at menarche, inside minute sacs called graafian follicles. These undergo characteristic cyclic changes and participate in the endocrine interactions of the menstrual cycle. Estrogens are produced by the theca interna cells of the maturing follicle, and progesterone by the mature follicle in small amounts just prior to ovulation and in larger amounts by the corpus luteum, which continues to produce estrogens.

The fallopian tubes are composed of involuntary muscle and lined with ciliated epithelium. They are about 7 to 12 cm. long and are curved to partly surround the ovary, from which the fimbriated extremity of the tube collects the ovum. Contractions of the muscle of the tube and the action of the cilia move the ova toward the uterus. The hypothalamus and pituitary glands, located at the base of the brain and connected by a stalk, share the complex function of regulating the menstrual cycle with the ovary.

Theory of Menarche

The changes associated with sexual maturation occur at a typical time for the species, and in humans maturation is triggered by a critical weight. Increasingly, more of the body composition of children is taken up by fat tissue in proportion to muscle. A girl's body composition during the adolescent growth spurt preceding puberty has a 5:1 ratio of muscle to fat, and by menarche this ratio has become 3:1. The critical weight, reflecting a body composition of 24 percent fat, is 94 to 103 pounds. This appears to serve a biological requirement by providing the female with adequate stored calories to sustain a pregnancy, even if she were to suffer malnutrition.[2] The mechanism by which critical weight provokes menarche is hypothesized to be through an alteration of hypothalamic sensitivity to circulating estrogen. The receptor for such steroids, which are located in the hypothalamus and exert endogenous control, seem to be extremely sensitive to circulating estrogen; increased estrogen causes decreased secretion of follicle-stimulating hormone (FSH) in prepubertal children. This negative feedback gradually diminishes as a higher set point for response to estrogen is established. That is, more and more circulating estrogen is needed to "turn off" the action of releasing factors.

Releasing factors then begin to flow from the hypothalamus to the pituitary, directing it to stimulate follicular growth and the ovarian production of estrogen. Secondary sex characteristics begin to develop, and gradually the ability to ovulate and the adult pattern of estrogen-progesterone secretion is attained. This all takes time, however, and the first few years after menarche tend to have frequent anovulatory cycles, as many as 55 percent. Menses may be irregular and of varying lengths and amounts. In the adolescent, the hypothalamic-pituitary-gonadal axis is easily disrupted by numerous emotional and physical factors.[3]

Interestingly, the average age of menarche has been falling by about 4 months per decade for the past 130 years. This is thought to be related to better nutrition, a trend which is consistent with the critical weight theory. The average age of menarche in the United States is between 12 and 13 years and the age of menarche seems now to be leveling off. Average ages for female prepubertal growth spurts, development of secondary sex characteristics, and menarche are presented in Table 4-1.

Endocrine Interactions in the Menstrual Cycle

The major actions of the endocrine glands central to menstrual physiology are the secretion of releasing factors by the hypothalamus, gonadotropins by the pituitary and gonadal steroids (estrogens, progestogens) by the ovaries (Figure 4-3). Gonadotropins are secreted with a pulsation every 90 minutes, whether at a low or a high level. Levels of both estrogen and progesterone are low during menses. The hypothalamus initiates the next cycle by secreting the FSH releasing factor which causes the pituitary to secrete FSH. Even as estrogen is decreasing at the end of the cycle, FSH has begun to increase and at day 1 of menses has risen to the point where it stimulates primordial follicles to begin developing. During its initial development, the follicle secretes little estrogen. Although several follicles begin to grow, by about day 6 one enlarges rapidly while the others regress. About day 6 or 7 estrogens begin to be secreted by the follicle, slowly at first, then more rapidly, by the theca interna cells.

As estrogen levels rise, there is a negative feedback to the hypothalamus which reduces the secretion of FSH releasing factor. Under estrogen influence, the endometrium undergoes proliferation, with a rapid increase in the depth and development of glandular and stromal cells, increasing from a thickness of 1 or 2 mm. to about 4 mm. There is a wide variation among women in the length of the follicular or proliferative phase of the menstrual cycle, and this phase can also vary at different times in the same woman; the normal range is from 4 to 26 days.

There is a sharp rise in estrogen just prior to ovulation that is thought to be responsible for stimulating the hypothalamus to secrete LH

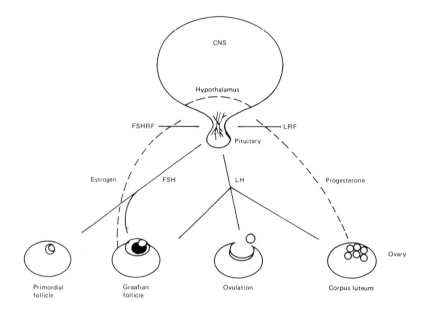

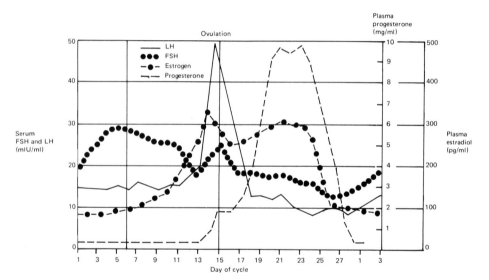

Figure 4-3. Endocrine interactions and fluctuations in hormone levels during the menstrual cycle. Prior to ovulation, estrogen—responding to the follicle-stimulating hormone (FSH)—predominates. The luteinizing hormone (LH) peaks just before ovulation, causing the progesterone level to rise rapidly. Following ovulation, progesterone predominates.

releasing factor which in turn causes the pituitary to release LH. This estrogen rise is followed by a marked LH surge and ovulation about 12 to 30 hours later. Under LH influence, the graafian follicle completes its development

and the ovum ripens. The distended follicle ruptures and the ovum is expelled into the abdominal cavity, to be picked up by the fimbriated end of the fallopian tube. A few drops of blood or follicular fluid may fall into the abdominal cavity and cause localized peritoneal irritation, producing the typical one-sided lower quadrant pain which lasts a few hours to a day and is known as *mittelschmertz.* The empty follicle fills with luteal cells which form the corpus luteum.

Following the LH peak, there is a relative drop in the estrogen for 2 to 3 days before it

Table 4-1
Growth Chart for Pubertal Changes and Menarche

Age in Years	Signs of Normal Growth
9-16	Menarche (average age 12 to 13)
9-10	Growth of the bony pelvis, budding of nipples
10-11	Spurt of growth in height, budding of breasts
11-12	Appearance of pubic hair, growth of external and internal genitals, changes in vaginal epithelium and increased leukorrhea
12-13	Pigmentation of areola, breasts filling in
13-14	Appearance of axillary hair
15-16	Acne, deepening voice
16-17	Arrest of skeletal growth

rises again. This slight withdrawal of estrogen support of the proliferative endometrium causes a light pink vaginal discharge in some women, called mittelstaining. The corpus luteum begins secretion of progesterone, which rises rapidly to high levels during the second part of the menstrual cycle. Cholesterol is the major precursor of progesterone. About 36 to 48 hours after ovulation, secretory changes begin in the endometrium under progesterone influence. Vacuoles appear in the glandular cells and increase in size, the glands increase and become tortuous, and the stroma becomes edematous. Glycogen and glycoproteins are secreted by the glands, which become tightly coiled and folded. There is an increase in leukocytes, around the small blood vessels, which also increase in size and become tortuous. The endometrium reaches a thickness of about 6 mm.

If conception and implantation do not occur, the corpus luteum begins to degenerate about 4 days before menses. High levels of progesterone after ovulation have caused a decrease in the secretion of LH releasing factor and LH, and, with degenerating corpus luteum function, the level of progesterone begins to drop. Estrogen, also secreted by the corpus luteum, falls at the same time. When estrogen and progesterone fall below a critical point, they no longer support the hypertrophied endometrium. Fibrin thrombi form in the venules, and small areas of necrosis at different places in the endometrium begin to bleed. These areas en-

large and finally become confluent. The menstrual endometrium has a histopathology resembling that of infarction, as blood vessels become distended and engorged with red blood cells, with increasing autolysis and destruction of the glands and stroma. Blood, mucus, and endometrial tissue fragments make up the menstrual discharge. Eventually most of the tissue fragments of the endometrium desquamate into the uterine cavity, leaving only the basal layer. Neoepithelization of the basal endometrium is completed by the fifth day of menstruation.

The length of the luteal or secretory phase of the menstrual cycle is fairly constant at 14 ± 2 days. Eventually the degenerating corpus luteum is replaced by scar tissue and called the corpus albicans. Menstrual bleeding lasts, on the average, 5 to 7 days, with the next cycle already initiated on the onset of bleeding, as FSH stimulates new follicles to begin developing. The processes which occur, should conception take place, are discussed in Chapter 5.

Types of Steroid Hormones

There are three major types of estrogen: estrone, estradiol, and estriol. Estradiol is the most estrogenic, and estriol the least. The development of female sex characteristics and the regulation of the menstrual cycle are primarily under estradiol influence; estriol is called the estrogen of pregnancy because it is increased the most during gestation; estrone is the major circulating estrogen after menopause. Estrogens are secreted by the ovary, the adrenal gland, and the placenta during pregnancy. Estrone can also be derived from peripheral conversion of androstenedione (a type of androgen) which is largely secreted from the adrenal gland. Adrenocorticotropic hormone (ACTH) stimulates adrenal production of androstenedione and ovarian release of estrogens.

Progesterone seems to have only one active endogenous form, with cholesterol as its major precursor. Numerous progestins have been identified, but none has any significant progestational activity. The corpus luteum and the placenta secrete progesterone. In addition to its effect on the secretory phase of the menstrual cycle and in pregnancy, progesterone has a number of metabolic influences. In effecting the regulation of salt and water metabolism, it has a natriuretic effect and acts as an aldosterone antagonist in the kidney tubule. In protein metabolism in nonpregnant women, progesterone causes specific protein synthesis in responsive tissue, urinary nitrogen excretion and amino acidemia, and a net catabolic effect. In protein metabolism of pregnant women, progesterone contributes to a positive nitrogen balance and to overall weight gain. In carbohydrate metabolism, progesterone seems to have the balancing effect of increasing plasma insulin response to a glucose load and producing a mild resistance to the hypoglycemic effect in insulin. It may also play a role in fat deposition in women. Respiratory dynamics are altered during pregnancy by progesterone, which causes a reduction in arterial pCO_2 and a steeper stimulus-response curve for inspired CO_2 at a lower threshold.[4] Progesterone also causes a rise in basal body temperature shortly after ovulation and stimulates lobular-alveolar growth in the breasts. Small amounts of progesterone are present during the proliferative phase and menopause, secreted by the adrenal gland under the influence of ACTH.

The female also produces androgens, though in small amounts under normal circumstances. Both the ovaries and the adrenal glands secrete testosterone, the most potent androgen. Androstenedione secreted by the adrenal glands can be converted peripherally to estrone or testosterone in response to ACTH. Luteinizing hormone seems to cause the ovary to secrete androgens. Androstenedione is involved in the regulation of gonadotropin secretion.

Psychophysiology and Variations

Variation seems to be the constant of the menstrual cycle, and although averages have been identified, there is a wide range of fluctuation within the limits of normal. Table 4-2 details the average characteristics of the menstrual cycle. Although each woman tends to have a fairly recognizable pattern, this too is subject to many influences. Age affects the characteristics of the cycle, for during the first few and last several years of menstruating there is more irregularity. Frequent anovulatory cycles contribute to skipped menses and heavy flow postmenarchally and premenopausally. As cycles become more regular during the late teens and 20s, the heaviest bleeding usually occurs on the first and second days of flow. The greatest regularity in cycles seems to happen when the woman approaches age 30, and for a few years the mythical 28-day regular cycle is as closely approached as ever. Nearing age 40, the woman's cycles become more irregular, a state which increases as she gets closer to menopause. Cycles as short as 18 to 20 days and as long as 40 to 45 days are within the normal range. Cycle lengths can vary from month to month in the same woman, for fewer than 13 percent of the women in one study had cycles which varied by less than 6 days.[5] A difference in the amount of flow is often noted by women over 30, who report one day of very heavy flow frequently preceded by a day or two of spotting. The mid- to late 40s are known for their heavy, lengthy menses which are called "flooding." Then there may be a gradual tapering off of flow and greater intermenstrual intervals up to menopause.

Menstrual discomfort also follows an age gradation in some cases. The first 2 or 3 years after menarche are characterized by painless bleeding, with an increase in dysmenorrhea from midteens to mid-20s, then a decrease thereafter. Premenstrual symptoms, however, seem to increase with age in those susceptible, and may get worse with each successive pregnancy.

The mood of women has been noted to fluctuate during different phases of the menstrual cycle, as have certain behaviors. It is assumed that this is in response to hormone levels although the situational and social-attitudinal context must be constantly kept in mind (Fig-

Table 4-2
Average Characteristics of the Menstrual Cycle

Menarche	Usually between 11 and 16, average age 12 or 13, range of normal 9 to 18 years
Interval	Usually 27 to 31 days between menses, but regular cycles as short as 17 or 18 days and as long as 40 to 45 days are considered normal if a constant pattern for an individual
Duration	Menstrual flow usually lasts 3 to 7 days, range of normal is from 1 or 2 to 8 or 9 days. Fairly constant for the individual, but wide variations among women
Amount	Average menstrual loss is 30 to 100 ml. per menses, but 200 to 300 ml. is still considered normal for some women. Amount varies among women and in the same woman at different times. Usually heaviest the first 2 days, but this pattern may alter with age. Use pads or tampons to estimate amount; the average pad or tampon completely saturated absorbs 20 to 30 ml.
Composition	Menstrual discharge is a mixture of endometrium, blood, mucus, and vaginal cells. It is dark red, less viscous than blood, and usually does not clot. Clots are an aggregate of red blood cells, mucoid substances, mucoprotein, and glycogen and usually occur when menses are heavy.

ure 4-4). According to one report, women feel more alert, happy and other-directed during the first part of the cycle when estrogen is increasing. At ovulation in midcycle, when estrogen peaks, self-esteem and self-confidence are at their height. Women also show more competitiveness at midcycle, which seems related to outward-striving, active, assertive qualities associated with greater confidence and self-esteem. During the second part of the cycle, under the dominant influence of progesterone, women become more passive and inner-directed. Just before menstruation, as both progesterone and estrogen fall abruptly from high levels, women feel more tense, anxious, depressed, and irritable. The premenstrual phase is also associated with feelings of helplessness, hostility, and yearning for love. Changes in sexuality are also identified at different phases of the cycle. There was surprising uniformity among respondents, as ovulation was associated with underlying optimism, and the premenstrual phase with pessimism. Other low estrogen states, during early postpartum and menopause, also correlate with depression. The rate of decline of estrogen is thought to be more significant than the absolute amounts, with a more rapid rate causing more severe symptoms.[6]

The paramenstrum seems associated with negative behavior changes as well as with mood differences. In another study, it was re-ported that more than half of the women who attempt or successfully commit suicide and newly convicted or disorderly female prisoners are in the four premenstrual and first four menstrual days of their cycles. Also, it was during the paramenstrum that about 50 percent of the women in the study reported sick at work, were admitted for psychiatric care, admitted for emergency care and acute medical and surgical problems, died of viral and bacterial infections, and brought their children to a clinic with minor colds.[7] There are no doubt several complex mechanisms involved in these events, and not simply the fluctuation of hormones. For example, hormonally-induced physiological changes can contribute to irritability, making a mother less able to tolerate a child's minor illness, or to lowered reaction time and increased sluggishness, making a woman more likely to get caught in misbehavior or criminal activities. However, women's attitudes and coping mechanisms are probably more significant determinants of behavior than psychophysiology, the vast majority of women continue to function normally and well during the paramenstrum.

There seems to be some evidence that women who have internalized the menstrual taboo and the concept of the wife-mother role identity as the only legitimate one for women have the most problems with menstruation. Viewing menstruation as totally negative could

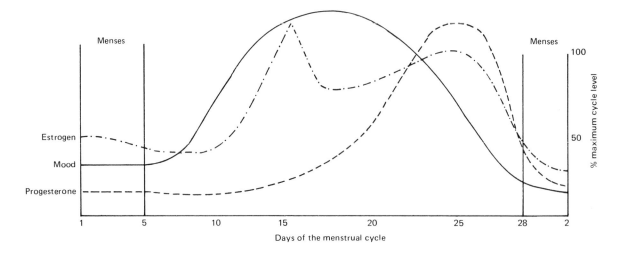

Figure 4-4. Hormonal and mood variations during the menstrual cycle.

conceivably exacerbate its associated physical changes and the woman's intolerance of these, with a snowballing effect of increasing severity. Women whose religions reinforced negative views of menstrual functions, such as the Jewish ban on sex during menstruation and cleansing rituals after or the Catholic belief that it is a woman's lot to suffer, expected to have more problems with menstruation. The more fully these women lived out the feminine role ideal with which they were brought up, the more frequent were their menstrual problems.[8]

MANAGEMENT OF MENSTRUAL PROBLEMS

When evaluating a woman presenting with a menstrual problem, the health provider must think hormonally. Although some problems have their roots in anatomical abnormalities, systemic diseases, or invasion by pathogens, the vast majority seen in ambulatory practice are due to some type of disturbance in the intricate hormonal system which regulates menstruation. As with other kinds of problems, the history is of prime importance.

Taking a Menstrual History

Specific information obtained from the history provides the key in establishing etiology. Whatever the nature of the particular menstrual problem, a thorough menstrual history is essential. Questions may be phrased as follows:

How old were you when you had your first period? About 80 to 85 percent of the patients will answer between the ages of 12 and 14, which is a good signpost of normal growth. If the patient says between 16 and 17, an endocrine problem involving growth alterations is suspect.

Were you prepared for it or was it a surprise? Cues are provided about attitudes toward menstruation, both of parents and the women. Lack of preparation and distaste, if expressed, might imply that emotional factors underlie her presenting complaint.

How long do you go between periods? Normal variation can be 18 to 45 days, which many women do not realize. If menses are reported as more frequent than 18 days, be sure to correlate with the nature of bleeding to rule out midcycle spotting from ovulation (mittelstaining). Note the age of the patient if cycle interval is greater than 45 days.

How long does the flow last? Average duration is 3 to 7 days, although menses of 7 to 9 or 1 or 2 days could be normal if constant for the individual. Also determine changes in the character of the flow over her menstrual span.

Is the flow light, medium, or heavy? There are many variations to this answer, and what is sought is a change in her usual amount or pattern. The best way to assess the amount of flow is to ask how many pads or tampons she uses in a day. The average tampon completely soaked absorbs 20 to 30 ml. of blood, but most women change before complete saturation.

Use of two pads with complete soaking in 1 to 2 hours indicates very heavy flow.

Do you have any clotting or cramping? Usually menstrual blood does not clot, and if clots are present it means there is heavy flow or vaginal pooling. Determine exactly when cramps begin, if prior to or after the onset of flow, how long they last, and how severe they are by the extent to which her usual activities are interrupted. Ask what she has done to relieve the pain, what makes it better, what makes it worse. Trace the natural history of menstrual cramping since this gives invaluable cues to rule out pathology versus functional dysmenorrhea.

Do you use birth control, and if so, what type? Oral contraceptives are a common cause of both amenorrhea and bleeding problems, and the IUD is associated with heavy menses and cramping. Inquire into her reliability in taking the pills or the possible loss of the IUD. If she is not using a birth control method and is sexually active, inquire into the possibility of pregnancy.

Have you had a recent pregnancy, abortion, or gynecological procedure? Depending on the nature of the problem, many diagnoses are suggested by a positive answer to one of these questions. Find out what happened, if there were complications, and the relation of the pregnancy or procedure to the onset of the present problem. Note pregnancy outcomes.

Have you ever had a serious disease or operation? A number of systemic illnesses can be related to menstrual problems. If the answer is positive, consider an exacerbation of the disease. Use the information given to gauge the general state of health and prior trauma to the body.

Are you currently taking any medications or drugs? Barbiturates (alcohol), opiates, corticosterids, chlordiazepoxide (Librium), phenytoin (Dilantin), and thioridazine (Mellaril) can cause amenorrhea. Ask if she was treated in the last 15 months with medroxyprogesterone (Provera) and what happened afterwards, as this can aid in the diagnosis of certain endocrine disorders.

Have you gained or lost weight recently? Both obesity and malnutrition can cause amenorrhea. Additionally, this could imply a systemic disease or endocrine disorder.

Did the problem with your menstrual cycle come on gradually or suddenly? Depending on the type of menstrual problem, certain cues are provided. Gradually lengthening cycles indicate failure of some component of the menstrual endocrine system, whether it be the ovary, pituitary, or thyroid or adrenal gland. Abrupt amenorrhea suggests pregnancy or functional anovulatory problems. Sudden heavy bleeding suggests abortion or unopposed estrogen effects on the endometrium. Gradually increased menstruation is characteristic of the latter part of the reproductive years.

Did any significant event occur around that time? Changes in marital status, relations, recent moves, a death in the family, financial stresses, or other emotional crises suggest the influences of psychological factors. These effects can cause either amenorrhea or unusual bleeding.

When was your last menstrual period and previous menstrual period before that, and were they normal? The date of the last menses helps to calculate the phase of the present menstrual cycle, the length of gestation or other amenorrhea, or unusually short intermenstrual time. Normality of the last two menses assists in determining whether they represent the usual pattern or are a deviation from it, suggesting diagnostic possibilities.

Amenorrhea

The absence of menses, or skipping periods, is a common problem seen in primary care. Some women may seek help after missing one menses; others may wait for many months. A careful menstrual history will suggest the most likely causes of amenorrhea, which can be confirmed by physical examination and laboratory tests. Most causes are benign, although occasionally endocrinopathies or significant pathology are involved.

AMENORRHEA WITH BREAST TENDERNESS, NAUSEA, AND URINARY FREQUENCY. If a woman between the ages of 18 and 45 presents with amenorrhea and associated symptoms including any combination of breast tenderness, nausea, urinary frequency, weight gain, fatigue, or changes in food tolerance (the smell of coffee can produce nausea in a regular coffee drinker), suspect pregnancy. The woman may have only missed one period, or three or four, and she may or may not be using birth control. Women do get pregnant with IUDs in place and while taking oral contraceptives, though with the latter there is usually a history of missing one or more pills. If diaphragms, jellies, or condoms are used, determine the frequency of use, for many women combine these with a rhythm method, using contraceptives only during what they think is the fertile time of the cycle. Obviously, with menstrual cycles so variable, it is easy to miscalculate ovulation and to have unprotected sex during the fertile time. If the woman denies sexual activity, another diagnosis must be entertained, unless for some reason she is not being honest with the provider. Young girls may deny intercourse, meaning actual penetration, but on careful questioning admit to sex play involving ejaculation between the thighs or near the introitus. Pregnancy can occur from migration of sperm in these situations, something many girls do not realize.

The physical examination consists of general inspection to determine the development of secondary sex characteristics or a chronically ill appearance and a pelvic examination, primarily to look for the changes of pregnancy or for ovarian masses. Positive Chadwick's sign (bluish discoloration of cervix and vagina), enlarged uterus with compressible isthmus and globular fundus (Hegar's sign), and the absence of ovarian masses strongly suggest pregnancy. However, these findings are generally not present until after 10 to 12 weeks gestation, and the uterine size and configuration of a 6 to 8 week pregnancy often differ little from the nonpregnant uterus. History is the best guide for early pregnancy.

Laboratory testing consists of one of the rapid pregnancy tests, such as Gravindex, Pregnosticon, UCG Slide Test, Pregnosis, or Twentisec. Based on urine samples, these tests are reliable after 42 days (6 weeks) following the last period. They can be performed in minutes. In early pregnancy, these tests are more reliable on a concentrated urine specimen, for an afternoon specimen tends to be dilute and to have a relatively lower concentration of human chorionic gonadotropin and thus may give a false negative. It is best to get a first-voided early morning specimen. Some providers think that the DAP test, based on blood instead of urine, is more reliable.

Treatment consists of discussing with the woman her desires related to continuation or termination of the pregnancy. Chapter 5 covers pregnancy and Chapter 7 covers abortion.

AMENORRHEA WITHOUT OTHER SYMPTOMS. If a regularly menstruating women presents with the absence of menses but has no other symptoms, then some malfunction of the hypothalamic-pituitary-ovarian axis is a likely cause (Table 4-3). First systemic conditions must be ruled out, particularly tuberculosis, diabetes, hyperthyroidism, hypothyroidism, and heart disease such as mitral stenosis. Use of oral contraceptives must be carefully explored, for this is a leading (and growing) cause of amenorrhea. Find out exactly how and when she is taking the pills, if any were missed, previous patterns of menses and skipping, or discontinuation of pills. Also determine her use of other medications which might cause amenorrhea. Here the provider is especially interested in stressful events in the woman's life, major changes, or conflicts.

Oral contraceptives cause amenorrhea through their actions on the hypothalamic-pituitary-ovarian axis and on the endometrium. Oral contraceptives suppress hypothalmic release of FSH and LH by providing a continuous exogenous source of estrogen and progestin which gives negative feedback. The endometrium also builds under the influence of the exogenous hormones, but it is atypical and does not progress through the usual proliferative and secretory phases. It does not attain the thickness of the normal endometrium, especially if the low estrogen pills are used. This accounts for the decreased menstrual flow most women experience when taking oral contraceptives. Occasionally the endometrium does not increase enough for sloughing after withdrawal of the exogenous hormones, and there may be only slight spotting or the absence of menses. Most oral contraceptives have literature which advises patients that skipping one period is common, but to be examined if they skip two.

Examination consists of inspection for systemic causes of the problem and a pelvic examination to rule out asymptomatic pregnancy and pelvic masses. Laboratory tests are usually not necessary unless pregnancy or other systemic problems are suspected.

Treatment includes discussing the functional causes of pill-related amenorrhea. If the patient is disturbed by the lack of menses, or very scant menses, she could be switched to a higher estrogen preparation. Many women desire regular menses as a sign of normal body

Table 4-3
Organic Causes of Secondary Amenorrhea

Sheehan's syndrome	Pituitary necrosis characterized by a history of hemorrhage postdelivery and never menstruating again. Look for loss of breast tissue, loss of axillary and pubic hair, dry vaginal mucosa, muscular weakness, perhaps premature aging and hot flashes.
Hyperthyroidism	About 70 percent of the women with Graves' disease have oligomenorrhea or amenorrhea. Signs and symptoms are tachycardia, palpitations, weight loss despite good appetite, heat intolerance, exophthalmos, enlarged thyroid, elevated PBI and BMR.
Galactorrhea	Leakage of fluid from the breasts, headaches, hearing or visual loss suggest pituitary tumor. Prolonged lactation can occur after normal delivery with or without nursing. In women who have never been pregnant galactorrhea may be of emotional origin.
Virilization	May be caused by adrenal, ovarian, or pituitary disease. In the Stein-Levanthal syndrome, the woman may be hirsute, but true virilization is uncommon.
Cushing's syndrome	Major signs are hypertension, diabetes, obesity of face and trunk with slender extremities, fat pad accumulation in cheeks and over cervical spine, florid complexion, hirsutism of face and chest, and male pubic hair distribution.

function, although a few women see the absence of menses as a boon.

Postpill amenorrhea occurs in a small but significant number of women. It does not seem related to how long the woman has been on oral contraceptives. After discontinuation of the pills, menses may not occur for 6 to 9 months or a year. The probable cause is that high levels of endogenous estrogen, almost in a rebound phenomenon, effectively suppress the release of FSH and LH. The source of this estrogen could be ovarian, such as a persistent follicular cyst. Also, once the exogenous supply of hormones is removed, it may take time for the estrogen levels to build adequately to trigger the LH surge responsible for ovulation. Whatever the mechanism, regular cycling should be restored in 6 to 9 months. If the woman is concerned, the causes can be further investigated as discussed below.

Hypothalamic amenorrhea is a term used to categorize the lack of menses in the absence of systemic illness or organic causes; it is thought to be emotional in origin. It is a diagnosis made by exclusion. There are four questions to ask in exploring the basis for hypothalamic amenorrhea:

1. Does the patient have an endometrium for estrogen/progesterone to act upon?
2. Does she have deficient estrogenic

"priming" of the endometrium either because the pituitary is incapable of secreting FSH or because the ovaries are incapable of estrogen secretion?

3. Is the patient's endometrium continually exposed to progesterone so that no withdrawal bleeding may occur, due either to pregnancy (which is ruled out as described above) or to a corpus luteum cyst (which will rarely cause prolonged amenorrhea)?

4. Is there a failure to ovulate, with a consequent absence of cyclic bursts of progesterone to act upon the estrogen-primed endometrium?[9]

Failure to ovulate is the most common cause of this type of amenorrhea. With a negative physical examination and history, one test can give the answer to three of the above questions:

The progesterone withdrawal test gives data about the woman's endometrium and ovarian estrogen secretion. Administer 10 to 20 mg. Provera by mouth for 5 days. If bleeding occurs in the next 3 to 5 days, it means that the woman has an endometrium which has been adequately primed by estrogen. Withdrawal bleeding would not occur from an endometrium under the influence of progesterone alone. Thus you know that the ovary has been secreting estrogen in adequate amounts. You also know that there must not be a continuous endogenous source of progesterone (from pregnancy or a corpus luteum cyst), otherwise the administration of exogenous progesterone would not have caused bleeding.

If the woman bleeds after the progesterone withdrawal test, the conclusion is that she failed to ovulate. There was adequate estrogen secretion by the ovary to develop a proliferative endometrium, but no release of LH to stimulate the corpus luteum to produce progesterone, thus completing the menstrual cycle. Or, LH was released, but the ovary could not respond to it. The first situation is a very common cause of amenorrhea, and is thought to be related to emotional factors. The second indicates that there is a thickening of the ovarian capsule which prevents ovulation, such as seen in the Stein-Levanthal syndrome (see Table 4-3). Obviously emotional factors are a much more likely cause, but if normal cycling did not resume after one or two progesterone withdrawal tests, then the Stein-Levanthal syndrome would be more likely.

Treatment is usually accomplished by administration of the progesterone withdrawal test, and normal cycling should resume. In discussing with the patient how and why emotions can interfere with her menstrual hormone flow, one can speculate about the biochemical effects of ACTH and other stress-triggered steroids. Since ACTH stimulates ovarian release of estrogens, unusually high estrogen levels may block the complete development of the graafian follicle or suppress the estrogen-hypothalamic feedback mechanism. If the hypothalamus does not receive the message to secrete LH releasing factor, whether by too much or too little circulating estrogen, the follicle cannot mature, rupture, and progress to the progesterone phase. Undoubtedly the mechanism involved is much more complex than this, but the general principles may be correct.

A persistent follicular cyst may also be implicated in this type of amenorrhea. Occasionally a graafian follicle does not rupture to release the ovum but remains enlarged and continues to secrete estrogen. These cysts may be felt during pelvic examination as an enlarged ovary. The ovary will usually feel between 6 to 8 cm., but in any case should be less than 10 cm. These are usually unilateral, frequently silent in that the patient experiences no pelvic symptoms, and they regress spontaneously. Most are never palpated or are found incidentally in a pelvic examination for other reasons. If amenorrhea is the presenting symptom, and the woman or health provider prefers not to wait for spontaneous regression and resumption of menses, the treatment is to use oral contraceptives for 1 or 2 cycles to cause involution of the cyst. The woman should be reexamined in 6 weeks, by which time the cyst should be much smaller or resolved. If the health provider has any doubt about the enlarged ovary, either because its size approaches 10 cm. or more or because its consistency is hard rather than cystic, consultation with a physician must be sought. A cyst which fails to resolve must be referred to the physician.

Suppose, however, that the woman does not bleed following the administration of the progesterone withdrawal test. The possibilities to be considered now are that no endometrium is present, the endometrium has not been adequately primed by estrogen, or there is a continuous endogenous source of progesterone. The next step is to use a combined estrogen/progesterone withdrawal test (E/P), in which ethinyl estradiol 0.02 to 0.05 mg. or Premarin 1.25 to 2.5 mg. is given orally for 21 days, followed by Provera 10 to 20 mg. orally for 7 days.

If the E/P test produces bleeding, the woman does have an endometrium, but it has not been adequately primed by endogenous estrogen. The likely causes of this are endocrinopathies such as primary ovarian failure (premature menopause), or hypopituitarism. In any case, this is a patient for the specialist, and the nurse practitioner would refer her to a gynecologist or an endocrinologist. If bleeding does not take place after the E/P test, there are several other possibilities, some of which can be confirmed by other tests or physical examination. Once again pregnancy must be ruled out, for it produces constant endogenous sources of estrogen and progesterone. Get another pregnancy test, and do another pelvic examination. Rarely, a corpus luteum cyst may provide a continuing source of endogenous progesterone. It should be felt on pelvic examination as a unilateral cystic ovarian enlargement of less than 10 cm. The usual treatment is to wait for the cyst to resolve, reexamining at different phases of the menstrual cycle at 1 to 3 month intervals. Eventually it should disappear with the resumption of menses. The nurse practitioner should probably manage this case in collaboration with a physician. A confirmatory diagnostic test is urinary pregnanediol levels which should be elevated to over 4 to 5 mg. in 24 hours.

Another cause of failure to bleed after the E/P test can be found on pelvic examination. Cervical stenosis may be present, in which case the endocervical canal cannot be sounded. This usually results from previous conization or cauterization which produced scarring and obstruction of the canal. Treatment consists of dilating the endocervical canal with Hegar dilators. A second traumatic cause of amenorrhea is more serious, for it implies destruction of the basal layer of the endometrium. Overzealous curettage is the most common cause, in which the bleeding postpartal or postabortion patient was given a D and C to stop the bleeding, with too deep scraping of the lush, edematous, and easily separated endometrium. The result is sclerosis of the endometrium with scarring, shrinking, and permanent amenorrhea. If no other causes can be found, and the woman has a positive history, this serious situation must be considered. A referral for confirmation to a gynecologist is indicated, with arrangements for supportive therapy or counseling. A final possibility is the rare TB endometritis, which would be confirmed by a TB skin test and by stain and culture of endometrial aspirate or biopsy. This case would be managed in collaboration with a physician.

Thus, in the woman who has been previously menstruating, the absence of menses for 6 months or more is called secondary amenorrhea, and the most likely causes, in probable descending order, are: pregnancy, hypothalamic (emotional) causes, oral contraceptives, other medications or systemic illness, functional cysts, trauma causing cervical stenosis or sclerosis of the endometrium, endocrinopathies, and TB endometritis.

PRIMARY AMENORRHEA. When a girl reaches 18 years of age, and has never menstruated, she is considered to have primary amenorrhea. Probably she would be brought to a health provider's attention before this time, either due to the mother's or the girl's concern about her not beginning to menstruate. Girls generally expect to menstruate by age 12 or 13, and it would not be unusual for the nurse practitioner to see a 15 to 17 year old with the complaint or amenorrhea. If the girl is 17 or below, she should be examined for normal growth signposts (Table 4-1). If these signposts are appropriately present, discuss with the patient and her mother or father the ranges of normal pubertal development. Family history can be significant, because girls tend to begin menses around the same age as their mothers and grandmothers. If any signs of physical abnormalities are present, or the girl is behind on normal development for her age, she should be referred to a pediatrician or endocrinologist.

On physical examination, the health provider should look particularly for imperforate hymen, vaginal or cervical obstructions, absence of the vagina or uterus, immature genitalia and breasts, scanty pubic hair, and presence of labial or groin masses. Positive findings indicate a physician consultation and probable referral. Table 4-4 summarizes the most frequent causes of true primary amenorrhea due to congenital, structural, and endocrine abnormalities.[10]

Short, Scant, or Frequent Menstrual Flow

Among the more common problems with menses for which women seek help are short and scant menses or frequently occurring menses. The first thing to determine is whether the bleeding represents cyclic or noncyclic flow, data which can be obtained from the menstrual history. If the bleeding occurs at regular intervals, it implies that ovulation is occurring; if it is irregular and unpredictable, the cycles are probably anovulatory. Usually scant or frequent menses are physiological variations and require little treatment.

Short, scant menstrual flow occurring at regular intervals is simply the normal pattern for some women. They may have spotting or light bleeding, which lasts only 1 or 2 days. If this represents a change from the usual pattern, however, other factors come into play. Oral contraceptives are a common cause of very light periods, as has been previously discussed. Also, some women continue to have menses after conception, and these tend to be lighter than the usual flow, occurring at the normally expected time. A pelvic examination can rule out ovarian masses and an enlarged uterus, and a pregnancy test may be indicated. If the cause is oral contraceptives, a higher-estrogen pill can be used if desired. If pregnancy and oral contraceptives are ruled out, and the decreased

Table 4-4
Causes of Primary Amenorrhea

Gonadal dysgenesis	Signs are shielded chest, webbed neck, arched palate, and short stature. Other tests show chromatin negative buccal smear, retarded bone growth, high FSH, and the diagnosis confirmed by finding XO or XX/XO chromosome pattern.
Congenital anomalies	Examination may reveal imperforate hymen, absent vagina or uterus, obstruction of the cervix or vagina.
Testicular feminization	Also called the androgen insensitivity syndrome. Signs are small nipples, scanty pubic hair, and presence of labial or groin masses (testes).
Prepubertal ovarian failure	The girl appears tall with immature genitalia and underdeveloped breasts. The buccal smear is chromatin positive and there is high urinary FSH.
Congenital adrenal hyperplasia	Signs include virilization, chromatin positive buccal smear, and elevated 17-ketosteroids. Clitoral hypertrophy may be present.
Hypopituitarism	May be normal appearing females or sexually immature, depending on the age of onset. Cause may be pituitary tumor or cyst apparent on X-ray examination of the skull.

flow is a change in the woman's normal pattern, she should be followed for several cycles to see if her normal flow resumes; and if it does not, she should be retested.

Frequent, regular menstrual cycles usually mean normal, frequent ovulation. If the woman says her periods are coming every 2 weeks, question her carefully about the character of the bleeding. She may report that one menses is lighter than the next and not preceded by premenstrual symptoms, and this is her regular alternating pattern. In this case, the likely cause is mittelstaining, the pinkish discharge of the midcycle estrogen dip (see p. 97). Or, the menses may have exactly the same premenstrual symptoms and character of flow but may occur as frequently as 17 to 20 days apart. In either case, you want to know if the woman is ovulating if frequent menses persist. If this is a one-time occurrence, it is reasonable to wait 2 or 3 weeks and then reevaluate.

There are three simple ways to assess whether or not the woman is ovulating: basal body temperature, the test for "ferning" of cervical mucus, and the test for *spinnbarkeit* of cervical mucus. To find her basal body temperature, the woman takes her temperature orally each morning before arising, leaving the thermometer in a full 5 minutes. It is recorded on a graph (see Figure 3-6) and plotted in relation to the menses for 2 to 3 months. Since progesterone causes a rise in basal body temperature, a characteristic pattern emerges if the woman is ovulating, in which there is a dip at midcycle just prior to ovulation, followed by a sustained rise of 0.5 to 1.0 degrees F. above the levels of the first part of the cycle. The woman should also note any other reason for temperature elevation, such as a cold, to avoid confusion. At the end of this time, a consistent biphasic curve, changing about 14 days before the onset of menses, is good evidence of ovulation.

The ferning test is done by figuring out the latest ovulation can occur according to the length of the woman's cycle, then taking a smear of cervical mucus after that time, allowing it to air-dry and looking under the microscope for the presence of typical ferning crystal patterns (Figure 4-5). If, for instance, the woman has a 20-day cycle, she should ovulate by day 6 or 7; therefore a specimen of cervical mucus taken on day 8, 9, or 10 showing an amorphous pattern without ferning strongly suggests the influence of progesterone, indicating ovulation. Cervical mucus under estrogen influence has a high concentration of salt and is quite viscous; thus it forms crystal patterns upon drying.

To do the spinnbarkeit test, also calculate the time of expected ovulation and do the test 2 or 3 days later to see if the cervical mucus shows estrogen or progesterone influence. Using a sponge (uterine dressing) forceps, take some cervical mucus out of the os. Then, watching it carefully, open the forceps, and if

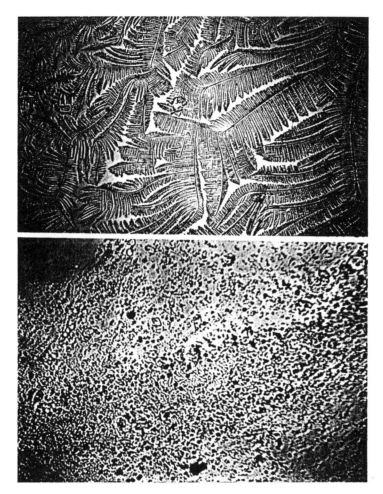

Figure 4-5. (Top) Typical ferning pattern of cervical mucus at midcycle under estrogen influence. (Bottom) Cervical mucus showing the effects of progesterone-producing, amorphous pattern after ovulation. Note absence of ferning, Beacham and Beacham, *Synopsis of Gynecology,* 1972.

the mucus pulls out into strings, it is under estrogen stimulus. If progesterone is present and dominant, however, the mucus does not form long strings but tends to form globs on the ends of the forceps. The absence of strings is a good indication of ovulation.

If the tests determine that the woman is ovulating, there is no reason for concern. Simply explain to her that she is having normal, though short, cycles and that this may be her pattern for a while, discussing the variations in menstrual patterns at different ages. If she is not ovulating, referral to a gynecologist is probably in order. Consult with physician colleagues first, bearing in mind the two major reasons for concern in this case: infertility and endometrial hyperplasia. Unopposed estrogen is the cause of endometrial hyperplasia, and almost all of the endometrial carcinoma seen in younger women (30 and below) is in those

who have been consistently anovulatory. Although this is very rare, it must be considered.

Cervical stenosis is another cause of very light menstrual periods. The usual pattern is the appearance of dark brown spotting, with cramping at the time menses are due. Strictures of the upper vagina, partial endometrial sclerosis, diabetes, starvation, thyroid problems, and excessive intake of vitamin A are also possible, though unusual, causes.

Heavy or Long Menstrual Flow

Heavy menses (hypermenorrhea, menorrhagia) may be normal for some women. Periods may last 7 to 9 days, and pads or tampons soaked every several hours without causing a problem with anemia. However, other symptoms must be explored to determine whether there is reason for concern. Especially if heavy bleeding is a change from the usual pattern, its cause should be sought and treated. Obtain a good menstrual history and determine if the bleeding is cyclic or irregular. Try to obtain an accurate picture of just how much blood is lost and of the character of the bleeding. Remember that an IUD can double a woman's menstrual flow, and is a common cause of heavy menses. If the bleeding is a great bother to her, the IUD may need to be removed. Before taking this step, however, the woman can be cycled on a low estrogen oral contraceptive for 2 to 3 cycles, which often causes enough endometrial atrophy to solve the bleeding problems for months or years, permitting the IUD to be left in place.

A single episode of heavy bleeding can indicate an early spontaneous abortion or ectopic pregnancy and must be carefully evaluated. Pregnancy tests at this point may be negative, for the fetus usually dies about 4 weeks prior to miscarriage and human chorionic gonadotropin levels would be low. On pelvic examination, check the cervical os carefully; if it is open, with tissue extruding, it is very suggestive of abortion and the tissue should be removed and sent to pathology. If the cervix is closed and the pregnancy test negative, it still does not rule out spontaneous abortion, which could be threatened, incomplete, or complete. Physician consultation should be sought if any indications of pregnancy are present in the history or physical examination.

Occasionally, women on oral contraceptives, with IUDs or postconization of the cervix have an isolated episode of heavy menstrual bleeding, or a sudden onset of heavy irregular bleeding. The cause is not always discernible, although anovulation with excessive proliferation of the endometrium is a prime suspect. Whenever the endometrium builds up under unopposed estrogen, the glands, stroma, and blood vessels do not undergo their characteristic changes under progesterone influence, and there are no proper controls for the breakdown of the endometrium as hormone levels drop. Thus when the levels of estrogen fall off, with no progesterone to regulate endometrial sloughing, bleeding tends to be sudden and profuse and often lasts longer than

menses. If this happens once, the most common approach is to wait for the bleeding to subside spontaneously unless the woman is actually hemorrhaging. If it happens repeatedly, then the cause must be investigated.

REPEATED HEAVY MENSES.   The woman with regular hypermenorrhea presents a typical history of "flooding," in which she bleeds through two pads or a super tampon and a pad, and worries about bleeding through to her clothes. It may be her normal pattern, and she is usually a hyperestrogen woman with large breasts and a considerable amount of premenstrual tension, and is somewhat overweight. She is commonly in the 30 to 45 age range, and wants something done about her heavy bleeding. It often is a problem which has come on over a span of several years, and she feels she has put up with it long enough.

The history should rule out systemic causes. The pelvic examination is important because it can help to rule out two common causes, uterine fibroids or adenomyosis. If fibroids are present, the uterus may feel nodular or irregular on its serosal surface; if they are interstitial or submucosal the only sign may be an enlarged uterus. Ulceration, hyperplasia, or venous dilatation and congestion of the endometrium in the area of the myomata are all causes of heavy bleeding. In adenomyosis, there are endometrial implants in the muscle of the uterus, which on examination should be freely movable, slightly enlarged, boggy, and tender, especially before menstruation. Findings suggestive of either of these should be corroborated with the physician and the therapy should be planned jointly.

If the findings of the pelvic examination are normal, anemia must be ruled out as this alone can perpetuate heavy menstrual bleeding. A hematocrit alone is often not enough to assess the presence of anemia properly, and a complete blood count with indices gives a better picture. Serum iron and iron-binding capacity tests may also be done to assess the woman's iron stores, for even with a reasonable hematocrit there may be no more iron stores, as evidenced by a low serum iron or a high iron-binding capacity. If hemoglobin drops more than 2 Gm. in a menstrual period, or serum iron is low and iron-binding capacity high, oral iron supplements can be given to correct iron deficiency anemia.

In the absence of the above organic problems, the treatment of the hypermenorrheic woman is aimed at producing relative atrophy of the endometrium. One way to do this is to use a low or balanced estrogen oral contraceptive with norethindrone (Norinyl, Norlestrin, Norquen, Ortho-Novum). These seem to have a better atrophy-producing effect on the endometrium than pills with norethynodrel (Enovid). Essentially these pills accomplish a "medical curettage," but may either be unacceptable to the woman or fail to work adequately to reduce the menstrual bleeding. A D and C may then be indicated and has been found effective in 60 percent of patients with simple hypermenorrhea, with effects lasting 6 months to 1 year, or perhaps permanently.[11] When a D and C is under consideration, referral to the physician is needed, with a discussion of benefits and risks. Another approach is to use Provera 10 mg. daily for 5 days at the end of cycle. Of course, a routine Pap smear would be done.

LONG MENSES WITH PARAMENSTRUAL SPOTTING. A change often noted by women aged 30 to 35 is a longer menstrual period, not necessarily heavier, but having a different quality of bleeding. There may be 2 to 3 days of spotting followed by 1 or 2 days of steady bleeding, which tapers gradually; or the onset of menses with usual steady bleeding will be followed by 2 to 3 days of spotting as menses end. This type of spotting either preceding or following the regular menstrual flow is characteristic of deteriorating corpus luteum functioning. The corpus luteum either dies too quickly or hangs on too long. Instead of the smooth, even decline of hormone levels usually occurring at the end of the menstrual cycle, progesterone falls in a "staircase" fashion, causing the intermittent sloughing which produces spotting.

In this age group, more serious causes of unusual bleeding must be kept in mind, and a thorough history and physical examination, including a Pap smear, and complete blood count should be done. Tests for ovulation are indicated to verify the presence of corpus luteum. If indeed deteriorating corpus luteum function is the final diagnosis, the treatment is to support the corpus luteum for about 4 days before the time menses is expected. This can be done by completely cycling the woman with oral contraceptives for 2 or 3 months, or more simply, giving the oral contraceptives for the last 4 or 5 days of her cycle. Alternately, oral progesterone alone can be used, Provera 20 mg. for 2 days or 10 mg. for 5 days preceding menses.

SYSTEMIC CAUSES. The history gives insight into possible systemic causes related to heavy menstrual bleeding. Among the drugs which can cause abnormal bleeding are the phenothiazines, hypothalamic depressants (morphine, reserpine), anticholinergics, anticoagulants, and thiazide diuretics. Blood dyscrasias such as thrombocytopenia and leukemia are also, though infrequent, causes.

Intermenstrual Bleeding

Bleeding or spotting in between menstrual periods is often a sign of an organic problem, although there are some physiologic or functional causes. It is important to ascertain whether the intermenstrual bleeding is occurring repeatedly in a cyclic pattern, or is noncyclic and completely irregular in its occurrence. Again, a thorough menstrual history is needed, with particular attention paid to the amount and character of the bleeding and any events or activities associated with it. A pelvic examination provides additional information which helps to confirm the diagnosis and to indicate treatment.

MIDCYCLE SPOTTING. Occasional or even repeated light spotting at midcycle is a common symptom reported by women. This is the mittelstaining associated with ovulation if the following additional characteristics are present: the woman is having reasonably regular menses, is ovulating (and often can describe mittelschmertz), the spotting is light pink and lasts for a few hours to a day or so, there are no premenstrual symptoms with the spotting, and the history is negative for other significant problems (see p. 97). With any kind of intermenstrual spotting, however, it is essential to take a Pap smear to screen for cervical carcinoma. Confirming that the spotting is indeed associated with ovulation can be reassuring to both the patient and the practitioner, and tests for ovulation such as basal body temperature, ferning, or the spinnbarkeit test of cervical mucus (see pp. 106 to 107) can be done.

Once mittelstaining is diagnosed and explained thoroughly to the patient, the therapy depends upon how disturbing she finds the spotting and whether she can live with it or not. As spotting tends to be intermittent and to occur only during some menstrual cycles, many women will be satisfied with understanding the phenomenon and will tolerate the day or so of light staining. Others, however, will want the spotting stopped; this can be easily accomplished by giving small amounts of estrogen such as diethylstilbestrol 0.25 mg. or ethinyl estradiol 0.02 mg. orally for about 5 days around the time of ovulation. To be effective, the time of ovulation must be calculated for the particular woman according to her length of cycle, and the estrogen should be started about 3 or 4 days before ovulation is anticipated.

Oral contraceptives can also cause spotting between menses, though the pattern is not as regular as in mittelstaining. This is called breakthrough bleeding or spotting and is a common experience among women on oral contraceptives. If it happens just occasionally and the spotting is light, then no action is indicated. The next cycle will probably be without spotting. If it happens repeatedly, then the woman is probably on an oral contraceptive with too little estrogen and should be switched. However, other causes should be ruled out, such as pregnancy and pelvic pathology.

IRREGULAR INTERMENSTRUAL SPOTTING. Depending upon the woman's age, there are a number of organic causes for spotting between menses which has no particular pattern. This can be a sign of potentially serious problems and must be carefully evaluated by history and examination. Most important here is to obtain a good description of exactly when the spotting occurs, what events immediately preceded it, what other symptoms might be related, and the character and amount of the spotting. Certain cues from her history can be confirmed by examination to substantiate a diagnosis, but sometimes only more extensive testing can reveal the cause. Pregnancy is still a leading cause in all women in the reproductive years and must be ruled out as discussed before.

Irregular intermenstrual spotting associated with increased vaginal discharge, itching, dysuria, or discomfort with intercourse suggests cervical or vaginal lesions or infections. A typical history would be the above symptoms associated with spotting following intercourse or douching. Or, there may be no other symptoms, just the spotting after intercourse or a douche. A pelvic examination may reveal erythema of the labia, vaginal walls, or cervix and a heavy white to greenish yellow vaginal discharge, indicating vaginitis. The treatment and diagnosis of vaginitis are discussed in detail in Chapter 9. There may be cervical eversion of varying degrees; perhaps some erosion or cervicitis causing the ectocervical columnar epithelium to be friable and to bleed easily. An endocervical polyp, tear-shaped and bright red, may be seen protruding from the os. Or, there may be lesions of the vagina or cervix not readily identifiable, discolored or thickened or irregular tissue which appears alien to the vaginal or cervical mucosa.

Any abnormal appearing cervical or vaginal lesion should be stained with Lugol's or Schiller's solution. With the speculum exposing the suspicious area, dip a vaginal swab in the solution and thoroughly paint the area and the surrounding tissue. If there is much cervical mucus or vaginal discharge, it will need to be swabbed out before applying the staining solution. The iodine in the stains is taken up by normal cervical and vaginal tissue, and the color becomes dark brown. Any cells that are deficient in glycogen, however, will not take up the stain and will appear pale in comparison to the surrounding tissue. The pale area is highly suspect for neoplasm, which depletes the cells' glycogen stores. Any pale area should then be biopsied with a punch biopsy or skin biopsy, placed in fixative, and sent to pathology for cytologic studies.

To do the punch biopsy, the cervix is grasped with a tenaculum for stabilization, and the biopsy instrument is aimed directly at the lesion and a tiny portion snipped, while traction on the cervix is provided by the tenaculum against the pressure of the biopsy forceps. All suspicious areas should be sampled. There is usually minimal bleeding from a biopsy, and it is easily controlled with pressure or the application of silver nitrate. Vaginal biopsies are done similarly, but without the tenaculum. In case the practitioner should be tempted to rely on Pap smear results alone, it must be pointed out that while Pap smears are highly effective for carcinoma *in situ*, the incidence of false negatives in gross lesions runs close to 20 percent. And, it may be very difficult to differentiate an extensive cervical eversion with erosion from carcinoma just by looking.

If the diagnosis is vaginitis or cervicitis by a wet prep and the identification of an infecting organism (see Chapter 9), specific treatment should be prescribed as indicated. Very friable eversion or extensive erosion may need to be treated by cryosurgery or cauterization. After biopsy of pale staining of suspicious lesions, the case should be managed jointly with the physician. Endocervical polyps can be removed in the office if their point of attachment can be seen. To do this, grasp the polyp with a sponge forceps at the very base of the stalk, close the forceps tightly and begin to twist it slowly. Continue to twist in the same direction, and the polyp will eventually come free. Place it in preservative and send it to pathology. Bleeding can be controlled by pressure, silver nitrate application or, if necessary, electrocautery.

Foreign bodies are another cause of intermenstrual spotting, though they are much more common in young girls than in adult women. However, it is possible for a woman to forget a tampon or a diaphragm in the vagina and to present some days to weeks later with such symptoms as lower abdominal cramping, increased vaginal discharge, spotting, foul-smelling discharge, pressure sensations, or reporting that their sexual partners felt something strange in their vagina (often mistaken for lumps or abnormal tissue). The foreign body is readily apparent on speculum examination and can be removed, and the cause of the symptoms explained. Vulvar lesions can also cause spotting, especially after intercourse, are often identified by the patient, and may be infectious, traumatic, or neoplastic. Again, suspicious lesions should be biopsied; infections and traumas should be treated.

IRREGULAR INTERMENSTRUAL BLEEDING. When a noncyclic discharge is heavier than spotting, its cause is usually different and again can be either organic or functional. Here the potential for serious problems is also increased, especially as a woman grows older. A careful history and physical examination are as important as before.

The sudden onset of heavy bleeding without any cyclic pattern and in the absence of premenstrual symptoms suggests anovulatory bleeding. The proliferative endometrium under estrogen influence begins uncontrolled sloughing, and there is no progesterone action to regulate the endometrial breakdown, as in normal cycles. When there is an unopposed estrogen effect upon the endometrium, it continues to proliferate and grow in depth, and the cells undergo hyperplasia to varying degrees. This type of bleeding can happen to menstruating women of any age, but it is more common during adolescence, when cyclicity and hormone flow are not yet well established, and toward the end of the fertile years, as ovarian function declines. Heavy bleeding with large clots is typical and may persist upward of 2 weeks. If it becomes necessary to stop the bleeding, this can be done by administering either estrogen such as Premarin 3.75 mg. per day orally or Provera 10 to 20 mg. per day orally for about 5 days. Usually the bleeding does stop in about 3 days, but either medication has its own effects, too. Estrogen will stop bleeding because it stimulates a proliferative endometrium to begin building up again, leaving the same problem of continuing endogenous estrogen influence which may eventually produce another episode of heavy bleeding. If estrogen is used, it should be followed by a progestational agent such as norethindrone acetate (Norlutate) or an oral contraceptive to produce a secretory endometrium and more controlled bleeding next time. With progesterone, the woman should be informed that she will start to bleed about 3 days after she stops the medication, and that the bleeding should be more controlled and counted as day one of her next menstrual period.

Most women with acyclic intermenstrual bleeding will eventually stop spontaneously; a few will have to be admitted to the hospital and given a D and C to halt the bleeding. If acyclic intermenstrual bleeding is a continuing problem, additional work-up is needed to search for more serious causes. After a good history to determine the characteristics of the bleeding, it is important to ascertain whether these are indeed anovulatory episodes of estrogen withdrawal bleeding. In addition to the tests for ovulation already discussed, endometrial biopsy is now an important diagnostic tool, particularly since endometrial hyperplasia is a danger. This office procedure is better done with an assistant holding an anterior vaginal retractor and with a weighted speculum in place to give good exposure (Figure 4-6). After a pelvic examination to determine the position and size of the uterus, the anterior lip of the cervix is grasped with a tenaculum, and the depth of the uterus is measured with a uterine sound. Then the endometrial biopsy instrument is introduced carefully through the

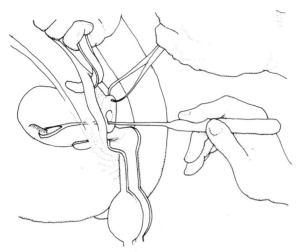

Figure 4-6. Technique for endometrial biopsy. After sounding to determine uterine size and position, you can insert the curette without danger of penetration. One swipe from back to front is needed.

cervix, inserted a little less than the depth sounded, and drawn from back to front in one swipe along the inferior surface of the endometrium. The specimen withdrawn in the loop of the biopsy instrument is preserved and sent to pathology.

If the endometrial biopsy is done in the latter half of the menstrual cycle, about days 21 and 22, it helps to evaluate the corpus luteum and to determine whether or not the patient is ovulating by the presence or absence of a secretory endometrium. It may also give evidence of neoplasia, but the results of the biopsy are not conclusive if they are negative. Only one small portion of the endometrium is sampled, and neoplastic tissue may be located in another area. Further diagnostic work-up is required to rule out carcinoma and should be undertaken in women over 25 who experience repeated irregular intermenstrual bleeding or spotting. The jet washer is a relatively new office technique used to screen for endometrial carcinoma. The device uses a syringe, a collecting tube with 35 cc. normal saline solution, and an irrigating tip with a rubber stopper which fits into the cervical os. By negative pressure, the jet washer bathes the endometrium with the saline solution, which cycles from tube to syringe. Cells and tissue fragments are dislodged as the solution washes through the endometrial cavity. The rubber stopper serves as a seal against the cervical os,

and the negative pressure almost totally eliminates the danger of spreading possibly malignant cells into the fallopian tubes. Generally anesthesia is not required, but for some women a local infiltration of the cervix may be indicated. In one study, the endometrial jet washer was found to identify endometrial carcinoma in 87 percent of the positive cases, and the endometrial biopsy identified carcinomas in only 63 percent of those cases.[12]

If the endometrial biopsy shows the endometrium to be proliferative in the latter part of the cycle, and the jet washer screen is negative for significant hyperplasia or carcinoma, the pelvic examination may give evidence of two other common causes of repeated intermenstrual spotting. Uterine myomata (fibroids) may be felt as irregularities or nodules on the corpus of the uterus, as a separate movable mass, or simply as an enlarged uterus. Endometriosis, the presence of endometrial implants in such areas as the ovaries, uterine ligaments, pelvic peritoneum, sigmoid colon, vagina or cervix, may be indicated by nodularity of the uterosacral ligaments on rectovaginal examination or a fixed ovary. If either of these is found or suspected, consultation with the physician is indicated. The work-up would also include a Pap smear.

Treatment of uncomplicated intermenstrual bleeding depends in part on the woman's age (Table 4-5). In the 15 to 25 age group, such irregular shedding of the endometrium is not uncommon and will usually correct itself with time. Irregular shedding and anovulation are most easily corrected by using an oral progestational agent; norethindrone compounds have a more atrophying effect on the endometrium, and such preparations as Ortho-Novum, Norinyl, or Norlestrin can be used for three cycles with generally good results. Only if the problem did not improve after this treatment would a D and C be considered. In the 25 to 35 age group, the administration of a progestational agent (Provera) during the last part of the cycle or a low-estrogen oral contraceptive for three cycles usually causes the woman to revert to normal cycling. When the woman reaches the age of 40 to 42, the risks of thromboembolic problems and hypertension with the use of oral contraceptives increase significantly, and many practitioners arbitrarily select this age as the cut off point for the pill. Lower amounts of estrogen are indicated, such as 0.625 to 1.25

Table 4-5
Most Common Causes of Abnormal Gynecological Bleeding by Age Group

Age 5-13	Age 14-25	Age 25-35	Age 35-45	Age 45+ (postmenopausal)
Foreign bodies	Pregnancy	Pregnancy	Pregnancy	Estrogen therapy
Self-inflicted lacerations	Oral contraceptives or IUD	Oral contraceptives or IUD	Anovulation	Endometrial hyperplasia or polyps
Vaginitis (non-specific)	Cervical eversion or cervicitis	Cervical eversion or cervicitis	Endometrial hyperplasia	Endometrial carcinoma
R/O UTI and rectal bleeding	Anovulation	Cervical polyps	Uterine fibroids	Uterine fibroids
	Vaginal lacerations or infections	Anovulation	Adenomyosis	Coital injuries
	Foreign bodies	Vaginal lacerations or infections	Endometriosis	
	Adenosis	Foreign bodies	Endometrial carcinoma	
	Cervical polyps	Uterine fibroids	Oral contraceptives or IUD	
		Endometrial hyperplasia	Cervical polyps	
			Other cervical and vaginal causes	

mg. conjugated estrogen, with a progestin added the third week. Another approach which gets around the estrogen problem is to use only progesterone to convert the estrogen-primed proliferative endometrium to a pregestational endometrium and to cause regular bleeding once a month. As the woman in this age group is not having predictable cycles and is bleeding irregularly from unopposed estrogen, a time can simply be selected, such as the first 10 days of each month, to administer the progesterone. Thus she will bleed once a month in a controlled manner, and the endometrium will not continue to build up.

Benign endometrial hyperplasia, caused primarily by anovulation and the resultant unopposed estrogen effect which stimulates the uterus to continue to build a proliferative endometrium, can be managed by the practitioner in primary care in the manner described above. However, the appropriate diagnostic tests must be performed to rule out other causes which require different management. If the cytological report confirms the presence of atypical cells, the case needs referral to a gynecologist. It is thought that the pattern which leads to well-differentiated carcinoma of the endometrium proceeds from benign hyperplasia to atypical hyperplasia, adenomatous hyperplasia, atypical andenomatous hyperplasia and, finally, carcinoma. This does not imply that any continued proliferative endometrium or benign endometrial hyperplasia should at once be referred for hysterectomy, but that

these conditions must be properly diagnosed and treated and followed for further progression. The health provider would collaborate closely with the physician in the management of these cases. In the types of irregular intermenstrual bleeding discussed here, if appropriate treatment with hormones did not restore regular cycles or if the unpredictable bleeding continued during treatment, then a diagnostic D and C would be necessary. Remember that the techniques used to test the endometrium do not sample its entire surface, and submucous fibroids and endometrial polyps may not be apparent except upon D and C, as may small areas of atypical hyperplasia or carcinoma.

Postmenopausal Bleeding

Any bleeding or spotting during the postmenopausal years must be looked upon with a high degree of suspicion. While there are some innocent causes, the incidence of carcinoma in women with postmenopausal bleeding is 30 to 40 percent. Malignancy must therefore be a prime suspect in this age group, and a thorough work-up should be undertaken. Because many of these patients will require a D and C and possibly a hysterectomy, the health provider would refer them to the physician early in the diagnostic work-up and would not assume the primary responsibility for these cases.

An accurate history of the bleeding, a menstrual history, and a family history are the first steps. The work-up also includes a complete blood count, physical examination, pelvic examination, Pap smear, and possibly jet wash or endometrial biopsy. When the Pap smear is taken, the lower vagina can be swabbed and a cornification index requested from the laboratory. This will provide an assay of estrogen levels because the vaginal mucosa undergoes typical changes under estrogen influence, and the cells reflect different levels of maturation. A cervical biopsy is often included also, even in the absence of suspicious appearing lesions, because of the risk of cervical cancer. Some physicians routinely proceed to a D and C, even if the endometrial biopsy and the jet washing screen are negative.

A considerable degree of judgment enters into the decision of whether or not to do a D and C, and the women's individual menstrual and postmenopausal history are central to this decision. Women who have had irregular periods during the perimenopausal stage, or previous postmenopausal bleeding, who are obese, hypertensive, or diabetic, or who have had problems with fertility are at higher risk for endometrial carcinoma. There is also a high familial incidence; some studies indicate as high as 26 percent. If the woman has already had a D and C for postmenopausal bleeding, and if the present work-up shows that there is an estrogen effect on the vaginal mucosa, then her risk of endometrial carcinoma also increases. Any positive findings on pelvic examination, such as an enlarged uterus or pelvic masses, indicate further work-up. In these circumstances, a D and C is indicated as the next step. Even without these findings, however, postmenopausal bleeding in which there is any question about etiology would probably also necessitate a D and C by the physician.

One of the most common causes of postmenopausal bleeding is injudicious use of estrogen by the practitioner. When hormone therapy is instituted in this group, the lowest dose that will control the symptoms should be used, beginning with 0.625 mg. conjugated estrogen (Premarin). It is usually recommended that estrogen be given cyclically rather than continuously, on a 3-weeks-on 1-week-off schedule, to permit the endometrium to regress periodically. Some think that this might increase the incidence of bleeding from estrogen withdrawal, but lower doses could probably prevent spotting. However, postmenopausal estrogen therapy is becoming more controversial (see Chapter 8).

Submucous fibroids and polyps can also cause postmenopausal bleeding. As the vaginal mucosa is thin and easily traumatized, infections and intercourse can cause bleeding, usually in the form of light spotting. Urethral and rectal bleeding must also be ruled out, common causes being cystitis, urethral polyps, hemorrhoids, and fissures. Local treatment by use of estrogen vaginal creams (Dienestrol, Premarin) can help thin and dry vaginal mucosa, but it must be kept in mind that a considerable amount of the estrogen in these cases can be absorbed, causing systemic effects. One indication of an excess of systemic estrogen is breast tenderness.

Bleeding in the Young Girl

In the young girl prior to menarche, vaginal bleeding is very uncommon. If this is the presenting symptom, it is important to determine if the bleeding is really vaginal. Staining on the panties may be assumed to have a vaginal source, but can easily be from the urethra due to urethritis or cystitis, or the rectum due to scratching from pinworms, rectal fissures, or intestinal parasites. When the bleeding is vaginal in origin, and the girl has a normal physical appearance for her age, the most likely cause would be the presence of a foreign object in her vagina. Young girls are likely to explore themselves and experiment sexually by introducing some object into the vaginal opening. Lacerations are also a common cause of vaginal bleeding in young girls and may be self-inflicted in sexual experimentation or may be accidental due to falls or fighting. Vaginitis can also occur, though it is much less frequent in young girls than in menstruating females. Increased vaginal discharge and itching often accompany vaginitis, and the type of infecting organism should be identified by smear (a Q-tip introduced into the vaginal orifice can often obtain an adequate sample), and the appropriate treatment should be given. While Trichomonas, Candida and gonorrhea need to be ruled out, the most common type of vaginal infection in young girls is nonspecific and is usually treated with estrogen cream, good cleaning habits with mild soaps, and the use of clean cotton underwear.

If a local cause of bleeding is not apparent, systemic causes must be considered. The cause may be a blood dyscrasia, such as leukemia, or it may be drug effects from agents like griseofulvin (used to treat fungal infections). Here a complete history is of the utmost importance. Rule out the use of oral contraceptives, which might unadvisedly have been given to a premenstrual girl or taken without medical supervision. If secondary sex characteristics are present too soon, think of precocious puberty. Ovarian tumor or uterine sarcoma may be causes without secondary sex characteristic development.[13]

Another cause to consider if the girl's mother has a history of threatened miscarriage of that pregnancy which was treated with diethylstilbestrol is vaginal adenosis. Diethylstilbestrol was thought to be helpful in preventing miscarriage some years ago and was frequently given to women who were spotting during early pregnancy. Now it is found that daughters born of such pregnancies have an increased incidence of a rare form of vaginal cancer (clear-cell carcinoma), the forerunner of which may be vaginal adenosis. Adenosis is usually located in the anterior vaginal vault and is difficult to see without special techniques using the colposcope. Any girl with a positive history, whether or not there are any symptoms, should be referred to a gynecologist or, preferably, to a medical center where special screening programs for vaginal adenosis are being conducted.[14]

Dysmenorrhea

Menstrual cramps are very real pain and not nearly enough is known about their causes or treatment. Dismissing dysmenorrhea as being merely a psychogenic complaint has been an all too common practice, probably growing out of the fact that most physicians are male and cannot personally experience or identify with such pain, and the lack of emphasis on this type of problem in medical education. Although the data are incomplete (reflecting a lack of research funds and interest in this woman's complaint), there is some interesting information about the phenomenon. Dysmenorrhea is one of the most common conditions for which women seek help from the health professional, and an estimated 80 percent of all women have discomfort associated with menses, while about 10 percent of these women are incapacitated enough to lose time from school or work.[15]

Discomfort with menses takes the form of a syndrome or perhaps several syndromes. Almost all women have some sense of awareness that their period is about to begin. The prodromal symptoms may vary from slight breast tenderness, abdominal heaviness and mild irritability to severe multiple symptoms, including combinations of the following: edema and weight gain; abdominal bloating with other manifestations of disturbed bowel function such as constipation, diarrhea, or cramping; headache and feeling of fullness in the head; mood alterations, including anxiety, depression, and irritability; and pelvic, perineal, or leg ache. These symptoms usually are worst just prior to the onset of menses and begin to subside after the flow starts, but they may last through several days of bleeding. Unrelated problems such as migraine headache, spastic colitis, and epileptic seizures may be aggravated during the premenstrual phase of a woman's cycle.

This type of problem has been called premenstrual syndrome, premenstrual tension, and premenstrual molimina. No single specific cause has been identified, though it is evident that the syndrome is related to cyclic fluctuations in ovarian hormones. It tends to be more severe in cycles with irregular or abnormal ovarian activity, such as heavy bleeding, and usually increases during the later reproductive years when ovarian function declines and more abnormalities are associated with the menstrual cycle. Because weight gain is frequently associated with menses, a generalized edema due to sodium retention (one effect of estrogen, which is sodium sparing) has been used to explain many symptoms ranging from lower abdominal pain and bloating to breast tenderness to central nervous system manifestations such as nervousness, depression, headache, and irritability. Progesterone has a natriuretic effect, however, and any disequilibrium in the sodium balance is quickly compensated for by the renin-angiotensin system, thus progesterone is thought to counteract the estrogen effects. If an excess of estrogen is the cause of premenstrual symptoms, giving exogenous progesterone should help to relieve them. Although this does occasionally help, it often has no effect or may even aggravate the symptoms. Also, if generalized edema is the underlying cause of the symptoms, giving a diuretic should help. Diuretics do in fact provide good relief in some cases, but in others, while there is weight loss through diuresis, the other kinds of symptoms, particularly mood changes persist and are unaffected. In theory, the use of tranquilizers would help the depression and nervousness if these were of psychogenic origin, and while such psychotrophic drugs sometimes do help they are not always effective. While the underlying mechanisms do seem to involve fluid and electrolyte balance and undoubtedly certain vascular phenomena, these mechanisms are not well understood at present.[16]

Symptoms compatible with hypoglycemia are experienced premenstrually by some women. These include fatigue, faintness, or shaking attacks that are relieved by eating sweets. Some women show a flattened glucose tolerance curve during the premenstrual phase which resembles that of functional hypoglycemia, a syndrome associated with the tense, anxious woman who also has gastric hypermotility and excess gastric acidity.[17] Some of the effects of progesterone on insulin secretion and increased glucose load suggest that this hypoglycemic response of some women would seem to imply a malfunctioning during the late luteal phase, associated with progesterone production and secretion or with autosensitivity to the effects of endogenous progesterone, or the failure of target organ response, or the lack of certain enzymes which mediate the actions of progesterone.

Treatment of the premenstrual syndrome remains largely symptomatic. For a complete assessment, a menstrual history and a physical examination including a pelvic exam are done. In the absence of abnormalities, treatment can be aimed directly at the predominant symptoms. If congestion and fluid retention are present, diuretics such as hydrochlorthiazide 50 mg. orally may be given once or twice a day for 4 to 5 days preceding menses. This diuretic has relatively few side effects if used in low doses for short times; however, it has been known to cause blood dyscrasias. Some practitioners may want to use tranquilizers such as Valium or Librium if irritability, depression and nervousness are the dominant symptoms, but a philosophy of use should be developed by each practitioner (see Chapter 15). Diarrhea and intestinal cramping can be treated with antispasmodics, and constipation can be treated with increased roughage in the diet, bulk producers such as Metamucil, or stool softeners such as Colase. Disturbances of the menstrual cycle attributable to ovarian causes such as anovulation and unopposed estrogen effect should be treated as discussed previously.

Painful menstruation, dysmenorrhea per se, can be associated with the premenstrual syndrome or can occur with relatively few or no prodromal symptoms. There are two types of dysmenorrhea, primary and secondary. Primary dysmenorrhea is the term used to denote painful menses without associated physical abnormalities or pathology. Typically, the onset of primary dysmenorrhea is shortly after menarche, although there may be a 1 or 2 year interval from menarche to the beginning of painful periods. It is thought that the absence of ovulation during the first year or two following menarche is the reason for this pain-free time. Anovulatory bleeding tends to be painless, but if such bleeding is very heavy and associated with clotting, the pain can be considerable. There seem to be two different types of primary dysmenorrhea which have characteristic patterns and types of discomfort. Spasmodic primary dysmenorrhea usually starts with cramping on the first day of flow and lasts for 1 or 2 days. The pain is sharp and comes and goes in waves and is located in the lower abdomen and inner thighs. It is most common between the ages of 14 and 25 and is usually markedly improved or absent after pregnancy; it is relieved by taking oral contraceptives. Incoordinate, severe uterine contractions are thought to underlie spasmodic dysmenorrhea possibly related to a type of prostaglandin present in the luteal phase endometrium. Pregnancy somehow desensitizes the woman to this, and oral contraceptives alter the character of the endometrium, with resultant effects on prostaglandin activity. The second type, congestive primary dysmenorrhea, is felt as a dull, aching pain that often begins before menses and has associated premenstrual symptoms. The areas involved in discomfort are the lower abdomen and back, breasts, wrists, ankles and feet, and forehead and lower face. Symptoms related to edema affect many of these areas, with the typical bloating, cramping, weight gain, breast tenderness, and headache. The symptoms usually improve after 1 or 2 days of menstrual flow and gradually decrease. This type of dysmenorrhea often does not improve with age but gets worse. Each successive pregnancy may cause increased symptoms, and declining ovarian function toward the end of the reproductive years also contributes to increased symptomatology. Menopause is the cure. The causes of congestive dysmenorrhea are probably the same as for the premenstrual syndrome.

In the management of primary dysmenorrhea, the history is used not only to obtain data about menstrual experiences and to rule out significant organic problems, but also to assess certain emotional factors which often heavily color a woman's response to menstrual discomfort. A family history is an important guide to both inherited physiological responses and environmental influences which might set up patterns of perception and coping. Experiences of the patient's mother, sisters, and female relatives with their menses may predispose her to the expectation of severe pain and disability or, conversely, to a painless menses which in no way affects her usual functioning. The role of a woman in her own particular family structure affects the extent to which secondary gain from menstrual symptoms may be a factor, whether as a ploy for attention, excuse from usual duties, expression of hostility, or exercise in self-pity. While manipulative motives no doubt are involved in the expression of pain with menses by some women, this should not be assumed unless the history gives evidence of dissatisfactions with feminine identity, permissible expressions of the woman's role, or conflicts and resentments in marital or familial relations.

A chronically anxious woman may tend to somatize and thus exaggerate all sorts of body discomforts, menstrual cramping included. Or, sexual conflicts may be involved that are related to the woman's own sexual identity as manifest in this cyclic expression of femaleness, or vis-à-vis the male's reactions to menstruation. If there are cues that sexual conflicts may be involved, a sexual history can further explore these possibilities (see Chapter 2). Remember, however, that we do not understand all the causes of menstrual pain, and it is possible that this phenomenon could be purely physiologic and without psychic overlay in some women. In order to plan the patient's therapy, it is also necessary to determine the extent of disruption caused by dysmenorrhea. Inquire whether the woman can continue her regular activities or must she lie down? How long does the pain last? What treatments has she tried and how did they work? What other symptoms bother her, and in what other ways

does her period interfere with her activities and relations.

With a negative history and physical examination to check for serious pathology, the treatment begins with a discussion of the sources of menstrual pain and the interplay of mind and body. Sources of tension and conflict are evaluated and patterns of coping are identified. Information and education regarding menstrual functioning and women's cyclic physiology can be provided, as well as a discussion of sexuality and related concerns. If there are symptoms of hypoglycemia, encourage the patient to follow a high protein, low carbohydrate diet. Mild analgesics can be suggested, such as aspirin, Tylenol, or Darvon. Aspirin seems to be more effective than the other two, perhaps because it has a special antiprostaglandin effect. Most of the over-the-counter drugs for menstrual cramps are also relatively effective, probably due to their aspirin content. The use of narcotics and barbiturates is controversial and probably should be avoided because dysmenorrhea is a repeated regularly occurring problem, and the danger of addiction is high. With symptoms of edema and fluid retention, diuretics can be used for 4 or 5 days premenstrually. In spasmodic dysmenorrhea, oral contraceptives can provide good relief, if their use is appropriate, but oral contraceptives are strongly contraindicated in early adolescence and in women with documented irregular menses.

Secondary dysmenorrhea is defined as the onset of painful menses after having an established pattern of relatively comfortable periods. Often the cause can be traced to organic problems, although no pathology may be found. In the latter case, the cause is thought to be changes in the hormone balance between estrogen and progesterone. When a woman presents with a history of previously pain-free menses and then either a gradual or a sudden onset of dysmenorrhea, pathology must be assumed until proven otherwise. The history and physical examination provide the evidence needed to determine the nature of the problem. An important cue is just when the pain is felt in relation to menstrual bleeding. The age of the woman and recent history of gynecological surgery or procedures are also significant. Vaginal infections, especially gonorrhea, may be implicated, as well as abnormal bleeding or recent childbirth with or without complications.

A woman in the 30 to 40 age range with low fertility may describe gradually increasing dysmenorrhea which begins a short time prior to or with the onset of menses then gradually diminishes. The pain is often a dull aching or cramping in character and frequently involves the lower back and abdomen. She may also have pain with bowel movements during menstruation and painful intercourse between menses. This is a classic presentation of the symptoms of endometriosis, a disease in which there are endometrial implants scattered through the pelvic cavity, perhaps on the ovaries, uterosacral ligaments, rectum, or cul-de-sac. The pelvic examination may reveal nodules on the uterosacrals or ovaries or that the uterus is tender. Consult with the physician in the management of endometriosis.

Another typical history is one of a gynecological procedure such as conization or cauterization of the cervix, with the onset, several months later, of gradually increasing dysmenorrhea. The pain usually begins after the onset of menses and increases through the menstrual flow, then gradually resolves. The flow itself may be scanty, typically some dark brown spotting for several days but no heavy bright red flow. These conditions indicate the presence of cervical stenosis caused by a build up of scar tissue in the endocervical canal as a result of trauma from the procedure. On pelvic examination, the cervix will resist the insertion of a uterine sound or probe. The treatment is to break up the scar tissue and dilate the endocervical canal. It is done in consultation with the physician.

Dysmenorrhea which follows a recent treatment for vaginal infections, particularly gonorrhea, is probably secondary to the spread of the infection causing endometritis or pelvic inflammatory disease. The woman will usually have an elevated temperature and feelings of general malaise. A pelvic examination may reveal that purulent material is draining from the cervical os. The most important finding is an exquisitely tender uterus, in which even light pressure during the examination causes intense pain. The adnexa may or may not be full and tender. The treatment is to administer systemic antibiotics, with hospitalization if indicated (see Chapter 11).

A less specific history may suggest other types of uterine pathology. The onset of dysmenorrhea is gradual, but the quality of pain and its location are highly variable. The cause may be adenomyosis or fibroids (see p. 113) confirmed by pelvic examination, or cervical or uterine polyps which may or may not be evident on examination.

If dysmenorrhea increases after childbirth and is associated with the premenstrual syndrome, it may be of the congestive type which was mild enough to be overlooked before. However, broad ligament tears may be involved, particularly if the woman also has dyspareunia on deep penetration. Also, if there was extensive laceration of the cervix during delivery, cervical stenosis due to scarring is also a possibility. These may be confirmed by examination although often laparoscopy is needed to diagnose broad ligament tears, and referral to the physician is in order.

The health provider's approach to dysmenorrhea needs to be thoughtful and sensitive. Emotional and physical factors must be carefully evaluated. Often the health provider's attitudes are as important as counseling and other supportive therapy for this most common of women's problems.

NOTES

1. P. Weideger, *Menstruation and Menopause: The Physiology and Psychology, the Myth and Reality* (New York: Alfred A. Knopf, 1976), pp. 85-113.
2. R. E. Frisch and R. Revelle, "Height and Weight at Menarche and a Hypothesis of Critical Body Weights and Adolescent Events." *Science* 169, 397 (July 1970): 397-99.
3. S. L. Romney, et al., *Gynecology and Obstetrics: The Health Care of Women* (New York: McGraw-Hill, Blakiston, 1975), pp. 126-27.
4. *Ibid.*, pp. 373-83.
5. L. Chiazze, Jr., et al., "The Length and Variability of the Human Menstrual Cycle." *JAMA* 203, 6 (February 5, 1968): 89-92.
6. J. M. Bardwick, *Psychology of Women* (New York: Harper & Row, 1971), pp. 32-39.
7. K. Dalton, *The Menstrual Cycle* (New York: Pantheon Books, 1971).
8. Weideger, *Menstruation and Menopause*, pp. 184-89.
9. "Secondary Amenorrhea: Why Has She Missed Six Cycles?" *Patient Care* (October 15, 1972): 64-71.
10. "Primary Amenorrhea: Why Haven't Her Menses Started?" *Patient Care* (October 15, 1972): 74-82.
11. "Abnormal GYN Bleeding: Diagnosis and Treatment During Childbearing Years." *Patient Care* (October 15, 1973): 20-60.

12. "Abnormal GYN Bleeding: When the Postmenopausal Woman Bleeds." *Patient Care* (December 1, 1973): 70-93.
13. "Abnormal GYN Bleeding: When a Youngster Bleeds Vaginally." *Patient Care* (November 1, 1973): 56-70.
14. "Are There Stilbestrol Babies in Your Practice?" *Patient Care* (November 1, 1973): 73-75.
15. Romney, et al., *Gynecology and Obstetrics*, p. 151.
16. *Ibid.*, pp. 166-67.
17. M. A. Friederich and A. Labrum, "Evaluation and Preferred Management of Premenstrual Tension: Pelvic Congestive Syndrome and Allied States." In *Controversy in Obstetrics and Gynecology*, D. E. Reid and C. D. Christian (eds.) (Philadelphia: W. B. Saunders, 1974), pp. 760-75.

5

Pregnancy

Most women will experience pregnancy in their lifetime. However, the choice to remain childless is both more readily made and more widely accepted now than in preceding decades. Pregnancy is a biological process invested with great social meaning and surrounded by values, customs, and laws in all human societies. Reproduction is a private act, but it is not a private affair; there are far-reaching social consequences of the choices individuals make concerning whether to bear children, at what age, and how many. The personal meanings of childbearing are influenced by pervasive social values, religious belief systems, governmental policies, economic and educational factors, and family or reference group traditions. Of growing importance in women's attitudes toward childbearing is the change now happening in women's roles and status. Pregnancy, motherhood, and the care of the family no longer need monopolize the majority of a woman's adult years; shared parenting responsibility and the move toward equality of opportunity for life choices have opened other vistas for women.

As a personal experience, pregnancy can be of central importance in several ways. It may be a time of growth, a developmental process leading to maturation in which challenge and learning, stress and mastery have pivotal roles. The fulfillment of various aspects of feminine identity is accomplished by pregnancy, in the realization of reproductive potential through the unique female generative function. Social reinforcement of femininity and positive recognition of worth are triggered by pregnancy in most cases—at least pregnancy which occurs in a socially acceptable context. Pregnancy can

be an expression of primal creativity, a thread of immortality, and a sign of generativity in service to the species. As an adventure into self-awareness, pregnancy can bring a woman into closer touch with her physical and emotional self. The many mood and body changes, the sensations and feelings accompanying pregnancy provide multiple opportunities for exploration, insight, and learning about individual response.

Ideally, pregnancy should only occur when it is planned and desired. In fact, many women are pregnant who do not want to be and bear children who are not wanted. In part this is due to conflicts in a time of transition in social values and cultural norms, in part to ignorance, and in part to shortcomings in contraceptive technology. Even with planned pregnancy there may be ambivalence, of course, because it is a commitment to a sequence of events with continuing impact on the lives of the parents. Thus many women have mixed feelings about being pregnant, for although the choices are wider today—with abortion available, less dominance of motherhood as the central theme of women's lives, and a changing ethic of shared parenting responsibilities—the burden of childrearing still remains with the woman. Attitudes change more rapidly than practices, and the necessary institutional supports which would enable women to realize their new options remain largely lacking.

GOALS OF REPRODUCTIVE CARE

Pregnancy has an interesting characteristic from the point of view of the health care provider: it is a part of normal physiology but represents an unusual state occurring only a few times during a woman's lifespan. Major changes take place in almost all body systems which are largely reversible, but which alter the function of these systems significantly while present. Patients generally diagnose the condition themselves, are prone to study it, and may be more knowledgeable in some areas than providers. They develop certain expectations about the care indicated and the conditions surrounding labor and delivery, and they usually attach great positive meaning to the event. Childbearing has only recently in human history moved from the domain of the family to the professional domain, and current ferment promises to bolster family involvement and control. The trend toward naturalism exerts a strong influence upon the nature of the health services provided. There is widespread use of prepared childbirth techniques which require the mother's full awareness during birth and the involvement of her partner and companions. Women and providers increasingly avoid the use of drugs during pregnancy and childbirth. There is an upsurge of interest and support for breast feeding, and increasingly parents request nontraumatic approaches to birth. Alternate maternity care, often including delivery at home or in special birth units resembling hotels more than hospitals, is gaining advocates. Parents and professionals are rediscovering the importance of continuous, close contact between mother and infant following birth if optimal bonding is to occur. Decreasing birth and fertility rates and increasing consumer power have combined to place the management of pregnancy in a new perspective (Table 5-1).

The goals of prenatal care include assuring the health of both mother and fetus during a normal gestation and parturition, reducing discomfort and danger, and minimizing any intrusion on normal birth and bonding. The provider is responsible for monitoring the progression of pregnancy and identifying problems and risks early. Information and education comprise a large part of prenatal care. Concurrent illnesses must be managed carefully and conservatively. Preparation for childbirth is largely the woman's responsibility, whether undertaken in a formal program or individually, but she should have professional support and reinforcement.

Significant problems in achieving good childbirth experiences still remain. Not all women and their families have access to quality prenatal care. Inequitable educational and economic levels affect both health-seeking behavior and opportunity. Reproductive care as practiced by providers may conflict with the needs and desires of their clients. Active medical intervention and management of pregnancy and labor may create more problems than it solves—not only client dissatisfaction, but also iatrogenic morbidity. It has been estimated that 80 to 90 percent of all women are perfectly capable of delivering themselves normally without any help from professionals and that there is a point of diminishing return in interfering with the delicately balanced biology of childbirth.[1] While medical technology is invaluable for many women with complicated pregnancies, for the vast majority of women undergoing a normal, natural process the professional better serves by "following" the pregnancy and standing by while the woman "delivers herself."

PHYSIOLOGY OF PREGNANCY AND RELATED SYMPTOMS

Most of the physiological changes that occur during pregnancy are obligatory. The organ systems must alter in order to respond to the increased demands of pregnancy. If an organ is damaged or diseased so that it cannot respond, decompensation and the signs and symptoms of impaired function will occur. Pregnancy, however, is not a parasitic state. Under normal circumstances, the changes that occur enable both the mother's and fetus's needs to be met, and the demands of the fetus are not met at the expense of the mother. Many changes do not produce appreciable symptoms of which the mother may be aware, but others cause the widely known and familiar signs and symptoms of pregnancy.

Hormone and Endocrine Changes

The pattern of circulating hormones changes markedly in a menstrual cycle in which fertilization takes place. Implantation of the blastocyst takes place about 7 days after fertilization, and by the seventeenth day true placental circulation has been established. Progesterone, instead of falling on about the tenth postovulatory day, rises steadily until the third or

Table 5-1
Reproductive Statistics

	1974 (final)	1975 (provisional)
Number of births	3,159,958	3,149,000
Birth rate (births/1000 population)	14.9	14.8
Fertility rate (births/1000 women age 15-44)	68.4	66.7
Maternal mortality rate (deaths/100,000 live births)	14.6	10.8
Infant mortality rate (deaths below one year/1000 live births)	16.7	16.1
Neonatal mortality rate (deaths below 28 days/1000 live births)	12.3	11.7

R. M. Pitkin and J. R. Scott (eds.), *The Yearbook of Obstetrics and Gynecology 1977* (Chicago: Yearbook Medical Publishers, 1977), p. 443.

fourth week of pregnancy when it falls temporarily. After the eighth week it rises again until term, falling slightly before the onset of labor. In the secretory phase of the menstrual cycle, plasma progesterone is 5 to 10 ng. per ml.; by the end of pregnancy the level approaches 150 ng. per ml. The corpus luteum is present throughout pregnancy but becomes much less active after pregnancy is well established. The placenta takes over the major production of progesterone, synthesizing it from cholesterol obtained from the maternal circulation.

Human chorionic gonadotropin (HCG) starts to rise rapidly about 10 days after ovulation. It is a glycoprotein consisting of an alpha (α) and a beta (β) subunit; the α subunit seems identical with luteinizing hormone (LH). Produced by the syncytiotrophoblast, HCG rises sharply after implantation and reaches a peak value about days 60 to 70 of gestation. After this, it gradually falls until the 120th day of gestation, when it remains at a constant lower level throughout pregnancy. The plasma level of HCG is 0.1 IU per ml. in early pregnancy, reaches peak values of 120 IU per ml. and plateaus at about 20 IU per ml. for the rest of pregnancy. Within 2 weeks after delivery, HCG disappears from circulation. In early pregnancy, HCG appears important for maintaining the corpus luteum, but its physiologic role in later pregnancy is not known. There may be an immunologic role through inhibition of lymphocyte response to "foreign placenta."[2]

Human chorionic somatotropin (HCS) is a protein hormone immunologically similar to human (pituitary) growth hormone (HGH). Also produced by the syncytiotrophoblast, it appears in the serum in very early pregnancy and rises steadily to peak levels of 6 to 7 mcg./ml. at term. Human chorionic somatotropin stimulates lipolysis, inhibits gluconeogenesis, and may have an anabolic effect on mother and fetus. It is thought partly responsible for the diabetogenic nature of pregnancy. The synergistic action of HCS with hydrocortisone and insulin in the development of the alveoli of the breast produces a lactogenic effect.

Plasma follicle-stimulating hormone (FSH) falls rapidly to very low levels around the tenth postovulatory day and remains low throughout pregnancy. The pituitary gland is relatively inactive, probably suppressed by steroids from the corpus luteum. It also secretes very little HGH during pregnancy. There is an increase in size, however, with the development of characteristic "pregnancy cells" of the anterior pituitary. The adrenal cortex produces increased corticosteroid-binding globulin, resulting in an increase in bound cortisol in response to increased estrogen levels. After the fifteenth week of pregnancy there is an increase in aldosterone secretion, causing the retention of sodium.

The thyroid increases in size during pregnancy, due to hyperplasia and increased vascularity. Estrogens cause an increase in thyroid-binding globulin, producing an increase in thyroid hormone but no major increase in free thyroxin, the biologically active form of the hormone. Because of these increases, thyroid function tests must be interpreted cautiously. Protein-bound iodine (PBI) values rise during pregnancy, as does radioactive iodine uptake and the clearance of inorganic iodine. Enlargement of the thyroid gland is often apparent (goiter of pregnancy). These changes reflect increased thyroid activity in compensation for the physiologic effects of increased thyroid-binding globulin. Although the basal metabolic rate rises in pregnancy, this is largely due to increased growth and oxygen consumption by the pregnant uterus, the fetus, and placenta.

Estrogens are produced by the syncytiotrophoblast, but the placenta is not a complete endocrine organ because it cannot synthesize estrogens from simple substances like acetate or cholesterol. Many of the precursors of estrogenic hormones come from the fetus. Estradiol is formed from both maternal and fetal precursors, estrone is elaborated by the placenta also, but estriol makes up a major proportion of urinary estrogen and is most useful in evaluating the function of the fetoplacental unit. Estriol is formed from precursors of maternal and fetal origin and is widely used as an index of fetal welfare. Urinary estriol values rise gradually throughout the course of a normal pregnancy, from microgram amounts in the nonpregnant woman to 1 mg. or more per 24 hours during early pregnancy. By the end of pregnancy urinary excretion of 30 to 40 mg. of estriol per 24 hours is usual.

The widespread organ system changes of pregnancy are mediated through the effects of estrogen and progesterone. Estrogen is concerned with the growth of the fetus, decidua, myometrium, and breasts, and it alters the functions of other endocrine organs. Progesterone causes proliferation of the decidua to meet the nutritional needs of the growing embryo, affects alveolar growth of the breasts, plays a part in maintaining fluid and electrolyte balance, and exerts significant effects on smooth muscles.

Weight Gain

There is wide variation in the amount of weight gained during pregnancy, but an average is about 24 to 27 lb. (10.0 to 12.3 kg.). Most women gain weight somewhat in excess of that contributed by the fetus, placenta, amniotic fluid, increased blood volume, and increased size of uterus and breasts. Much of the additional weight is due to the increased deposition of fat and is thought to be a protective mechanism to provide a readily available source of energy, should the fetus need it. There is an increased protein need of about 500 Gm. for the fetus and placenta and an additional 500 Gm. for increases in maternal uterus, breasts, and blood (Table 5-2).

WATER BALANCE. There is an average increase in total body water of 6.8 L. during pregnancy, in the absence of clinically apparent edema. Until 30 weeks gestation this increase is attributable to the fetus, placenta, amniotic fluid, uterus, breasts, and increased maternal blood volume. Closer to term there is an additional 1 to 2 L. of extracellular fluid, amounting to about 7,500 gm. in women without edema. This rises to 7,880 Gm. with leg edema and 10,830 gm. with generalized edema. About 40 percent of pregnant women have dependent edema in the ankles and lower legs, which usually disappears after rest, and is rarely present in the morning. This edema is due to fluid retention under hormone influences and venous pressure in the iliofemoral veins, intensified by standing for long periods. Elevation of the legs improves return circulation, and moderate sodium restriction may retard edema formation. Diuretics are contraindicated and may be dangerous. Generalized edema involving hands and face may be an ominous sign of toxemia.

Carbohydrate Metabolism

Changes occur in carbohydrate metabolism, with pancreatic beta-cell hyperactivity beginning toward the end of the first trimester and reaching its maximum at term. Circulating insulin is increased but seems less effective in lowering blood sugar, either due to cellular resistance to the effects of insulin or increased destruction of insulin. Mean blood glucose levels remain within the normal nonpregnant range, but glycosuria occurs in about 10 percent of pregnant women. The renal threshold for excretion of glucose is lowered due to an increased glomerular filtration rate without an increase in tubular reabsorption of glucose. The urine normally contains glucose postprandially in pregnancy, and there may be spilling with blood glucose of 120 mg. per dl.

Genital Organs

UTERUS. During pregnancy the uterus increases remarkably in size, and its volume is increased by 500 times. Its weight increases from 50 to 1000 Gm. and its capacity from 2 ml. to 5000 ml. This is accomplished mainly through hypertrophy of individual muscle cells, each fiber becoming ten times longer and five times thicker. There is also the formation of some new muscle cells and the development of fibroelastic tissue around muscle bundles. The contractility of the uterus also increases,

Table 5-2
Components of Weght Gain in Normal Pregnancy

Component	Amount (gm.) gained at:	10 Weeks	20 Weeks	30 Weeks	40 Weeks
Fetus		5	300	1500	3300
Placenta		20	170	430	650
Amniotic fluid		30	250	600	800
Uterus		135	585	810	900
Breasts		34	180	360	405
Maternal blood		100	600	1300	1250
Total gain of pregnancy (rounded)		320	2100	5000	7300
Total gain of body weight		650	4000	8500	12500
Weight not accounted for (total gain of body weight minus total gain of pregnancy rounded)		330	1900	3500	5200

R. C. Benson, *Current Obstetric & Gynecologic Diagnosis & Treatment* (Los Altos, Calif.: Lange Medical Publications, 1976), p. 69.

and the contractions that can be felt after the first trimester become progressively stronger as term approaches.

The uterine shape changes from its nonpregnant flattened, triangular configuration and may at first enlarge asymmetrically with bulging over the site of implantation. It loses its firmness and resistance and becomes globular in shape until about the sixth month. After this time the uterus becomes ovoid and during the third trimester rotates to the right (dextrorotation) because the rectosigmoid colon is on the left. Changes in uterine consistency are noted beginning the sixth week past the last menstrual period with softening of the isthmus and easy compressibility. The cervix still is relatively firm as is the fundus, and the softened isthmus produces a sensation of the detachment of the fundus from the cervix (Hegar's sign). The cervix softens about the eighth week (Goodell's sign) and is often patulous enough at term to admit a fingertip. The fundus also softens.

During the first 8 weeks of gestation, the uterus remains a pelvic organ, but by the ninth week it can be palpated above the symphysis pubis. By the twelfth week it has become an intraabdominal organ and can readily be palpated externally. The top of the fundus is halfway between the symphysis and the umbilicus at 16 weeks, reaches the umbilicus at 20 to 22 weeks, and is at the xyphoid and costal margins at 36 weeks. With the engagement and descent of the fetal head into the true pelvis, fundal height decreases by 2 cm. (lightening). This usually occurs in the last week or two of pregnancy in primigravidas and with the onset

of labor in multigravidas. The coiled uterine arteries gradually straighten and permit better circulation to the enlarged uterus, and there is greatly increased venous drainage. Blood flow through the uterine vessels progressively increases during pregnancy and is about 500 ml. per minute at term. This flow is markedly diminished during contractions.

CERVIX. As pregnancy progresses, the cervix becomes more congested and soft. Hypertrophy of the endocervical glands results in the increased production of cervical mucus which normally does not form a fern pattern. The endocervical columnar epithelium proliferates and is thrown into large folds, frequently everting into the visible portion of the cervix. Thick, tenacious mucus accumulates within the cervical canal to form the mucus plug which is expelled at the onset of labor with the disruption of the cervical vasculature, causing the bloody show. The cervix becomes somewhat effaced and slightly dilated as term approaches, particularly in multigravidas.

VAGINA. The increase in vascularity and in congestion causes a bluish discoloration of the vaginal mucosa at about 6 to 8 weeks (Chadwick's sign). There is a considerable loosening of connective tissue to permit greater distensibility, and hypertrophy of smooth muscle cells. The vaginal walls increase in length. An increased amount of glycogen in the epithelial cells normally occurs. Vaginal secretion is increased, causing a leukorrhea which is high in glycogen. This stimulates the growth of vaginal bacilli, leading to an increased lactic acid content that reduces vaginal pH to 4.0 to 6.0. Although this keeps the vagina relatively free from pathogenic bacteria, Candida grow well in this environment.

OVARIES AND OVIDUCTS. The ovaries are large and white, without active follicles except the corpus luteum of pregnancy. On the surface there may be friable, pink, papillary excrescences which are patches of decidual reaction in response to progesterone. Ovarian vasculature hypertrophies. The oviducts become elongated, but no actual hypertrophy occurs. The epithelial lining remains low, with occasional decidual reactions.

BREAST. Tenderness, tingling, and engorgement of the breasts occur from the first few weeks of pregnancy to about 2 months. They increase in size and become more firm, due to an increase in the alveoli. Superficial veins enlarge and become noticeable, and there is increased blood supply. The nipples become larger, darker, and more erectile. The hypertrophy of the sebaceous glands in the areola produces tiny protrusions (Montgomery's tubercles). The areola becomes more pigmented and enlarges. Colostrum may be expressed in midpregnancy but is more common as term approaches.

Blood and Cardiovascular System

Blood volume begins to increase after about 8 to 10 weeks gestation, averaging about 1,500 ml., of which 450 ml. are red cells and 1000 ml. is plasma. Maximum volume expansion of 25 to 60 percent is reached by 35 to 36 weeks, where it remains constant until after delivery, returning to prepregnancy levels within 4 weeks. Several physiologic events contribute to this increase, including progesterone-induced generalized smooth muscle relaxation, arteriolar dilatation, and increased capacity of the vascular compartment. Progesterone is also natriuretic, causing a mild hyponatremia. This activates the renin-angiotensin system, leading to increased vascular tone and to aldosterone production and antidiuretic hormone (ADH) release. These hormones reduce the renal excretion of salt and water, thus increasing intravascular volume and electrolyte content.

There is increased erythropoiesis during pregnancy, but relatively more plasma is produced, so normally there is a decline in hemoglobin concentration and hematocrit. Hemoglobin decreases from an average in the nonpregnant woman of 13.3 Gm. per dl. to an average of 12.1 Gm. per dl. in the pregnant woman, reaching its lowest point at 32 to 34 weeks. The increase in red cell count requires about 500 mg. iron, and additionally about 800 mg. are needed for the production of blood in the fetoplacental unit. The normal rate of excretion of iron accounts for another 200 mg. needed during pregnancy. Thus, the amount of iron needed to meet physiologic demands during pregnancy is about 1.5 Gm. The stored iron available in the mother is only about 500 mg., and although absorption of iron seems increased in pregnancy, the total amount of iron available from storage and intestinal uptake usually does not provide an adequate supply, especially during the second half of gestation. Exogenous iron supplementation is required, particularly in late pregnancy.

Plasma fibrinogen and factors VII, VIII, IX, and X are increased in pregnancy, and there is an increased platelet count. However, there is a decrease in prothrombin time and partial thromboplastin time in late pregnancy, and no significant increase in intravascular coagulation problems has been noted. This paradox is not understood. Total protein concentration falls moderately mainly due to decreased albumin. Plasma oncotic pressure is lowered, erythrocyte sedimentation rate (ESR) raised, and the albumin/globulin ratio reversed. Plasma lipids (cholesterol, phospholipids, free fatty acids) rise gradually; alkaline phosphatase and SGOT rise markedly. There is generally a leukocytosis during pregnancy, with a white blood cell count between 10,000 and 12,000 per mm.

Cardiac output increases by about 30 percent during the first and second trimesters and remains elevated until delivery. The maximum is reached after about 28 to 32 weeks. The output of the heart is increased primarily by increased stroke volume, although some is due to a faster pulse rate (seldom more than a 10 percent increase over the value found in nonpregnant women). Systolic blood pressure remains essentially unchanged, with a slight decrease in diastolic blood pressure as a result of decreased peripheral resistance. There is no change in venous pressure in the upper body, but it is markedly increased in the lower extremities when the woman is supine, sitting, or standing. In these positions, venous pressure rises 10 to 30 cm. of water. The pressure of the enlarged uterus on pelvic veins and the inferior vena cava causes retardation of return blood flow from the extremities to the heart, decreased cardiac output, a fall in blood pressure, and edema. This predisposes the woman to varicosities of the legs and vulva, to edema, and to faintness from hypotensive effects. The supine position aggravates these problems.

The increased blood flow occurs mainly in the uterus, kidneys, and skin, but there are slight increases to the breasts and intestines also. An increased cutaneous flow serves to dissipate the excess heat generated by increases in metabolism. The heart is displaced upward and to the left because of the elevation of the diaphragm by the enlarging uterus. This causes a left axis deviation on the ECG. Systolic murmurs over the pulmonary valve and at the apex are common. An increase in cardiac volume of about 10 percent has been noted in normal pregnancy, probably due to cardiac dilatation. Palpitations are frequently felt by women during pregnancy.

Respiratory System and Ear, Nose, and Throat

Oxygen consumption increases by almost 20 percent during pregnancy. This is accomplished by an increased tidal volume and a slightly increased respiratory rate. Ventilation rate rises to about 10 L. per minute, or an increase of 40 percent. The diaphragm is displaced upward due to the enlarging uterus, and in compensation there is an expansion of the rib cage, permitted by a relaxation of costosternal and costovertebral ligaments. Vital capacity does not change significantly. However, expiratory reserve, residual volume, and functional residual capacity are decreased. This, together with the increased tidal volume, allows a more effective mixing of gases so that the alveolar ventilation increases by about 65 percent. As a result, there is a decrease in alveolar pCO_2 and in blood bicarbonate, but no or little change in blood pH. Pulmonary resistance is decreased, and airway conductance increased. Mild dyspnea on exertion is consistently noted, especially in late pregnancy. Deep respirations or sighing may be more frequent.

The tissues of the respiratory tract and nasopharynx exhibit hyperemia and edema. There may be engorgement of turbinates with nasal stuffiness and mouth breathing. Nasal and sinus secretion is increased, nosebleeds more common, and vocal cord edema may cause changes in voice. Hypertrophy of the gums and hyperemia often occur (pregnancy epulis), appearing in about the second month. Occasionally an increased vascularity of the tympanic membranes and decreased hearing due to the blockage of the eustachian tubes may be reported.

Urinary System

A generalized atony and dilatation of the urinary system is characteristic of pregnancy, and results in the retention of urine and a susceptibility to infection. Both the renal plasma flow (RPF) and the glomerular filtration rate (GFR) increase in early pregnancy and remain elevated by 50 percent and 25 percent respectively. Position is important, with both GFR and RPF decreased when the woman is standing. Pregnant women produce less urine during the day and more at night. Frequency of urination is experienced early in pregnancy due to the displacement of the bladder as the uterus changes size and position. After the fourth month, vascular engorgement and hormonal changes lead to urinary statis, with residual urine in the bladder, and to the incompetency of the vesicoureteral junction, with ureteral urinary reflux. The ureters become elongated, somewhat tortuous, and dilated—especially above the pelvic brim—and displaced laterally. The right side is more affected due to dextrorotation. Calyceal dilatation also occurs, due to pressure and smooth muscle relaxation. The ureterocalyceal capacity is about twice that of the nonpregnant woman by the end of pregnancy, and a considerable increase in dead space in the collecting system predisposes the pregnant woman to cystitis and pyelitis. Asymptomatic bacteriuria occurs in 5 or 6 percent of pregnant women. All changes related to gestation resolve within 4 to 6 weeks of delivery. Acute pyelonephritis is one of the most common medical complications of pregnancy, with a 2 percent incidence (see Chapter 10, Urinary Problems).

Gastrointestinal System

The smooth muscle throughout the gastrointestinal system becomes more atonic during pregnancy. This creates the greatest number of pregnancy symptoms which women report.

Relaxation of the cardiac sphincter permits esophageal reflux of gastric contents, causing heartburn (pyrosis). Gastric emptying time is prolonged, perhaps contributing to nausea. Acid and pepsin production are decreased. The motility of the large bowel is diminished, often explaining the gaseous distention and constipation so frequently noted.

Nausea and vomiting are the most common complaints of early pregnancy; no doubt the problem has an endocrine basis related to high levels of HCG and progesterone and their effects upon smooth musculature. Although more common in the morning, nausea may occur throughout the day and is often associated with certain odors. Dehydration is seldom a concern unless vomiting is severe and persistent. This problem usually disappears around the end of the third month.

Heartburn is frequent throughout pregnancy because of acid changes, delayed gastric emptying and reflux. Temporary hiatal hernia occurs in 20 to 30 percent of pregnant women and contributes to this problem. Varices appear in the distal two-thirds of the esophagus in the second half of pregnancy, an effect of hypervascularity. The decrease in large bowel motility results in constipation, a common complaint. The colon retains its absorptive capacity, and delayed transit of fecal material causes increased dehydration of the fecal mass with increased solidarity and more difficulty in evacuation. The cecum is progressively displaced laterally as the uterus enlarges, moving also upward and posteriorly. This changes the anatomic situation of the appendix, and signs of appendicitis during pregnancy may not be localized to the right lower quadrant as anticipated otherwise.

Ptyalism, or excessive salivation, is not frequent but does occur in a small number of women and is very troublesome. Pica is the ingestion of substances with no food value, such as clay and laundry starch. It is probably not due to physiologic craving but is a folkway or custom in some subcultural groups, especially those located in the southeastern United States. Pica can be harmful when it interferes with good nutrition by substituting nonnutritious bulk.

Hemorrhoids are frequent and cause considerable discomfort during pregnancy. The pressure of the uterus on the venous return from the lower extremities is a major factor in causing hemorrhoids, as it is with varicose veins. Constipation and hard stools also contribute to this problem. Swelling, pain, and rectal bleeding are common symptoms. Most hemorrhoids which develop during pregnancy resolve after delivery, but intermittent problems with these anal varices may persist.

Liver function seems unchanged during pregnancy. There is some bile stasis both in the liver and the gallbladder, and cholestatic jaundice may occur particularly in late pregnancy. Gallstones are more common in multigravidas.

Skin

Melanin is increased during pregnancy due to the greater activity of melanocyte-stimulating hormone. Hyperpigmentation occurs as a streak in the abdominal midline (linea nigra) and in the nipples and areola, and there is often irregular mottling of the cheeks and forehead (mask of pregnancy). The skin may also be darkened over bony prominences, the labia majora, and the perineum and perianal area. Preexisting nevi may become larger and more intensely pigmented, and new nevi appear. Recent scars generally become more pigmented. These resolve, in varying degree, after pregnancy.

Vascular changes are expressed cutaneously, including a diffuse vasodilation or blushing, thought to be due to elevated circulating estrogen. This vasodilation also produces spider angiomas in 10 to 15 percent of pregnant women, primarily in the distribution of vessels draining into the superior vena cava (upper chest and extremities). Stasis of blood flow is also involved in this sludging effect and consequent telangiectasia. These appear after 2 to 5 months of gestation, and most disappear postpartally. Localized areas of erythema of the fingers and fingertips, and irregular mottled palmar erythema are part of this vascular phenomenon.

The hair tends to straighten with occasional hair loss in the frontal and parietal regions. Rarely, there may be an increase in facial hair and body hair between the umbilicus and the symphysis; this increase is thought to be related to increased androgens and corticotropic hormones. Increased sweating from exocrine glands is common and usually occurs in the first trimester and postpartally. Pruritis, either localized or widespread, is a leading skin complaint which is perhaps due to estrogen effects. Women with pruritis of pregnancy frequently develop pruritis also when taking oral contraceptives.

Musculoskeletal System

During pregnancy the fibrocartilage which lines pelvic articulations becomes thick and softens, and the ligaments which bind the pelvic joints also soften, producing increased mobility of the symphysial, sacrococcygeal and sacroiliac synchondroses. Although this does not visibly enlarge pelvic diameters, it does permit slight gliding and rotating movements. These changes are responsible for the high incidence of backache during pregnancy, usually localized in the sacroiliac and lumbar areas. As the enlarged uterus presses forward on the abdominal wall, there is a compensatory muscular distention, and the pelvis tilts forward, creating an increased lumbar lordosis. This is compensated for by accentuated dorsal kyphosis and cervical lordosis to maintain balance. Slumping of the shoulders is increased by the downward pull of the enlarged breasts. Cervical spine and thoracic pain are also frequent discomforts. Pelvic and postural changes may produce a waddling gait.

Leg cramps in pregnancy may be due to an elevation of serum phosphorus with a diet of substantially increased milk intake. Phosphorus binds calcium, which is consumed in proportionately smaller amounts, and may deplete muscular stores in order to achieve a serum balance. However, correlation between calcium levels and muscular cramps has not been well established. A variety of discomforts and sensations in the legs is attributed to nerve compression. Numbness in the lateral femoral area may be due to the compression of that nerve beneath the inguinal ligament, and medial thigh sensory changes may be due to the compression of the obturator nerve against the pelvic sidewall. Periodic numbness and tingling of the fingers affects at least 5 percent of pregnant women; it is a brachial plexus traction syndrome due to drooping shoulders. The discomfort is most common at night and early in the morning and may progress to partial anesthesia and impaired manual function. Carpal tunnel syndrome is caused by the compression of the median nerve due to the physiologic changes in fascia, tendons, and connective tissue in pregnancy. It is characterized by a paroxysm of pain, numbness, tingling or burning in the sides of the hands and fingers (thumb,

second and third fingers, lateral side of the fifth finger). Skilled movement of fingers may be impaired.

Abdominal pain of varying degrees frequently occurs, and its causes can range from bowel distention and cramping to tension and traction of uterine ligaments, particularly the round ligament. Serious intraabdominal disease must be ruled out. Sometimes rupture of connective tissue as the abdominal wall distends, vigorous kicking of the fetus, and muscle strain can be the cause. Increasing pelvic pressure and aching from congestion occur in later pregnancy.

PSYCHOLOGICAL PROCESSES OF PREGNANCY

Pregnancy is one of the developmental crises of the human life cycle. Like puberty and menopause, pregnancy is a time which involves profound endocrine and general somatic changes, as well as important psychological changes. Pregnancy is developmental in that it is a biological and social event which serves to move the woman and her partner and family from one point in the life cycle to another; such as from mate to parent, from family of three to family of four. Pregnancy is a crisis because the woman's steady state is disrupted and the demands for adaptation are different from those she has known in other situations before. The impact of this event is so great that parents' and families' usual modes of coping with stress are often inadequate, resulting in a state of disequilibrium. In seeking new ways of adapting, they may experience some disorganization and confusion, and resort to earlier forms of behavior. Pregnancy thus constitutes a biologically determined developmental crisis which involves significant physical and psychological changes. It signifies a turning point from one developmental phase to the next (Figure 5-1).

There appear to be specific psychological tasks connected with bodily and emotional changes which the woman works through during pregnancy. The tasks involve a process of incorporation, differentiation, and finally separation of the fetus from the mother. Initially the woman must accept the fetus as present in and a part of her body (incorporation), then she must realize that although the fetus is within her it actually has its separate identity (differentiation), and finally she must prepare to give up the fetus and to enter a different relation with the newborn (separation).[3] The psychological timetable of pregnancy is not as precise as the physiological one, but there is an orderly progression of changing themes in pregnant women's interests and concerns.

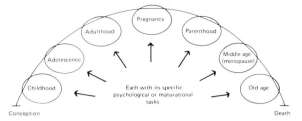

Figure 5-1. Developmental stages accompanying critical life changes.

Tasks of Early Pregnancy

The realization that pregnancy is a fact and not just a possibility carries considerable psychological impact. Whether conception was planned or desired or not, most women are ambivalent initially. They have both positive and negative feelings toward their pregnancy and experience increased anxiety. Although the woman knows she is pregnant, it is not yet apparent. She may share the information selectively, watch people's responses, seek internal and external reinforcement that her body is really different now. In the first trimester, women have an increased awareness of bodily changes and tend to focus inward. There are often mood swings, with marked fluctuations from euphoria to sadness, occurring rapidly and without connection to external events. Hypersensitivity and overreaction are often reported, causing women some embarrassment.

Pregnant women become concerned with their relation with their own mother toward the end of the first trimester. This is a complex task laden with guilt and conflict and is one of the most withdrawn phases of pregnancy. The relation is opened for reexamination; old problems surface again, and new resolutions or perspectives are sought. The pregnant woman must form her unique mothering identity, separate and apart from that of her own mother, and the outcome of this effort is critical to her future feelings about herself as a woman and a mother.[4]

Feelings of dependency and vulnerability increase, and the woman needs to receive nurturance and support from others. Social customs provide many ways in which pregnant women receive extra consideration, recognizing them as people needing special protection. Appetites may change regarding both food and sex. Nausea may decrease appetite, or certain foods may seem repugnant and others particularly appetizing. Some women have increased sexuality, enjoy sex more and seek it often. They are often more aware of sensuality in a broader sense, with heightened perceptions and response to stimuli. Other women have decreased sexual desires, or may fear injury to the fetus.

Through directing large amounts of psychic energy inward, examining implications for the self, ruminating over childhood experiences, and focusing on numerous bodily changes, the pregnant woman merges the pregnancy and fetus into her self-concept.

Tasks of Midpregnancy

The most impressive experience of the second trimester is feeling the baby move. Women are alert to early flutterings, try to differentiate movement from gas bubbles, and take delight in talking about the sensations of quickening. There often seems a sense of vital inner potential, a comradery with the otherness within. Babies begin to take shape in the woman's mind, and the individuality of the fetus is gradually perceived. Women have emotional responses to the fetus, liking or disliking it, wondering how it feels, being thankful when it is "cooperative." Although the baby is seen as small and needing protection, it still represents a powerful force, with the ability to make many changes in her life. She may realize for the first time she cannot control these changes and so feel frightened. Worries about how her family will respond to her pregnancy often develop.

An emotional shift occurs as alienation and uncertainty disappear; the pregnancy is apparent and accepted, and early discomforts such as nausea also disappear. Planning is mostly in the form of fantasies, and information about children and mothering is sought though specific actions, such as preparing a room or a layette, are often put off. The woman's psychic life is rich, with fears and dreams taking on great significance. Almost all women are haunted by the fear of producing an abnormal baby, and there is some preoccupation with danger, damage, and death, particularly related to children. Fears are usually rather magical and tend to alternate with positive images.

Because many of the events of pregnancy are beyond the woman's control (kicking of the fetus, dreams and moods, bodily changes), her weight becomes intertwined with her need to exert influence and to counteract the feeling that her body and emotions are running away with her. Some women use dieting as a means of exercising their sense of control, while others may overeat to assert themselves against authority represented by the provider's admonitions about weight gain.

Midpregnancy is often a time of heightened sexuality, increased sense of potency as a person, and sense of being more alive than ever before. Many women feel more erotic, perhaps having satisfying sex for the first time or experiencing their first orgasm. Physiological changes, including increased pelvic vascularity and vasocongestion, contribute to this phenomenon. Emotional relations are very important, especially with her partner. With pregnancy firmly established but the child not yet imminent, it is a good time to examine key relationships.

Tasks of Late Pregnancy

During the third trimester, the fetus is very real to the mother, and she thinks in terms of "her baby" with a concentration of energy upon preparations for its arrival and caretaking. Activities become goal-directed, with specific preparations such as childbirth classes, getting the baby's room ready, gathering the necessary equipment, planning for family adaptations. There is anxious anticipation of labor, with fear of the unknown and a sense of danger. Time becomes burdensome, particularly as her delivery date approaches, with a strong desire to have the pregnancy over with. Partly this is because pregnancy has become very uncomfortable, with many physical discomforts such as backache, difficulty in sleeping, frequency of urination, dyspnea, and leg cramps. The woman usually feels awkward and unattractive. Women also may resent the baby's strong kicking, pounding away at her vital organs and causing discomforts. Negative feelings, fears, and conflicts may be discharged through complaints about these physical symptoms.

Concern over labor and delivery is very ap-

parent, and the centrality of this theme suggests that it poses a psychological task of only slightly less importance than a safe outcome for the baby. This is an aspect of pregnancy over which the woman can have some control, and many pursue specific techniques vigorously. There may be some sadness about separation which delivery symbolizes—some sense of loss or emptiness when the baby is no longer inside and is able to survive on its own. A spurt of activity during the last month may be accelerated by the fears and anxieties surrounding labor, depressing feelings about the possible loss of the baby, and worries about increased responsibilities.

Women need reassurance and support, especially from their partners, as they may feel ugly and sloppy and must contend with increasing anxieties. Although heightened sexuality continues into the third trimester, physical or emotional factors may curtail or prevent sex. Some couples draw closer during pregnancy, but for others it accentuates sex role differences. Some cultures provide for support systems through female relatives and friends.

The final task of pregnancy is for the woman to prepare for the baby's separation and to lay the foundation for the assumption of mothering and care-taking. The discomforts of pregnancy and the anxieties surrounding labor and delivery make the woman eager to move on to the next phase. Information is gathered and preparations are made for the baby's arrival. The baby has become a real person and the woman is ready to establish a new nurturing relationship.[5]

Psychological Processes and the Father

Pregnancy has an impact upon the father and triggers a sequence of concerns somewhat analogous to the mother's. The discovery of his partner's pregnancy may be accompanied by mixed feelings. There is often a sense of pride in having made the woman pregnant, a sense of enhancement of his masculinity or proof of his potency. Some concern about paternity may exist, an ancient dilemma for men. His fulfillment of social or family expectations often brings him positive feedback. Many men have a desire for children to carry on the family name, deriving from a primal force to establish some continuity or link with immortality. The increased responsibility of paternity may cause the father worries about his competence as a provider for his family and their future security. In early pregnancy the man must contend with his partner's changing body and emotions, with responses which range from delight to repulsion. His relation with his own mother may be heightened, and old conflicts reawakened. His feelings and responses may be repressed, either as part of his masculine style or because the woman's feelings are more obvious and take precedence.

Feeling the baby move through the woman's abdomen confirms the pregnancy for the father and makes it more real for him. He may have an increased need to touch and feel so that he can establish a relation with the fetus. The woman's changing sexual appetites in midpregnancy may be gladly accepted or they may pose a threat. The man's own sexual feelings may be affected by changes in the woman's body. An increased dependency and passivity in his partner may be difficult for the father. Some men seem to have increased needs to be creative when their partners are pregnant. Toward the end of pregnancy, fathers often become involved in childbirth classes and in making preparations for the baby. They may become concerned about changes in family structure and roles after the baby arrives. Fathers fantasize about older children when they rehearse for the future and have trouble in conceptualizing a newborn and establishing a relation with an infant. For the man there are also fantasies and fears about labor, the possible loss of his partner or the baby, and what his role during labor will be. Some men seek involvement in assisting their partners during labor; others prefer not to be involved, and other family members assume this supportive role.

Although men rarely admit that pregnancy is a profound emotional experience for them, there is a higher incidence of physical symptoms among men whose partners are pregnant. About one man in ten experiences weight gain, nausea, stomach distress, loss of appetite, toothache, or abdominal bloating. There is an element of rivalry in pregnancy for the man, and his relation with his partner undergoes stress.[6] The emotional needs of the father, though not as obvious as the mother's, deserve consideration and attention during pregnancy.

PRENATAL MANAGEMENT

Most women know, or strongly suspect, that they are pregnant when contact with the health care provider is made. The confirmation of their pregnancy and the ongoing monitoring of the status of mother and fetus are sought, in addition to information, detection and treatment of problems, and assistance and support through labor and delivery.

The History

The initial prenatal work-up includes a thorough history, a physical examination, and laboratory tests comprising a prenatal panel. Most health facilities utilize a prenatal form to summarize their data which acts as a flow sheet for regular visits throughout pregnancy. The history includes questions about menstrual cycles, present pregnancy, previous pregnancy, past medical problems, family health history, social factors and habits, and pregnancy plans (Table 5-3).

When was your last menstrual period? Was it normal or abnormal? The date of the woman's last menstrual period (LMP) is important in calculating the expected date of confinement (EDC) and in ascertaining the duration of gestation. If the LMP was normal in onset, character, and duration, it can generally be used to determine the EDC by Nägele's rule: count back 3 months from the first day of the LMP and add 7 days. Forty weeks from LMP the pregnancy is considered at term. If the LMP was abnormal, such as shorter and lighter, later than expected, consisting of spotting, or any other differences, the woman may have conceived previously. Some women experience implantation spotting about the time their next menses would be due. Others continue to bleed lightly from the endometrium for several cycles after they are pregnant. Ask if the previous menstrual period (PMP) was normal and, if so, calculate the EDC from then. Women with longer cycles, such as 35 days between menses, would suggest an EDC 7 days later than that calculated by Nägele's rule.

What symptoms make you think you are pregnant? The common symptoms of pregnancy help establish the diagnosis and may include any combination of nausea, vomiting, breast fullness or tenderness, nipple tenderness, frequency of urination, abdominal bloating, fatigue, sleepiness, lassitude, constipation.

Is this pregnancy planned or not? Were you using any contraceptive? Assessing how the woman feels about the pregnancy helps in anticipating problems or exploring alternatives. Particularly in the first few weeks, the woman

Table 5-3
Diagnosis of Pregnancy

Presumptive Manifestations		Probable Manifestations		Positive Manifestations
Symptoms	Signs	Symptoms	Signs	Signs
Amenorrhea	Bluish coloration	Same as	Abdominal	Fetal heart tones
Nausea, vomiting	of vagina, cervix	presumptive	enlargement	Palpation of fetal
Mastodynia	Softened		Uterine	outline
Quickening	uterocervical		contractions	Sonography of
Urinary symptoms	junction		Ballottement of	gestational sac
Fatigue	Irregular softened		object in	or fetal shape
Constipation	fundus		abdomen	Fetal electro-
Weight gain	Uterine		Uterine souffle	cardiogram
	enlargement		Agglutination	Radioimmunoassay
	Breast changes		pregnancy tests	for HCG
	Skin changes			X-ray examination
	Basal body			of fetal skeleton
	temperature			
	elevation			
	Gingival			
	hypertrophy			

may want to consider abortion for a pregnancy which resulted from contraceptive failure or was accidental. Some are happy to be pregnant whether or not it was planned, or even if it was not planned desire to continue the pregnancy for various reasons. Asking if the pregnancy occurred at a good time for the parents can often lead to a discussion of concerns, stresses, or problems of the family.

Have you had any problems with this pregnancy? Specifically, ask about bleeding or spotting since conception, for these might indicate a threatened abortion. Colds, flu, urinary tract infections, exposure to x-rays, and use of medications should all be noted and the date of occurrence recorded.

How many previous pregnancies have you had, and how long were they? A history of previous pregnancies provides cues to potential problems in the present one. If there were premature deliveries, ascertain how many months the pregnancy progressed. If there was an early abortion (called miscarriage by most patients), was it spontaneous and complete or was a D and C performed? Were there any previous therapeutic or induced abortions? Repeated midtrimester spontaneous abortions may indicate an incompetent cervix. Note also if any pregnancies went more than 2 weeks beyond the EDC.

The term gravida refers to the total number of pregnancies, regardless of their duration. Para means the number of viable infants (weighing more than 500 Gm. or achieving at least 20-weeks' gestation) the woman has borne, whether live or dead at birth. This is often subdivided into term and premature births. Early abortions are listed separately. Thus, a woman who is pregnant for the fourth time, has had two term births and one abortion at 2 months would be: G4, P2, Premature 0, AB 1.

What were the birth weights and conditions of the babies? Children of the same parents tend to be of similar birth weight, usually increasing slightly with successive offspring. Birth weight can aid in determining the duration of the previous pregnancy. Excessively large babies (above 9 lbs.) suggest the possibility of diabetes mellitus in the mother. The condition of the babies gives cues about congenital anomalies, pregnancy complications, and childbirth complications.

How long was each previous labor? Was it spontaneous or induced? What type of delivery? Very short or long labors could be repeated. The reasons for induction might indicate problems which could affect the present pregnancy. Breech presentations tend to recur, and the previous use of forceps might indicate a narrow outlet. If a cesarean section was done, the reasons should be explored. Type of analgesia and anesthesia are noted, and the patient's reactions to these.

Were there any complications during previous labor, delivery, or postpartum? Signs or symptoms of toxemia, episodes of vaginal bleeding, concurrent diseases requiring medical or surgical treatment are of importance in anticipating the course of the present pregnancy. Also note previous dystocia, eclampsia, heavy bleeding in labor, postpartum hemorrhage, infection, or other problems.

Have you had any serious illnesses, operations, or hospitalizations? Preexisting disease of the cardiovascular, endocrine, gastrointestinal, or musculoskeletal system may be aggravated during pregnancy. Prior blood transfusions may have introduced antigens leading to hemolytic disease of the newborn. Prior gynecological surgery, especially uterine or pelvic floor repair, may contraindicate vaginal delivery. It is important to be aware of a history of appendectomy, especially should abdominal pain occur.

Do you have any present health problems or take any regular medicines? Noting minor illnesses or conditions alerts the practitioner to potential hazards as well as annoyances during pregnancy. Medicines are to be minimized or, preferably, avoided. Need for care in addition to prenatal management can be determined, and referrals made as indicated.

In your family is there any history of. . . .? Pregnant women may be at increased risk if parents, siblings, or other relatives have had major illnesses such as diabetes, tuberculosis, renal disease, heart disease, hypertension, congenital anomalies, seizure disorders, psychiatric problems, or multiple births. Specific inquiry should be made about these diseases, and positive responses should be followed up, with appropriate further exploration and testing.

Are you allergic to any medications? Do you have any other allergies? This is a standard question necessary for safe treatment with medications. A history of other allergies such as to foods or pollens alerts the health provider to the possibility of allergies in the baby.

Do you smoke or use alcohol or drugs? Problems with fetal growth and well-being have been associated with substances abuse, and it is important to determine early whether these factors must be considered in planning prenatal care. Significant use would place the pregnancy in a high risk category.

What is your home situation, and how does your family feel about the pregnancy? Information about the woman's social situation is a help in understanding her needs for support, the inclusion of others in care, stresses and conflicts, and responses to treatment. Initiation of referrals to community health or social welfare agencies can be done when the need is present.

Do you have any requests, questions, or desires related to childbearing? Asking if the woman has thought about the method of feeding, natural childbirth, anesthesia for delivery or analgesia for labor, partner involvement, rooming-in, or other practices provides insight into the woman's attitudes and knowledge. Many women are well informed and will express their intent to use a prepared childbirth method such as Lamaze or Bradley, to breast feed, to have the baby born via the LeBoyer technique, to put the baby to breast immediately, to have rooming-in, or to have early discharge. Others may not have thought about such details and will need a considerable amount of information about their options. Some women still request sedation and need education about the necessity of minimum medication. Knowledge of community resources enables the provider to make referrals for the type of program best suited to the woman's or couple's needs.

Physical Examination

A thorough physical examination is performed as part of the prenatal work-up. Usually examination forms are more detailed for the abdominal and pelvic portions. Of particular importance in pregnancy are the following:

HEAD AND NECK. Cervical and other lymph nodes are palpated for disorders of the lymphatic system. Nasal and oral mucous membranes may exhibit hyperemia and some bogginess, and the thyroid gland is normally slightly diffusely enlarged. No changes are usually noted in ears.

CHEST AND HEART. Lungs should be clear, and any rales, wheezes, or ronchi are abnormal findings. The heart should be in regular rhythm without murmurs, although occasionally a functional murmur of pregnancy may be present. Murmurs should be referred for further evaluation, as should persistent arrythmias.

BREASTS.   Palpation for masses or nodules is important, as cancer growth may be accelerated by pregnancy. Because of increased size, ductal development, and congestion, breasts are often difficult to evaluate. Questionable nodules can be reexamined a week later, but any definite mass must be referred for further evaluation. Nipples should be evaluated for adequacy for breast feeding. Gentle, repeated traction can be used to evert nipples which are inverted. Clear fluid is often expressed from nipples in later pregnancy.

SKIN.   The pigmentation and circulatory changes typical of pregnancy can be noted. Pallor, jaundice, and other skin lesions need diagnosis and treatment.

EXTREMITIES.   Deformities or limitations in the motion of arms, legs, and back are noted as these may influence the conduct of labor or inherited problems. Varicosities of the lower extremities can be a source of major discomfort during pregnancy and can lead to embolism, particularly postpartally. Edema should be carefully assessed; pretibial and presacral edema may be early signs of fluid retention, and the edema of face, arms, or hands may be indicative of cardiac, renal, or preeclamptic problems. Deep tendon reflexes are elicited and recorded. Hyperreflexia and clonus, combined with other signs, can indicate preeclampsia.

ABDOMEN.   An inspection of the abdomen can provide information about the position of the fetus after the thirtieth week. With longitudinal lie, the uterus is ovoid, and with transverse lie it appears rounder, low, and broad. In posterior positions a saucerlike depression is seen below the umbilicus. If the pregnancy is beyond 12 or 14 weeks, the height of the fundus is measured using McDonald's technique. With a flexible tape measure, the distance from the upper margin of the symphysis pubis to the top of the fundus is measured, draping the tape measure over the uterus. This distance in centimeters multiplied by 2 and divided by 7 gives the approximate duration of pregnancy in lunar months. For the duration of pregnancy in weeks, multiply the distance by 8 and divide by 7.

In determining the presentation of the fetus in a pregnancy beyond 30 weeks, Leopold's maneuvers are used (Figure 5-2). The first three maneuvers are done with the health provider standing at the patient's side facing her, and the last one is done with the provider facing her feet. Using the pads of the fingers, the examiner moves the hands smoothly over the abdomen without lifting them and uses gentle pressure to avoid stimulating a contraction. The patient is recumbent for this examination, and flexing her legs at the knee helps to relax her abdominal musculature. The fundus is palpated first, and if the fetal head is present it will feel harder than the breech, round and smooth, and will move independently of the trunk (ballottement), producing the sensation of a hard object bouncing back and forth between the examiner's fingers. The breech is softer, less smooth and regular, and when moved the entire trunk, located lower in the uterus, moves also. The second maneuver locates the fetal back, using palmar pressure. One hand is used to steady the uterus and to press the fetus toward the examining hand. With gentle pressure or circular motions of the finger pads, the examiner searches for a smooth, hard, resistant place which would be the fetal back. If the small parts are felt, these feel knobby and irregular and tend to recede or move with pressure. If the back cannot be palpated and small parts are evident over a wide area, a posterior position is probable. The third maneuver determines if the head is at the pelvic inlet and whether it is mobile. The examiner grasps the lower pole of the uterus gently between thumb and fingers of one hand. The head feels round, hard, and smooth. If not engaged, it can be ballotted readily, but if it has settled into the pelvis, its mobility will be limited. The fourth maneuver, done facing the patient's feet, provides more information about the fetal presenting part. The examiner places the hands on either side of the abdomen and moves them downward and inward. If the fingers converge easily just above the symphysis, the fetal presenting part is not engaged. If the fingers flare outward instead of converging, some descent into the pelvis has occurred. On one side, a prominence may be noted just above Poupart's ligament, which represents the brow of the fetus in an occiput presentation with good flexion. If this cephalic prominence is very easily palpated, feeling as if it were just under the skin, a posterior position of the occiput is suggested. The location of the cephalic prominence also indicates how far the head has descended.

The abdominal examination also includes

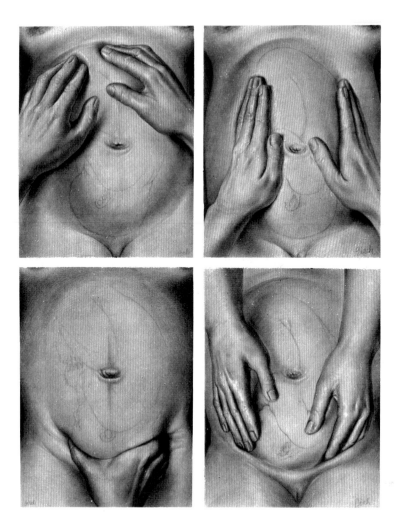

Figure 5-2. Abdominal palpation for fetal presentation (Leopold's maneuvers). (Top, left to right) First maneuver and second maneuver. (Bottom, left to right) Third maneuver and fourth maneuver.

palpation for masses and any enlargement of the liver, kidney, or spleen. In more advanced pregnancies little except the uterus may be felt. Auscultation for bruits and bowel sounds is done if the uterus is small enough to permit it. After about the twentieth week of gestation, fetal heart tones are also auscultated, and are heard best over the area of the fetal back. Generally a fetascope, which provides sound conduction both by bone and by air, is used. A rate of 120 to 140 beats per minute is usual, and may be obtained by counting for 15 seconds and multiplying by 4. Uterine and occasionally funic (umbilical cord) souffle may be heard. If there is any question whether the sounds heard are fetal heart tones or uterine souffle, the mother's pulse should be taken simultaneously. With an ultrasonic monitor (Doptone) the fetal heart can be picked up as early as the tenth week.

PELVIC EXAMINATION. Both speculum and bimanual examinations are carried out to identify signs of pregnancy, determine length of gestation, ascertain pelvic characteristics, identify abnormalities, and obtain a Pap smear, gonorrhea culture and other specimens, as indicated. The diagnosis of early pregnancy (below 16 weeks) is described in Chapter 7, Induced Abortion.

On speculum examination, the characteristic bluish discoloration of mucosa is noted (Chadwick's sign). As pregnancy progresses, there is increased leukorrhea which is white or greyish and mucoid, with a musty odor. The cervix is congested, softened, and often somewhat patulous, and an eversion of the endocervical columnar epithelium may be pronounced. Cervical mucus does not fern upon drying but shows a granular pattern. The vagina is long and congested, with increased rugae.

On bimanual examination, the cervix feels soft and may admit a fingertip. By 10 to 12 weeks, the uterus has assumed a globular shape and is diffusely softened, often making the fundus hard to identify. As pregnancy progresses the uterus becomes more ovoid longitudinally. After about 30 weeks the fetal presenting part may be felt vaginally in the lower uterine segment. Up to 14 to 16 weeks uterine size can best be estimated by bimanual examination, with gestation in weeks approximating the number of centimeters of longitudinal uterine size. After this point, abdominal measurements as described before provide good data by which to estimate the length of gestation. Up to approximately 32 weeks, the number of centimeters which express the distance from the symphysis to the top of the fundus roughly corresponds to the number of weeks of gestation.

A clinical evaluation of the bony pelvis is generally carried out, although current thinking holds that even with apparently small pelves a trial of labor is necessary to see whether fetal accommodation can occur. Diameters of the inlet, midpelvis, and outlet are measured during the bimanual examination. Of course, these measurements are only estimates, and x-ray pelvimetry is necessary for an accurate determination of pelvic configuration. This should not be done routinely, but only near term or during labor for suspected fetopelvic disproportion.

The pelvic outlet can be adequately measured clinically by noting the angle of the pubic rami. This is done by palpating the rami from the symphysis to the ischial tuberosities and estimating their angle. A subpubic angle of less than 90 degrees indicates an inadequate outlet. The intertuberous (biischial) diameter is frequently measured by fitting the fist between the ischial tuberosities, and knowing the measurement across the knuckles. A distance of more than 8 cm. is usually adequate for delivery. A Thoms's or Williams's pelvimeter can also be used to measure biischial diameter.

The midpelvis cannot be measured precisely by physical examination, but certain indicators of adequacy or narrowness are available. The ischial spines are felt, and their prominence and relative closeness noted. Flat, dull, or blunt spines contribute to greater diameter; sharp or pronounced spines reduce it. If the walls of the pelvis seem to converge, if the curve of the sacrum is straightened instead of hollow, or if the sacrosciatic notches are unusually narrow, this indicates a small midpelvis, and its adequacy is in question.

The anteroposterior diameter of the inlet is measured by obtaining the diagonal conjugate, the distance from the sacral promontory to the inner surface of the symphysis pubis. This is measured by sweeping the examining fingers along the curve of the sacrum and following it upward, trying to reach the protrusion of the sacral promontory. The thumb is pressed against the symphysis, which serves as an anchor. The examiner must know the distance from the tip of her or his middle finger to the insertion of the thumb, usually from 11 to 12 cm. If the promontory is reached, the diagonal conjugate is less than this distance, indicating a small inlet. If the promontory cannot be reached, which is the usual case in an adequate pelvis, the diagonal conjugate is recorded as greater than 11 or 12 cm. To obtain an estimate of the true conjugate, 1.5 cm. is subtracted from the measurement for the diagonal conjugate (Figure 5-3).

A clinical appraisal of whether the pelvis is adequate or narrowed in the inlet, midpelvis, or outlet is usually recorded. For any accurate further characterization of pelvic configuration, x-ray pelvimetry is needed.

The adnexa are palpated for masses, and the condition of the ovaries is noted if these can be felt.

Laboratory Tests

The prenatal panel of laboratory tests includes serological testing for syphilis (VDRL), a complete blood count including hematocrit and hemoglobin, ABO blood type and Rh factor, antibody screening, rubella titer, routine urinalysis, Pap smear, and a gonorrhea culture (GC). In some areas, or depending upon history, toxoplasmosis titer or Tine test/PPD may be done. Screening urine cultures may also be included, using one of the new dehydrated, miniaturized culture media (Microstix Reagent Strips). The father's Rh factor may be obtained

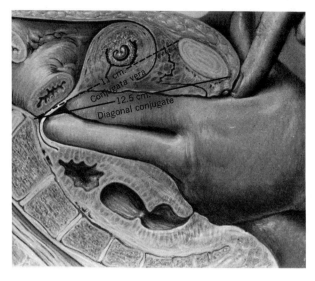 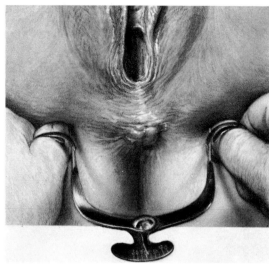

if the woman is Rh negative; and Rh antibody titers taken regularly throughout pregnancy.

Continuing Care and Return Visits

After the initial prenatal work-up, women are seen once a month until the seventh month, every two weeks during the seventh and eighth months, and weekly during the ninth month until delivery. If problems arise, visits are more frequent. Return visits include the following:

PHYSICAL EXAMINATION. The woman's weight, blood pressure, fundal measurements, and fetal heart tones are taken each visit. Weight gain is plotted, and significant deviations above or below expected amounts are explored. Blood pressure should remain essentially unchanged; any rises must be carefully watched. The abdomen is examined as described before for fetal presentation and location of fetal back, the fetal heart tones taken and recorded, and the fundus measured by McDonald's technique. A fundal height that does not correspond to gestation as calculated from the woman's history requires further investigation. If too small, an error in dates may be the reason or intrauterine growth retardation may be suspected. If too large, multiple pregnancy or hydramnios could be present, or dates may have been miscalculated. The average height of the fundus at various stages of gestation is shown in Figure 5-4.

The degree and location of edema is noted, if present. Ankle edema is common, and some patients have swelling of hands and fingers

Figure 5-3. Clinical pelvic measurements. (Left) Method of obtaining diagonal conjugate diameter. (Right) Method of measuring tuberischii or intertuberous diameter of outlet using the Williams's pelvimeter. The measurement is made on a line with the lower border of the anus.

making it difficult to wear rings. More generalized edema, especially facial and orbital, may indicate preeclampsia and particular note must be made of blood pressure, weight gain, proteinuria, and hyperreflexia. Other areas are examined according to symptoms or suspected problems. Vaginal examinations are usually not repeated until the last month as the patient approaches term, for assessing the status of the cervix, presentation, and the degree of engagement.

HISTORY. Inquiry is made into the woman's general health and feeling, and any symptoms mentioned explored fully. Depending upon physical findings (i.e., excessive weight gain, glycosuria) specific related questions are asked.

LABORATORY TESTS. Repeat urine testing is done on each visit for protein and glucose. The hematocrit is repeated at 32 to 34 weeks. If the woman is Rh negative, antibody titers are measured at least twice more during pregnancy. Titers greater than 1:16 should be repeated and the patient referred for evaluation of Rh incompatibility. Repeated spilling of glucose or high levels in the urine raise the suspicion of diabetes, and a 2-hour glucose tolerance test is indicated. More than a trace of

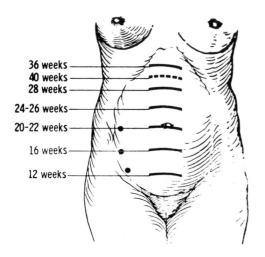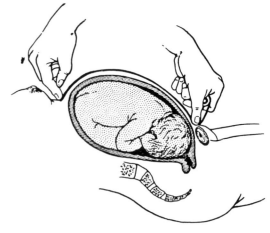

Figure 5-4. (Left) Fundal height and weeks of gestation. (Right) McDonald's measurement of fundal height. R. C. Benson, *Current Obstetric & Gynecologic Diagnosis & Treatment* (Los Altos: Lange Medical Publishers, 1976), p. 486.

protein in the urine may be a sign of developing preeclampsia, and other parameters should be carefully assessed.

Education During Pregnancy

It has long been known that women who are well informed about pregnancy and childbirth, who have learned techniques to cope with labor, and who have positive attitudes about the reproductive experience have few physical and emotional problems, as a general rule, and are able to cope well with the demands and stresses of these events. Although there is a strong trend toward the childbearing couple's (or individual's) taking responsibility for this learning process, many women still do not take the initiative or, for various reasons, do not place a high priority upon perinatal education. Certain areas of key information can be identified by providers and discussed in short educational sessions during the several months of prenatal care. A form or check list attached to each patient's chart is a handy way to assure that all topics have been covered and to order the topics systematically in relation to the progression of the pregnancy (Figure 5-5).

Initially, it is important to cover the routine of prenatal visits and what the woman may expect from her prenatal care. Information about the physical and emotional changes of

pregnancy enables the woman to anticipate these events and reduces her concerns over normality. Gaps in information about reproductive anatomy and physiology can be filled and explanations provided for the patient's particular problems, such as vaginitis, varicosities, or negative Rh factor. Habits which could affect the fetus should be discussed early, including smoking, drug use, and alcohol use. Smoking has been associated with lower birth weight and a smaller head circumference and length of infants. This effect is related to how many cigarettes are smoked daily, with a gradient from heavy (greater than 15 cigarettes per day) to light smokers. It is known that smaller infants have an increased rate of perinatal complications, but the direct effect of smoking on infant mortality is uncertain. It appears that the major mechanism by which smoking affects infant birth weight is through a diminished maternal food intake, with less weight gain during pregnancy. Maternal vascular effects or placental transfer of toxic substances probably have only minor roles.[7] Pregnant women should be encouraged not to smoke, but if this creates too much stress, they might attempt to reduce the number of cigarettes per day and to increase their food intake and weight gain. Drugs are to be minimized during pregnancy because they all cross the placental barrier to some degree and some have either proven or suspected teratogenicity or other adverse fetal or neonatal effects (Table 5-4). Maternal drug addiction presents additional dangers, including infection, growth retardation, and withdrawal symptoms in the baby after

Date   Initials

———— ————   Prenatal history and physical examination results discussed.
———— ————   Prenatal laboratory panel results discussed.
———— ————   Medications and teratology discussed.
———— ————   Nutritional counseling.
———— ————   Preferred weight gain ————————.
———— ————   Smoking discussed.
———— ————   Activity, exercise, travel, working discussed.
———— ————   Sexual activity discussed.
———— ————   Prenatal classes discussed.
              Enrolled in class: date ———————— type ————————————
———— ————   Hospital arrangements discussed (visit and register).
———— ————   Breast versus bottle feeding discussed.
              Type selected ————————. Breast care taught ————————.
———— ————   Management of labor and delivery discussed.
              Anesthesia/analgesia ————————————————
              Prepared childbirth ————————————————
———— ————   Partner in delivery room discussed. Yes ———— No ————
              Minor problems discussed:
———— ————   Constipation and/or hemorrhoids
———— ————   Backache
———— ————   Leg cramps
———— ————   Stretch marks
———— ————   Difficulty sleeping
———— ————   Ankle edema
———— ————   Nausea and vomiting
———— ————   Heartburn
———— ————   Signs of labor discussed, when to go to hospital.
              Instructed on what to do about:
———— ————   Rupture of membranes
———— ————   Bleeding
———— ————   Fever
———— ————   Fetal monitoring equipment discussed.
———— ————   Contraception discussed. Plans: ———— birth control pills, ———— IUD, ———— diaphragm,
              ———— foam and condom, ———— tubal ligation, ——— vasectomy, ———— rhythm or ovu-
              lation, ———— none.
———— ————   Baby care and circumcision discussed.
———— ————   Special requests related to birth ————————————————.
———— ————   Medications prescribed ————————————————.

FIGURE 5-5. Prenatal Check List

birth. Alcohol consumed in small amounts apparently has no adverse effects, although babies of chronic alcoholics often show withdrawal symptoms after birth and may be malnourished.

Daily routines and activities as affected by pregnancy are also discussed. A balance between exercise and rest is encouraged. Walking, swimming, and other sports which do not pose the danger of falls or injuries promote well-being during pregnancy. Generally, the woman may continue with any activity to which she is accustomed as long as it is not dangerous. Travel does not adversely affect pregnancy, but does remove the patient from her health provider should a problem develop. Distances should be small close to term, or throughout pregnancy if the woman has a history of abortion or of vaginal bleeding during this pregnancy. Bathing poses no problem because bath water does not enter the vagina. Douching is generally not recommended, and the use of a hand syringe may be harmful. Necessary dental fillings or extractions may be done, preferably with local anesthesia. Pregnancy has no detrimental effects on the mother's teeth and does not withdraw calcium.

Clothing during pregnancy should be loose

Table 5-4
Effects of Drugs in Pregnancy

Drug	Proven Fetal or Neonatal Effect
Aminopterin	Abortion, various anomalies
Busulfan (Myleran)	Various anomalies
Chlorambucil (Leukeran)	Various anomalies
Colchicine	Various anomalies
Cyclophosphamide (Cytoxan)	Abortion, various anomalies
Methotrexate	Malformations of skull, face, extremities
Radioiodine	Anomalies if early, congenital hypothyroidism if late
Diethylstilbestrol	Vaginal adenosis or clear cell carcinoma in daughters after puberty
Alkyl (methyl) mercury	Cerebral palsy, microcephaly
Diphenylhydantoin	Cleft lip and palate, microcephaly, heart defects
Tetracyclines	Stained teeth, enamel hypoplasia, cataract
Warfarin	Nasal hypoplasia and stippled epiphyses
Progestins	Masculinizaton of female fetus
Oral contraceptives	Anomalous genitalia, limb reduction defects
Barbiturates, opiates	Respiratory depression
Heroin, methadone	Withdrawal symptoms
Streptomycin	Deafness
High doses ascorbic acid	Withdrawal scurvy
Synthetic vitamin K	Kernicterus

Drug	Suspected Fetal or Neonatal Effect
Lithium	Various anomalies
Coumarins	Various anomalies
Quinine	Limb reduction defects, deafness
Reserpine	Lung cysts
Alcohol	Microcephaly, maxillary hypoplasia (rarely)
Trimethadione	Various anomalies
Vitamin D (massive doses)	Aortic stenosis, elfin facies, mental retardation
X-ray (diagnostic)	Increased risk of leukemia before age 10
Chlordiazepoxide (Librium), diazepam (Valium), meprobamate (Equanil, Miltown)	Various anomalies from exposure during first 6 weeks only
Meclizine (Bonine), cyclizine (Marezine), chlorcyclizine (Perazil), phenmetrazine (Preludin)	Isolated case reports of anomalies
Isoniazid (INH)	Isolated case reports of anomalies

Benson, *Current Obstetric & Gynecologic Diagnosis, & Treatment* p. 536.

fitting and comfortable, and many women continue with regular clothes until uterine enlargement progresses enough to require maternity clothing. A well-fitting support brassiere promotes good posture, reduces shoulder traction, and protects the muscles of the breast. Maternity girdles are infrequently used, unless there is abdominal wall weakness or considerable back pain. Women are advised against panty girdles, garters, and other constricting clothing because these interfere with circulation in the legs. Low-heeled shoes will not aggravate postural changes.

Women who work often desire to continue employment during pregnancy, and this is discussed as an individual choice. Positions demanding excessive physical activity, such as physical education teacher, probably cannot be continued as long as more sedentary types of work. Many women continue to work until they go into labor, and if they are capable of carrying out their job responsibilities without undue stress and fatigue, there is no reason to stop during the third trimester. It is advisable to plan a leave of 2 to 6 weeks after the baby's birth to allow time for the recovery of full strength and for working out a schedule with the new baby and family.

Sexual activity can be continued during pregnancy according to the couple's patterns and desires unless the woman is bleeding, threatening premature labor, or has ruptured membranes. Intercourse poses no threat to pregnancy under normal circumstances; this is information that is important for couples to have. Sensations for the woman may change, and techniques may need to be altered, especially during the last month or two because of the large uterus and increased pelvic pressure. In the absence of complicating factors, there is no reason to advise abstinence before the onset of labor.

Information should also be provided about hospital admission and routine, signs and symptoms of labor, and the process of labor and delivery. Childbirth classes are often invaluable in providing more education to the parents than the provider has time for and in equipping them for participant childbirth and the care of the new baby.

Nutrition and Weight Gain

Good maternal nutrition is a major determinant of normal fetal growth and development. The woman's nutritional status at conception may well be as important as nutrition during pregnancy, but this is a set factor. Women with low prepregnancy weight and those who gain little weight during pregnancy are more likely to have low birth weight babies (2500 Gm. or less), with higher infant morbidity and mortality during the first week of life. A severely inadequate nutritional status of the mother is believed associated with lower DNA content of fetal brain cells and a decrease in their number. Overnourished women predispose their infants to obesity, because there is increased subcutaneous fat and possibly an excessive number of fat cells in the infant.

The quality of nutrition is much more important than simply caloric content, and this is best approached by stressing what foods should be eaten instead of what foods to avoid. Each day the woman should eat foods from the milk group, protein group, dark green and deep yellow vegetables, fruits or other foods high in vitamin C, and from the bread-cereal group, and water or liquids. Providing a sheet with typical foods in each category and how many servings per day gives the patient a continued source of information about diet (Table 5-5). Certain minerals and vitamins need to be supplemented, including calcium, iron, and folic acid. One quart of milk per day provides nearly all the pregnant woman's calcium requirement, but if this is not feasible alternate sources can be used (cheese, yogurt, spinach, calcium tablets). Iron supplementation is necessary because most diets are not rich in this mineral, and the absorption of iron from foods is only 10 to 20 percent of their iron content. Maternal iron stores will be depleted, especially in late pregnancy, if iron is not supplemented. From 30 to 60 mg. of elemental iron is needed, which can be obtained from ferrous sulfate 300 mg. 3 times a day. Enteric-coated iron tablets are not advised, as absorption is markedly reduced. Ferrous gluconate provides less than half the elemental iron of ferrous sulfate. A daily supplement of 1 mg. folic acid is also needed to prevent folic acid deficiency, the second most common cause of gestational anemia. Pernicious anemia is very rare in the pregnancy age group, and there is little danger from routine folate treatment. Daily multiple vitamins are usually given.

Moderate weight gain during pregnancy is associated with the lowest incidence of low birth weight infants and neonatal mortality, and this avoids the problems of obesity and more complications of pregnancy that come with excessive weight gain. Women with low weight gain should be considered high risk. As the average weight gain is 24 to 27 lb., a range between 20 and 30 lb. would be in the moderate category. The relation between excessive weight gain and toxemia is questionable, and the declining incidence of toxemia in the United States is probably due in part to better nutrition. There is no advantage to dietary restriction during pregnancy, and indeed there may be risks for the fetus. A more liberal attitude on weight gain prevails presently, and certainly no woman should try to lose or maintain her weight during pregnancy. The gain should occur smoothly through pregnancy, averaging about 2 lb. per week though there may be larger jumps at certain points. With larger

Table 5-5
Foods Needed During Pregnancy

Foods Needed Every Day	Amounts
Milk— whole milk, nonfat milk, evaporated milk, nonfat dry milk, cheddar and Monterey Jack cheeses (1 slice = 1 cup milk), cottage cheese	
Pregnant woman over 18 years old	1 quart (4 cups)
Pregnant woman under 18 years old	1¼ quarts (5 cups)
Meat/protein group—meat, fish, fowl, cheese, beans, peanut butter. A serving is:	2 servings
2-3 oz. cooked meat, fish, fowl	
½ cup cottage cheese	
1 cup cooked dry beans or peas	
4 tbs. peanut butter	
Eggs—one daily or another serving of the meat group	1 serving
Dark green and deep yellow vegetables and fruits—broccoli, greens, spinach, sweet potatoes, yams, yellow squash, pumpkin, carrots, cantaloupe, dry apricots	½ cup
Citrus fruits or other vitamin C foods—oranges, grapefruits and their juices, greens, broccoli, green peppers, brussels sprouts, tomatoes, strawberries	½ cup
Other fruits and vegetables—white potato, cabbage, corn, green beans, green peas, apple, banana, prunes, raisins, lettuce, and others	2 servings (1 cup)
Bread and cereal group—whole grain or enriched bread and cereals. A serving is	
1 slice bread	
1 tortilla	
½ cup cooked cereal	
½ cup grits	5 servings
½ cup macaroni or spaghetti	
¾ cup dry cereal	
½ cup rice, enriched or converted	
Coffee or tea in moderation	As desired
Margarine, butter, salad dressing, dessert	As desired if not overweight

Foods to Minimize or avoid	
"Empty calories" which contain little or no food value such as soft drinks, candy, potato chips, cake	Small amounts unless overweight
Foods whose sugar or carbohydrate content outweighs their food value such as ice cream, pies, sweetened cereals, some beverages and juices, popcorn, various chips, pastries	Small amounts unless overweight

weight gains, the patient should be checked for edema.

Moderate amounts of salt or foods containing sodium are not harmful in a normal pregnancy, and there has recently been a deemphasis on sodium restriction. The requirement for sodium is increased slightly in pregnancy, and when there is a reduction in intake a mechanism for increased sodium reabsorption and retention is activated, which can lead to hypovolemia. Particularly in combination with diuretics, sodium restriction can be dangerous. Advising against heavy use of dietary salt is appropriate because this can increase problems with fluid retention and edema. However, sodium restriction is not justified unless there is sudden weight gain or the development of preeclampsia.

Management of Common Problems

NAUSEA AND VOMITING. Assisting the woman to tolerate mild to moderate nausea and occcasional vomiting is the best approach. Understanding that there is very little danger and that the problem will disappear by the end of the third month usually enables the woman to live through this phase. Dietary changes may help, such as eating dry toast and jelly or crackers just upon arising, having six small dry meals per day, and drinking liquids separately. Foods with pungent odors or which are rich or fatty should be avoided. If severe enough to warrant medication, dicyclomine HCL (Bendectin) is an approved antiemetic for pregnancy. Usually two tablets are taken at bedtime, with one tablet at 10 A.M. if necessary. Bendectin is an antihistaminic preparation.

HEARTBURN.   When this is a problem, very little fatty food should be included in the diet. However, with gastric hypoacidity and delayed emptying time, it is a common complaint and may be managed with antacids containing magnesium hydroxide and aluminum hydroxide, 1 tbs. every 2 to 3 hours p.r.n. Sodium bicarbonate should be avoided since its benefit is brief, and it may contribute to excessive sodium intake.

CONSTIPATION.   This problem may often be prevented with a diet containing fresh fruit and raw vegetables, whole grain breads, and cereals, and large fluid intake. Adding such foods, particularly whole bran cereals, can relieve constipation. If this is not adequate for relief, a stool softener such as dioctyl sodium sulfosuccinate 50 to 240 mg. daily can be used. Mild laxatives such as Milk of Magnesia may occasionally be needed, but purgatives are contraindicated. Mineral oil also should not be used, as it absorbs fat-soluble vitamins from the gastrointestinal tract, and lack of vitamin K could cause hemorrhagic disease of the newborn.

HEMORRHOIDS.   Pregnancy often precipitates hemorrhoidal varicosities which can cause a considerable amount of discomfort. Keeping the stool soft, establishing regular bowel habits, and avoiding the need to strain at stool help to prevent or minimize hemorrhoids. Standing for long periods of time may aggravate them. When hemorrhoids have developed, they can be treated with hot sitz baths three times a day, local application of astringent compresses (witch hazel, Epsom salts), or topical anesthetic suppositories or creams (Anusol, Americaine, Nupercainal).

VARICOSE VEINS.   The familial tendency toward varicosities is often first realized during pregnancy. Both vulval and lower extremity varicosities can be precipitated, causing varying degrees of pain. The aim of the treatment is to collapse the large, distended, and tortuous superficial veins but to continue to ensure good circulation. Avoiding garters, garter belts, girdles, stockings, or other constricting clothing is essential and is advised for all pregnant women. Once varicosities develop, they can be treated by frequent elevation of the legs or by wearing elastic stockings. Supportive pantyhose or thigh length hose are available in different thicknesses and often provide good relief. For vulvar varicosities, a perineal pad wrapped in a plastic film, held snugly by a menstrual pad belt or T-binder and elastic pantyhose, can be effective. Surgery or injection is usually not done during pregnancy. Obesity and excessive weight gain serve to aggravate varicosities.

EDEMA.   Ankle swelling and edema of the lower extremities not associated with toxemia develops in about 2 out of 3 women in late pregnancy. Sodium and water retention due to steroid hormones and increased venous pressure cause this edema. Although common, this type of edema is not a serious problem and does not cause much discomfort. The treatment consists of having the woman elevate her legs frequently, sleep in a slight Trendelenburg's position if feasible, and avoid excessive salt in her diet. This can be done by advising the woman to salt food in cooking, but not to add table salt for herself, and by giving her a list of high sodium foods to avoid.

LEG CRAMPS.   Cramping or knotting of muscles of the calves, thighs, or buttocks may occur suddenly after sleep or recumbency or upon sudden shortening of leg muscles by stretching with the toes pointed. Immediate treatment consists of massaging the contracted muscle, flexing the foot, and applying local heat. To prevent cramps, the woman should walk leading with the heel and avoid pointing her toes when stretching her legs. Vibratory shaking of the legs from hip to foot, especially before going to sleep, may reduce leg cramps. Dietary treatment aimed at reducing phosphorus intake and increasing calcium intake also can be used. Limiting meat to one serving and milk to one pint daily reduces phosphorus intake, and taking 8 ml. of aluminum hydroxide gel orally before each meal eliminates excessive phosphate absorption. Calcium intake can be increased by giving calcium lactate 0.6 Gm. (or equivalent) orally before meals. It is hard to find dietary sources high in calcium that are not also high in phosphorus (see Chapter 8, Menopause).

ACHES, PAINS, AND PRESSURES. Particularly in later pregnancy, women suffer a variety of musculoskeletal discomforts. Aching in the areas of the symphysis and sacroiliac articulations is due to pelvic instability, and a firm girdle or frequent bed rest may provide relief. Backache due to lumbar lordosis and muscle strain is common and can be helped by good posture, avoiding excessive weight gain, a maternity girdle to support the abdomen, shoes with 2-inch heels to keep the shoulders forward, local heat and back rubs, and exercises to strengthen the back muscles. Pelvic heaviness and a dragging pressure is due to the weight of the uterus on the pelvic support muscles and the abdominal wall. Resting in the supine or lateral recumbent position is recommended. Tenderness and some pain in the mid and lower quadrants, usually to the left, are due to round ligament tension and traction. Treatment consists of local heat and rest.

Flatulence, distention, and bowel cramping are also common, due to dietary practices which include large meals, fats, gas-forming foods and chilled beverages. Correcting the diet, maintaining regular bowel habits and adequate exercise with frequent changes in body position often relieve this problem. Braxton-Hicks contractions can often be painful in later pregnancy, but no specific treatment except use of breathing and relaxation techniques is recommended. Pain, numbness, tingling or burning of hands or fingers due to brachial plexus traction can be improved by maintaining good posture and elevating the arms slightly away from the body. If such symptoms are caused by carpal tunnel syndrome (diagnosed by eliciting pain upon tapping the median nerve at the wrist, Tinel's sign; or by hyperextension or hyperflexion of the hand), elevation of the arms and splinting the hand in the neutral position may help. Later, surgery may be necessary to free the median nerve to achieve complete relief.

HEADACHE. Most headaches during pregnancy are caused by muscle tension or sinus congestion. Migraines are much less common. Emotional tension and stress produce a constant bandlike, occipital type of headache. Vascular engorgement of the turbinates with sinus blockage produces headaches with pressure sensations over sinuses or behind orbits. This type can be treated with nose drops for nasal decongestion. Analgesics must be used with caution and minimally. Helping the woman to find ways to relax and avoid tensions and stresses is preferable. As with any other musculoskeletal discomfort, explaining their basis and confirming that they do not pose serious dangers is often enough to enable the woman to tolerate them. Persistent, severe headache may suggest toxemia when combined with other findings.

LEUKORRHEA AND VAGINITIS. Heavy vaginal discharge without itching, burning, yellow-green discoloration, or foul odor is simply due to excessive cervical and vaginal secretions. An explanation is provided, and the woman may wear a perineal pad if she desires. With any additional symptoms, however, vaginal infection is likely and should be diagnosed by wet prep and KOH mount (see Chapter 9, Vaginal Discharge and Itching). Trichomonas vaginalis can be found in 20 to 30 percent of pregnant women, but only 5 to 10 percent are symptomatic. Treatment with metronidazole (Flagyl) is contraindicated during pregnancy because of possible fetal damage. Alternative treatments that are safe and helpful include AVC cream, Vagisec suppositories, and trichofuron cream. Candida albicans is present in the vaginas of many pregnant women, but only about half of these women have symptoms. The changes in vaginal pH, hyperemia, and increased cellular glycogen predispose pregnant women to Candida infections. The treatment is with nystatin (Mycostatin) vaginal suppositories or a miconazole nitrate cream preparation (Monistat). Nonspecific vaginitis is treated with sulfa cream. With vulval swelling and burning, cortisone creams applied locally often give good relief.

Genital herpes infections during pregnancy pose a serious threat to the fetus and if suspected or diagnosed consultation should be sought. Maternal herpes in early pregnancy is associated with an increased incidence of spontaneous abortions and congenital anomalies; in later pregnancy fetal viremia can occur which usually leads to fetal or neonatal death. With maternal herpes at term, delivery by cesarean section within 4 hours of rupture of membranes is recommended, but this does not guarantee against fetal infections (see Chapter 11, Venereal Disease).

URINARY TRACT INFECTIONS. Whether symptomatic or not, urinary tract infections during pregnancy must be treated. An increased incidence of premature delivery and perinatal mortality has been found with these infections during pregnancy. Microscopic urinalysis indicating bacteriuria or pyuria must be followed with a culture or else routine screening cultures must be done. Asymptomatic bacteriuria occurs in 5 to 7 percent of all pregnant women, mostly caused by *Escherichia coli*. Pyuria may be absent in over 50 percent of women with asymptomatic bacteriuria and if not treated intercurrent pyelonephritis can be expected in about 30 percent of these women. If a culture reveals more than 100,000 colonies per ml., a broad spectrum antibiotic such as ampicillin is used for 2 weeks, or a sensitivity test is done and the patient treated with the appropriate antibiotic. Sulfisoxazole, nitrofurantoin, penicillin, and cephalexin (Keflex) are often used. Caution must be exercised in the use of antibiotics, however, as tetracycline affects fetal long bones and teeth, chloramphenicol may cause the neonatal "gray syndrome," and sulfonomides during the last few weeks of pregnancy can interfere with neonatal bilirubin transport and possibly cause kernicterus. A repeat culture is done 1 month after treatment, and if a urinary tract infection is still present, a second course of specific medication is given. If the infection fails to clear, continuous therapy with sulfisoxazole may be necessary, up to several weeks from term. Resistant organisms which persist after antibiotic treatment may be controlled with methenamine mandelate 4 to 12 Gm. daily with minimal risk to the patient.[8] Symptomatic infections are diagnosed by culture, sensitivity tests are made, and treatment with a specific appropriate antibiotic is given, as above. Chronic pyelonephritis, a major cause of death in older women, often follows recurrent urinary tract infections during successive pregnancies. If symptomatic or asymptomatic bacteriuria occur during pregnancy, the patient should undergo a renal work-up after the postpartum period. This further investigation often reveals significant upper urinary tract abnormalities in the majority of these women (see also Chapter 10, Urinary Problems).

ANEMIA. Iron deficiency anemia occurs in about 20 percent of pregnant women in the United States and about 95 percent of all anemias occurring in pregnant women are due to iron deficiency. Although there is a physiologic decrease in hematocrit (HCT) and hemoglobin (Hgb) concentrations in pregnancy, values less than 12 Gm. per dl. Hgb and 35 percent HCT represent true anemia, which should be treated. Iron deficiency usually causes a microcytic hypochromic anemia, although in about 20 percent of iron deficiency anemias the red cells are of normal size and nearly normochromic. The hemoglobin concentration may fall as low as 3 Gm. per dl., but the red cell count is rarely below 2.5 million per cu mm. The reticulocyte and platelet counts are normal or high, and the white count is normal. Serum iron is low, usually less than 30 mcg./dl. (N = 90−150 mcg./dl.); total iron-binding capacity is elevated to 350 to 500 mcg./dl. (N = 250−350 mcg./dl.). Saturation is 10 percent or less. When anemia is found, inquire about a history of blood loss or a diet low in iron, and perform stool guaiac test for occult gastrointestinal bleeding. Consider infection and hemoglobinopathy in the differential. With the above described laboratory values, the treatment is usually undertaken without further diagnostic work-up in pregnant women. Oral iron therapy of ferrous sulfate 300 mg. with meals is the standard treatment. After the initiation of this treatment, maximal reticulocyte response can be expected within 5 to 10 days, then a gradual rise in hemoglobin concentration, with a return to normal levels in 2 to 3 months. If this response does not occur, either the woman is not taking the medication as prescribed, or the cause of anemia is not purely iron deficiency. Parenteral iron therapy may be necessary if intestinal disease precludes the use of oral iron, if the patient cannot tolerate oral iron or it is not being absorbed, if continued blood loss occurs, or if there is a failure of response to iron given orally. Iron dextran injection (Imferon) is given intramuscularly (IM). The dosage is calculated at 250 mg. per Gm. of hemoglobin below normal (i.e., 12–16 Gm.). Imferon 50 mg. per ml. is administered IM, usually 1 ml. initially then 2 to 2½ ml. per week until the total dosage has been given. It should be injected deeply using a 2-inch needle and the Z tech-

Table 5-6
Identification of High Risk Pregnancy: Factors Association with Increased Risk

Maternal Characteristics
Age less than 15 or over 35
Lower socioeconomic status
Unmarried
Family or marital conflicts
Emotional Illness or family history of mental
  illness
Persistent ambivalence or conflicts about the
  pregnancy
Stature under 5 feet
20 percent underweight or overweight
Inadequate diet

Reproductive History
Parity greater than 8
Two or more previous abortions
Previous stillborn or neonatal death
Previous premature labor or low birth weight
  infant (<2500 Gm.)
Previous excessively large infant (>4000 Gm.)
Infant with isoimmunization or ABO
  incompatibility
Infant with congenital anomaly, genetic disorder,
  or birth damage
Preeclampsia or eclampsia
Uterine fibroids >5 cm. or submucous
Abnormal Pap smear
Infertility
Prior cesarean section
Prior fetal malpresentations
Contracted pelvis
Ovarian masses
Genital tract abnormalities (incompetent cervix,
  subseptate or bicornate uterus)

Substances Abuse
Drugs
Alcohol
Heavy smoking >2 packs/day

Medical Problems
Chronic hypertension
Renal disease (pyelonephritis, glomerulonephritis,
  polycystic kidney)
Diabetes mellitus

Medical problems, continued
Heart disease (arotic insufficiency, pulmonary
  hypertension, diastolic murmur, cardiac
  enlargement, heart failure, arrhythmia)
Sickle cell trait or disease
Anemias with hemoglobin <9 Gm. and hematocrit
  <32 percent
Pulmonary disease (tuberculosis, COPD)
Endocrine disorders (hypo- or hyperthyroidism,
  family history of cretinism, adrenal or pituitary
  problems)
Gastrointestinal or liver disease
Epilepsy
Malignancy (including leukemia and Hodgkin's
  disease)

Complications of Present Pregnancy
Low or excessive weight gain
Hypertension (mean arterial pressure >90, BP
  140/90, increase >30 mm. Hg systolic or >20
  mm. Hg diastolic)
Recurrent glycosuria and abnormal FBS or
  glucose tolerance test
Uterine size inappropriate for gestational age
  (either too large or too small)
Recurrent urinary tract infections
Severe varicosities or thrombophlebitis
Recurrent vaginal bleeding
Premature rupture of membranes
Multiple pregnancy
Hydramnios with a single fetus
Rh negative with a rising titer
Late or no prenatal care
Exposure to teratogens (medications, x-ray,
  radioactive isotopes)
Viral infections (rubella, cytomegalovirus, herpes,
  mumps, rubeola, chickenpox, shingles,
  smallpox, vaccinia, influenza, poliomyelitis,
  hepatitis, Western equine encephalitis,
  Coxsackie B virus)
Syphilis, especially late pregnancy
Bacterial infections (gonorrhea, tuberculosis,
  listerosis, severe acute infection)
Protozoan infections (toxoplasmosis, malaria)
Postmaturity

nique to prevent leakage and staining of the skin. Improvement following parenteral iron is only slightly more rapid than with oral iron.

Folic acid deficiency anemia is most common in multiparas over age 30, and is the second most common type of anemia during pregnancy. The incidence of this deficiency is between 1 per 40 to 1 per 200 deliveries, oc-

curring most often when dietary resources are inadequate. It is associated with malnutrition, alcoholism, and protracted vomiting, and it may also be seen with multiple pregnancy, toxemia, sprue or sickle cell disease. Epileptic patients on long-term primidone (Mysoline), phenytoin (Dilantin) or barbiturate therapy often have folic acid deficiency anemia. The

Table 5-7
Tests of Fetal Status

Urinary estriol—Assesses function of maternal-fetal-placental unit. Serial determinations done in later pregnancy, estriol rises progressively. Twenty-four hour urine samples should contain levels of 10 to 20 mg. estriol/24 hours. Low or decreasing values (40 percent less than the mean of three previous values) indicate fetal deterioration or impending death.

Ultrasonic determination of fetal biparietal diameter—Ultrasound B scan provides a two dimensional representation of the fetal skull, and the A scan produces unidirectional measurements for fetal cephalometry. This method of measurement does not have the hazards of x-ray examinations. A fetal biparietal diameter of 8.5 cm. indicates gestation of 36 weeks or more.

Lecithin/sphingomyelin ratio (L/S)—Lecithin is a major component of pulmonary surfactant, a substance which prevents collapse of alveoli with each breath. Comparison of the amount of lecithin present in amniotic fluid to the amount of sphingomyelin enables evaluation of fetal lung maturity. Mean concentrations of these do not differ until about the thirtieth week of gestation. An increase of lecithin at 35 weeks indicates pulmonary maturity. About 5 cc. of amniotic fluid is removed and chromotography performed in a laboratory requiring several hours. An L/S ratio equal to or more than 2:1 signifies fetal maturity with no respiratory distress syndrome likely upon delivery. A transitional ratio of 1.5 to 1.9:1 indicates the possibility of mild to moderate respiratory distress. A ratio of 1.0 to 1.4:1 usually means relatively immature lungs with respiratory distress a distinct possibility if the infant is delivered.

Shake test (rapid surfactant test)—A rapid test for surfactant in amniotic fluid can be performed outside a clinical laboratory. Amniotic fluid is withdrawn and diluted after centrifuging in two test tubes 1:1 and 1:2 with normal saline and ethanol. After vortexing, the tubes are set upright for 15 minutes. A complete ring of bubbles around the meniscus in both tubes indicates mature lungs; a complete ring in the 1:1 dilution only is intermediate; and no complete ring in either dilution indicates immaturity.

Amniotic fluid creatinine and bilirubin—Rising concentrations of creatinine in the amniotic fluid are correlated with gestational age, with concentrations of less than 1.8 mg./dl. prior to the thirty-sixth week and greater than this value after the thirty-sixth week. After 37 weeks, creatinine concentration is 2 to 4 mg./dl. Bilirubin in amniotic fluid decreases as term approaches (only used for nonisoimmunized patients) by spectrophotometric analysis. Levels above 0.01 occur in gestations less than 35 weeks; 0.0 levels at 36 weeks.

Oxytocin challenge test—Decelerations in fetal heart rate with uterine contractions usually indicate fetal hypoxia. Weekly challenge tests during late pregnancy allow an index of fetal condition. Using an external fetal monitor and tocohynamometer for uterine contractions, a baseline is first obtained of FHT and uterine activity. Then intravenous oxytocin is given at gradually increasing doses until there are three contractions per 10 minutes. With no late decelerations for 30 minutes, the test is negative. Positive tests are combined with other data to make decisions about terminating the pregnancy.

---

hematologic findings are similar to those of true pernicious anemia (vitamin B^{12} deficiency). The hemoglobin may be as low as 4 to 6 Gm. per dl., and the red cell count below 2 million per cu. mm. in severe cases. The red cells may be normocytic or macrocytic, with the most constant change being macroovalocytosis. If there is a coexistent iron deficiency, the cells may be hypochromic. The mean corpuscular volume is normal or increased. Peripheral white cells are often hypersegmented. As a rule, the reticulocyte count is normal, and the platelet count normal or slightly decreased.

Nucleated megaloblastic red cells are difficult to demonstrate on peripheral smear but are found mixed with normoblastic cells if a bone marrow aspiration is done. Serum iron values are high, and serum vitamin B^{12} is normal. Free gastric hydrochloric acid is present in normal amounts. Treatment is with folic acid 5 to 10 mg. per day orally until the anemia improves. Iron is also given orally with a high vitamin, high protein diet. Use of vitamin B$_{12}$ even in high doses is generally not helpful. Megaloblastic anemia during pregnancy is usually not severe unless associated with systemic infections or toxemia. Inclusion of folic acid in prenatal vitamins or in prophylactic dosage of 1 mg. per day is now common practice.

IDENTIFICATION OF HIGH RISK PREGNANCY

The extent of involvement of the nurse practitioner or other primary care provider in the management of high risk and complicated pregnancies will vary by setting. Specialty practitioners in the area of obstetrics and gynecology will probably assume more shared responsibility in such cases, although physician referral and management is mandatory. Discussion of diagnosis and treatment of high risk pregnancy is beyond the scope of this text, but Table 5–6 highlights the identification of pregnancies at high risk and Table 5–7 outlines tests for fetal maturity and condition.

NOTES

1. P. M. Dunn, "Obstetric Delivery Today: For Better or for Worse?" *The Lancet* (April 10, 1976): 790-93.
2. R. C. Benson, *Current Obstetric & Gynecologic Diagnosis & Treatment* (Los Altos, Calif.: Lange Medical Publications, 1976), p. 68.
3. G. L. Bibring, D. S. Huntington, and A. F. Valenstein, "A Study of the Psychological Processes in Pregnancy and of the Earliest Mother-Child Relationship." *Psychoanalytic Study of the Child* 16 (1961): 1-24.
4. A. D. Colman and L. L. Colman, *Pregnancy: The Psychological Experience* (New York: Herder and Herder, 1971), pp. 31-40.
5. L. M. Tanner, "Developmental Tasks of Pregnancy." In *Current Concepts in Clinical Nursing*, vol. 2, B. S. Bergersen, et al. (eds.) (St. Louis: C. V. Mosby, 1969), pp. 292-97.
6. Colman and Colman, *Pregnancy*, pp. 96-144.
7. R. M. Pitkin and J. R. Scott (eds.), *The Yearbook of Obstetrics and Gynecology 1977* (Chicago: Yearbook Medical Publishers, 1977), p. 37.
8. S. L. Romney, et al. (eds.), *Gynecology and Obstetrics: The Health Care of Women* (New York: McGraw-Hill, Blakiston, 1975), pp. 800-01.

6

Labor, Delivery, and Postpartum

Women approach labor with both fear and excitement, with dread and anticipation. It is an unparalleled psychophysiological event, the culmination of an inexorable process that, once begun too subtly to perceive, will be realized by the timeless workings of the female body in the service of procreation. Few physical states are as all-consuming as labor, when the woman's emotional and cognitive functions are so totally focused on the sensations which accompany her body's physiology. Involvement is complete; the woman is in another space and time, and the external world recedes from her concern. For these several hours her body is her world, and she moves with its rhythms until the cellular commands are completed. Some women are terrified passengers on a journey in which they really want no part, and from which they futilely cry for escape. Others greet the challenge as an athlete greets a match—physically and emotionally prepared—and often undergo almost transcendent experiences in a wild communion with biology. Labor and delivery can be a high point in life or one of its horrors. And for some, no doubt, it is only a difficult task.

The institution of widespread prenatal care and hospital deliveries undoubtedly contributed to the marked decrease in maternal and neonatal mortality that is characteristic of the twentieth century. However, the influence of improved maternal nutrition and the declining birth rate might be even more significant factors. Professional norms surrounding childbearing have replaced cultural traditions, and folk wisdom has been lost. Attempts by health providers to replace the traditional supports have often been ineffective or have led to additional problems. Physician control of pregnancy, "leading" the woman through childbearing rather than "following" her, and "delivering" her rather than having the woman "deliver herself" have led to infantilization of women at a time when they should be most mature and in control. It is widely known that "civilized" women have more protracted, painful, and difficult labors. Changing the laboring location from the comfortable and familiar home to the dispassionate and alien hospital environment was one source of added stress. Going through labor and delivery lying flat with legs tied up in stirrups, prevented women from seeking the most advantageous position to maximize the force of gravity and the efficiency of uterine contractions. The loss of opportunity to learn about childbearing through personal exposure while growing up has contributed to the fear and uncertainty many women experience. While sedation has been a boon in relieving pain, it has also led to depressed newborns and mothers with impaired perception, to increasing infant mortality and morbidity, and to risking faulty mother-infant bonding.

Values change, and both women and health providers desire less interference in the labor and delivery process. Women increasingly want to be awake and involved, fathers to participate, and health providers to facilitate a natural, comfortable childbirth experience. More

149

judgment and courage are required to stand back and wait than to intervene, and an orientation toward pathology makes it easy to see abnormality in what really may be physiology.

Normal labor and delivery will be covered in this chapter; complications and abnormalities are beyond the scope of this text. Postpartum management and treatment of common problems will also be included.

DIAGNOSIS OF TERM PREGNANCY

Term pregnancy is reached when the fetus has developed to the point of maximum opportunity for extrauterine survival. Although this is thought of as a particular day, the expected date of confinement (EDC), based upon calculations from the woman's last menstrual period (LMP), it is actually a period of time. Term is the season of optimal maturation, beginning about the thirty-seventh week of gestation and extending to the forty-second week. By this time the fetus usually weighs more than 2500 Gm. (5 lb. 8 oz.), is about 45 cm. long from crown to heel, and has a head circumference of 33 cm.

If the EDC seems reasonably accurate by history, labor within 2 weeks before or after this date is normal. If there is any question about dates, or if the pregnancy has progressed beyond the EDC, or the mother and practitioner seek signs by which labor may be anticipated, other data can be used to evaluate whether the pregnancy is at term and the fetus mature. If the presence of fetal heart tones has been auscultated for 20 weeks by stethoscope, the pregnancy is approximately 40-weeks gestation, as fetal heart tones are usually first auscultated at 20 weeks. Adding 24 to 26 weeks to the date at which the woman first reported fetal movement gives the date of fetal maturity, as quickening is usually felt after 14- to 16-weeks gestation. Lightening usually occurs 2 to 3 weeks before delivery in primigravidas; it is the time when the fetus descends into the pelvic cavity and the height of the uterus decreases. Women may report easier breathing, less pressure upon the stomach with fewer digestive symptoms, and increased pelvic pressure and vaginal discharge. Fundal measurements (taken by McDonald's technique) decrease by 1 or 2 cm. from the thirty-sixth to the fortieth week. The uterus becomes more prominent and protrudes

forward (Figure 6-1). In multiparas this is more pronounced due to their less firm abdominal muscle tone. The fetal head, as a rule, does not become engaged in multiparas until labor begins. The mechanism of lightening includes the widening of the symphysis pubis, the sagging of the relaxed pelvic floor by as much as 4 cm., and the stretching of the lower uterine segment to permit the fetus to sink further down inside the uterus.

Cervical changes often begin as term is reached but prior to labor. The cervix shortens as it is drawn up and merged into the lower uterine segment. It tends to move forward from the posterior position typical of early pregnancy to a more anterior location in the vagina. Softening of the cervix means term is near, and effacement often begins. In primigravidas, noticeable effacement starts after about 36 weeks, and the cervix may thin almost completely and dilate 1 or 2 cm. by 38- to 40-weeks gestation. In multiparas, effacement is not as pronounced, but the external os is often dilated 1 or 2 cm. and patulous. There is often an increase in the frequency and intensity of Braxton-Hicks contractions near term, and many women mistake these for true labor contractions. Urination may become more frequent as bladder capacity is reduced due to descent of the fetal head.

PHYSIOLOGY OF LABOR AND DELIVERY

Normal labor occurs when the fetus is born at term, in vertex presentation, and when the process is completed spontaneously by the natural efforts of the mother within 24 hours and without complications. The onset of labor is the result of a combination of factors whose interrelation is not fully understood. Because the pregnant uterus is a contractile organ and has the ability to expel its contents at any time, pregnancy is able to continue through factors suppressing or inhibiting the uterus from performing at its effective working potential. Thus, the onset of labor should be thought of as a process in which there is a gradual release of inhibition, rather than one which is triggered by the appearance of a new substance which initiates a new event.[1]

The fetal endocrines, maternal endocrines, placenta, and uterus all seem to have important roles in the onset of labor. The fetal hypothalamus stimulates the secretion of corticosteroids which increase placental production of estrogen and prostaglandin precursors. Prostaglandins are effective in inducing uterine contractions and may cause pituitary release of oxytocin. Progesterone influence at some point diminishes, and its calming effects on the uterine muscles decrease. Oxytocin levels increase, particularly during the second stage of labor, and the uterus is more sensitive to its effects, possibly through a drop in levels of its inhibitor, oxytocinase. The contractility of the uterus increases as pregnancy advances; it is associated with an increased uterine volume which outgrows the influence of progesterone and placental inhibition during the last month of pregnancy. The pressure of the presenting part on nerve endings in the cervix may also play some role. The symbiotic relationship between mother and fetus during pregnancy is eventually disrupted, probably mediated by prostaglandin, and vigorous uterine muscle activity ensues.

The First Stage

The onset of labor to complete cervical dilatation comprise the first stage of labor. The average duration is 12 hours in primigravidas and 6 hours in multigravidas, with wide variations. Uterine contractions begin which are rhythmic and regular, occurring at decreasing intervals and with increasing intensity. In early labor, contractions are short and mild, 10 to 15 minutes or more apart, and may resemble menstrual cramps. As labor becomes more active, contractions occur every 3 to 5 minutes, last 50 to 70 seconds, and are very strong and often painful. Contractions usually start in the fundal region and spread downward. They are stronger and persist longer in the upper uterus, with fundus and midzone remaining hard throughout. In the lower segment, contractions are weaker (fundal dominance), permitting the cervix to dilate and the strongly contracting fundus to expel the fetus. Polarity is the term for this neuromuscular harmony between upper and lower uterine segments in which both poles (segments) act cooperatively. The upper pole contracts strongly and retracts, while the lower pole contracts slightly and dilates. Dystocia occurs if this polarity is disorganized.

Retraction is a special quality of the uterine muscle by which its fibers retain some con-

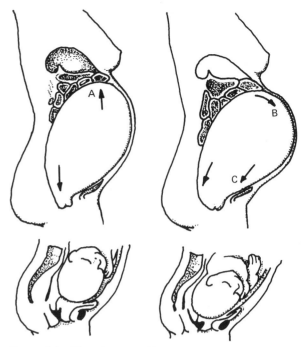

Figure 6-1. The changes which take place in lightening. (A) Pressure exerted on diaphragm before lightening. (B) Pressure relieved by falling forward of uterus. (C) Descent of head causes pressure on pelvic structures, particularly bladder.

traction instead of becoming completely relaxed after each labor contraction. The fibers become progressively thicker and shorter, enabling the upper segment of the uterus to decrease in size and to diminish its cavity. As the upper segment shortens, the lower segment stretches, aided by the force of the descending head. A ridge, the retraction ring, forms at the border where the thick upper segment meets the thin lower segment. In normal labors this ring is not visible abdominally and is a natural occurrence. In obstructed labors, where the fetus cannot descend to pass through the cervix, the lower segment must stretch excessively to accommodate it and a depressed ridge running transversely or obliquely across the abdomen above the symphysis can be seen. This abnormal retraction ring is called Bandl's ring[2] (Figures 6-2 and 6-3).

Cervical effacement progresses during the first stage as the muscle fibers surrounding the internal os are drawn upwards by the retracted upper segment. The shortened cervix merges into the lower uterine segment as its canal widens to form a funnel, with the external os

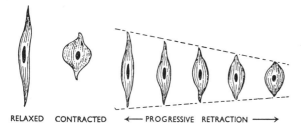

RELAXED   CONTRACTED   ←— PROGRESSIVE RETRACTION —→

Figure 6-2. Retraction of muscle fibers of upper uterine segment. M. F. Myles, *Textbook for Midwives* (Edinburgh: Churchill Livingstone, 1975), p. 232.

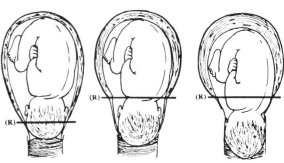

Figure 6-3. Rising retraction ring (R) during normal labor. As the upper uterine segment contracts and retracts the lower uterine segment has to "thin out" to accommodate the descending fetus. This continues until the cervix is fully dilated and the fetus can leave the uterus. The retraction ring rises no further, unless labor is obstructed. Miles, *Textbook for Midwives*, p. 212.

as the narrowed portion. Dilatation of the external os gradually occurs from 1 to 2 cm. at the onset of labor to 10 cm. at the end of the first stage. Upward traction helps draw the external os open, but downward pressure from the force of uterine contractions on the fetus and the action of a tightly fitting presenting part against the os are central to effective dilatation (Figure 6-4).

The interaction of the amniotic sac and uterine contractions affects the first stage. While the membranes are intact, the pressure of uterine contractions is exerted on the fluid and equalized throughout the uterus. When the

membranes rupture and the fluid escapes, the placenta is compressed between the uterine wall and the fetus during contractions, and the fetal oxygen supply is further diminished. There may be some physiologic advantage for membranes remaining intact through most of the first stage, although rupture is usually known to increase the force of uterine contractions. With an intact sac, normally there is detachment of the chorion from the lower segment as it stretches, and the loosened sac bulges downward into the dilating internal os. If the well-flexed fetal head fits snugly into the cervix, the fluid in front of the head (forewaters) is cut off from the remainder (hind-

Figure 6-4. Cervical effacement and dilatation. (Top, left) At beginning of labor; no effacement or dilatation. (Top, right) About one half effaced, but no dilatation. (Bottom, left) Completely effaced, but no dilatation. (Bottom, right) Complete dilatation.

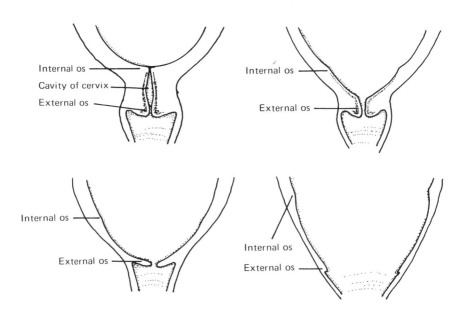

Internal os
Cavity of cervix
External os

Internal os
External os

Internal os
External os

Internal os
External os

waters). Thus the pressure of the contractions is not exerted as much on the forewaters and they remain intact, acting as a dilator by burrowing into the cervix (Figure 6-5).

A blood-stained mucoid discharge occurs a few hours before, or within a few hours of the onset of labor. Called the bloody show, it is composed of the thick, tenacious mucus which formed the cervical plug during pregnancy and blood from ruptured capillaries from the decidua where the chorion has become detached and from the dilating cervical canal. It is small to moderate in amount and may be dark or bright red. A variable amount of bloody vaginal discharge occurs during the first stage, especially as cervical dilatation nears completion. This is due to slight cervical or upper vaginal wall lacerations caused by tissue stretching. Once the membranes have ruptured, amniotic fluid continues to trickle out of the vagina, and it may be pink-tinged, clear, or milky with white flecks of vernix. Heavy bleeding is abnormal.

The Second Stage

Lasting from complete cervical dilatation to the expulsion of the fetus, the second stage of labor is about 45 minutes to 1 hour in the primigravida and 15 to 30 minutes in the multigravida. Uterine contractions are stronger and more frequent. The upper uterine segment continues to shorten and thicken, and the lower segment is completely thinned out and pulled up, so that the cervix cannot be felt in front of the fetal head. The upper vagina is stretched, and pressure is exerted on the rectum, initiating reflexive pushing by the woman. The fetal spine tends to straighten and elongate the fetus, so that the height of the fundus remains well above the umbilicus, although the head is on the pelvic floor.

During each contraction the uterus lifts forward and the force of the contraction is transmitted via the long axis of the fetus toward the birth canal. Early sensations of rectal pressure make the woman want to push or bear down, but this should not be done until cervical dilatation is complete. Using the muscles of the abdomen and the diaphragm, women augment the force of the contractions in expelling the fetus. Once the fetal head has reached and distended the pelvic floor, pushing is involuntary. The posterior segment of the pelvic floor is pushed downwards in front of the presenting

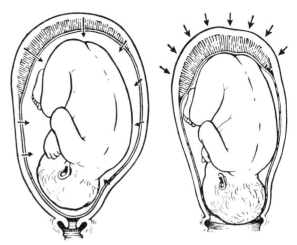

Figure 6-5. Interaction of amniotic sac and uterine contractions. (Left) General fluid pressure. The pressure of the uterine contractions is exerted on the amniotic fluid and equalized. The placental circulation is only interfered with slightly. (Right) Fetal axis pressure (*aids expulsion of the fetus*). The membranes have ruptured and much of the fluid has drained away. The pressure of the abdominal muscles and diaphragm is exerted on the buttocks and body of the fetus. The placental circulation is interfered with during contractions. Miles, *Textbook for Midwives*, p. 216.

part and the rectum is compressed. Any fecal contents present will be expelled, and the anus pouts and gradually gapes until the anterior rectal wall shows. The triangular perineal body is flattened out, becoming thin and almost transparent and increasing in length from about 4 to 10 cm. The thinned perineum lengthens the posterior wall of the birth canal and causes the vaginal opening to be directed upward.

The *mechanism of labor* is a series of passive movements of the fetus as it passes through the birth canal, accommodating itself to the diameters of the pelvis in different planes. The movements are brought about by the expulsive actions of uterine and abdominal muscles and by the resistance offered by the pelvis, cervix, and pelvic floor. *Descent* begins with engagement and progresses further during the first stage. As the head meets resistance, *flexion* is increased and the smaller occipitobregmatic (9.5 cm.) diameter of the head presents. This makes the occiput the leading fetal part by presenting a wedge which, being short and steep on one side, meets less resistance and thus descends more rapidly (Figure 6-6). *Internal rotation* is a turning forward of the occiput when it reaches the pelvic floor. This is brought

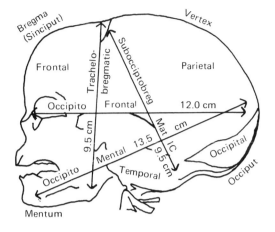

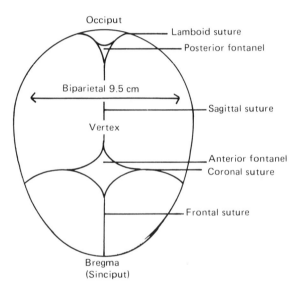

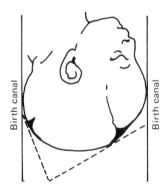

Figure 6-6. Diameters of fetal skull and occipital wedge in birth canal.

about by passive recoil of one lateral half of the pelvic floor. In the left occiput anterior (LOA) position, for example, the occiput stretches the left half of the pelvic floor during contractions, pushing it downward and outward. When the contraction eases, the pelvic floor recoils, and the occiput glides back along the left side of the pelvis, turning gradually anteriorly. The gutter shape of the pelvic floor directs the occiput toward the front, where it passes through the weakened area of the pelvic floor (vaginal opening) and under the pubic arch. With a deflexed head, both sides of the pelvic floor are contacted, and rotation does not take place. Occasionally the occiput rotates posteriorly, making extension more difficult.

Extension occurs with the occiput in the anteroposterior position, as the nape of the neck pivots on the lower border of the symphysis while the bregma (sinciput), face, and chin pass over the thinned perineum. As pressure is exerted downward, the pelvic floor and perineum offer resistance and push the head forward and upward through the area of less resistance, the vaginal opening. The occipitofrontal diameter of the fetal head (10 to 12 cm.) sweeps the perineum. Restitution then occurs, as the head moves to align with the shoulders, correcting the twist that occurred during internal rotation. From this movement it is apparent whether the baby is in LOA or right occiput anterior (ROA) position. Next the *internal rotation of the shoulders* occurs, bringing them into anteroposterior position. This should occur with the next contraction after the head is born. Accompanying this is *external rotation* of the head to maintain alignment. There is lateral flexion of the fetal body to conform to the birth canal, and the anterior shoulder escapes under the symphysis, then the posterior

Figure 6–7. Mechanism of labor. (Top, left) Before labor, showing the uterus relaxed with the cervix closed and thick pelvic floor. (Top, right) First stage of labor. Rhythmic contractions of the uterus aid the progressive effacement and dilatation of the cervix and the descent of the infant. (Center, left) Full dilatation: cervix high, head deep in birth canal, membranes intact. (Center, right) Second stage of labor. Top of infant's head begins to appear through the vulvar opening. (Bottom, left) Head extends upward, pelvic floor retreats. (Bottom, right) Birth of shoulders. (Dickinson-Belskie models, Cleveland Health Museum)

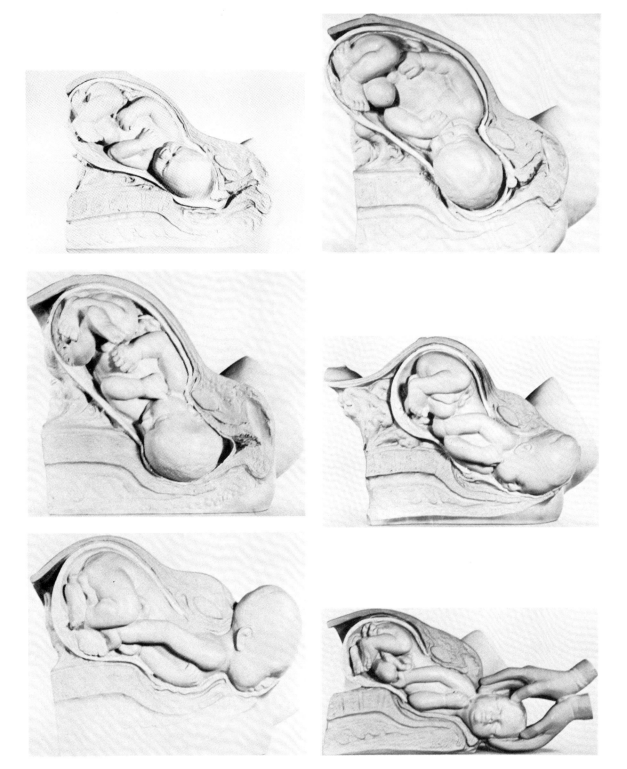

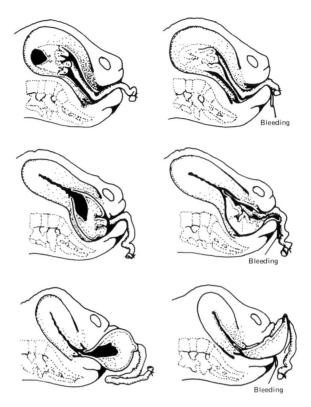

Figure 6-8. Successive stages of expulsion of placenta. (Left) Schultze's mechanism. (Right) Duncan mechanism.

shoulder passes over the perineum. *Expulsion* of the rest of the baby's body follows quickly. Figure 6-7 illustrates the mechanism of labor.

The Third Stage

The period from delivery of the baby to expulsion of the placenta and membranes is the third stage of labor, and it lasts about 15 minutes in both primi- and multigravidas. The uterus forms a firm, globular mass about the level of the umbilicus. Shortly after, it relaxes and assumes a discoid shape. These contractions and relaxations and the reduced size of the placental attachment site cause a buckling and separation of the placenta. Bleeding into the placental folds expedites separation. There is often a gush of blood from the vagina and the umbilical cord descends. The placenta is expelled with a few additional pushes by the woman, appearing either inverted, with the glistening fetal membranes presenting, or

rolled, with the maternal surface outermost (Figure 6-8).

The Fourth Stage

The first hour postpartum is often considered the fourth stage of labor in order to stress the importance of close observation for hemorrhage and other problems. During this time there is a restoration of physiologic stability. This time is also important for the initial formation of the mother-child relationship and for the consolidation of the family unit.[3]

CONDUCT OF NORMAL LABOR

Women are instructed to notify their birth attendant and come to the hospital or birth center when they think labor has begun. Guidelines for determining the onset of labor include regular contractions approximately 5 to 7 minutes apart which gradually increase in intensity and come closer together; the rupture of the membranes, either by a gush of fluid or a trickle; and the appearance of the bloody show. Upon arrival at the labor area, the woman is evaluated to determine whether she is in true or false labor and how far labor has progressed. Although there is a trend toward home births, particularly in certain areas of the country, the conduct of home births is beyond the scope of this book.

The Labor History

The woman is asked when regular contractions began, how frequently they are coming, and where she feels discomfort or sensations. Backache may be the only symptom of early labor, or varying degrees of pain may be felt in the lower abdomen, often wrapping around toward the lower back. Some women describe initial labor pains as similar to menstrual cramps, which continue to become more intense. It is important to distinguish when stronger, regular contractions began, as opposed to Braxton-Hicks's contractions. These intermittent, usually milder pains may be called labor pains by the woman, who might report that she has been in labor for 3 days. False labor is not included in the recorded time of true labor.

The presence of the bloody show, and when it was noticed, is part of the history. Show often appears a few hours before labor but is less in multiparas and may not appear until the first stage is more advanced. The woman may report bleeding, which, upon obtaining details about its character and amount, actually is show. Inquiry is made about rupture of the membranes, and the woman may be uncertain at times, confusing this with urinary incontinence. Usually if there has been a small tear in the membranes, fluid will continue to leak intermittently even after the bladder is empty. When rupture of the membranes is in question, litmus paper can be used to test vaginal drainage, for amniotic fluid is alkaline and urine and vaginal secretions are acidic.

The time of the woman's last meal is recorded, and what she has consumed since then. Intercurrent infections or other illnesses are noted. The record of prenatal care, including visits, examinations (especially pelvic measurements), laboratory reports, and any treatment given is reviewed. If the woman's prenatal record is not available, a pregnancy history must be taken and the standard laboratory tests obtained. Whether the woman has been able to sleep and get enough rest for the last week or several days is also important because this provides information about her energy reserves to cope with labor.

Initial Examination and Procedures

GENERAL EXAMINATION. Vital signs are taken, including temperature, pulse, respirations, and blood pressure. These normally do not rise significantly during labor, except that the pulse rate increases during contractions and the blood pressure may rise as much as 10 mm. toward the end of the first or during the second stage. An elevated temperature suggests infection or dehydration, and unless the woman's history reveals an obvious cause, such as mild upper respiratory infection, consultation should be sought. A rapid pulse may indicate blood loss, and the amount of bleeding should be carefully explored. It is extremely helpful to have baseline blood pressure readings during pregnancy because this makes the recognition of blood pressure elevation in labor much easier. A woman may present in labor with a BP of 120/80, which appears normal, but with a prenatal average of 90/60, this represents a significant elevation. Preeclampsia can be absent during pregnancy, and the urinalysis negative for protein on admission, but eclamptic convulsions may nevertheless occur during labor. A blood pressure of 130/80 or above indicates the need for physician consultation.

The woman's general appearance is noted, particularly for dehydration, exhaustion, and disorientation. Her extremities and face are examined for edema. A clean-catch urine specimen is obtained to check protein and glucose levels. A trace of protein after the membranes are ruptured is not significant. Ketones and pH may also be noted.

If an infectious or contagious disease is suspected, the woman must be isolated. If there is evidence of complications, physician consultation or referral is indicated.

ABDOMINAL EXAMINATION. The abdomen is palpated to determine the fetal presentation, position, and engagement, and the level of the most dependent part. The size of the uterus gives some information about the length of gestation, and a small uterus combined with labor beginning more than 2 weeks before the EDC suggests premature labor. Breech presentation should be readily identifiable by the presence of the fetal head in the uterine fundus, and referral is necessary. Transverse lie can also be detected by abdominal examination, as the transverse diameter of the uterus is greater than the longitudinal, and the head can be felt in the mother's right or left flank. Whether or not the head has engaged or is well descended is important, for failure of descent can either indicate cephalopelvic disproportion or alert the practitioner to the danger of umbilical cord prolapse when the membranes are ruptured.

The fetal heart tones are counted and recorded by the standard method of the given institution. Whether auscultated by a stethoscope or an electronic instrument (e.g., Doptone), the fetal heart tones should fall within the normal range of 120 to 160 per minute. Rates above or below this require further monitoring for possible fetal distress.

Uterine contractions are palpated for frequency, intensity, duration, and regularity. Frequency is timed from the beginning of one contraction to the beginning of the next. The duration of a contraction is timed from the initial tightening of the uterus until it relaxes. Intensity may be mild, moderate, or strong and is determined by the hardness and resistance of the contracted uterus to pressure by the examiner's hand. A strong contraction has a feeling of woody hardness, and at its height the uterus cannot be indented by pressure. In a moderate contraction, the uterus feels firm but not completely hard, and there is slight indentation of the uterus to pressure. Mild contractions cause some increased tenseness of the uterus as compared to its resting state, but this is slight, and the uterus yields easily to the examiner's pressure.

Mild contractions in early labor are often 10 to 15 minutes apart and last 20 to 25 seconds. Most women are not uncomfortable with these, and report mild backache or cramping and a sense of uterine tightness. Moderate contractions occur in the early active phase of labor, may be between 3 and 10 minutes apart, and last 45 to 60 seconds. These produce more discomfort or pain, depending upon many individual variables such as pain threshold, tension, and use of childbirth techniques. Hard contractions occur during normal, active labor and are 2 to 3 minutes apart and last 45 to 60 seconds or slightly longer. These contractions have a consuming intensity, often described as the most severe pain ever experienced, and demand the woman's full concentration. Again, response differs according to many factors. Well-prepared women use childbirth techniques to focus sharply inward, no longer sociable between contractions but resting quietly and conserving energy to meet the next contraction. Diaphragmatic breathing or rapid shallow costal breathing, along with the partner's coaching and encouragement, are usually included. Unprepared women, however, may panic as contractions become hard, crying out and thrashing about during contractions, grabbing at attendants and pleading to be relieved of their pain. Some unprepared women can be reached before the intense contractions begin and taught simple breathing techniques in earlier labor. Teaching them to breathe slowly and evenly during early contractions, then more rapidly and shallowly as labor gets harder, may provide them with a method of coping with labor pain. They must often be reminded not to hold their breath but to keep breathing during contractions, and they need the encouragement of an attendant constantly at the bedside coaching and reassuring them.

If the woman describes rectal pressure and the need to empty her bowels or bear down, she may be entering the second stage and an immediate pelvic examination is indicated. Some women experience these sensations before full dilatation, however, and need instructions not to bear down as this is ineffective, wasteful of their energy, and can lead to an edematous lip of the cervix.

VAGINAL EXAMINATION. The vulva and vaginal opening are inspected for bleeding or loss of amniotic fluid. If amniotic fluid is leaking, note the amount, its color, and character. If greenish, this indicates meconium is present in the amniotic fluid, a sign of fetal distress unless there is breech presentation. As amniotic fluid is normally amber or pinkish due to the normal slight bleeding from cervical dilatation, dark pink or red discoloration of the fluid indicates more bleeding than is normal. Dark yellow fluid may imply the presence of bilirubin and an incompatibility problem. Foul-smelling amniotic fluid usually means amnionitis, and it should be carefully assessed after the membranes have been ruptured for several hours. Heavy bleeding is a complication also needing referral. When checking for

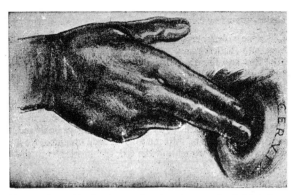

Figure 6-9. Vaginal examination for cervical dilatation. Cervix is 4 cm. dilated. Miles, *Textbook for Midwives*, p. 249.

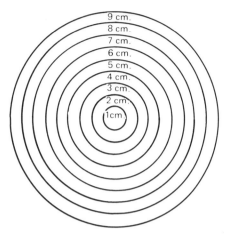

Figure 6-10. Chart for visualization of cervical dilatation. Representation of dilatation is in centimeters to scale.

the presence of amniotic fluid, litmus (Nitrazine) paper turns from its usual yellow (acid) to deep blue-green (alkaline) if amniotic fluid is present. The presence of blood, which is also alkaline, creates a false positive.

An aseptic vaginal examination is done upon admission to determine the degree of dilatation and effacement of the cervix, to identify the presenting part, and to determine descent through the birth canal (station, position) (Figure 6-9). Any abnormalities of the soft tissues of the birth canal are also identified and consultation sought. The vaginal walls should feel soft and dilatable; when firm and rigid a longer labor is likely. The presence of scar tissue in the lower vagina may cause delay during the perineal phase of the second stage because of a lack of elasticity, and the perineum is more

liable to tear. Fecal mass in the rectum may be felt.

The dilatation of the cervix is expressed in centimeters indicating the diameter of the cervical opening. This is estimated by feeling the cervix with the vaginal-examining fingers, and imagining how large the cervical opening is. The width of one fingertip is slightly more than 1 cm., and the combined size of two fingertips is about 3 cm. (Figure 6-10 and Table 6-1).

The effacement of the cervix is estimated by feeling vaginally the length and thickness of the cervix and comparing it to an uneffaced cervix which is 2 to 2.5 cm. long. Effacement is expressed in percentage, with 0 percent

Table 6-1
Estimation of Cervical Dilatation

Centimeters	Approximate Fingers
1	One fingertip, tight
2	One finger, loose
3	Two fingers
4	Three fingers
5	Four fingers, or double the width of the two examining fingers. Cervix is halfway dilated.
6	The examining fingers are spread to touch each cervical border, or are held together and swept around the edge of the cervix. It is more helpful now to imagine a cervical chart for comparison (Figure 6-10).
7	Same technique as above. Cervix three-fourths dilated.
8	Examining fingers can find only a 2 cm. rim of the cervix.
9	Examining fingers can find only a 1 cm. rim of the cervix.
10	No cervix can be felt. Full dilatation.

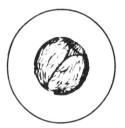 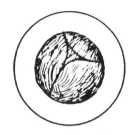 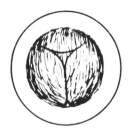

Figure 6-11. Determination of position by vaginal examination.

being uneffaced and 100 percent representing complete effacement when a cervix is less than 0.25 cm. thick. The estimation is based upon imagining the thickness of the cervix as felt by the examining fingers compared to approximately the 2 cm. thickness of an uneffaced cervix. Primigravidas and secundagravidas can have a cervix which is tissue-paper thin upon complete effacement, and often the examiner's fingers slip over the edge without detecting it, leading to the incorrect assumption of full dilatation. Also, in primigravidas effacement may be complete before dilatation has progressed beyond 2 or 3 cm., and the cervix may be posterior and high in the vagina. This makes the cervical opening hard to reach, and the thinness leads the examiner again to mistakenly think that there is complete dilatation. These situations should be suspected if the examiner cannot feel any cervix but the woman does not show signs of the second stage of labor.

The position of the presenting part is determined by the relation of the fetal occiput (in cephalic presentations) to the mother's right or left side. To do this, the sagittal suture is palpated, and the anterior and posterior fontanels located, if possible. The location of the posterior fontanel is the guide, and is expressed as OA (occiput anterior) when the fontanel is directly anterior, LOA (left occiput anterior) when the fontanel is toward the mother's left and up (Figure 6-11), LOP (left occiput posterior) when it is toward the mother's left and down, and so on for ROA and ROP. Breech presentations can usually be identified by the relative softness and irregularity of the presenting part, in contrast to the smooth, regular, and hard head. In face presentations, the hard, angular chin is a prominent and identifiable landmark. Brow presentations may be more

difficult to identify, but the larger anterior fontanel may be more easily felt than the posterior fontanel. These are considered abnormal presentations and should be referred.

The term station is used to describe the location of the presenting part in its progress through the birth canal. The distance of the fetal head from the ischial spines of the mother's pelvis is the determinant of station. If the head is at the level of the spines, it is at zero station; if above or below the spines, this distance is estimated by centimeters from the spines. Distances above the spines are stated as −1 cm., −2 cm., −3 cm. and floating, below the spines as +1 cm., +2 cm., +3 cm., and on the perineum (Figure 6-12). The degree of *moulding* of the fetal head is also assessed, primarily through the amount of overlapping of the skull bones. Excessive or pronounced overlapping, especially if the head is not well engaged, suggests fetal death or intracranial injury. A large *caput* may cause the station to be interpreted as lower than the actual location of the fetal skull.

The status of the membranes is also ascertained by vaginal examination. With very scanty forewaters, the membranes are difficult to feel because they lie close to the fetal scalp. The scalp, when covered with mucus, has the same smooth, slippery feeling as the membranes, but during a contraction the membranes often become tense and bulge slightly. Usually the forewaters are shaped like a wristwatch crystal, but if the fit of the head is not tight into the pelvis, some hindwaters are forced forward during contractions, and the forewaters protrude more through the cervix. The presence of a bag of waters after the membranes have been reported to be ruptured usually means that a tear higher in the membranes has been closed off by the descent of the fetal head or that only the outer layer has been ruptured, with the escape of chorionic fluid (Table 6-2).

Preparation for Labor and Continuing Care

After it has been determined that the woman is in true labor, she is admitted to the hospital labor unit or the birth unit. The perineum is usually prepared by cleansing and shaving of the vulvar hair. Use of this "miniprep" is now common, with the removal of hair only on the perineum and lower labia, leaving the hair over the mons pubis. If delivery is not imminent, the lower bowel is emptied with an enema or suppository. This promotes a clean field for delivery and stimulates labor contractions. With a multipara in active labor and dilated more than 6 cm., the enema is often withheld if the fetus is well descended because it can lead to precipitous delivery.

A woman in early labor need not remain in bed if the membranes have not ruptured, she is not bleeding, and has not received sedation. Small amounts of clear fluids are given, but no solid food. To prevent tracheal irritation in case of vomiting, small amounts of antacids may be given to reduce gastric acidity. This also reduces the likelihood of serious pulmonary complications in the case of aspiration of vomitus. The approach to the routine use of intravenous fluids varies by setting. If labor is prolonged or dehydration is present, a continuous IV drip of 5 percent glucose is indicated. The woman is encouraged to empty her bladder regularly to prevent distention, which can interfere with the progress of labor. Urine is

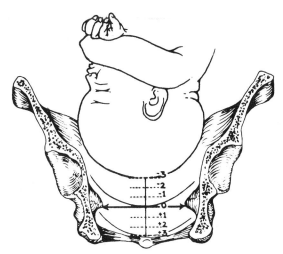

Figure 6-12. Stations of the fetal head. R. C. Benson, *Current Obstetric & Gynecologic Diagnosis & Treatment* (Los Altos, Calif.: Lange Medical Publications, 1976), p. 574.

tested frequently for protein, ketones, and glucose.

CONDUCT OF THE FIRST STAGE. The frequency, length, and strength of uterine contractions are noted regularly, about every 15 to 30 minutes. The descent of the presenting part can be followed primarily by abdominal palpation, noting the downward movement of the occipital prominence. The location of the maximal volume of the fetal heart tones can be

Table 6-2
Differentiating True Labor from False Labor

True Labor	False Labor
Contractions	*Contractions*
Occur at regular intervals	Occur at irregular intervals
Intervals gradually shorten	Intervals remain the same
Intensity gradually increases	Intensity remains the same
Located in lower abdomen and back	Located chiefly in abdomen
Intensified by walking	Walking often gives relief or has no effect
Bloody show	*Bloody show*
Usually present	None
Cervix	*Cervix*
Effacement is present and progresses	Effacement is no greater than during later pregnancy, does not progress
Dilatation is present and progresses	Dilatation (may be around 2 cm.) does not progress
Membranes feel tense during a contraction	Membranes do not become tense during a contraction

marked on the abdomen, and its movement downward also can be used to follow descent. Pulse and blood pressure are also recorded every 15 to 30 minutes and temperature hourly after the membranes have ruptured. The bladder should be emptied every 2 to 3 hours, and if the woman is unable to do so in 6 to 8 hours or if the bladder is distended, catheterization is necessary. The perineum and vulvar region must be cleansed before and after pelvic examination, after voiding and bowel movements, or when covered with vaginal drainage. The character of vaginal discharge and bleeding is also frequently checked. The woman's partner or coach may be constantly present, providing support and encouragement, or the labor staff may have to assume this role.

Fetal heart tones are taken and recorded every 15 minutes. Practices vary regarding the method of taking these heart tones. Some settings utilize the stethoscope unless there are signs of fetal distress or the pregnancy is high risk. Others prefer external ultrasonic monitors, either intermittently every 15 minutes or continuously by attaching the monitor with a belt around the mother's abdomen. The fetal heart tones should be taken both during and after contractions in order to note the variations in rate. At the acme of a contraction, the fetal heart tones often drop to 100 to 120 beats per minute, beginning to slow after the onset of the contraction and picking up again about 10 to 15 seconds before it ends. This physiologic bradycardia is thought to be due to the compression of the fetal skull by the partially dilated cervix, and it appears most often between 4 and 8 cm. dilatation. If the fetal heart tones drop below 100, or if the bradycardia lasts more than 30 seconds after the end of a contraction, this is no longer physiologic and the physician should be notified. Internal monitoring of fetal heart tones and intrauterine pressure is usually done when there are signs of fetal distress or with a high risk pregnancy. The use of internal monitors is covered in other sources.[4]

The number of vaginal examinations should be minimized because of the potential of introducing infection. In early labor, hourly examinations are adequate and may be done less frequently when contractions remain of mild intensity. As labor progresses, more frequent examinations are usually required. On vaginal examination, dilatation and effacement of the cervix, station and position of the presenting part, or presence of any abnormality are noted. The possibility of prolapse of the umbilical cord must always be kept in mind, particularly when the head is not well engaged and the membranes have ruptured. Cervical dilatation follows a pattern in normal labor which is similar for primigravidas and multigravidas. There is first a *latent phase*, from the beginning of labor contractions until the cervix is dilated about 2 cm., during which contractions are mild to moderate and less frequent than during active labor. This phase lasts about 5½ hours in multiparas and 8 hours in primiparas. Next follows the *acceleration* phase, in which labor becomes active, with strong, regular contractions. This may last from 1 to 2 hours and is shorter in multiparas. Cervical dilatation progresses to about 3 cm. The *phase of maximum slope* occurs after this, in which dilatation is quite rapid and progresses from 3 to 8 or 9 cm. in about 1 hour. Contractions are intense, long, and hard. The pace slows somewhat with the *deceleration phase*, as the cervix completes the process of dilating. Another 30 minutes in multiparas and 1 hour in primiparas are needed to move from 8 or 9 to 10 cm. (Figure 6-13).

ANALGESIA. The use of medication for relaxation or pain relief during labor is primarily the decision of the woman. If she desires no medication, this must be respected. Women who are prepared by various techniques for coping with labor contractions often require no or minimal medication. Other women may desire maximum sedation, or are willing to accept whatever is suggested. In any case, the trend is to give as little medication of any type as possible. Obviously, decisions about specific drugs, dosages, and routes are the prerogative of the health provider. Discussing various types of analgesics, their advantages and drawbacks, prior to labor contributes to a compatible provider-patient partnership.

The woman in early labor who is tense, apprehensive, or exhausted often benefits from a hypnotic which will induce a few hours of sleep. This relaxation can often permit good labor to become established and can refresh the patient. Barbiturates commonly used for this purpose are sodium pentobarbital (Nembutal), sodium secobarbital (Seconal), and sodium amobarbital (Amytal). Oral or intramuscular doses of 100 to 200 mg. are given.

A.

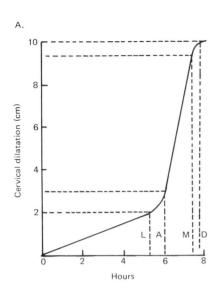

B.

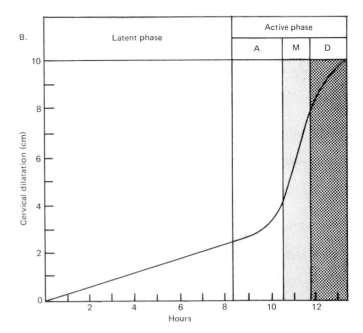

Figure 6-13. Dilatation of cervix at various phases of labor. (A) Multiparas. (B) Primigravidas. (A, acceleration phase; L, latent phase; M, phase of maximum slope; D, deceleration phase.)

The preferred analgesic in many settings is meperidine (Demerol), 50 to 75 mg. intramuscularly or intravenously. To potentiate its effect, tranquilizers such as promethazine (Phenergan) or promazine (Sparine) may be given concomitantly. These drugs are also effective antinauseants and reduce anxiety. If analgesics are given, they should not be administered too frequently. Intervals of 2 to 4 hours between doses is advised, and they should not be given immediately before anticipated delivery because of their depressive effects on the infant. Also, an analgesic, if given too early in labor, may prolong the latent phase. The progress of labor may be slowed at more active phases if an analgesic is given in excessive amounts.

Regional analgesia can be obtained during labor by a paracervical block, the transvaginal injection of 5 to 10 ml. of 1 percent lidocaine at the 4–6 o'clock and 6–8 o'clock positions of the cervical-vaginal junction (Figure 6-14). Sensory nerve fibers from the uterus fuse at these points, and a paracervical block can relieve substantial amounts of pain for 45 to 60 minutes. It can be done when the cervix is dilated 4 cm. or more. A 5- or 6-inch needle with a guide or lead shot affixed to it is used, which allows the point to be inserted 0.1 to 0.2 cm. into the tissues. Five ml. of lidocaine is injected about 2 cm. lateral to the cervix in the area described above. Transient fetal bradycar-

dia has been noted to follow paracervical block; the incidence is reported at 20 to 25 percent.[5] This is thought to be due to the rapid absorption of the medication from the very vascular cervical area. There usually is no continuing effect, and this method is relatively safe for both fetus and mother. Infrequently, there are serious complications, including maternal trauma and bleeding, fetal trauma and direct injection causing fetal death, and maternal convulsions resulting from inadvertent intravascular injection.

Pudendal nerve block is another method of regional analgesia or anesthesia used for second stage labor and delivery (Figure 6–14). The pudendal nerve approaches the ischial spines on its course to innervate the perineum. The injection of 10 ml. of 1 percent lidocaine on each side near the spines will achieve analgesia for 30 to 45 minutes in about 50 percent of the women who are injected. Variations in innervation may cause other women to require a more extensive injection in order to obtain good lower vaginal and perineal analgesia. The ischial spines are palpated vaginally. Using a 5- to 6-inch needle with a guide, 5 ml. of med-

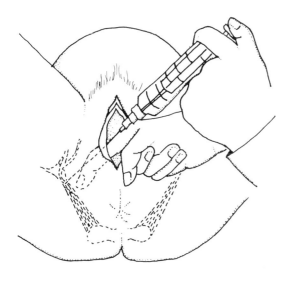

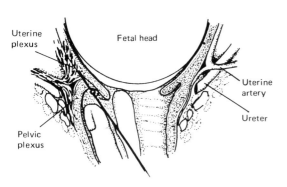

Uterine
plexus

Fetal head

Uterine
artery

Ureter

Pelvic
plexus

Figure 6-14. (Top) Pudendal block. (Bottom) Paracervical block.

ication is injected below each spine, after aspirating to be certain that the needle is not in a vein. If additional areas need to be anesthetized, the syringe is refilled and redirected as above, first toward the ischial tuberosity, where 3 ml. is injected near the center of each tuberosity to anesthetize the inferior hemorrhoidal and lateral femoral cutaneous nerves. Then, to block the ilio-inguinal and genitocrural nerves, the needle is advanced toward the symphysis almost to the clitoris, keeping it about 2 cm. lateral to the labial fold and 1 to 2 cm. beneath the skin. Complications include maternal trauma, bleeding, and infection and, rarely, convulsions.

Discussion of other regional anesthesia, including epidural and caudal blocks, is beyond the scope of this text.

CONDUCT OF THE SECOND STAGE. During the second stage, constant attendance by the health provider is necessary. The transition from first to second stage is not always clearly defined, and the only positive sign is complete dilatation on vaginal examination. There are at least five probable signs, however, which alert the provider. 1) The woman has expulsive contractions, during which she involuntarily bears down. If the head is deeply engaged, the rectum loaded, or the occiput posterior, the woman may have a strong urge to bear down during late first stage. 2) A sudden increase or trickle of blood occurs which is due to the slight lacerations of the cervix when it is stretched to full dilatation. However, the amount of bleeding during cervical dilatation is variable, and there may be no noticeable changes, or some women may not bleed although the cervix is fully dilated. 3) There is a tenseness between the anus and the coccyx which is felt upon pressing this area deeply; it is due to the pressure exerted by the descending head on the rectum and pelvic floor. Pouting and gaping of the anus occur when the head has reached the pelvic floor, though they may occur in late first stage in a multipara with the head deeply engaged and a lax pelvic floor. The woman's urgently requesting a bedpan for a bowel movement may also be a sign. 4) The gaping of the vulva is a more reliable sign in primigravidas, and the bulging of the perineum is a good later sign which usually means delivery is imminent. 5) The appearance of the head at the vaginal opening is usually an excellent sign but, rarely, with excessive moulding, a large caput may be visible during a contraction even though the head may be above the ischial spines and the cervix not fully dilated.

The second stage is relatively short, and there should be evidence of constant progress. In multiparas it often is less than 15 minutes; if beyond 30 minutes, consultation should be sought. Primigravidas may usually be allowed to spend 1 hour in second stage before concern is aroused, unless no progress in descent is occurring. Observations on contractions, blood pressure, and pulse are made every 10 to 15 minutes, and the fetal heart tones auscultated before, during, and after each contraction if an ultrasonic or electronic monitor is not being used. Bladder distention should be prevented by voiding as needed or by catheterization if the woman is unable to void a full bladder.

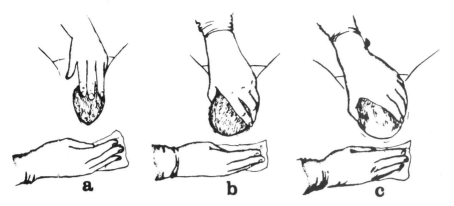

Figure 6-15. Delivering the head. (A) Controlling the crowned head. (B) Grip altered to extend the head. (C) Widest diameter distending the perineum. Miles, *Textbook for Midwives*, p. 276.

The woman is often encouraged to push with each contraction to aid fetal descent. Although the dorsal position is most commonly used, some women may prefer lying on one side with rounded back, semisitting with back supported, kneeling, or squatting. Bearing down efforts can be augmented if the woman is in the dorsal position by raising her head and shoulders slightly with good support, flexing her thighs on her abdomen with her hands grasped just below her knees, taking a deep breath as soon as the contraction begins and, with breath held, bearing down in a long sustained push. Crying out or grunting will cause much of the expulsive force to be lost. Pushing can be maintained as long as the uterus is contracted, but the woman should not push between contractions because this can overstretch the transverse cervical ligaments and predispose her to uterine prolapse. Two or three sustained pushes with quick breaths between can generally be done with each contraction.

Delivery should be anticipated when the head reaches the pelvic floor, depending upon the rate of progress and whether the woman is a multipara or a primigravida. As the perineum is distended, the head bulges forward with each contraction and tends to recede slightly afterwards. Crowning occurs when the biparietal diameter of the head distends the vulva and the head does not recede after contractions. As crowning occurs, the woman is asked to stop pushing, and the advancement of the head is controlled by spreading the fingers uniformly over the vertex, with their tips pointing toward the bregma, in order to restrain any sudden expulsive effort. The speed of delivery is slowed as necessary to avoid pudendal lacerations or the unexpected extrusion of the fetal head

because marked variations in intracranial pressure may cause cerebral hemorrhage. The sinciput is allowed to glide slowly over the perineum at the end of a contraction (Figure 6-15). The extension of the head may be aided, if necessary, by pressure applied from the mother's coccygeal region upward. The fingers should not be inserted into the birth canal or the rectum to facilitate delivery because trauma or infection may occur. The perineum may be gently drawn downward with two fingers, if needed, to allow the head to clear the perineal body (Figure 6-16). The chin is freed by slipping the index finger under the side of the jaw and sweeping it below the chin and out at the other side, as needed.

Once the face and chin are delivered, the neck should be checked for the presence of the cord. In about 15 to 20 percent of deliveries, the umbilical cord is wrapped around the baby's neck, though rarely tight enough to cause hypoxia. If present, the cord is loosened cautiously, and pulsations are checked. If the cord is pulsating well, there is no need to hasten delivery. If there is enough slack, the cord may be removed by hooking a finger around the cord and gently slipping it over the baby's head. Strong traction must not be used as there is a danger that the cord might break. If the cord cannot slip over the head, the cord is clamped with two forceps and cut between them. As this cuts off the baby's oxygen supply, delivery should not be delayed.

The infant's airway is cleared by pressure on

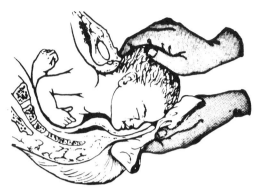

Figure 6-16. Aiding extension of the head (modified Ritgen maneuver). Benson, *Current Obstetric & Gynecologic Diagnosis*, p. 580.

the trachea and nose. Fluid is wiped from the nose and mouth, and then the nasal and oral passages are aspirated with a soft rubber suction bulb or a small catheter attached to a DeLee suction trap. Before external rotation and the birth of the shoulders, the head is usually drawn back toward the perineum. In the contraction following the birth of the head, the anterior shoulder rotates forward so that the shoulders are in the anteroposterior diameter of the outlet. This is evident by external rotation. The infant is supported manually through the rest of delivery. It is important not to hurry this stage, as there is an adaptive advantage to the baby in the slow delivery of the body. The baby's face will look reddish blue, but such congestion is a necessary stimulus to respiration. If, however, the color becomes dark blue delivery should be expedited.

To facilitate the expulsion of the anterior shoulder, the head can be gently depressed downward toward the mother's anus. The shoulder will gradually appear. It is better not to extract the arm by bringing it down under the pubic arch because to do so would increase the danger of fracturing the humerus. Traction on the head should be minimal and should not make the neck twist or bend sideways because of the risk of injury to the brachial plexus (Erb's paralysis). Hematoma of the neck or a fractured clavicle can also occur from excessive traction or attempts to extract the anterior shoulder. When the anterior shoulder is free, the head is guided upward toward the mother's symphysis, so that the posterior shoulder can escape over the perineum (Figure 6-17). The body and legs are delivered gradually by easy traction after the shoulders have been freed.

Perineal lacerations cannot always be avoided, but these can often be minimized by careful technique. The principles of this technique are to have the smallest possible diameter of head and shoulders emerge and distend the vulval opening and to control the birth of the head and shoulders so that this takes place slowly and without expulsive force. By maintaining the flexion of the head and prohibiting too rapid extension, the smallest diameter will distend the vulva. The actual extension of the head should take place in a gliding motion, with the woman panting or breathing rapidly to avoid pushing. The head should be born at the end of a contraction or between contractions. If, during a contraction, there is too much force the tense perineum can rupture more readily. Applying pressure to the perineum with hands or fingers can cause bruising, thins it more, and is conducive to tearing. The provider's hands should always control the advancing head because an unexpected cough, push, or sudden move by the mother can cause sudden extrusion and tearing. The shoulders must also be delivered carefully and slowly; allowing the anterior shoulder to escape first presents a smaller diameter. External rotation of the head must occur before the shoulders are delivered, signifying internal rotation; otherwise, they will rotate while passing through the vulva and strain the perineum. After both shoulders are born and the baby carried upward, the arms should be grasped alongside the body; if the body is grasped under the arms their outward thrust puts additional strain on the perineum. Signs of probable perineal tear include a long edematous perineum, trickling of blood from the vagina when the head is on the perineum, a bluish appearance in the perineal midline which later becomes white, shiny, and transparent, and a tear in the fourchette before the head is crowned.

Episiotomy may be necessary to enlarge the vaginal orifice, particularly if the perineum is long or rigid, the head is disproportionate to the vaginal opening, or there is a need to hasten delivery (Figure 6-18). It is usually advisable to infiltrate the perineum with lidocaine (Xylocaine) in the area the perineum is to be cut. Two fingers are inserted into the vagina to separate the perineum from the fetal scalp. During a contraction, the needle is introduced on the midline of the inner edge of the fourchette and directed subcutaneously for about 3 cm. to the

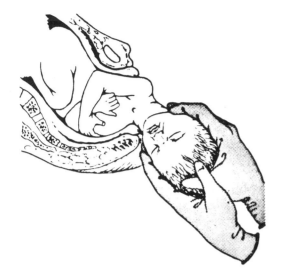
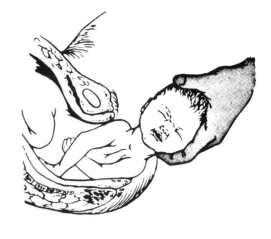

Figure 6-17. Delivering the shoulders. (Left) Anterior shoulder. (Right) Posterior shoulder. Benson, *Current Obstetric & Gynecologic Diagnosis*, p. 582.

right or left. After aspirating, the medication is injected while the needle is slowly withdrawn. About 3 ml. are given, then the needle is redirected 1 cm. from the first injection and another 3 ml. deposited in the same way. This may be repeated again 1 cm. in the other direction.

After waiting 1 or 2 minutes, the fingers are again inserted between perineum and fetal head, and the episiotomy made with a single snip, during a contraction. It is placed in the center of the anesthetized area, and should be about 3 cm. long. Median or mediolateral episiotomies are more commonly done. Consultation should be sought in performing or repairing episiotomies.

Oxytocics are used after delivery to reduce blood loss and prevent subinvolution of the uterus. Pitocin or Syntocinon (almost pure oxytocin) is used in doses of 0.5 ml. (5 IU of extract) with, or immediately after, delivery of the infant and repeated in the same dose after the placenta is removed. Methergine 0.2 mg. IM can be given immediately after the placenta is delivered.

CONDUCT OF THE THIRD STAGE. Placental separation usually occurs within 5 minutes following delivery, although up to 15 minutes is considered within the range of normal. If the placenta has not been expelled within 30 minutes, this indicates a complication such as incomplete separation or placenta accreta. Considerable blood may be lost if the third step is prolonged, and the placenta's remaining in the

uterus prevents the contraction and retraction of muscle fibers around the large torn placental sinuses. Expulsion of the placenta was probably intended by nature to be accomplished by gravity, with the mother in a squatting position. When this occurs in the dorsal position, assistance is usually needed to shorten the time of expulsion.

After the birth of the baby, the fundus is about 2.5 cm. below the umbilicus. As the uterus contracts and becomes smaller, it changes in shape from discoid to globular. A slight gush of blood or lengthening of the cord may signify separation. When the placenta is ready for expulsion, it will present at the cervical os and may dilate the cervix slightly. If the placenta can be palpated by vaginal examination at the cervical os or in the vagina, then gentle cord traction can help to remove it. The method used for the recovery of the placenta is the Brandt-Andrews maneuver (Figure 6-19). Pressure is placed on the abdomen, with the fingers just above the symphysis in order to elevate the uterus into the abdomen and at the same time to express the placenta into the vagina. The cord may be grasped with a forceps or by hand, and gentle traction guides the placenta through the birth canal. Traction is steady while there is a contraction; if the uterus relaxes, it is stopped temporarily. As the placenta moves down, pressure is exerted with

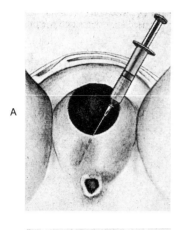

A

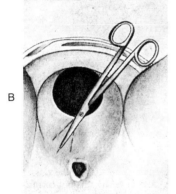

B

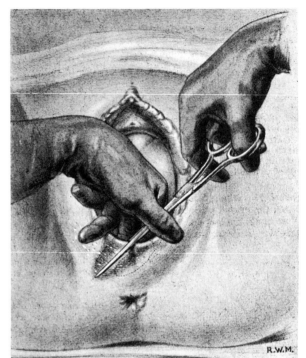

C

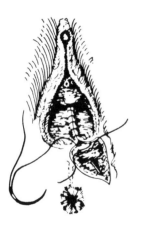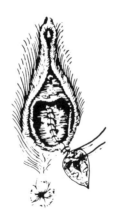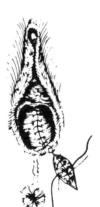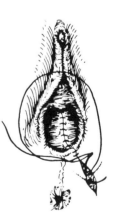

D

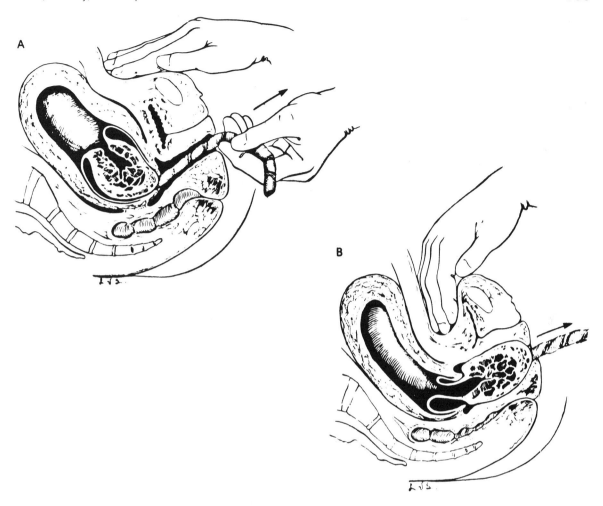

Figure 6-19. Recovery of the placenta. (A) Abdominal pressure, traction guiding placenta through birth canal. (B) Abdominal pressure being exerted between symphysis and fundus, forcing uterus upward and placenta outward.

the abdominal hand between the symphysis and the fundus, forcing the uterus upward and the placenta outward, as cord traction is continued.

Both fundal pressure and cord traction are dangerous and should never be combined because uterine inversion can result. The safety of the Brandt-Andrews maneuver lies in bracing back the uterus while cord traction is applied. The placenta is carefully inspected to be sure that there are no missing cotyledons and that membranes have been totally recovered. When the placenta is laid flat, all the cotyledons should be present and fit together. The

Figure 6-18. Episiotomy performance and repair. (A) Injection of local analgesic. (B) Making the incision. (C) Fingers protecting fetus. (D) Episiotomy repair. Miles, *Textbook for Midwives*, pp. 560-561 and Benson, *Current Obstetric & Gynecologic Diagnosis*, p. 588.

membranes should be stretched and should appear large enough to have contained the fetus and amniotic fluid. The placenta is inspected for infarcts or other abnormalities, and the number of vessels in the cord is noted.

The uterus is palpated and elevated at the completion of the third stage. Firm compression of the uterus may express clots and stimulate contraction, which reduces blood loss. If the uterus remains flaccid, causing persistent bleeding, gentle fundal massage and oxytocics can be used. If bleeding cannot be controlled by these methods, postpartum hemorrhage is occurring and immediate consultation should be obtained. This is a grave danger to the mother and a leading cause of perinatal maternal mortality. Average blood loss during and immediately after the third stage is 120 to 240 ml. (without episiotomy).[6]

IMMEDIATE CARE OF THE INFANT. Just after delivery, the infant's head is held slightly lower than the body to facilitate the drainage of mucus, and the air passages are cleared with a bulb syringe or other means of suction. Placing the baby on a stand or a table below the level of the delivery table allows blood to drain from the placenta and cord to the newborn, amounting to 30 to 90 ml., before the cord is clamped and the placenta separates. As soon as pulsations in the cord cease, it must be clamped. A sterile cord clamp, tie, or rubber band is used to clamp the cord at about one cm. from the skin reflection.

It is important to protect the baby from chills, but it is also important for the mother, and father, if present, to see the baby. A table with radiant heat from above is often used and placed close to the mother's eye level so that she may readily watch the baby. Some prefer to place the baby on the mother's abdomen immediately after birth and shortly afterwards beneath the radiant heat. The baby can also be dried with a warm towel, making sure that the head and hair are dry, and wrapped in a warm blanket.

Close observation of the newborn is essential in order to ascertain the adequacy of air passages. Apgar ratings are done at 1 and 5 minutes (Table 6-3). Resuscitative measures are immediately begun if there is any evidence of respiratory distress. A general physical examination of the infant is done, noting any gross abnormalities or congenital anomalies on the record. Weight, length from crown to heel and crown to rump, shoulder circumference, head circumference, and cranial diameters are also recorded. Time of birth is noted and identification placed on the infant. The eyes must be treated with silver nitrate or penicillin ophthalmic ointment (according to individual state law), and this is usually done in the immediate postdelivery period. However, the significance of maternal-infant eye contact to bonding (see below) suggests that treatment of the eyes be postponed until after the first hour.

It is common practice to transfer the newborn to the nursery within 15 to 30 minutes of birth. In some instances the mother is allowed to hold the infant or put him to breast briefly before his transfer to the nursery. In light of current information on the importance of the first hour after birth to the parental attachment process and its long-term implications, it seems critically important to leave the baby with his parents during this time unless the mother's or infant's condition precludes it.[7]

CONDUCT OF THE FOURTH STAGE. The first hour after the expulsion of the placenta is often called the fourth stage of labor in order to stress the importance both of careful monitoring for physical complications and of encouraging family interaction during this period. Hemorrhage is the ever-present danger to the mother, and the contraction of the uterus and the amount of bleeding must be carefully monitored. The uterus should remain firmly contracted and in the midline, about the level of the umbilicus. If flaccid or enlarged, a blood clot may be present in the uterine cavity and should be gently expressed by pressing and squeezing the uterus between both hands, holding it up and backward to avoid prolapse. Routine massage of a well-contracted uterus is not necessary and may cause trauma. The perineal pad is checked frequently for the amount of bleeding and changed as needed. Blood pressure and pulse rate are taken frequently and should remain stable. A pulse of over 90 may indicate excessive blood loss, as may falling blood pressure. Some women may exhibit toxemia during this stage, and a rising blood pressure needs consultation.

Liquids are given and the bladder checked for distention. Voiding is encouraged, if the bladder fills, and the amount voided is measured. If the woman is unable to void, catheterization is necessary. The fourth stage of labor is usually conducted in a recovery room, prior to the mother's transfer to the postpartum unit. Usually the baby has already been sent to the nursery, and the father may or may not be present. As this first hour is central to the family's incorporation of the new member, it is important that this time be made available for them to be with the infant. A private setting with as few interruptions as possible is ideal, so that mother, father, and baby can begin their process of attachment.

Table 6-3
The Apgar Scoring Chart

Sign	0	1	2
Heart rate	Absent	Slow (less than 100)	Over 100
Respiratory effort	Absent	Slow, irregular	Good, crying
Muscle tone	Flaccid	Some flexion of extremities	Active motion
Reflex irritability	No response	Weak cry or grimace	Vigorous cry
Color	Blue, pale	Body pink, extremities blue	Completely pink

MATERNAL-INFANT BONDING

There is strong evidence that a unique period exists in the human shortly after birth that is essential for mother-to-infant attachment. This period lasts only a short time, and complex interactions occur between mother and infant which help to bond them together. Following normal labor and a delivery without oversedation, a state of heightened awareness and receptivity exists in both mother and baby. In one study, mothers who lay skin-to-skin with their infants under a heat panel for 45 minutes immediately after leaving the delivery room were compared to mothers separated from their babies after birth, but after 12 hours brought together under a heat panel for identical contact. A third group was separated after birth and reunited after 12 hours, but without privacy and skin-to-skin contact. Observations made 36 hours after birth by an observer who did not know which group the mothers were in revealed that the mothers who had immediate contact with their infants after birth showed significantly more attachment behaviors (en face or looking intensely full face into the baby's eyes, talking to the baby, fondling, caressing, kissing, and smiling at the baby) (Figure 6-20). A progression in attachment behaviors was evident from the early skin-to-skin contact group to the two groups with later contact.

Mothers with early and frequent contact with their babies in the first several days were found in various studies to show more attachment behavior, to have fewer problems with feedings and adaptation to the child, to nurse longer, to have fewer episodes of infection, and to have babies gaining nearly 1½ more pounds by 6 months of age than control groups without such contact. It has also been observed that

paternal caregiving in the first 3 months of life was greatly increased when the father undressed his infant twice and established eye-to-eye contact for 1 hour during the first 3 days of life. Thus, the first few minutes and hours after an infant's birth appear optimal for parent-infant attachment.

The infant has six states of consciousness, ranging from deep sleep to screaming. In the quiet, alert state, the infant's eyes are wide open and he is able to respond to his environment. Infants may spend as little as a few seconds in this state at a time. During the first hour after birth, however, the infant is in this state for a period of 45 to 60 minutes. He will turn his head to the spoken word and show visual preferences for the full human face during this time. The infant is ideally equipped for the critical first encounter with his parents. After this hour, he goes into a deep sleep for 3 to 4 hours. Mothers have intense interest in looking into their baby's eyes and often feel the baby is alive and real after eye contact. The baby's gaze in return is a reward or signal giving important feedback to the mother. An infant's eye-to-eye contact seems to be one of the innate releasers of maternal caretaking responses, having powerful effects even on nonrelated persons.[8]

During the first few days, mother and baby are intimately involved with each other on a number of sensory levels, and their behaviors complement each other and serve to bond the pair together. These behaviors do not occur in a chainlike sequence but have a rippling effect on many levels. The mother touches the infant in a characteristic sequence, progressing from fingertip exploration of extremities and face to palm contact including massaging, stroking, and encompassing the trunk. Separation and prematurity delay the progress of maternal

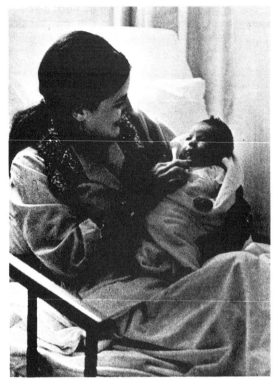

Figure 6-20. Mother and baby in the *en face* position. M. H. Klaus and J. H. Kennell, *Maternal-Infant Bonding* (St. Louis: Mosby, 1976), p. 71.

touch. Mothers speak to babies in a higher-pitched voice than they use for everyday conversation, and babies respond preferably to speech in the high-frequency range. While mothers are talking to their babies, the configuration of moving parts of the baby's body becomes coordinated with the points of change in the mother's sound patterns. Only natural, rhythmic speech elicits these synchronous movements. With this synchronization between mother and baby, the infant reestablishes his biorhythmicity after undergoing disruption and disequilibrium during birth. This is established by following a steady routine in the baby in colostrum and breast milk, includ-this dyad can be impressive indeed. The baby's synchronized responses (entrainment) are important feedback or response signals to the parents which help to form a close bond. The mother also passes many of her antibodies to the baby in colostrum and breast milk, including high concentrations of IgA and T and B lymphocytes, which may line the gastrointestinal epithelium and protect the baby against

enteric pathogens. Also, the mother colonizes the infant's respiratory and gastrointestinal tract with benign normal strains of bacteria which prevent pathogenic bacteria from establishing themselves and causing infections. Mother and infant respond to each other's unique odor, and the mother's body provides warmth for the baby. The baby's cry can increase the blood flow to the mother's breasts and trigger the milk letdown reflex, while nursing initiates the secretion of maternal oxytocin, which stimulates uterine contractions and reduces bleeding, and prolactin, which induces the alveoli of the breasts to secrete milk.

Many practices in hospitals today seriously interfere with or impose burdens on the process of maternal-infant bonding, and often the advantages of early contact are lost. To enhance attachment, Marshall Klaus and John Kennell in their book *Maternal-Infant Bonding* suggest:

1. During the birth and postpartum period, the mother have a companion of her choice for labor, be provided privacy for extended periods of father-mother-infant contact, and be given complete responsibility for care of her baby with a nurse or midwife as consultant.
2. Eye medications (i.e., silver nitrate) be delayed until after the mother has had an extended period with her infant the hour after birth.
3. The mother, father and infant have a period alone together in privacy after the placenta is delivered (and episiotomy sutured). An overhead heat lamp is used, the baby kept nude, and the mother encouraged to hold him against her bare chest. Nursing can also occur.
4. Mother and infant should be kept together continuously, or have long periods together in the days after birth. The mother has control over the baby and professionals act as consultants.
5. Family visits be encouraged so the mother can have contact with the father and other children. The father may visit often and care for the baby.[9]

POSTPARTUM MANAGEMENT

The postpartum period is the time required for involution of the genital organs following pregnancy. Traditionally it extends through the sixth week after delivery, by which time the reproductive organs have virtually returned to their normal nonpregnant state; most non-lactating women resume menstrual cycles at this time or shortly after.

Physiologic Changes

The many changes which occurred during pregnancy are reversed. The *uterus* decreases from the size of a 20-week pregnancy to a 12-week pregnancy by the end of the first postpartum week (Figure 6-21). It weighs 1 kg. immediately after delivery and 100 Gm. by 6 weeks postpartum. This rapid catabolism after birth is demonstrated by the release of about 20 Gm. of nitrogen and an increase in the urinary excretion of creatinine and urea. Myometrial force and intrauterine pressures are higher in early puerperium than before delivery due to decreased uterine volume, and contractions greater than 150 mm. Hg are common. These afterpains occur the first 2 or 3 days after delivery and are more noticeable in multiparas.

Constriction and occlusion of underlying blood vessels occurs at the placental site, accomplishing hemostasis and some endometrial necrosis. Involution occurs by the extension and downward growth of marginal endometrium and by endometrial regeneration from glands and stroma in the decidua basalis. This process is completed by the end of the third postpartum week, except at the placental site, where involution is not complete until 6 weeks. Subinvolution with incomplete obliteration of placental site vessels causes persistent lochia and brisk hemorrhagic episodes. *Lochia rubra* is the bloody uterine discharge including shreds of tissue and decidua which lasts about 3 days. The discharge gradually becomes serous and paler, is called *lochia serosa*, and lasts from 10 to 14 days. During the second postpartum week the lochia, now called *lochia alba*, becomes thicker, mucoid, and yellowish-white with a predominance of leukocytes and degenerated decidual cells. Lochial secretions usually cease about 4 weeks postpartum as healing nears completion.

The *cervix* closes, and the external os is converted into a transverse slit, often with scarred notches at the site of tears. The thinned *vaginal wall* thickens, and there is increased cervical mucus production; however this is delayed in lactating women. The *abdominal muscles* are lax and stretched, and diastasis of the rectus muscle may have occurred, taking about 6 to 7 weeks for involution. Rupture of the elas-

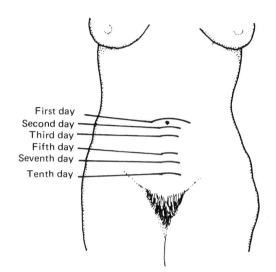

First day
Second day
Third day
Fifth day
Seventh day
Tenth day

Figure 6-21. Postpartum involution.

tic fibers of the cutis and persistent striae may remain during this time if the abdominal wall was overdistended.

Plasma levels of *estrogen* and *progesterone* decline rapidly after delivery, and estrogens do not reach follicular phase levels until 19 to 21 days postpartum in nonlactating women and longer in those who are lactating. Follicle stimulating hormone levels are low in all postpartum women for 10 to 12 days, then increase to follicular phase concentrations during the third week. *Prolactin* reaches its peak concentration around the time of delivery, then declines erratically over 2 weeks in nonlactating women. It increases during nursing and is followed by breast engorgement and milk letdown in early puerperium; however, this diminishes later. It is thought that prolactin can suppress ovulation for several weeks postpartum, but there is great variation in its capacity to do so due to individual differences in the strength of the suckling stimulus and to partial weaning by formula supplementation. The *first menses* after delivery usually follows an anovulatory cycle or one with inadequate corpus luteum function. About 10 to 15 percent of nonnursing mothers ovulate by 6 weeks, and 30 percent within 90 days postpartum. The earliest documented time is 33 days postpartum, with ovulation before the tenth week unlikely in nursing mothers.[10] Approximately 70 percent of nonlactating women reestablish menstruation by the twelfth postpartal week, while this same percentage is not reached until the thirty-sixth week among women who are lactating.

At least six pituitary hormones play a role in *lactation* and mammary development. They are: prolactin, adrenocorticotropic hormone (ACTH), human growth hormone (HGH), thyroid-stimulating hormone (TSH), follicle stimulating hormone (FSH), and luteinizing hormone (LH). In addition, human chorionic somatotropin (HCS) and steroid hormones secreted by the adrenal glands, the ovaries and placenta play a part. The onset of lactation appears to be due to a combination of elevated prolactin, a fall in steroid concentration (particularly estrogen), and the onset of suckling. Lactation is blocked by the administration of estrogens, but this does not cause a fall in prolactin levels; estrogen thus appears to act at the level of the breast epithelium. Women given estrogens for lactation suppression often undergo transient breast engorgement. In breast feeding women, colostrum is secreted for 2 or 3 days after delivery, and with regular suckling milk production begins on the third or fourth day. The color of breast secretion changes from clear yellowish to bluish white, and the breasts become larger, firmer, and often more tender. This congestion usually subsides in 1 or 2 days with regular nursing. Milk production continues at a constant rate and can be stored in the gland duct system for 4 to 6 hours before fluid pressure reduces the rate of production. Milk is moved from the acini toward the nipple by contractile myoepithelial cells, stimulated by oxytocin release in response to nursing (milk letdown). Stress inhibits the letdown reflex, and suckling aids in the maintenance of milk secretion by stimulating the release of prolactin, TSH and ACTH. Sustained production of milk can be achieved by most women in 10 to 14 days, with a yield of 120 to 180 ml. per feeding by the end of the second week. Human milk is generally adequate nourishment for infants until they are 4 or 5 months old. Weaning is accomplished by gradual or sudden cessation of breast feeding, and usually does not cause any significant engorgement or discomfort.

Diuresis occurs about 2 to 5 days after delivery when the fluid retained during pregnancy is lost. Two L. are excreted during the first postpartum week and an additional 1.5 L. during the next 5 weeks. Most women lose about 9 pounds during the puerperium. Mild proteinuria and glycosuria often occur in early postpartum. The total *blood volume* decreases from 5 to 6 L. during pregnancy to 4 L. by the third week after delivery. Normal vaginal delivery causes a blood loss of about 400 ml., and the blood volume and hematocrit postpartally are determined by the quantity of blood loss at delivery. A rise in hematocrit usually occurs 3 to 7 days after vaginal delivery, but hemodilution occurs in women who lose 20 percent or more of circulating blood at delivery. A rapid and short-lived reticulocytosis occurs as a result of sudden blood loss during delivery, and marked leukocytosis (up to 25,000 white blood cells per μl.) extends into early puerperium in response to the stress of labor. The increased concentration of *clotting factors* which occurred during pregnancy provides a reserve for the rapid consumption of these factors during delivery and promotes hemostasis postpartum. The fibrinolytic activity of maternal plasma, which was reduced during late pregnancy, increases rapidly after delivery, returning to nonpregnant values in 3 to 5 days. This provides a dynamic equilibrium with the loss of factors promoting coagulation. There is, however, a secondary increase of some clotting factors in the first postpartum week, and this, along with immobility, sepsis, or trauma during delivery predisposes women to the increased thrombosis seen postpartally.

Early Postpartum Care

AMBULATION AND REST. Early ambulation after delivery hastens the involution of the uterus, improves uterine drainage, and lessens the incidence of postpartum thrombophlebitis. It also promotes a sense of well-being and normality. Most women prefer to rest after the excitement of delivery and greeting the infant. In the absence of complications, the woman may ambulate as desired and should be up and about within 24 hours of birth. Alternating exercise with periods of rest is preferable. It is important that the mother have time to learn about and become comfortable in the care of her new baby, and therefore her responsibilities for other aspects of family and home management should be minimized.

DIET. Many women are quite hungry after labor and delivery and are able to eat a full diet at once. Others may have some decreased appetite until they recover fully from the effects of analgesics and anesthetics. Protein foods, vegetables, and fruits, milk products, and a high fluid intake are recommended, especially for breast feeding mothers. Lactating women probably require not more than 2600 to 2800 calories per day. Continuing with vitamin supplementation is not necessary in most cases, especially oral iron for women with normal postpartum hematocrit and hemoglobin concentrations. With normal blood loss, there is often a moderate excess of red blood cells after delivery, which may lead to an increase in iron stores. A diet with adequate bulk and fluid helps to prevent or relieve postpartum constipation.

BOWEL FUNCTION. Constipation is common postpartum due to a mild ileus which follows delivery, fluid loss, and perineal discomfort causing a tendency to delay evacuation. If an enema was given prior to delivery, the woman is unlikely to have a bowel movement for 1 or 2 days after birth. Milk of Magnesia, 15 to 20 ml. orally on the evening of the second postpartum day, will usually stimulate a bowel movement the next morning. Stool softeners such as dioctyl sodium sulfosuccinate (DOSS) help to reduce the discomfort of early bowel movements. Rectal suppositories such as bisacodyl may also be given if the above are not effective. Discomfort from hemorrhoids is common after delivery, and is treated with suppositories and sitz baths. These gradually resolve and rarely need additional treatment unless there is marked thrombosis.

BLADDER FUNCTION. The bladder mucosa is edematous as a result of labor and delivery, and overdistention and incomplete emptying with residual urine are common postpartum problems. The marked polyuria during the first few days after delivery causes the bladder to fill in a relatively short time; thus it is important that the woman be able to void completely shortly after delivery. If she cannot empty her bladder or there is significant residual urine, catheterization is necessary about every 6 hours until spontaneous voiding is reestablished. Intermittent catheterization is preferable to an indwelling catheter because there is less risk of urinary tract infection. If the bladder fills to more than 1000 ml., however, at least 2 days of decompression by retention catheter is generally required to regain bladder tone and to establish voiding. If urinary tract infections develop these must be treated with specific antibiotics.

BATHING. The woman may shower as soon as she is ambulatory. Most women prefer to take showers postpartum because of the usually heavy lochia, but a sitz or tub bath is most probably safe if the tub is clean because bath water will not gain entrance into the vagina unless directly introduced. Vaginal douching is contraindicated during early postpartum. Breast feeding mothers are often advised not to use soap on their nipples because it removes natural oils, which may lead to drying and cracking.

CARE OF THE PERINEUM. The perineal area is gently cleansed with plain soap one or two times a day and after voiding and bowel movements. This is often done by the patient, using a squeeze bottle and directing the flow of the solution from the vulva toward the anus. Dry heat applied to the perineum with an infrared lamp for 20 minutes three times a day helps relieve discomfort and promote healing. The perineum heals rapidly and has a remarkable resistance to infection, considering the difficulty of avoiding the contamination of this area. An episiotomy, if present, is inspected daily, but a vaginal or rectal examination is not done unless a hematoma or infection is suspected. If an examination is done, aseptic technique must be used. Local heat and irrigation are used for mild episiotomy infections, but if the response is not immediate antibiotics are necessary. Episiotomy pain is usually relieved by simple analgesics.

OXYTOCICS. It is not routine to use oxytocic agents beyond the immediate puerperium because the administration of such preparations for extended periods of time has a questionable value in hastening uterine involution. The possible disadvantages of these medications include the inhibition of prolactin release and ergot poisoning from prolonged therapy. Specific indications for oxytocic therapy include postpartum hemorrhage or endometritis, for which preparations such as methylergonovine maleate (Methergine) 0.2 mg. orally every 6 hours are used.

BREAST CARE AND NURSING. Breast feeding is most successful when the mother is motivated, relaxed, and not under stress and when the baby remains with her and can be fed on demand. Initially the frequency of feedings may be irregular, about six or seven times per day, but after 1 to 2 weeks a reasonably regular 4 to 6 hour pattern usually emerges. It is important to nurse from both breasts at each feeding because the letdown reflex affects both breasts simultaneously and leaving one unempted may lead to engorgement and reduced milk output. If the baby is sleepy and does not nurse well at first, the mother is taught to empty the breasts after each feeding (usually manually) to stimulate milk production. The breasts and nipples should be cleansed only with water. To begin the breast feeding process, the baby should nurse at each breast on demand about every 3 to 4 hours, for 5 minutes' total nursing time (2½ minutes per breast). This is increased by 1 minute per day up to a total of 7 minutes. The average baby obtains 60 to 90 percent of the milk it can ingest in 4 minutes of nursing, thus suckling longer is not necessary to satisfy the baby's hunger and may cause maceration and cracking of the nipples. The nipple should be placed well into the baby's mouth so it rests against the palate, and the periareolar area can be compressed with the baby's jaws. The baby's nostrils must be kept clear, often by the mother's depressing her breast with her fingers just under his nose. To get the baby to take the breast, softly touch his cheek on the side you want him to turn toward. It is also helpful to express a small amount of colostrum or milk into the nipple. This is done by compressing the edge of the areola between thumb and fingers. To remove the infant from the breast, suction must be broken by slipping one finger beneath the lip and jaw in the corner of the baby's mouth. Otherwise, his considerable suction will cause traction and trauma to the nipple.

The prevention of breast infection depends upon cleanliness and good hygiene. If a fissure of the nipple develops, a nipple shield should be used. The most common symptoms of *mastitis* are a painful erythematous lobule in an outer quadrant of the breast, usually during the second or third week postpartum, and fever. High fever should never be ascribed to simple engorgement. Treated early with frequent hot showering and continued nursing, engorgement usually disappears. Inflammation of the breasts seldom begins before the fifth postpartum day. Treatment for acute mastitis includes discontinuation of nursing, application of local cold (or heat), a well-fitted brassiere, and appropriate antibiotic treatment. The organism is usually coagulase-positive Staphylococcus aureus, and frequently the infant will also be found to have furunculosis.

IMMUNIZATION. Rho (D antigen) immune globulin (RHoGAM) is administered after delivery to Rh negative women who are previously unsensitized if the baby is Rh positive, and if the result of a Coombs's test of the cord blood is negative. The RhoGAM is cross-matched to the mother's red blood cells to ensure compatibility, and 1 ml. (300 mcg.) is given intramuscularly within 72 hours of delivery. Women who have never had rubella, as demonstrated by a negative rubella titer (1:8 or less), can safely be immunized with attenuated virus postpartally because it is not communicable. Nursing mothers need not be excluded.

EXERCISES. Postpartum exercises (Figure 6-22) to strengthen the muscles of the back, pelvic floor, and abdomen can be started about 3

Figure 6-22. Postpartum exercises. First day: lie on your back with your body and legs straight. Inhale slowly, expanding your chest. Pull your abdominal muscles in and press the lower part of your back to the floor. Hold, then relax. Repeat 5 to 10 times. Second day: raise your head from the floor, bringing it as close to your chest as possible. Try not to move any other part of your body. Repeat 5 to 10 times. Third day: put your arms straight out at your sides, then raise them over your head until your hands meet. Keeping your arms stiff, lower them again until they rest at your sides. Repeat 10 to 15 times. Seventh day: bring one leg up over your body until your foot touches your buttocks. Straighten and lower it, then repeat the exercise with your other leg. Repeat one more time each day. Seventh to tenth day: if ordered by your physician, turn on your stomach and raise your body so that your knees and chest are close together. Your chest should be against the floor, and your legs about a foot apart. Hold this position for two minutes. Without using your hands, raise one leg at a right angle to your body. Repeat using the other leg. Later when you are stronger, raise both legs at once. Repeat 5 to 10 times. Fourteenth day: lying on your back, cross your arms on your chest and raise your body upright, keeping your legs close together on the floor. Later, when you are stronger, sit up while clasping your hands behind your head. Repeat one more time each day. Next, bend your legs almost to a right angle and raise your body, supporting it on your shoulders. Press your knees together, but keep your feet apart. Contract the muscles of your buttocks at the same time. Repeat one more time each day.

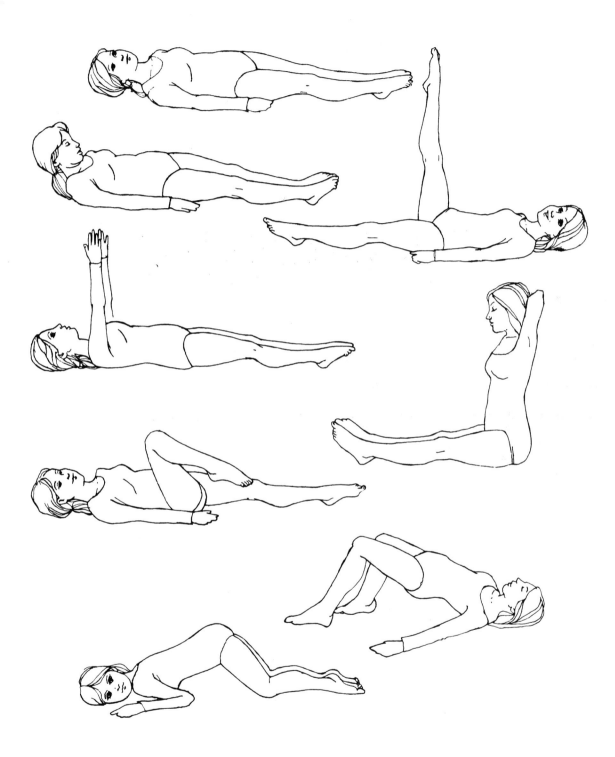

weeks after delivery. The woman begins with a single exercise performed 5 times and repeated several times a day. A new exercise is added each day. Strenthening the back and abdominal muscles helps to correct lordosis and the diastasis of the rectus muscles caused by pregnancy and will improve posture.

SEX AND INTERIM CONTRACEPTION. Once the lochia has ceased and the episiotomy is well healed, sexual intercourse may be resumed. The woman should gauge her readiness by perineal discomfort and sexual excitement. A relative state of hormone deprivation exists postpartally, and vaginal lubrication may not be so effective as it was before pregnancy. Since the couple may have refrained from sex in the form of intercourse for a few weeks before delivery, it is difficult to continue abstention until 6 weeks postpartum, particularly when the woman's body is almost back to normal and the desire is great. Probably a more realistic estimate of when to resume intercourse is about 2 to 3 weeks after delivery. Most women are having intercourse when seen at 6 weeks. It is therefore important to discuss contraception before the woman leaves the hospital and to emphasize that although it is unlikely, it is possible to ovulate and conceive before 6 weeks. Vaginal foam and a condom are recommended as interim contraceptives from delivery until the 6-weeks' checkup. There are drawbacks or dangers with the other methods during this time: the diaphragm cannot be properly fitted; the pregnancy, expulsion, and removal rates are highest for IUDs inserted within 2 to 4 weeks postpartum; and oral contraceptives may cause increased thromboembolic risks and continued hypothalamic-pituitary axis suppression.

POSTPARTUM INFECTIONS. There is often a slight rise in temperatire following delivery, but an elevation of 100.4°F (38°C) when oral temperature is taken indicates an infection. The majority of patients with puerperal infection have endometritis, with associated signs of tachycardia, uterine tenderness, and malaise. The lochia is often profuse and has a foul odor. The most common pathogens are anaerobic nonhemolytic streptococci, coliforms, bacteriodes, and staphylococci. Puerperal sepsis caused by group A beta-hemolytic streptococcus is much reduced now, but when it oc-

curs there is rapid lymphatic spread of infection, with bacteremia and toxicity. Lochia is often scanty and free of odor. Serious complications include parametritis, pelvic peritonitis, abscess formation, pelvic thrombophlebitis, disseminated intravascular coagulation, septic shock, and subsequent infertility. Consultation is necessary for the managmnt of infections.

Six-Week Postpartum Examination

A follow-up visit is scheduled for 6 weeks postpartum to assess the process of involution and the woman's adaptation to motherhood. Occasionally earlier visits are scheduled, or the mother may be seen in family practices when the baby comes in for its 2 week check. The woman's weight and blood pressure are recorded, and a breast and pelvic examination done. If she is breast feeding, this is discussed, and her nipples are examined for fissures. Masses or inflammation require follow-up and referral. On vaginal examination, the amount and character of discharge is noted. Profuse discharge is usually not present unless there is vaginitis, and bleeding should have ceased. Nursing mothers often show a hypoestrogenic condition of the vaginal epithelium, and local dryness and coital discomfort can be relieved by local use of estrogen cream. If cervicitis is present, it may be treated with sulfa vaginal cream. The episiotomy incision and repaired lacerations are inspected, and the adequacy of pelvic and perineal support is noted. For mild relaxation, Kegal's exercises should be taught (contracting perineum and rectum with enough force to stop a stream of urine, repeated 100 times 3 or 4 times daily).

On bimanual examination, the size and position of the uterus are noted. It should be of normal multiparous nonpregnant size, usually increasing slightly in size with many pregnancies. There is often some degree of retrodisplacement of the uterus at the postpartum exam that soon corrects itself. Asymptomatic retroposition is not considered abnormal. The uterus should be firm and nontender. The adnexa are palpated and the ovaries should be of normal size, with no undue tenderness. There should be no adnexal fullness or masses. On rectovaginal examination, hemorrhoids may still be apparent, though they are usually smaller than immediately after delivery. Pap smear and gonorrhea culture may be repeated, depending upon policy.

Contraception is discussed, and the method is selected, and once it is determined appropriate for the particular woman, it is instituted. Inquiry is made into the woman's and the family's adjustment to the new baby, including such areas as her energy level, rest and exercise, diet, satisfaction with feeding, accomplishment of household chores, relations with relatives and friends, sexual relations, and physical symptoms and functioning. Any problems which are identified are further explored, and appropriate treatment or referral is initiated.

Weight may be a concern, for most women will retain about 60 percent of any weight in excess of 24 pounds gained during pregnancy. A suitable reduction diet and other weight control measures can be advised. The woman can usually resume full employment or activities after 6 weeks postpartum if there have been no complications and she is psychologically ready. Some women return to work much sooner—about 2 to 3 weeks after delivery. This is an individual decision which is up to the woman's personal judgment and desires.

Depending upon the type of contraception, return visits are scheduled as necessary. The woman is advised of routine health maintenance needs according to her age, including regular breast examination and Pap smear.

NOTES

1. S. L. Romney, et al., *Gynecology and Obstetrics: The Health Care of Women* (New York: McGraw-Hill, Blakiston, 1975), pp. 321-22.

2. M. F. Miles, *Textbook for Midwives* (Edinburgh: Churchill Livingstone, 1975), pp. 212-13.
3. S. S. Rising, "The Fourth Stage of Labor: Family Integration." *American Journal of Nursing* 74 (May 1974): 870-74.
4. S. Reeder, L. Mastrioanni, and L. L. Martin, *Maternity Nursing*, 13th ed. (Philadelphia: J. B. Lippincott, 1976), pp. 318-24; and R. C. Benson, *Current Obstetric & Gynecologic Diagnosis & Treatment* (Los Altos, Calif.: Lange Medical Publications, 1976), pp. 521-23.
5. *Ibid.*, p. 552.
6. Miles, *Textbook for Midwives*, p. 297.
7. M. H. Klaus and J. H. Kennell, *Maternal-Infant Bonding* (St. Louis: C. V. Mosby, 1976), pp. 12-14 and 50-66.
8. *Ibid.*, pp. 38-85.
9. *Ibid.*, pp. 95-96.
10. Benson, *Current Obstetric & Gynecologic Diagnosis & Treatment*, pp. 703-4.

SELECTED READINGS

Arms, S. 1973. *A Season to Be Born*. New York: Harper Colophon Books.

————. 1975. *Immaculate Deception*. Boston: Houghton Mifflin Co.

Brook, Danaii. 1976. *Naturebirth*. New York: Pantheon Books.

Doering, S. G., and Entwisle, D. R. "Coping Mechanisms During Childbirth and Postpartum Sequelae." *Primary Care* 3,4 (December 1976): 727-40.

Ewy, D., and Ewy, R. 1975. *Preparation for Breast Feeding*. New York: Dolphin Books.

————. 1972. *Preparation for Childbirth*. New York: Signet Books.

Leboyer, R. 1975. *Birth Without Violence*. New York: Alfred A. Knopf.

Milinaire, C. 1974. *Birth*. New York: Harmony Books.

Paschall, N. C., and Newton, N. "Personality Factors and Postpartum Adjustment." *Primary Care* 3,4 (December 1976): 741-50.

Seiden, A. M. "The Maternal Sense of Mastery in Primary Care Obstetrics." *Primary Care* 3,4 (December 1976): 717-26.

7

INDUCED ABORTION

Women have used induced abortion as a means of fertility control since antiquity. In diverse cultures throughout recorded history, abortions have been sought with varying degrees of success, whether the society approved or proscribed the practice. The reasons for permitting or restricting abortions grow out of sociocultural, ecological, and economic factors, ranging from food supply and population balance to maintaining the authority structure of the society. Attitudes concerning abortion have by no means been universal and must be viewed within the particular social, cultural, and historical context. Even when techniques for inducing abortion are primitive and there are considerable physical dangers or social consequences, the widespread and longstanding practice of abortion speaks to the determination of women to terminate unwanted pregnancies at any cost when they deem it necessary.

It is clearly evident that women will seek abortion when this is seen as a solution to unwanted pregnancy. Accurate abortion statistics are difficult to obtain, particularly when the procedure is illegal. Recent estimates of the number of pregnancies terminated each year throughout the world range from 30 to 55 million. While these data are speculative because of variations in reporting legal abortions and the need to estimate illegal abortions, they point toward a worldwide abortion ratio of between 260 to 450 abortions per 1000 live births. In the United States, abortion ratios have been reported as high as 435 per 1000 live births in the Pacific Census Division and 537 per 1000 live births in the Middle Atlantic Cen-

sus Division. Ratios in other areas of the country, particularly the southern and mountain regions, tend to be considerably lower.[1]

Induced abortion in the United States constitutes a significant portion of women's health care. Most early abortions are done in outpatient facilities or with minimal hospitalization, and frequently the nurse practitioner will be involved in preabortion evaluation and work-up, as well as postabortion follow-up. As a result of the removal of legal restrictions and increased public awareness, the great majority of abortions are done during the first trimester of pregnancy. Despite the now widespread and growing availability of abortion, many health professionals decline to participate due to personal ethics, and several organizations continue to oppose legal abortion and work to restrict this practice. Feminist groups and organizations concerned with population and fertility control continue their support of legal abortion, collection of data, and dissemination of information.

THE 1973 SUPREME COURT DECISION

On January 22, 1973, the U.S. Supreme Court announced its decisions on two landmark cases related to abortion. These cases questioned the constitutionality of the existing Texas and Georgia abortion statutes. Generally, state abortion statutes made the termination of pregnancy a crime unless abortion was justified on the grounds that 1) continuation of pregnancy would gravely impair the physical or mental health of the mother; 2) the pregnancy was a result of rape, incest, or other felonious intercourse; or 3) there was a substantial risk that the child would be born with a grave physical or mental defect. Many states proscribed abortion altogether, unless it was necessary to save the life of the pregnant woman. Other requirements generally included were that abortions be performed in licensed hospitals and be approved by a hospital committee or by two or more physicians certifying the circumstances which justified abortion.[2]

The Supreme Court ruled that the statutes in Texas and Georgia, and thus in most other states, were unconstitutional. Under the 14th Amendment, which protects people against the deprivation of life, liberty, or property without due process of law, the protection of the right to privacy is also included. The Court held that a woman's right to personal privacy includes her decision on whether or not to have an abortion. The word "person" as used in the 14th Amendment does not include the unborn, according to the Court, because the fetus represents "only the potentiality of life." The right to privacy is not absolute, however, and may be restricted by state regulation if there is a compelling government interest which makes this necessary.[3] Additionally, the Court ruled that the state may not require that an abortion be performed in a hospital during the first trimester, and that at no stage may the state require approval by a hospital committee or the concurrence of two or more physicians, since this was not required of other medical or surgical procedures. Furthermore, the state could not impose residency requirements for obtaining abortions.[4]

Essentially, the Supreme Court made the abortion decision a matter between a woman and her physician, within certain time limits. For the purpose of protecting the health of the mother, the state is empowered to set reasonable regulations on the performance of abortions once pregnancy has proceeded to the point where there is a substantial increase in the risks of the procedure (i.e., during the second trimester). Once the fetus has reached the stage of viability, the state may proscribe abortion except when it is done to preserve the mother's life or health. Thus, states may not have laws which restrict a woman's access to abortion, except during the third trimester of pregnancy, and may only regulate second

trimester abortions to make the procedure safe. In summary, the Supreme Court's 1973 decisions established that:

1. Prior to the end of the first trimester of pregnancy (about 12 weeks) the abortion decision and how it is carried out are left to the judgment of the pregnant woman and her physician.
2. During the second trimester of pregnancy (up to 24 to 26 weeks) the state, in promoting its interest in the health of the mother, may, if it chooses, regulate the abortion procedure in ways reasonably related to maternal health.
3. After the fetus achieves viability (24 to 26 weeks and after) the state, in promoting its interest in the potentiality of human life, may, if it chooses, regulate or proscribe abortion except when it is necessary to preserve the life or health of the mother.

MOTIVES FOR ABORTION

Women seek abortions for a variety of reasons, basically growing out of their conclusion that they have begun an unacceptable or unwanted pregnancy. The meaning of the pregnancy, and of abortion as an option, involves societal norms and values, economic factors, personal goals, sexual mores, women's status, and the influence of the woman's interpersonal system. Pregnancy is an event with many positive implications involving the woman's self-concept and society's valuation of her, and the decision to terminate a pregnancy cannot be undertaken without some conflict. Even if the outcome of a pregnancy, the child, is completely unwanted, there is a multitude of factors having individual significance which contribute to ambivalence and emotional distress in making the decision to have an abortion.

Powerful forces, many of which are unconscious, may have contributed to the pregnancy's occurring. A woman may desire to be pregnant for a variety of reasons, but not wish to have a child. Or, pregnancy may be truly accidental, with no hidden motives, as in the case of contraceptive method failure. Whether the conception was in some way motivated or not, the woman may decide that the completion of the pregnancy is unacceptable to her and that termination by abortion is the solution to the problem for any one of a number of reasons. For example, the pregnancy may be an untimely event in her life, interfering with her goals or creating significant interpersonal or social conflicts. The pregnancy of an unwed teenager is both embarrassing and a cause of real hardship for the girl and her parents. The violation of parental values and society's disapproval of premarital sex may be involved. The young teenager's immaturity makes her unfit to be a parent, and her economic dependency makes it impossible for her to assume the responsibility for raising a child. There are often questions of paternity, or the father may be uninvolved, and frequently he is also an adolescent. While forced marriages were once seen as the necessary solution to the unplanned teenage pregnancy, many people now recognize the unfortunate consequences of this demand as it is reflected in divorce, desertion, child neglect, and child abuse. In this situation, abortion is often seen as the most reasonable choice by the girl and her parents, as well as by the father, if he is involved.

Women may find pregnancy untimely in other circumstances. Whether the woman is married or not, a pregnancy may interfere with educational or professional goals which have a high priority at this point in her life. Pregnancy may follow marriage too closely, and couples may opt for abortion out of the needs in their relation for growth or development, or because other pursuits have primacy. Some couples decide to remain childless, and a pregnancy occurring even after many years of marriage is not acceptable. Contraceptive failure can lead to an untimely pregnancy for which the woman and her partner are not emotionally prepared. Particularly when efforts have been made to prevent pregnancy, it is difficult to accept accidental conception.

Pregnancies occurring in too rapid succession are a frequent reason for abortion. Most women feel unable to cope with another pregnancy and child when they are postpartum or have a young infant. Couples may desire to space their children for economic reasons or because of the emotional or time resources available for childrearing, and they may want to abort another pregnancy occurring too soon in their time framework. Economic pressures are frequently cited as a reason for seeking abortion. Aspirations for a higher standard of living, unwillingness to subject themselves or already existing children to material deprivation, and goals for the social betterment of the family and the children prompt couples to choose abortion for undesired pregnancies. Women are realizing that a number of other choices are open to them when they have fewer children, and that delaying their first pregnancy allows them more years to devote to their education or job training. Having the capacity to earn a better income may enable a woman or a family to move out of poverty or to improve their socioeconomic status. For many of these same reasons, a pregnancy occurring after the desired family size has been achieved may be aborted. A woman who has borne as many children as she wants or feels she can adequately care for may choose not to burden the family with an unwanted child, either for economic or emotional reasons, or both.

Pregnancies involving the violation of the woman's integrity as a person are also frequently terminated. Rape is the prime cause of this type of unwanted pregnancy. Incest is also considered felonious intercourse, and pregnancies resulting from either rape or incest have traditionally been included among those for which abortion is justifiable, even under restrictive statutes. However, only a very small number of abortions are done because of rape or incest.

Women may seek abortion for eugenic reasons, even when a child is desired. Pregnancies which carry a high risk of congenital malformation, such as rubella infection during the first trimester or the use of known teratogenic drugs, may be terminated out of concern for the immediate and long-term impact of a deformed child on the parents, family, and society. The woman's perceptions of the type of life a child with serious mental or physical defects would be able to lead also affect her decision. As techniques of prenatal diagnosis advance, increasing numbers of genetic abnormalities can be detected early enough in pregnancy for abortion to be feasible. At present, amniocentesis and fetal cell culture can diagnose Tay-Sachs disease, hemophilia, Down's syndrome, and a number of other chromosomal disorders. In couples at high risk for genetic abnormalities, prenatal diagnosis can identify an affected fetus and often leads to the decision for abortion. Considerable anguish can be spared the couple and their family, and both personal and societal costs can be reduced in the custodial and medical care of these usually short-lived defective children. Genetic screening programs serve to identify the population at risk and to provide prenatal diagnosis when appropriate and are completely voluntary at every phase. The couple may choose to be screened or not, to have an amniocentesis or not, and to abort or not. The necessary information is provided to reach a knowledgeable decision.

FACTORS INFLUENCING THE ABORTION DECISION

Every woman lives within a network or system of persons, places, institutions, and ideas. Her life is a continuum of events and experiences, with its history, present reality, and future hopes and dreams. An abortion cannot be seen as an isolated happening in her life but must be viewed in the context of the multiple influences and complex feelings that converge at the moment of decision to shape her behavior. These influences include her feelings about herself as a woman, her fertility and sexuality, her emotional relation with the man who is a partner to the conception, his attitudes toward this pregnancy and toward abortion, her family's response—whether expressed or imagined—her own and her family's religious convictions, the norms and values of her culture, societal attitudes and practices regarding abortion, and the particular meaning of this pregnancy to her. Some of these factors will encourage the continuation of the unwanted pregnancy, and others may contribute to the desire to terminate it.

Cultural Factors

The laws of a country usually reflect the opinion of the majority of its citizens, and those who break the laws fear not only criminal prosecution, but condemnation by their peers and community. When abortion is illegal, the woman taking this action against society's values is in a vulnerable and dangerous position, with a high potential for emotional distress. Physical danger is ever-present when abortions must be performed illegally, due to poorly trained or amateur practitioners operating in rudimentary facilities without backup services in the event of complications. The need for secrecy prevents any evaluation of the quality of the services. Infection, hemorrhage, impaired future reproduction, and death are always significant risks when abortions must be obtained illegally.

The behavior of health providers is affected by national policies on abortion. When abortion is prohibited or restricted, health providers may be caught between their obligation to conform to the law and their assessment of the individual needs of the patient. The person who diagnoses the pregnancy often exerts a powerful influence on the woman's decision, how she carries it out, and how she feels about it. Drawn between the preservation of life and the alleviation of suffering, the physician may break the law by performing the abortion, refer the woman to an abortionist, or try to dissuade her. The wealthy usually have access to well-trained and sympathetic professionals for abortions, either in secret in their own country or by traveling to another country with less restrictive laws.

When laws change, there is usually a lag in general attitudes. Time is required for facilities to develop and professionals to become interested in providing legal abortions. More progressive communities move more rapidly, often causing women to travel to these areas for abortions. As more women accept abortion as an alternative to unwanted pregnancy and as the service becomes more available and health providers more understanding and sympathetic, the stress and trauma associated with abortion decreases.

Cultural attitudes toward family size influence the abortion decision. Over the last decade, the concern in the United States about ecology and natural resources has provided a strong force toward "zero population growth," promoting the desirability of the two-child family to achieve a stable population. Some segments of the population continue to value a large family, however, with children viewed as economic assets, social security for the parent's old age, testimony to the sexual potency of the male or reinforcement of the wife's maternal role, or an expression of religious beliefs.

Religion is a shaper of dominant societal values, and the laws tend to reflect the beliefs of the majority religion in a country. Countries in which Catholicism is a strong influence generally prohibit abortion, with Judaism and Islam promoting restrictive policies. Despite religious precepts and proscriptive laws, women still seek abortion in these countries. Countries with Protestant religions or those under socialism or communism tend to have more liberal policies toward abortion. In the United States, with its mixed religious heritage, the influence of religion is mainly personal. It can be strong enough to make abortion out of the question even if a pregnancy is unwanted or hazardous, or it can act to create varying degrees of guilt and remorse if a woman carries out her choice of abortion.

Personal and Interpersonal Factors

The woman's age, state of emotional and physical health, pursuits and life goals, marital status, financial situation, relation with her sexual partner, family situation, and relation with her parents and siblings all exert influences upon her decision to terminate an unwanted pregnancy. The very young woman may have become pregnant to feel grown up or mature, as a proof of fertility, to enhance her self-concept as a woman, as an outgrowth of romantic ideals of motherhood, or as an accidental byproduct of sexual experimentation. Women may become pregnant at any age to overcome a sense of inferiority or inadequacy, or to assuage doubts about their femininity. Older women may try to deny menopause and the end of reproductive function or sexual attractiveness by conceiving. To desire pregnancy, however, is not to want a child and the ongoing obligations a child entails. Finding themselves pregnant, women who consciously or unconsciously sought pregnancy for these reasons often decide that abortion is their only reasonable choice.

Women in poor physical health recognize that pregnancy is a risk to their life and a diversion of energies needed elsewhere. Emotional illness, crises, or ongoing stresses often cause women to feel unable to cope with the demands of pregnancy and childrearing. When pregnancy is seen as interfering seriously with other life goals and pursuits, or as leading to financial problems, abortion may be sought.

Marital status can be a determinant of the abortion decision, with many unmarried women feeling incapable of bringing a child into the world alone and caring for a child outside of marriage. There are, however, increasing numbers of single parents and a growing social acceptance of this situation; thus marital status per se may not be a significant factor. The woman's relation with her partner or husband is probably a critical factor. Pregnancy may have been desired to test his commitment or as a pressure for marriage, to bolster a shaky union or deepen the man's involvement, for the romantic ideal of creating a new life that is part of both of them, or to please the man by enhancing his masculine potency. If the pregnancy does not produce the desired effect, conflict develops, as what was once welcomed and thought to be a solution becomes a burden and an added source of regret.

Some women find a disintegrating marriage or relation a strong motivator for abortion, while others may want to continue the pregnancy to meet their need to be loved or to replace the partner's loss. Women from deprived backgrounds may desire a baby to have something to call their own. When the reality of the difficulties to be faced in continuing the pregnancy and bearing the child dawns on them, conflicts develop within the women, and considerable stress accompanies the abortion decision.

When the relation is stable but the husband is opposed to abortion, significant conflicts develop, with consequences for the future of the marriage. Decisions jointly made to have an abortion offer much support to the woman during the process and decrease the stress on her. Family attitudes also come into play, as does the quality of the woman's relation with her parents and siblings. Pathologic relations within the family correlate strongly with unwanted pregnancy. When parental disapproval of abortion is anticipated, the woman may conceal her pregnancy to avoid strife, although this also removes a possible source of support. When parents or siblings can understand and accept the choice of abortion, resolution is made easier and stresses are decreased. Conversely, the important people in the woman's life may pressure her to have an abortion against her wishes. This is especially true of adolescent girls, who may have negative feelings about those who coerced them, regret the loss of the pregnancy, feel guilty and depressed, and not infrequently become pregnant again.[5]

PREABORTION PROCEDURES

When the woman initiates contact with the primary health provider, she may be reasonably certain that she is pregnant or she may only suspect that she is. In some instances she has had a pregnancy test performed elsewhere which was positive. Confirmation of pregnancy, assistance with decision-making, referral to abortion services, discussion of options, or implementation of abortion may be the goals of her seeking health care.

Diagnosis and Sizing of Pregnancy

The history ascertains the date of the woman's last menstrual period and the menstrual period previous to that and whether these were normal menses. If the last menstrual period was lighter and shorter than usual, conception may have already occurred, and the previous menstrual period, if it was normal, is a more accurate starting point in estimating gestation. A menstrual history is obtained, including the age of onset, interval between menses, duration and character of flow, and irregular or abnormal bleeding. This is often helpful in determining whether the two most recent menses are a deviation from the usual pattern. Use of contraceptives is important in ascertaining possible time of conception and in gaining some understanding of the woman's circumstances leading to her unwanted pregnancy. A brief pregnancy history and a determination of significant illnesses, operations, medications, and present health problems are included.

Signs and symptoms of pregnancy are explored, including nausea and vomiting, urinary frequency, breast tenderness, fatigue or sleepiness, or other signs which the woman associates with pregnancy. It is often instructive to ask the woman if she feels pregnant, for many women are tuned to subtle differences and recognize pregnancy quite early. Because amenorrhea may be due to illness or to emotional factors, questions should include whether the woman has any other symptoms or feels sick, and whether she has been experiencing stresses recently. Lower abdominal pain or unusual discharge may signify pelvic inflammatory disease rather than pregnancy as a cause of amenorrhea.

A social history is helpful for understanding the woman's situation and relation to significant persons in her life, for these can affect her motivation for and response to abortion. The topic must be approached with acceptance and tact; it is not the provider's responsibility to judge the woman's choices but to assess fully all the factors influencing the patient's physical and mental health. The husband's or partner's feelings about the pregnancy and abortion or the parents' attitudes, in the case of a young adolescent, are very important. Pressure may be exerted to continue the pregnancy or to have the abortion against the real desires of the patient. Other factors in the home situation, such as childrearing responsibilities, economic concerns, interpersonal conflicts, work or educational commitments, may also figure in the woman's reasons for seeking an abortion.

The initial physical examination is aimed at confirmation of pregnancy and the determination of the length of gestation to date. A more thorough examination is carried out later, either as part of the abortion work-up or for the provision of prenatal care. The abdomen is inspected for changes of contour and palpated for suprapubic uterine enlargement. If the top of the fundus can be palpated just above the symphysis pubis, the pregnancy is of 12-weeks gestation; if it is midway between the symphysis and the umbilicus, the pregnancy is at 16 weeks, and if it is at the level of the umbilicus the pregnancy is at about 20 weeks (see Figure 5-4). Palpation is carried out to discover any abdominal masses or enlargement of the liver, kidneys, or spleen. In most pregnancies of less than 12-weeks gestation, the fundus cannot be felt on abdominal examination.

A speculum and bimanual pelvic examination is carried out and specimens obtained, usually including a Pap smear, gonorrhea culture, and other slides as indicated. On speculum examination, the characteristic vaginal and cervical signs of pregnancy (bluish discoloration of the vagina and cervix, increased leukorrhea) may or may not be present. Although reliable signs, these are not diagnostic. On bimanual examination, a softening of the cervical tip may be felt as early as the fourth week, but the cervix may also feel firm and indistinguishable from that of a nonpregnant woman. The softening of the uterocervical junction is an extremely valuable sign of early pregnancy that occurs in two stages. First, there is a softened spot anteriorly in the midline at about the sixth week (Ladin's sign), then a widened zone of softness develops by the seventh or eighth week, accompanied by easy compressibility of the uterocervical junction (Hegar's sign) (Figure 7-1). If these changes can be felt, they are highly suggestive of pregnancy even if the uterus does not appear enlarged. In some women it may be impossible to identify these

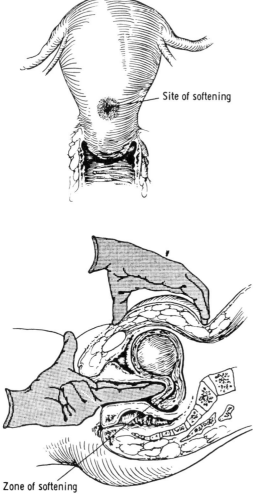

Site of softening

Zone of softening

Figure 7-1. Changes in uterocervical junction of early pregnancy. (Top) Ladin's sign. (Bottom) Hegar's sign.

should be able to identify an enlarged uterus at about 8 weeks. The isthmus should feel softened and compressible, the fundus softer and somewhat more globular than pear-shaped, and the size conceptualized at about 8 cm. From the point at which pregnancy can be identified (or at least presumed, on the basis of signs and symptoms) progressive enlargement of the uterus is estimated by centimeters corresponding in number to the approximate number of weeks of gestation. It is important to estimate gestation at least within 2 weeks accuracy, and within 1 week is preferable.

Getting the feel of early uterine enlargement in pregnancy takes practice and experience. It is helpful to have a reference point in mind; for instance, have in mind what a 12-week pregnancy feels like, and compare the smaller or larger uterus to it for purposes of estimation. The 16-week pregnancy is easy to identify because the uterus is markedly enlarged, soft, and halfway between the symphysis and umbilicus, whether palpated bimanually or measured abdominally. The findings of the pelvic examination are described according to the estimated time of gestation, for instance, uterus not clinically enlarged, uterus enlarged compatible with 9- to 10-weeks gestation, uterus enlarged compatible with 16-weeks gestation.

Accurate sizing of the pregnancy by estimating the number of weeks of gestation is extremely important because decisions about what type of abortion procedure is to be used are based upon the length of gestation. The critical time is 12 weeks; up to that time the simpler and less dangerous suction curettage can be used, but from that point on abortion is usually done by intraamniotic instillation of hypertonic saline or prostaglandins which initiate labor and expulsion and have a considerably higher rate of complications than does curettage. Many providers will not perform abortions beyond the twentieth week, and the law may restrict abortions beyond 24 or 26 weeks to only those necessary to save the life or health of the mother.

PREGNANCY TESTS. It is standard procedure to have all early pregnancies confirmed by a pregnancy test before an abortion is performed. This is particularly important when there is no or equivocal uterine enlargement. Most of the pregnancy tests currently used in ambulatory

early changes, whether due to obesity, abdominal guarding, or the subtlety of the changes themselves.

Changes in size and contour of the uterine corpus allow an estimation of gestation. Up to about 6 or 7 weeks, the uterus usually does not feel enlarged, and its shape has not changed sufficiently to be identified. As pregnancy progresses, the corpus enlarges and becomes diffusely softened until, by 10 weeks, it is double its nonpregnant size and globular in shape. In a patient of average weight, without undue abdominal guarding, and in the absence of a markedly retroflexed uterus, the practitioner settings are based upon the presence of human chorionic gonadotropin (HCG) in the urine. During the transport of the fertilized ovum through the oviduct and around the time of implantation, HCG is secreted by the trophoblast to nourish the corpus luteum, which then maintains the pregnancy until the placenta is well developed and functioning at about the ninth or tenth week of gestation. Human chorionic gonadotropin is excreted in the urine and becomes detectable 9 to 16 days after ovulation, or about 40 days from the last menstrual period. Tests use a sample of urine and are based upon the finding that HCG is a polypeptide with antigenic properties. Direct or indirect agglutination of sensitized red cells or latex particles is utilized to identify urine in which HCG is present. Peak levels of HCG occur from 50 to 90 days after the last menstrual period.

Indirect Tests	Direct Tests
Gravindex, Pregnosticon, HCG test, Pregnosis, UCG, Placentex, Gest-State Pregnant (positive test)—no agglutination Nonpregnant (negative test)—agglutination occurs	DAP Test-Macro Pregnant (positive test)—agglutination occurs Nonpregnant (negative test)—no agglutination

The rapid slide tests that can be done in 2 minutes utilize latex particles but are less sensitive than the 2-hour test and are reliable only after 41 days. The 2-hour test is more sensitive and is reliable after 38 days. Using a first morning-voided specimen increases the likelihood of detecting HCG; later, more dilute specimens may give a false negative, particularly in early pregnancies. Other causes of false negatives include error in interpretation, pregnancy too early or too late, urine stored too long at room temperature, threatened abortion, missed abortion, ectopic pregnancy, and too much antiserum. False positives can be due to error in interpretation, proteinuria, hematuria, persistent corpus luteum cysts, tuboovarian abscesses, psychotropic drugs (phenathiazines, antidepressants, antiparkinsonians, anticonvulsants), detergent residue on glassware, less than 10 days postpartum, and perimenopause. Some cancers and thyrotoxicosis can also cause a false positive pregnancy test.

Some of the immunological pregnancy tests in common use are as follows:[6]

	Time Required	Stability in Refrigerator
Tube Tests		
Pregnosticon accuspheres or tube (Organon)	2 hours	1 year
Placentex (Roche)	90 minutes	1 year
UCG test or Lyphotest tube (Wampole)	2 hours	18 months to 1 year (cool, dry)
Slide Tests		
Pregnosticon dri-dot slide (Organon)	2 minutes	2 years (shelf)
Pregnosis slide (Roche)	2 minutes	1 year
Pregnosticon	2 minutes	1 year
UCG slide (Wampole)	2 minutes	1 year
DAP-test-Macro (Wampole)	1 minute	1 year
Gest-state (Lederle)	2 minutes	1 year
Gravindex slide (Ortho)	2 minutes	1 year

A serum test for pregnancy which detects HCG by radioimmunoassay is the most sensitive method and can detect pregnancy as early as the fifth week, or about 1 week after the first missed menses. Radioimmunoassay can be used to measure HCG at very low concentrations, and a recent advance in serum testing identifies the β subunit of HCG, diagnosing pregnancy before the first missed period. This test does not cross-react with luteinizing hormone and is thus more accurate than radioimmunoassay for HCG itself. These tests are not yet widely available and require radiation in order to be read, necessitating special laboratory equipment.[7]

Counseling and Decision-Making

Once the pregnancy has been verified and the length of gestation determined, counseling about the type of abortion and assistance in exploring all the alternatives is carried out. Basically there are only three choices for the woman: to have an abortion, to continue the pregnancy and place the baby for adoption, or to continue the pregnancy and keep the baby. Some women may never have considered more than one choice, however, or thought through what meanings the other choices may hold for them. In this exploration of options, indications of how the woman feels about her pregnancy are sought, and what other factors are wielding influence. Often the woman's feelings will be confused, ambivalent, and conflicting. It is critical for the practitioner to stress that this decision is the woman's to make, and that she must not be pressured by others into a choice that is wrong for her.

For some women the decision comes more easily than for others. If she has no beliefs or attitudes that abortion is wrong, if she has a strong individualistic philosophy and goal orientation, or if she has pressing practical reasons for termination, there will be little difficulty with the decision to abort. There is a growing philosophy among women that control of the use of their bodies and reproductive functions is their basic right. The option of abortion for an unwanted pregnancy is part of that right, to be exercised freely within the individual's particular value system. If concerns for the feelings and attitudes of others are strong, if she struggles with principles of right and wrong, or if she is highly ambivalent about wanting or not wanting the pregnancy, the

woman's decision will be painful and difficult. Fear may be a strong motivating factor, blown up irrationally by the knowledge that time is sharply limited. Some women may maturely consider all alternatives, while others may never think beyond their distressing first reaction that they must not now be pregnant.

Exploring alternatives realistically limits and clarifies the situation. The woman can be helped to think through the meaning of each choice if she is having difficulty in deciding. If she continues the pregnancy, how will it affect her relations with the people who are important to her? How will it affect her plans and goals? Can she imagine going through pregnancy, labor, and delivery and giving the baby up? If she keeps the baby, how will she provide for its needs? Is she ready for the demands of motherhood? Can she imagine future years of raising a child? Where will her partner or parents stand if she continues the pregnancy? Who can she count on for continued help? If she chooses abortion, how will this decision affect the people who are important in her life? If they do not know about the pregnancy, does she think it is a good idea to keep it from them? Does she have anyone she can talk to about it? Can she live with her decision? Has she thought about going back to things the way they were before she became pregnant? Does she want to? And, if she is beyond the twelfth week of pregnancy, is she prepared to undergo the labor and delivery that are part of this type of abortion? Can she imagine how she will feel in 5 years if she terminates or continues the pregnancy?

Not all women need assistance in exploring their options and in decision-making. With the growing acceptance of abortion and more widely available facilities which provide abortions, many women present with firmly grounded decisions to terminate their pregnancy and with the expectation that health providers will facilitate this decision and implement it with minimal questioning. In this situation, it may be enough to ask, "Have you considered abortion carefully and decided that it is the best choice for you?" The opportunity for further discussion, if the woman feels the need, is present in the preabortion work-up and explanation of the type of abortion procedure.

The majority of abortions are done by suction curettage or surgical (sharp) curettage. It can be explained to the patient that suction curettage is a method of emptying the contents of the uterus, after the cervix has been slightly dilated, with a small suction apparatus. It is usually done with local paracervical anesthesia and sedation. Most patients are not admitted to the hospital, and the procedure is done in specially equipped outpatient facilities or through a special arrangement with hospital operating and recovery rooms. After a few hours in the recovery room, the woman is able to leave for home, provided that she is not bleeding too heavily or having other complications. Some uterine cramping is felt with this procedure, but it is usually not severe. Surgical (sharp) curettage is less often used, because general anesthesia is required and the rate of complications is somewhat higher than with suction curettage. If the health provider is not familiar with the suction method or the facility is not equipped for it, surgical curettage may be used. Overnight hospitalization may be necessary, or the patient may simply spend a longer time in the recovery room coming out of the general anesthetic before leaving for home. Both of these procedures are used only before the twelfth week of pregnancy.

Midtrimester abortions are done by the induction of labor with intraamniotic instillation of hypertonic saline, prostaglandins, or urea. This method requires hospitalization for several days because the complication rate and need for care and observation are much greater than with suction curettage. After local anesthetization of an area of the abdomen, a large needle is inserted into the amniotic cavity, some fluid withdrawn, and the agent to induce labor is introduced. The needle is then removed, and the patient waits for labor to begin—usually within 12 to 72 hours. Labor lasts a variable amount of time, ranging from a few hours to 24 or more, during which time sedation is usually given. The patient is usually not moved from her hospital room during the process. Expulsion of the fetus occurs rapidly once dilatation of the cervix is sufficient. The fetus is almost always dead at the time of expulsion and is well formed by this age. Scopolamine is often given during expulsion to induce amnesia because this type of abortion is usually very stressful emotionally for the woman.

Abortions after 16- to 20-weeks gestation are more distressing for all parties involved. One source of the stronger emotional impact on the woman is that fetal movement may have been felt and the fetus perceived as being real and alive. Additionally, the woman undergoes a painful labor and expulsion process without the positive connotations of childbirth. If the woman sees the aborted fetus, this can be another source of distress. Women whose pregnancy has progressed beyond 12 weeks before seeking abortion tend to have certain characteristics. Typically the very young adolescent has a late abortion due to her denial of the pregnancy and fear of telling her parents. Ambivalence and indecision can delay seeking abortion in any age group, and sudden changes in life situation (death of spouse, separation, illness, financial crisis) can underlie other late decisions. Health providers generally have greater difficulty in dealing with late abortions because the fetus has progressed considerably in its development and the conflict between saving life and ending life is even more pronounced. Some physicians refuse to perform late abortions, even though they might be willing or supportive in performing early terminations of pregnancy. The nursing staff in hospitals in particular have difficulty in providing bedside care for women laboring during late abortions and usually bear the brunt of the burden of managing the expulsion and disposition of the fetus. Performing abortions on maternity units is especially difficult because the procedure is alien to the goals, values, and attitudes which set norms of behavior on a maternity unit.[8] Special abortion units to which sympathetic staff can be recruited seem more appropriate. Health providers have, of course, the right to refuse involvement in abortions, early or late, if it is contrary to their beliefs and principles; they are, however, obligated to make a referral to another source so that the patient may seek the care to which she is entitled.

Work-up for Induced Abortion

After the confirmation and sizing of a pregnancy and after counseling, in which the woman has freely elected to have an abortion as the best choice for herself, a complete physical examination and additional laboratory testing are done. The work-up is usually done the day before the procedure is scheduled, and a laminaria is inserted to begin the dilatation process.

The physical examination follows the usual format for any operative procedure, with special attention to cardiovascular and respiratory systems and signs of infection. A standard history accompanies the physical in order to identify significant health problems, past medical history, family history, and previous operations and hospitalizations. During pelvic examination the size of the uterus is again checked, and a gonorrhea culture and Pap smear are obtained if they have not been done before. The laminaria insertion is done as a sterile procedure. After cleansing the vulva, a sterile speculum is inserted and the cervix is exposed. It is prepped with Betadine or another antiseptic solution, then grasped on the anterior lip with a tenaculum. A uterine sound may be inserted for the distance of the endocervical canal. The laminaria is then grasped firmly with sponge forceps and inserted into the endocervical canal until about 1 to 2 cm. is left extruding from the os. This may produce a cramping sensation which soon subsides. Occasionally, the laminaria is immediately expelled, in which case it is reinserted. The tenaculum is removed; some health providers prefer to pack the vagina with sulfa gauze while others do not follow this practice. Laminarias are made of hydophilic wood and dilate to twice their diameter at the time of insertion in about 2 to 3 hours. In some situations, the abortion work-up may be done a few hours before the procedure is carried out, and the laminaria inserted at that time will have enough time to dilate the cervix before the procedure is done. If sulfa gauze is not inserted into the vagina, the woman should be told that the laminaria may fall out in a few hours, and if it does so not to be concerned because this means that it has done its work of dilating the cervix.

In addition to a pregnancy test, laboratory tests include culture for gonorrhea and Pap smear, urinalysis, hematocrit or complete blood count, Rh typing, VDRL testing, and in some facilities blood typing and cross-matching. If the woman is Rh negative, part of her postabortion care includes the administration of RhoGAM unless it is known that the woman is already sensitized, that the father is Rh negative, or that the woman will have no further pregnancies. Five to 10 percent of Rh negative women will become sensitized to the Rh antigen following induced abortion if RhoGAM is not given.[9]

Patient instructions include telling her when and where the abortion is to be performed and when to arrive at the facility. She is to be NPO after midnight in most cases, although if local anesthesia is used she may take fluids. Local paracervical block is preferred in abortions before the twelfth week, as it avoids the complications possible with a general anesthesia. However, if the woman is very apprehensive and the physician thinks that she will not tolerate the procedure well under local anesthesia, most hospital-based facilities will administer a general. There is usually some sedation given when a local is used. The woman is also warned of the signs of complications after laminaria insertion—although the incidence is very low—including heavy vaginal bleeding, severe pain, and fever, which might indicate hemorrhage or infection.

The consent to perform the abortion to terminate pregnancy is obtained from the woman. Although some states have passed laws requiring the consent of the husband, or of the parents of an unmarried pregnant minor before terminating a pregnancy, these laws have been invalidated by the U.S. District Court in Miami, and its decision has been affirmed by the Fifth United States Circuit Court of Appeals. In its decision the Miami Court said:

> The State has no authority to interfere with a woman's right of privacy in the first trimester to protect maternal health nor can it interfere with that right before the fetus becomes viable in order to protect potential life. It follows inescapably that the State may not statutorily delegate to husbands and parents an authority the State does not possess.... A State which has no power to regulate abortions in certain areas simply cannot constitutionally grant power to husbands and parents to regulate in those areas. Therefore, husbands and parents cannot look to the State to prosecute and punish the physician (or other participants) who performs an abortion against the wishes of the husbands and parents.[10]

TYPES OF ABORTION TECHNIQUES
Methods Before 12-Weeks Gestation

SUCTION CURETTAGE. Also called vacuum aspiration or dilatation and evacuation (D and E), suction curettage is the most efficient and widely used method of terminating pregnancies of up to 12-weeks duration. In the United States about 75 percent of induced abortions are performed by this method, and it is widely used throughout the world. Suction curettage takes about 2 minutes to perform, is usually done under local anesthesia, and usually involves less than 30 to 50 ml. of blood loss. Premedication with diazepam (Valium) or analgesics is used in conjunction with a paracervical block for anesthesia. The cervix is progressively dilated until the diameter in millimeters corresponds to the number of weeks of the pregnancy, using Hegar or Pratt dilators. This process is aided by preabortion laminaria insertion. A suction curette of corresponding size is inserted into the uterine cavity, the electrically operated vacuum pump is switched on, and negative pressure in the range of 30 to 50 cm. Hg utilized, according to gestation (Figure 7-2 and Table 7-1).

Following aspiration, a sharp curette or ovum forceps is often used to check the completeness of the evacuation. Sharp curettage, if used, must be done very lightly to avoid damage to the basal layer of the endometrium which could produce sclerosis, formation of synechiae, or predisposition to subsequent placenta accreta. The tissue removed is sent for pathological examination for presence of products of conception. When the procedure is completed, the patient is observed in the recovery area for at least 2 hours and until vital signs are stable. In the absence of complications, the patient is discharged to home.

Suction aspiration is superior to surgical (sharp) curettage because it empties the uterus more rapidly, minimizes blood loss, reduces the likelihood of uterine perforation, and does not require general anesthesia. However, if the suction tip remains over the placental site too long, rapid and excessive blood loss can occur. If perforation does occur and is not recognized, serious damage to other abdominal organs can result. Careful and slow minimal dilatation of the cervix is necessary to avoid injury which can lead to later cervical incompetence or cervical stenosis. When performed properly, suction curettage is associated with a very low failure rate and a complication rate under 2 percent for infection, about 2 percent for excessive bleeding, and under 1 percent for uterine perforation. The mortality rate is less than 2 per 100,000[11] (Table 7-2).

SURGICAL CURETTAGE (D AND C). Surgical, or sharp curettage is also used for first trimes-

ter abortions and is basically the same procedure as the traditional D and C. It takes about 5 minutes to perform, results in about 100 to 200 ml. of blood loss, and usually requires general anesthesia. The cervix must be dilated more than for suction curettage, and the danger of damage to the cervix and uterus is increased. Once the cervix is dilated to the appropriate size, an ovum forceps is initially used, followed by the sharp metal curette, to empty the uterine cavity. Curettage must be carefully done, particularly as pregnancy progresses, in order to avoid damage and perforation. Despite its disadvantages, about 5 percent of the abortions done in the United States are still performed by sharp curettage. Its advantage is in its familiarity; D and C is a traditional and widely used technique known to anyone trained in obstetrics and gynecology.

The follow-up care for suction curettage and for D and C includes instruction about complications before the woman leaves the facility and where and how to contact health providers should complications occur. Signs and symptoms of infection such as fever and chills, foul-smelling vaginal discharge, and abdominal cramps; heavy bleeding persisting over several hours in which pads are rapidly soaked; and severe abdominal pain with nausea and vomiting indicate complications. The woman should avoid the use of tampons and refrain from intercourse for 2 weeks. She should also avoid douching to reduce the chance of infection. Normal activity can usually be resumed in 1 or 2 days. Discussion of contraception is initiated; in some instances an IUD may be inserted at the time of the abortion (although the perforation and expulsion rates are increased) or a prescription for oral contraceptives may be given, to be started 1 week after the abortion. Otherwise, contraception is provided at the 2-week follow-up visit.

MENSTRUAL INDUCTION. Very early abortions performed on an outpatient basis 5 to 7 weeks after the last menstrual period by the aspiration of the endometrium are variously called menstrual regulation, menstrual extraction, endometrial aspiration, minisuction, miniabortion, and interception. The procedure is simple and relatively atraumatic, with the use of a 4 to 6 mm. flexible plastic cannula and a syringe or other low pressure suction, requiring little or no cervical dilatation or anesthesia.

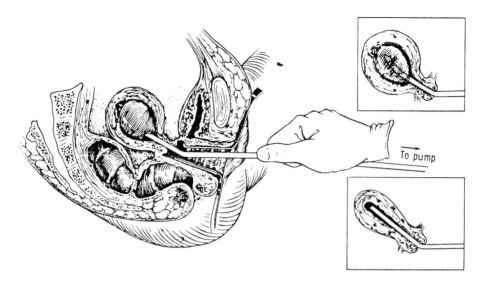

To pump

Figure 7-2. Suction curettage method of terminating pregnancy up to 12 weeks gestation.

Women who have missed one menstrual period and suspect that they are pregnant are candidates for menstrual induction, but the philosophy differs among health providers on other indications and requirements for the procedure. One approach is to fulfill criteria including amenorrhea of 7 to 21 days beyond the date of the expected menstrual period, sexually active or at least one unprotected intercourse since the last menstrual period, positive urine pregnancy test, uterus not clinically enlarged, and the woman's belief that pregnancy was possible or probable based upon her menstrual pattern and symptoms. Other providers do not require a positive pregnancy test, because false negatives are often obtained in early pregnancy, and there are advantages to some women who would have a problem of conscience in undergoing menstrual induction should pregnancy be confirmed. In the case of pelvic pathology or infection, the procedure is contraindicated.

The extent of the preliminary work-up differs, but generally it includes a pertinent history and physical examination and a gonorrhea culture and Pap smear as a minimum. Particularly if confirmation of pregnancy is a criterion, additional laboratory studies are included, consisting of a complete blood count or hematocrit, VDRL, urinalysis, blood grouping and Rh typing.

The procedure is done in the office, and most patients receive an analgesic or diazepam for premedication. Aseptic technique and sterile equipment are used, although gowns and masks are dispensed with. After exposing the cervix with a speculum, the vagina and cervix are cleansed with iodine solution and, in most cases, a paracervical block with 1 percent carbocaine is given. A nonperforating or single-toothed tenaculum is used to grasp the cervix, and the uterus is sounded, depending upon individual approach. Some providers think that sounding the uterus is unnecessary because the sound itself can be a cause of perforation, and the soft collapsible cannula will follow the uterine contour and is unlikely to perforate. Dilatation is usually not necessary, and a 4 to 6 mm. Karman cannula is inserted; the selection of its size is based upon the number of days from the last menstrual period (i.e., 4 mm. up to 40 days, 5 mm. for days 40 through 50, and 6 mm. for days 50 through 70). The cannula is attached to a 60 cc. hand-held syringe with a locking device or to an electric suction pump, and negative pressure from 50 to 75 cm. Hg is applied. The suction is carried out for about 2 minutes while the cannula is moved back and forth and rotated, until the grating feeling typical of the myometrium is felt. Generally, if the patient is not pregnant, only 2 to 3 ml. of aspirate is obtained; if she is pregnant the volume increases to 7 to 15 ml.[12]

The woman remains in the waiting room in the office for 1 hour after the procedure, and those with Rh negative blood who are not sen-

Table 7-1

Weeks of Gestation from Last Menstrual Period	Dilatation of Cervix (mm.)	Size of Suction Curette (mm.)	Vacuum (cm. Hg)	Expected Blood Loss (ml.)
1-4	4-5	4	30-40	10
5-8	8-9	8	30-40	10-30
9-10	10-11	10	40-50	30-80
11-12	12-13	12	40-50	80-200
13-14	14-15	14	50+	200-400

sitized are given RhoGAM if the patient consents, because fetal megaloblast bearing the Rh antigen has been found as early as 7 weeks from the last menses.[13] The aspirate is usually sent for pathologic diagnosis. The proportion of histologically confirmed pregnancies varies from 58 percent at less than 33 days after the last menstrual period to 95 percent at 45 days.[14] Although few reports show more than 65 percent confirmed pregnancies, if all criteria are fulfilled, including a positive pregnancy test, results as high as 98.2 percent pregnancies have been obtained.[15]

Complications are minimal with about 1 percent infections usually secondary to retained products, between 1 to 5 percent continuing pregnancy and requiring a second procedure, and from less than 1 to 6 percent excessive bleeding. No mortality has been reported. The major complication rate is considered to be less than 1 percent. Some providers think that an average of 35 percent of the patients who undergo menstrual induction and are not pregnant represents a large number of patients who have an unnecessary procedure. Waiting for a positive pregnancy test could certainly reduce this number, although the advantage of immediate action and avoiding ethical conflicts would be lost. For economic reasons and principles of safety this approach would seem appropriate, although as one physician put it:

> ... to insist that pregnancy be confirmed before endometrial aspiration is performed smacks unpleasantly of the arguments that we (mostly male) physicians formerly engaged in regarding the number of children a woman had to have before she was eligible for a tubal ligation. I really hope that those days of female coercion are gone.[16]

For women who are very anxious, who do not wish to know if they are pregnant, or who think that they cannot wait for a variety of reasons, menstrual induction offers a simple, safe, and low-cost solution to a possible un-

Table 7-2
Morbidity and Mortality Rates for Common Methods of Induced Abortion

Type of Complication	D and C	Suction	Saline	Hysterotomy
Hemorrhage	1.0	0.5	4.0	3.7
Infection	0.9	0.8	5.4	11.0
Perforation	1.9	1.3	0.2	5.1
Anesthesia	0.1	0.1	0.1	0.7
Shock	—	—	0.2	0.7
Retained products	0.5	0.5	14.7	1.5
Lacerated cervix	0.3	0.2	0.1	0.7
Other	0.3	0.3	1.0	4.4
Unspecified	0.1	—	0.2	—
Total morbidity*	5.1	3.7	28.3	27.8
Total mortality†	2.8	1.2	22.9	235.3

*Complications per 1000 abortions
†Deaths per 100,000 abortions

wanted pregnancy. Although this procedure has been taught and used in womens' groups, it is not a safely done self-administered operation. It is appropriate, however, for health providers other than physicians, who have been trained in this technique to perform the procedure.

Follow-up care includes instructing the woman on the signs and symptoms of infection and hemorrhage, to avoid tampons, sex, and douching, and to return for reexamination in 2 weeks. At the 2-week visit, an early morning urine sample is tested for HCG, an examination done to determine uterine size, and contraceptives are provided. If the pregnancy test is positive and the uterus is not clinically enlarged, a repeat menstrual induction can be done. If the uterus has enlarged, a standard suction curettage or D and C is indicated. When it is thought that patients might not return for a follow-up, an IUD may be inserted at the time of the procedure or oral contraceptives given, to be started 1 week later. In case of a positive pregnancy test without uterine enlargement, ectopic pregnancy must be ruled out, although its incidence is very low.

PROSTAGLANDINS. The name prostaglandins has been given to a group of fatty acids derived from semen, with the highest concentration found in the seminal vesicle fraction of the split ejaculate rather than the prostate fraction. Two of these acids, PGE_2 and $PGF_{2\alpha}$ have been found capable of inducing delivery at any stage of gestation. Prostaglandins are potent oxytocics, but this property alone does not make them effective abortifacients; exactly how they effect delivery is unknown. The mechanism is thought to be disruption of the implanted ovum rather than lysis of the corpus luteum. Certain of the 15 methyl analogues, $15(S)MeE_2$ and $15(S)MeF_{2\alpha}$, are also effective in terminating pregnancy. The main problem with prostaglandins is their side effects, including vomiting, diarrhea, fever, and shaking, which occur commonly when doses high enough to be effective are used. Oral administration is impractical, due to the side effects, but vaginal, intramuscular, and transcervical instillation show promise in terminating early pregnancies. The need for repeated doses and the relatively long time required for abortion to occur are the disadvantages of this method compared to suction curettage.[17]

Vaginal administration of $15(S)MeF_{2\alpha}$ in 0.5 or 1.0 mg. suppositories at 3-hour intervals for a total dose of 2.5 to 5 mg. resulted in the onset of bleeding within 9 hours in 90 percent of the pregnant patients, an average duration of bleeding of 8 days, and termination of 100 percent of the pregnancies. The women were from 31 to 43 days past their last menstrual period and of the 37 percent who were not pregnant all experienced bleeding—most within 9 hours of prostaglandin therapy. The amount of bleeding was similar to the patient's usual menses, with heaviest flow on the third and fourth days, and there were no complications necessitating further treatment. Episodes of nausea, vomiting, or diarrhea were minimal.[18] The direct administration of 5 mg. $PGF_{2\alpha}$ or 1 mg. PGE_2 in solution or pellet form through a transcervical catheter resulted in uterine bleeding in 3 hours, with the discharge of tissue fragments and blood 2 days later. Bleeding continued for about 1 week, and no serious complications have been reported. In women with amenorrhea up to 14 days after a missed period, this prostaglandin impact technique has a success rate of 97 percent, and is done in an office setting, with minimum premedication and no cervical dilatation.[19] The question of whether or not to diagnose pregnancy before therapy also arises with these early prostaglandin techniques; if not diagnosed, there will no doubt be a large proportion of nonpregnant patients treated. Because serious complications are rare and the side effects appear mild with the newer techniques, prostaglandin termination of pregnancy before 12 weeks will no doubt increase in clinical use.

Methods After 12-Weeks Gestation

AMNIOINFUSION. Intraamniotic instillation of a substance to induce labor is the most commonly used method for midtrimester abortion. Hypertonic saline has been used for several years, but now prostaglandins have become the most frequently used agent because delivery occurs more rapidly and there are fewer complications. This procedure requires hospitalization throughout, usually for 2 or 3 days, with the standard admission history and physical examination and laboratory tests. For effective amnioinfusion, pregnancy must be at least 16-weeks gestation. For pregnancies beyond 20 to 24 weeks, state laws and hospital policies must be taken into account.

The procedure is done with sterile supplies and aseptic surgical technique. No premedication is necessary. The patient's bladder should be empty. With the patient supine, the lower abdomen is prepped with iodine solution and draped with sterile towels. The skin is infiltrated with a local anesthetic over the injection site, then an 18-gauge spinal needle is inserted into the intrauterine cavity and a flow of clear amniotic fluid obtained. Usually a small amount of amniotic fluid is removed (not more than 200 ml.), standard infusion tubing attached to the needle, and the agent used introduced by syringe injection or by gravity drop. A small test dose is first given, then if there is no reaction within 5 minutes, the remainder is instilled over a 15-minute period. If a saline solution is used, the dosage is 200 ml. of 20 percent NaCl; the prostaglandin used is 40 mg. $PGF_{2\alpha}$. After instillation, the spinal needle is removed and the patient is returned to her room.

With hypertonic saline solution, the fetus and placenta usually die within 1 to 2 hours, and labor begins within 48 hours. About 97 percent of women abort in 72 hours, 85 percent abort in 48 hours, and only 22 percent abort in 24 hours. The complication rate is about 20 percent including, most often, hemorrhage, infection, and retained placenta. The injection-to-abortion time can be shortened with augmentation of labor by using pitocin, but the risks of a ruptured uterus, cervical lacerations, and water intoxication increase. The mortality rate is about 18 per 100,000 abortions. The injection of the saline solution into the placental site or maternal vessels produces hypernatremia which can cause cerebral edema, cardiac failure, and death. Amniotic fluid embolism and disseminated intravascular clotting with afibrinogenemia and bleeding are infrequent but serious complications. Necrosis of the myometrium can occur if the saline solution is injected into the uterine muscle.

Using intraamniotic prostaglandins, the onset of labor is sooner, and 93 percent of women abort in 48 hours, with 64 percent aborting within 24 hours. Medication can be used to attenuate the side effects of vomiting and diarrhea. Potentially serious complications are rare; those related to the drug per se include bronchospasm, arrhythmias, other cardiovascular changes, and grand mal seizures. These complications are more common with sys-temic administration of prostaglandins, thus to ensure the intraamniotic placement of the drug reduces the incidence of these complications. Hemorrhage, infection, uterine rupture, and cervical laceration are infrequent complications. The advantages of prostaglandins over saline solutions include fewer cardiovascular changes with more rapid resolution, no significant changes in clotting factors, no sodium load and danger of hypernatremia, and less myometrial damage when accidentally injected; the disadvantages include a higher proportion of second injections, more gastrointestinal side effects, and the greater cost of the drug, although this may be offset by shorter hospitalization.[20]

Follow-up care includes the administration of RhoGAM to unsensitized Rh negative women, instruction on signs and symptoms of infection and hemorrhage, avoidance of sex, tampons, or douches for 2 weeks, and reexamination in 2 weeks. Some depression is not uncommon, similar to that following term pregnancy and delivery, and the woman can be prepared for this before hospital discharge. At the 2-week check-up, uterine size should be back to normal and bleeding resolved. Contraception can be initiated at this time, according to the woman's needs and desires.

INTRAMUSCULAR PROSTAGLANDINS. The pregnancy of between 12 and 16 weeks poses a difficult problem in termination. Although suction curettage can be done up to 14 weeks, the risks are increased; and intraamniotic saline solution or prostaglandins are usually not effective until 16 weeks. Serial intramuscular injections of the 15 methyl analogues have been highly successful in terminating pregnancies of between 10 and 17 weeks without serious complications, though with the usual prostaglandin side effects. Abortion was completed in 96 percent of patients with intramuscular injections of 5 to 10 mcg. 15(S)MeE$_2$ every 2 hours until aborted, or for 24 hours of therapy. A high level of uterine activity occurred within 40 minutes of the first injection, and the mean abortion time from first injection to expulsion was 9.52 hours; with 76 percent of the patients aborting within 12 hours and 96 percent within 24 hours. Only 10 to 15 percent of the patients experienced gastrointestinal side effects, but nearly all had a temperature elevation of 2°F or higher, and one-fourth reached 102°F or above. Shaking and chills occurred in some. There was no irritation or inflammation at the injection site. In another series, $15(S)MeF_{2\alpha}$ was also found to be very effective in gestations of 17 weeks or less, but doses about 20 times higher were required. Gastrointestinal side effects occurred in 85 percent of the patients, but only 23 percent had a temperature elevation of more than 1°F. Thus the $F_{2\alpha}$ prostaglandins have a more specific effect on gastrointestinal motility, while the E_2 compounds affect temperature regulation more.[21] Intramuscular prostaglandins are managed as an inpatient procedure. Follow-up care is the same as for other types of midtrimester abortions.

HYSTEROTOMY. About 1 percent of the abortions done in the United States are performed by hysterotomy, a miniature cesarean section. The operation can be done abdominally or vaginally, requiring the usual preoperative preparation for surgery and general or spinal anesthesia. There is considerably greater morbidity and mortality than with other midtrimester techniques, with the risk of impairment of future reproductive function. An additional disadvantage is the delivery of a live fetus, while advantages include concomitant sterilization or treatment of preexisting pelvic disease.

CONSEQUENCES OF INDUCED ABORTION

Abortion during the first trimester carries considerably less risk of death than does pregnancy; the risk is comparable to that of IUD and oral contraceptive use. The risk of death for midtrimester abortion is equal to that for pregnancy (Table 7-3).[22] The overall complication rate for all types of abortions is 7.2 per 1000 abortions, with the incidence increasing the longer the gestation.[23] Data from other countries indicate that some long-term sequelae of abortion were subsequent infertility, spontaneous second trimester abortion, premature delivery, and infants with low birthweight. These findings may have been related to earlier abortion techniques; in the United States, the data clearly indicate that prematurity rates are declining, as reflected by a significant fall in infant mortality.[24] It is not known if decreased fertility is related to a

changed life style or to pelvic damage secondary to infection or trauma. Readily available, safe, legal termination of pregnancy has been shown to result in decreased maternal mortality rates and fewer medical problems in young women.[25]

The emotional consequences of abortion are largely determined by the woman's personal value system, events surrounding the pregnancy and abortion, and her cultural and interpersonal environment. Feelings of guilt, depression, and anger, when these occur, seem confined to the immediate postabortion period, and they have decreased in intensity and duration with growing social acceptance. Recent studies indicate that feelings of relief outweigh sadness and guilt and that the majority of women electing abortion feel positive about their decision. The reported incidence of serious regrets following induced abortion is less than 5 percent.[26] Women have fewer regrets and guilt when they feel that they have made the decision themselves, without undue influence by others. Those experiencing more difficulties with abortion include women with psychiatric problems, very young adolescents, women who believe abortion is wrong, who are involved in life crises, who seek abortion against their true desires or have significant ambivalence, and those without good support systems.[27]

There is a very high demand for abortion services from women with diverse characteristics. Single women seek abortion about twice as often as married, and first pregnancies are most frequently aborted, although the rates for second and third pregnancies are also quite high. More abortions are performed on women in the 20 to 30 age range than in any other, and women below age 20 constitute the second largest group having abortions. These are also the ages with the highest overall incidence of pregnancy. There has been an increasing utilization of abortion by nonwhite and lower socioeconomic women, reversing a prior pattern and showing that those groups (nonwhite, poor) with higher rates of excess fertility are now having higher abortion rates. This is a typical pattern as well in other countries with liberal abortion laws; when abortions are readily available, women in the lower socioeconomic groups who are not successful in controlling birth through contraception make the greatest use of abortion.[28]

Table 7-3
Risk of Death for Women Age 15-54

Pregnancy	16/100,000 live births	Curettage abortion	2.6/100,000 abortions
		Amnioinfusion	18.3/100,000 abortions
Oral contraception	0.3-3/100,000 women		
IUD	0.3-1.5/100,000 women		

Repeat Abortions

Little research has been done on repeat aborters, but rates ranging from 13 to 24 percent have been reported. Many providers thought of abortion as a one-time measure for women in trouble and advised women against having more than one abortion. It now appears that for some women, abortion is a new primary method of birth control. This is a deeply disturbing development for some health providers, raising new questions and conflicts. The average woman who used abortion as a primary means of birth control would have 1 or 2 abortions a year over her 30 years of sexual activity and fecundity. New techniques promise to make abortion in early pregnancy the safest birth control method, however, and if one abortion is acceptable why is it wrong to have more? Concerns involve the ethics and emotional dynamics of repeated abortions, which are seen as self-destructive on the part of women and sadistic on the part of men. A type of sexual game-playing may be involved in which risk and danger are necessary components of sexual satisfaction, or abdication of responsibility or need for complete spontaneity are part of the sexual set. A lack of respect seems implicit in the repeated casual removal of even early fetal life from a woman's body. Since a woman could really control her body through contraception, the acceptance of repeated abortions may represent society's ultimate lack of respect for the woman as well as her ultimate lack of respect for her moral and social self.[29]

THE ABORTION CONTROVERSY

Abortion continues to be an emotionally charged issue, with prolife groups promoting a constitutional amendment to prohibit abortion and working within state legislatures for specific laws affecting various aspects of abortion practices. Elective abortion is a difficult issue because there is much truth in the arguments and principles of both proponents and opponents. The basic moral-ethical issues involved are the sanctity of life, the beginning of human life, and fundamental human rights. Other questions revolve around the equal application of the law and due process of law. Belief systems and philosophies enter deeply into the debate, raising questions of freedom of religion and universal truths versus situational ethics. Social morality evolves and changes, as does a society's sense of justice and human rights; the issues surrounding abortion must also be viewed in the perspective of the times.

The Feminist Perspective

Proponents of abortion may view the issues within a feminist perspective which holds that one of woman's fundamental human rights is to control her reproductive powers and to decide how her body is to be used. The availability of abortion on demand is a necessary guarantee to this right. The struggle to assure this guarantee is part of woman's larger struggle for recognition as a person in the fullest sense—an equal member of humankind with the same legal, political, and economic rights as men. Women have suffered the consequences of unwanted pregnancy most severely, and the inability to fully control reproduction has been central in women's historic subjugation to men. Impregnation is often an accident of nature which shapes the life of the mother, conflicting with her needs and strivings in many instances and subjecting her to social mores and laws contrived, for the most part, by men. The underlying motivations for compelling women to be pregnant are the reinforcement of male potency, the perpetuation of female dependency and male superiority, and the continuation of the infrastructure of a society that is based upon sex-linked social roles, with all its implications for limiting personal freedom and maintaining the current relation between economics and power.

Because the biological event of pregnancy carries such social and personal implications, many women regard abortion as a fundamental human right so immediate and profound in its effects that to deny their access to abortion negates their rights to freedom, individual liberty, self-determinaton, and the security of their person and families. To force a woman to carry a pregnancy against her will is seen as an immoral act—a rape by civil authority in the same way that an actual rape can force a woman to conceive against her will. Men have been in almost exclusive social control, making the rules for the application of moral principles in such a way that male domination is assured. The truly moral question is whether half the human race can continue telling the other half what it may and may not do; whether women can compel men to divest themselves of the prerogatives they have assumed, and recognize women as people.

Some of the most vociferous opponents of voluntary abortion have been women themselves. One possible motive for their vehemence is the tremendous threat posed to their identities when motherhood is rejected as the central purpose and function of femininity. If motherhood is not the central element in the assignment of value to women, then their self-concept is reduced because they have not developed their identities and egos in any other spheres of human endeavor. Motherhood in the feminist view, however, is an avocation that should be actively sought and desired by a woman, not arbitrarily assigned to her by social coercion. Compulsory pregnancy therefore is both immoral and an infringement upon a woman's basic freedoms.

The Pronatalist Perspective

The views of many opponents to voluntary abortion involve a prolife stance in which the fetus is believed to be a human being from conception onward. The life force that sets in motion and directs the activities of the zygote is the same life force that animates the baby and every human, and all forms of human life are to be absolutely respected without discriminating among them on a scale of relative value. Both Judeo-Christian theology and a "natural metaphysic" affirm that life is sacred, either because God has invested life with sanctity or because of the primordial experience of the elemental sensation of vitality and the primal fear of its extinction. As life is all we are capable of knowing, then the decision for death is not safe for humanity.

Considering human life sacred has survival value for the species and is particularly important for fringe groups who might be out of favor with those in power. Once society enters the arena of deciding which subgroups of humans do not have full rights and protection of the law, then the possibility is opened that any other group can also be so defined. Placing the fetus in a subhuman group of beings which can legally be destroyed is thus seen as the prologue to such practices as euthanasia, infanticide, the destruction of the mentally or physically defective, the aged, or any group deemed nonproductive or unnecessary.

Emphasis is placed on the equal rights of all lives to protection, and the embryo is given a status of full equality—contrary to the tradition of formal and common law which has historically not extended the full rights of citizenship to the unborn. Thus, no reason short of saving the life of the mother is adequate justification for abortion. Even hard cases such as rape do not permit abortion, because if the fetus is a person then its destruction is not the sparing of suffering by the sacrifice of a principle but by the sacrifice of a life. If abortion for rape were permissible, then all involuntary or unwanted pregnancies could be seen as analogous because they too cause suffering and emotional distress. Any judgment preferring an interest less than human life is out of balance with true priorities; the woman's distress, her rights to personal autonomy, societal interests in economics or population control, all must be subordinate to the right of the fetus to life.

Conflicting Rights

Obviously the right of the woman to control her body and to determine her own life is in conflict with the right of the fetus to survive. There are dangers inherent in the taking of any form of human life, and there are dangers in the denial of human freedoms. The taking of life has always been part of the human experience, and most societies have had some sanctioned form of killing, such as "just" wars, self-defense, and capital punishment. As people are responsible for all human decisions, even over life and death, the question to be answered is how such decisions can be carried out with the greatest safety and fairness. If there is no accommodation for the impact of circumstances and if inviolable principles which are not categorically universal are upheld, then there is a dehumanization of living persons.

Life may be viewed in several different contexts, such as the survival of the species, the preservation of bodily life and integrity, person-life or the integrity of personal choice and self-determination, and family life or the survival of family lineages and subgroups. Each type of life has its sanctity, and no one type has absolute dominance over the others. At times species-life may prevail over bodily life or person-life, such as in times of famine or war. In the situation of abortion, the bodily life of the fetus is in conflict with the person-life of the woman, and must be weighed in the light of other ethical principles such as least suffering or lesser evil.

Beliefs about the beginning of human life also differ, and not everyone accepts nidation as the point at which full human rights and considerations should be applied. From the developmental viewpoint there are various forms and stages of human life from potential to fully realized to death. How much development is needed to be considered truly human is unclear, but many people do not regard the embryo or early fetus as human. Although some form of human life begins at conception, full value need not be assigned at once, thus allowing the weighing of comparative values and recognizing dilemmas in conflicting rights.

Religiocultural practices in baptism and funeral rites, as well as legal requirements for death certificates, do distinguish between early and late fetal development. The time for formal recognition of the existence of a person in this sense is about 4½- to 5-months gestation. Justifying abortion does not lead to treating human beings as expendable, for it has not been demonstrated empirically that liberalized abortion practices threatens the meaning and value of life in other areas. Apparently there has been no general devaluation of human life in countries with widespread legal abortion, probably due to the different reasons and moral meanings of individual abortion decisions.

Therefore, in approaching conflicting rights in abortion decisions, a broad perspective is necessary. Ultimately, a very personal and individual decision must be made by the woman involved, her partner or family, and the health provider. As expressed by Catholic lay theologian Daniel Callahan:

> Nothing less than a wholly impersonal calculus of rights, rigidly identified and unalterably ordered independently of individual human choice, responsibility, and circumstance, could conclude that the taking of fetal life in all circumstances constituted in principle a disrespect for life.... If the right to life of the fetus is inviolable, then all other human rights become endangered by the need to preserve that one.[30]

NOTES

1. C. Tietze, "Incidence of Legal Abortion." In A. R. Omran, ed., *Liberalization of Abortion Laws: Implications* (Chapel Hill, N.C.: University of North Carolina, Carolina Population Center, 1976), pp. 1-4.
2. L. Lader, *Abortion* (Indianapolis: Bobbs-Merrill, 1966), pp. 75-84.
3. *Roe* v. *Wade*, 410 U.S. 113, 157, 158 (1973).
4. *Doe* v. *Bolton*, 410 U.S. 179 (1973).
5. M. Gispert, "Psychosocial Aspects of Abortion." In Omran, ed., *Liberalization of Abortion Laws*, pp. 74-102.
6. R. A. Hatcher, et al., *Contraceptive Technology 1976–1977*, 8th ed. rev. (New York: Irvington Publishers, Halsted Press Division of John Wiley & Sons, 1976), pp. 21-23.
7. "Stat Answer to 'Am I Pregnant' "? *Patient Care* (January 1, 1977): 110-12.
8. R. Zahourek, "Therapeutic Abortion and Culture Shock." *Nursing Forum* 10,1 (1971): 8-17.
9. S. L. Romney, et al., eds., *Gynecology and Obstetrics: The Health Care of Women* (New York: McGraw-Hill, Blakiston, 1975), p. 579.
10. "Malpractice Decisions You Should Know About: Is a Husband's Consent Necessary for Abortion?" *Medical Times* 104,10 (October 1976): 160-62.
11. R. C. Benson, *Current Obstetric & Gynecologic Diagnosis & Treatment* (Los Altos, Calif.: Lange Medical Publishers, 1976), pp. 839-40.
12. R. P. Bendel, P. P. Williams, and J. C. Butler, "Endometrial Aspiration in Fertility Control." *American Journal of Obstetrics and Gynecology* (June 1, 1976): 328-32.
13. *Ibid.*
14. W. E. Brenner, et al., "Suction Curettage for 'Menstrual Regulation'." *Advances in Planned Parenthood.* Proceedings of the Annual Meeting, American Association of Planned Parenthood Physicians 9 (1974).
15. K. R. Irani, et al., "Menstrual Induction: Its Place in Clinical Practice." *American Journal of Obstetrics and Gynecology* 46, 5 (November 1, 1975): 596-98.
16. Bendel, Williams, and Butler, "Endometrial Aspiration." pp. 328-332.
17. W. E. Brenner, "The Current Status of Prostaglandins As Abortifacients." *American Journal of Obstetrics and Gynecology* 123:3 (October 1, 1975): 306-28.

18. M. Bygdeman, et al., "Outpatient Postconceptional Fertility Control with Vaginally Administered 15(S)15-methyl-PGF$_{2\alpha}$-methyl ester." *American Journal of Obstetrics and Gynecology* 12:5 (March 1, 1976): 495-98.

19. K. F. Omran, "Clinical Implications of Legalizing Abortion." In Omran, ed., *Liberalization of Abortion Laws*, pp. 136-43.

20. Brenner, "Prostaglandins As Abortifacients," pp. 306-28.

21. N. H. Lauersen, N. J. Secher, and K. H. Wilson, "Midtrimester Abortion Induced by Serial Intramuscular Injections of 12(s)-12-methyl-prostaglandin E$_2$-methyl ester." *American Journal of Obstetrics and Gynecology* 123:7 (December 1, 1975): 665-70.

22. Hatcher, et al., *Contraceptive Technology*, pp. 77-85.

23. S. Shindell, J. C. Salloway, and C. M. Oberembt, *A Coursebook in Health Care Delivery* (New York: Appleton-Century-Crofts, 1976), p. 68.

24. Hatcher, et al., *Contraceptive Technology*, p. 84.

25. Benson, *Current Obstetric & Gynecologic Diagnosis & Treatment*, p. 842.

26. *Ibid.*

27. *Ibid.*; Gispert, "Psychosocial Aspects of Abortion," pp. 96-97; and Romney, et al., eds., *Gynecology and Obstetrics*, pp. 581-82.

28. B. Sarvis and H. Rodman, "Social and Cultural Aspects of Abortion: Class and Race." In N. Ostheimer and J. M. Ostheimer, eds., *Life or Death—Who Controls?* (New York: Springer, 1976), pp. 104-18.

29. G. A. Geyer, "Repeat Abortions: The New Primary Method of Birth Control?" *Los Angeles Times*, April 28, 1977, 2:7.

30. D. Callahan, *Abortion: Law, Choice, and Morality* (New York: Macmillan, 1970), pp. 430-31.

8

Menopause

The "change of life" is a universal event among women. It is a natural process which is as much a part of their biological rhythms as menarche and pregnancy. Yet, this physiological occurrence is surrounded by myths and permeated with fear because of cultural attitudes woven tightly into the fabric of women's status and definitions of femininity in this society. Many women find it hard to think beyond their reproductive years; somehow their roles and concepts of self do not extend beyond the time of childrearing and home-tending. Once such a view was realistic, for in 1900 women experienced menopause at age 40, while their life expectancy was 49 years. Now with menopause occurring about age 50, a woman's life extends well into the mid-70s. Middle age, which once was a matter of a few years spent in declining health, today is the longest phase of a woman's life. With children raised and on their own and a husband settled down and established in his career, the average middle-aged woman can look forward to 20 years of good health, vigor, attractiveness, and newfound freedom and independence. Usually, nothing in her past has prepared her for this time, however.

Menopause is defined as the age of the last menstrual period and refers specifically to the cessation of menses. It is commonly used to include the 1 to 2 years of most noticeable decline in ovarian function, the phase of irregular menses which gradually become further apart and lighter in amount. During this time women are termed "menopausal" or are said to be "going through menopause." A broader term, "climacteric," describes the transition occurring over a period of 15 to 20 years between the biological states of middle age and older age. The climacteric encompasses the mid-40s to the mid-60s, and menopause is only one event among the many body changes happening during these years. Why menopause occurs when it does is not known. Gradually diminishing ovarian function is the cause, with the woman's body receiving decreasing amounts of estrogen and progesterone from the ovaries. Some estrogen continues to be produced, its primary source of precursors being the adrenals, for many years after menopause. Age at menopause seems to be an inherited characteristic, with a range of normal genetic variation from 35 to 60 years.

There are approximately 21 million women in America age 41 to 60, and they are facing an uncharted future. As the middle years begin, women experience menopause and an end to the cyclicity which has characterized their biological functions. They must undergo a transition in role from the familiar and socially approved version of femininity to another status in which fertility and motherhood do not figure. The character of many of their relations with friends, partner, children, and their own parents are changing. Personal values are reexamined in the light of many years of living, and often reordered or substantially altered. Old age, with its declining functions and increasing health problems, and the meaning of approaching death become ever more real concerns.

Middle age is a new territory for woman; it is the least definable and most poorly structured stage of her life. She must fulfill a "role without a script," as Janet Harris describes in

The Prime of Ms. America: The American Woman at 40. The woman of this generation reaching her middle years is a "completely new species," but one with a unique new hope:

Was it possible for a woman—in the absence, for the first time in her life of demands, values, and rewards established by others—to find herself in the scattered pieces of all the parts she had played and in effect to create herself and a life to be lived on her own terms?[1]

PSYCHOLOGICAL PROCESSES AND MIDDLE AGE

Each phase of life brings its own stresses and satisfactions and the challenge of psychological tasks to be accomplished in attaining a different level of adaptation and viewing the self and life from a new plane. Having passed through the phases of infancy, childhood, adolescence, and young adulthood, the person entering middle age faces new adaptive tasks which are often very different from those of the young adult. Both the problems confronted and the solutions possible in middle age are generally different for women and men. Shared by both sexes are the physical changes of aging which decrease strength and stamina, the increased incidence of illness, the loss of relations through the death of friends and relatives, changing goals and values and the impact of societal changes, and body image changes due to the aging process. Men face particular problems in the work arena; they are threatened by young competitors, aware that they are now at the apex of their career and any dreams not accomplished may be forever out of their reach, uncertain of their staying power, and ambivalent about retirement. Concerns over sexual capacity are common, and proof of potency may be sought in affairs with younger women. The drive for missed experiences before it's too late may be strong. Even self-actualized and powerful men must begin to face the waning of certain capacities and contemplate the next phase of life—old age. Despite these factors, a continuity in life style is characteristic for men.

Women in middle age, however, encounter marked cultural discontinuities. Social institutions which have provided guidance and spelled out expectations for motherhood and the role of the wife are now found to be lacking for such events as menopause and widowhood. Women not only outlive men, but they also outlive their culturally assigned functions: after age 45, they are no longer needed as childbearers and tenders of children, may be replaced by younger sex objects, face fewer demands as housewives, and find themselves ill-equipped as workers. In a male-oriented and youth-dominated society, older women are seen as unattractive, unneeded, and dispensable. They are often bewildered by their apparent irrelevance.[2]

Images of the Middle-Aged Woman

From the turn of the century up to the 1920s, the American woman occupied a position of worth in her middle years, for she was essential and important to her husband and family. In magazines she was pictured as mature, full-bosomed and wide-hipped, with beauty of heart and mind. Youth was seen as frivolous, vacuous, and a bit pitiable. In a time of high infant mortality, she was the preserver of new life. By teaching child care to her daughter, she preserved the continuity of life. She was an educator, the guardian of morality, the uplifter of taste who assisted men to value the finer things of life. The World War I woman was also pictured as adventuresome and courageous, a deeply religious self-realizer whose life had many responsibilities and accomplishments.

With the advent of the 1920s, following the shock of war and the upheaval of American values which caused a general "loss of innocence," the broad-hipped mother-of-the-race was replaced by the "child-woman." Morality changed radically, a devil-may-care attitude prevailed, the fast living created the flapper and the jazz-age baby. The woman of the '20s was an eternal child, a sprite who would never grow old, a sexy toy who viewed life as transitory and to be savored for the moment. The technological changes of the industrial age modified men's roles toward conformity and consumerism. No longer needing to tame the elements and face challenges, men were not heroes; thus, they did not need heroines for wives. This, along with the shrinking nuclear family, urbanization and smaller houses, and the new housekeeping technology, obviated many aspects of the woman's role.

The depression following the 1929 stock market crash again changed woman's image. The child-woman was a frivolous luxury;

women now had to be resourceful adults sharing the burden of living with men. Clothes became conservative, and women entered the job market in increasing numbers. But this new image conflicted with the persisting ideal that a man should have a "little woman he could take care of." Screen heroes asserted that men wore the pants, while their "girls" were scatterbrained darlings. World War II again placed demands for adulthood on women as they replaced the millions of soldiers at essential jobs and faced serious questions and national dangers. While Rosie and Riveter alternated with the Betty Grable pinup, women in the movies often achieved the smart, sophisticated image of the successful career woman, worldly-wise, independent, and capable of functioning on her own.

During the last half of the 1940s, the "feminine mystique" took over. Men returning from the war felt the pressure to make up for lost time, to relieve loneliness and fear, to re-create the home of their childhood, to establish a family and a career. Women also felt an urgent desire for the homes, children, and husbands they once feared they might never have. There was a great rush to marriage and motherhood. The woman's goal was now to support her husband while he finished his education and established his business or profession. Women were particularly susceptible to the feminine mystique because of the fear, loneliness, and deprivation of war: the price of a career or interests outside the home was to give up love, home, and children.[3]

There were many reasons why women succumbed to the feminine mystique, including the economic pressure to free jobs for men returning from the war, the sexual-sell that advertising was beginning to use to promote consumerism, and the return to old-style values that promoted women's secondary role to men. But the lack of any consistent role models and women's constantly changing image contributed to this process for "goals, values, life styles for women in American society change just often enough to prevent each new generation of women from identifying with any previous ones."[4]

Today's middle-aged women were the brides and young mothers of the '40s. They are the casualties of the feminine mystique, the disposable homemakers whose purpose in life is now gone. They lived by the dicta "A woman's place is in the home," "Find a good man and take care of him," and "Women don't compete with men." They invested their energies and drives into husband and children; gloried in the successes of husbands and the accomplishments of children; provided constant physical care, guidance, direction and support; made a science of motherhood, with advice from the experts; outran labor-saving appliances in the kitchen in their pursuit of the gourmet cult and in the washroom by their daily attack on loads of mildly dusty clothes; and they eschewed the external world because they didn't have time to read the newspaper. The activities of Little League and Girl Scouts filled their days; they entertained to promote their husband's business interests.

What of their other goals and purposes in life? What of their need for achievement, recognition, adventure, challenge, power, realization of their talents and abilities? These were simply turned away, or held in abeyance. Women lived vicariously through their men and their children and found self-expression in self-renunciation. If the children were doing well at school and had many friends, the woman was happy; if her husband was successful in his work she was satisfied. Thinking about her own needs made the woman feel guilty—as though she had trouble in giving to her family. When feeling dissatisfied or restless, she would plan to do all the things she wanted to do when the children were grown. But that future was far away, and all those "things" never well defined. Women did not realize that after deferring their own needs and living a life of service to others for so many years, they would be ill equipped for self-direction:

> The fact remains that the girl who wastes her college years without acquiring serious interests, and wastes her early years marking time until she finds a man gambles with the possibilities of an identity of her own. . . . It is not that easy for a woman who has defined herself wholly as wife and mother for ten or fifteen years to find a new identity at thirty-five or forty or fifty.[5]

MIDDLE-AGED WOMEN AND THE MEDIA. The middle-aged man today has many positive images in magazines, movies, and television. Whether a business executive or rugged outdoorsman, the tanned, virile, dignified 50- or

60-year-old man with silvery temples projects an image of success, self-satisfaction, and sexual potency. Usually a slender, nubile, lovely young woman in her 20s gazes up at him admiringly or hastens to serve him. But the middle-aged woman has no such positive images. Drug ads show close-ups of her lined, harassed face, while promising relief from her sufferings. Disdain and pity are communicated in vignettes portraying her as a silly clubwoman, inept housekeeper, incessant shopper, ridiculous dieter, nagging wife, nosey mother-in-law, meddling mother, a sexless, castrating female. In what is perhaps her least objectionable image, the middle-aged woman is a kindly neighbor advising young housewives about the proper brewing of coffee and unstopping of plugged sinks. Maude, television's most notable middle-aged woman, exhibited a curious mixture of initiative, independence, sarcasm, domesticity, emotional dependence, courage, and the biting tongue of the typical midyears carp. Perhaps her excursions into the world from a (relatively) safe home base are more characteristic of today's middle-aged woman than most would like to admit.

Images of women in general, as well as of middle-aged women, are, of course, changing. This is largely due to the Women's Movement and to the demands for more realistic and positive portrayals of women in the media. Occasionally one may glimpse the accomplished middle-aged woman, successful in her business or profession and presenting a trim, attractive, though mature, appearance. Older people are receiving better treatment also, with aged faces communicating pleasure and satisfaction. Magazines like *Ms.*, *Working Women*, and *Savvy* will continue to improve women's images, at least to their largely female readership.

The Fertility-Menopause Dichotomy

Menopause is a double blow to the culturally conditioned American woman. It signals both the end of fertility and the imminence of aging—events which carry strong negative connotations in our culture. When women are defined by their sexual functions and their value is derived therefrom, their status plummets with the curtailment of their reproductive capacity. When youth is idolized and glorified, then aging is regarded with sorrow and death with dread. The interplay of these pervasive values creates a mythical aura around the

young, fertile woman, who is seen as a combined sex-goddess and madonna, embodying the secret of generation and the affirmation of male sexual potency. What little privilege women have comes from this imagery; male deference and desire are based upon it.

The golden glow is threatened by signs of aging. All will be lost when age comes; fertility will be gone, the woman cast aside, and her lot will be uselessness and physical ailments. The rewards of glowing feminine fertility are granted at the expense of privilege with the coming of menopause. When youth and fertility, with their limited timetable, are the only rewards for women, then menopause is indeed a life crisis. This one distinct event, able to be identified clearly in time, marks the end of youth and the end of fertility.[6] No wonder menopause is so feared!

Men have no such clear mark of aging. Their loss of fertility as well as the decrease in their sexual potency occur gradually over a long period of time. Because men have many other ways of self-definition and identity, diminished reproductive capacity is not a significant concern. Men can continue to grow and realize their goals in the middle years; in fact they are often at the height of their esteem and achievement at the time when their female contemporaries are facing the end of their lives as meaningful and productive members of society.

The Crisis of Menopause

Women's crisis during the time of menopause is essentially one of lost identity. Although much of the mothering obligation decreases, many women manage to extend their caretaking role through an involvement with their children's families. Time becomes a problem, with empty hours to fill. Purpose and direction are lacking; what difference does the middle-aged woman's activities make? Many turn to volunteerism, but not so much due to a belief in and commitment to the cause as to friends' advice about "getting involved." The fear of widowhood, however, portends the gravest crisis. The loss of her husband means the loss of a woman's major mode of self-definition and self-esteem. With no clearly defined role for the later years, with her socially approved channels for establishing her value gone, with her guideposts for identity moving away, the middle-aged woman sees menopause as a symbol of profound loss. The crisis is heightened by widespread negative attitudes, often biased and erroneous:

> Without estrogen, the quality of being female gradually disappears. The vagina begins to shrivel, the uterus gets smaller, the breasts atrophy, sexual desire often disappears and the woman becomes completely desexualized.
> —Dr. David Reuben in *Everything You Always Wanted to Know About Sex but Were Afraid to Ask,* 1971.
> Woman is a pair of ovaries with a human being attached; whereas man is a human being furnished with a pair of testes.
> —Virchow in *Woman: An Historical, Gynecological and Anthropological Compendium,* 1935.

DEVELOPMENTAL TASKS OF MIDDLE AGE. Superimposed on the specific problems of menopause are the more general developmental tasks that every middle-aged person faces in moving from one phase of life to another. Methods of accomplishing these tasks vary, depending upon whether the middle-aged adult is married, single, or divorced; has children or is childless; and on previous life experiences and coping styles. Most tasks are carried out without conscious awareness or recognized acceptance. Good adaptation produces a secure person who can continue to grow and change; poor adaptation can occasion such responses as depression, suicide, anxiety, and physical and psychosomatic illness. The general tasks of middle age include the following:

1. *Reexamination of values and aspirations.* The experiences and knowledge gained through many years of living often provide a different perspective on the goals and values of youth. Questions are raised about certain assumptions and directions that have guided life through young adulthood, with a focus more on "what's really important to me" instead of "what is expected of me by society and others." Internal values become more important, and there is a renunciation of objectives that are no longer suitable or are now thought to be unattainable. This taking stock may lead to grieving over lost hopes and dreams, but when resolved it frees the person to pursue new values with vigor. Some values will be reinforced in this reexamination and will provide even stronger guidance to middle-aged living. A renewed belief in social institutions and tradi-

tions often produces a swing toward conservatism, as the merits of old values are reaffirmed.

2. *Maintenance of family supports and boundaries.* The middle-aged adult must change relations with both children and parents—a process involving separation and redefinition. The parenting of married children requires judgment and tact as a delicate balance between support and independence is sought. As their own parents age and no longer are strong and supportive, the middle-aged adult assumes a different attitude toward them and may move into a nurturant role. Often the middle-aged adult faces heavy demands from both young married children and elderly parents alike for emotional and financial help. Conflicts may arise or resurface. The goal is to be appropriately independent and secure, to set limits and meet one's own needs, yet to maintain the integrity of family relations.

3. *Redefinition of the self.* Both men and women have to seek different self-definitions that can include physical, interpersonal, and status changes as they grow older. Adults become quite self-oriented in the middle years, often undergoing a crisis of identity in the search for answers to the question, "Who am I?" The woman's unique problem of menopause has been previously discussed, as has the man's need to see himself in the latter years of his career. The numerous changes in the body for both sexes demand a readjustment of self-concept, as do the frequent health problems of this period. There is often a preoccupation with one's image, worries about appearance, sexual performance, relations with others, economic security. By developing self-awareness, examining assets and limitations, and working on interpersonal relations, the middle-aged adult can increase in self-esteem and move toward a positive redefinition of self.

4. *Planning for the future and aging.* Reality dictates that the middle-aged adult cannot continue in the same life mode for the entire foreseeable future. Preparation for retirement, the end of occupational work, and a change in daily patterns occupies people at this time. There may be a renewal of other interests set aside during the years of intense work, or the emergence of new sources of enjoyment. Without such shifts in energies, retirement is a sentence to empty days and boredom. The use of leisure time provides challenges and opportu-

nities for the older population, and planning must begin in the middle years. The existential dilemma of death now also confronts the mature adult with a new urgency. Parents and friends die, and although in midlife losses tend to be replaced by acquisitions, some time after 50 losses are no longer compensated. To discover methods of coping with loss is a huge task.[7]

Emotional Symptomatology of Menopause

Menopause is accompanied by a number of affective symptoms, and it is not clear whether these are primarily related to psychological processes and conflicts which accompany the middle years, or if they are precipitated by hormonal imbalances. In a study of 638 women aged 45 to 54, it was found that 30 to 50 percent experienced dizziness, palpitations, insomnia, depression, headache, and weight gain. Multiple symptoms were the usual case. These symptoms increased in the group menstruating regularly over the group with irregular menses, and there was no one age peak at which symptoms clustered. There was also no one age group at which the frequency of discomfort diminished.[8] The symptoms menopausal women frequently experience are as follows.

EMOTIONAL LABILITY. Rapid mood swings are as characteristic of the menopausal woman as they are of the pregnant woman, for both are experiencing times of marked change in hormone levels. Crying one moment and laughing the next, the woman and family may wonder if she is going crazy—an old wives' tale about menopause. Mood changes are often unpredictable and not related to external events.

ANXIETY. Tenseness and nervousness are often experienced by women in the middle years. The anxiety may have no apparent reason that the woman can identify. Women have heard that the change of life causes nervousness, and they attribute their feelings to this change. Anxiety may be nothing new for the woman, but simply more pronounced at this time. Many factors may underlie anxiety, but clearly the crisis of menopause could exacerbate or precipitate this feeling of diffuse fear (see Chapter 15, Nervousness and Fatigue).

INSOMNIA. Difficulty in sleeping plagues the menopausal woman, even after a long and tiring day. At times this is related to hot flushes in which she awakens to find herself drenched in sweat; at times it may accompany anxiety or depression.

DEPRESSION. Feelings of sadness, worthlessness, hopelessness, being blue or down characterize depression. It is a normal part of the grief reaction to any loss, and thus it can be expected in menopausal women contemplating the end of fertility and perhaps even of femininity. Chronic depression preceding menopause is common among middle-aged women, however, and it is related to the negative aspects of women's role. Menopause only serves to deepen the depression. Women with overprotective and overinvolved relations with their children and families tend to have the highest incidence of middle-aged depression.

FATIGUE. The classic hallmark of depression, feelings of tiredness and a lack of energy, may be recognized by women more readily than a depressed emotional state. Insomnia and anxiety contribute to fatigue by draining off energy, until some women cannot keep up with their normal activities. Although this dragged-down feeling always raises the question of organic illness, by far the commonest cause of fatigue is depression (see Chapter 15, Nervousness and Fatigue).

PALPITATIONS AND DIZZINESS. Sensations of the heart pounding, racing, or doing "flip-flops" are frequent accompaniments of anxiety. Likewise, dizziness may be related to hyperventilation or anxiety states. It is possible that these symptoms may be due to vasomotor instability, secondary to hormone imbalances, or to a combination of this and anxiety.

HEADACHE. Tension is a known cause of headaches, but there is also a vascular basis for headaches via constriction and dilatation of the arteries. Thus menopausal headaches may be either part of a vasomotor instability or related to anxiety. It would be important to ascertain the woman's previous headache pattern.

About 10 percent of all women have severe, incapacitating menopausal symptoms. It has been noted that women who manifest severe psychological reactions during this time have often had earlier emotional problems which have not been resolved. However, some women who are considered to be well adjusted also develop severe symptoms, particularly if their self-esteem had been based primarily on childrearing and on reproductive capacity.[9]

PHYSIOLOGICAL CHANGES OF AGING

Aging is essentially a regression in the size, structure, and functioning of many body organs. Although the changes which occur in the body with age are well known, the questions of why these changes occur and exactly how they are brought about remain unanswered. Undoubtedly there is a complex interplay of factors, some intrinsic and some external, which bring about the changes of aging. Certain common conditions of the elderly, such as skin wrinkling, atherosclerosis and osteoporosis, previously thought to be inevitable, are now recognized as having significant external determinants. Much skin wrinkling is actually pathologic and due to excessive exposure to the sun in light-skinned people. Skin with more pigmentation, such as black and yellow skin, is more protected from solar rays and less subject to skin wrinkling with age. Atherosclerosis, although present in the majority of older Americans, is predominantly due to several external factors such as diet, exercise, and smoking and is not an inevitable accompaniment of aging. Likewise, recent-memory impairment in older persons is related to hypertension and cerebral hypoxia; mental function in healthy elderly persons is not impaired. While some bone demineralization seems inevitable with aging, significant osteoporosis is related to such external factors as a diet relatively low in calcium, inactivity, and early or precipitous estrogen deficiency.

Presently a general biological theory of aging remains elusive. Some of the phenomena of aging observed in humans and mammals include the inability to resist stress (heat, cold, infection), the decreased ability to react to stimuli such as sounds, and the decreased ability of the body to buffer and absorb internal fluctuations such as in the pH of the blood. One of the best-documented general changes of aging is the accumulation of aging pigments (lipofuscins) in the cells. These increase proportionate to age and vary from cell to cell. The autointoxication theory of aging is based on this phenomenon; cells are thought to poison themselves due to their inability to remove these waste products. However, no cellular dysfunction has been demonstrated for the accumulation of lipofuscins in any cell type.

Another general change of aging is the alteration of mechanisms which govern hormones, including gonadotropins, adrenocorticotropic hormone (ACTH), thyroid-stimulating hormone (TSH), and growth hormone, and the regulation of the autonomic nervous system. Control of these hormone mechanisms may ultimately be traced to the brain. It is known that there is a loss of nerve cells from the brain with age, although not all regions show a major loss of neurons. As there is both specificity and generality in aging changes, there may be a "cascade effect" during aging in which a change in one body component triggers another change, which in turn alters body clockwork. The cascade effect would necessitate a complex theory of aging, with a chain of influences from one cell type to another. At certain stages in the aging process there may be a dominance of physiological mechanisms involving hormones and neuroendocrine control mechanisms, while at a later time aging pigment accumulation and its effects may dominate.[10]

General Changes of Aging

SKIN AND SUBCUTANEOUS TISSUE. After age 45, there is a diminution of subcutaneous fatty tissue, particularly from the periphery of the body. Multiple factors influence this loss, including body type and obesity; the more fat one starts with the less obvious is the loss. Fat loss makes bony markings more prominent and deepens body hollows. The collagen and elastic fibers of the skin decrease, the epithelial layer shrinks in thickness, and sweat glands diminish in number. The net effect is skin that is thin, dry, and inelastic. Regulation of body temperature is affected, with elderly people more prone to heat exhaustion and more sensitive to cold. There is cellular loss of melanocytes (pigment cells) and a decrease in superficial blood vessels, leading to skin pallor and greying of the hair. There is a thinning of scalp hair and hair loss from axilla, pubis, and extremities. Changes in the androgen-estrogen ratio in older women may cause the growth of bristly facial hair.

Wrinkles are permanent infoldings of epithelium and subepithelial tissues and are due to repeated stresses on the skin produced by muscular activity and the effects of gravity. Atrophic changes in subcutaneous tissue may lead to a myriad of fine wrinkles in a crisscross pattern. Exposure to the sun is the single most important factor in producing wrinkles. Wrinkles follow linear or curvilinear patterns and are especially noticeable on the front of the neck, above the eyebrows, at the corners of the eyes, and radiating outward from the lips in a pursestring effect. Gravity also pulls the earlobes and jowls downward.

EYES. Corneal opacities, cataracts, often begin in the 50s. Fatty material is deposited around the periphery of the cornea, forming a white arcus senilis. Though common with age, this can form in people in their 20s and 30s. The pupil becomes smaller and occasionally irregular, due to the long-standing effects of parasympathetic tone. Upper lids may droop and become everted, and there is decreased lacrimal gland activity, leading to dryness of the eyes. The lens loses its elasticity and cannot accommodate well to close vision.

HEARING. Diminished hearing in aging people is caused regularly by degenerative changes in the cochlea. However, these changes apparently do not occur in areas of the world where there is little noise; hearing loss is known to be aggravated by acoustic trauma, both long- and short-term.

MUSCLES. Striated skeletal muscle shows a decrease in the number of fibers, as well as a reduction in size and strength with age. Microscopically there is a shrinkage of individual cells with the infiltration of connective tissue and fatty cells. As muscle mass decreases there is weakness, producing postural changes of the spine, sagging shoulders and loss of strength.

SKELETON. Loss of bone mineral and mass begins in women at about the age of 35 and continues progressively; similar but less pronounced changes happen in men. There often is bowing of the vertebral column, especially in the thoracic region. The fibroelastic discs between the vertebrae undergo shrinkage. These factors combine to shorten the spine, and a decrease in height of ½ to ¾ inch can be noticed by ages 50 to 55. Elderly women may lose up to 2 to 4 inches in height.

Osteoarthritis is very common, in which there is proliferation of bone around the joints. In the spine these bony growths, osteophytes, produce a lipping at the intervertebral surface that may advance until a bridge is formed between vertebrae. This can seriously limit motion. Another readily visible form of osteoarthritis is the thickening of the distal finger joints, called Heberden's nodes. More common in women, this generally appears in the forties and has a hereditary component. Osteoarthritis in the hips and knees can be disabling if severe. Obesity aggravates these bony changes.

ARTERIES. Arteriosclerosis is an accompaniment of aging in which there are two processes: deposition of fatty materials in the intima of the artery (atherosclerosis), and calcification of the middle coat of the vessel (Mönckeberg's sclerosis). Calcification does not interfere with blood flow in the way that obstructive atherosclerosis does, but it causes the elongation and increased tortuosity of arteries throughout the body. More pronounced changes accompany hypertension. During their reproductive years, women have lower plasma lipids, especially triglycerides, than do men, but postmenopausally there is a rise in cholesterol, triglycerides, and phospholipids to levels indistinguishable from those of men. Blood pressure increases moderately with aging up to age 65, where it stabilizes.

BRAIN. Older people have lighter brains than the young, often with flattening of the gyri and sulci and an increase in the size of the ventricles. It is estimated that about 50,000 to 100,000 brain cells are lost daily beginning in the mid-20s and continuing steadily thereafter. Despite this rather large cellular loss, the number of functioning cells remains enormous, and many brain cells which seem to have no identifiable function may serve as a contingency reserve. This loss of neurons goes on for decades with no apparent interference of function.

OTHER ORGANS. The weight of the liver, pancreas, and kidneys decreases with aging. In old age not complicated by cardiovascular disease, the heart is much smaller than in youth. It is clear that with aging there is a loss of functioning tissue from all vital organs and that this is replaced by fat, a more primitive type of tissue.[11]

Changes in the Reproductive System

ENDOCRINES. Because there is a decrease in follicular maturation and formation of the corpus luteum, estrogen concentration decreases. The pituitary, losing its estrogen feedback mechanism, dramatically increases follicle stimulating hormone (FSH) secretion, which continues at high levels into advanced age. Estrogens continue to be produced for many years after menopause, but their source is apparently the conversion of circulating androstenedione (from the adrenals) by peripheral adipose tissue into estrone and to estradiol. It does not appear that the ovaries or adrenals produce estrogens themselves. There is a wide variation in individual postmenopausal estrogen levels, depending upon the amount of androstenedione produced and the rate of peripheral conversion. Corticoid production decreases slowly after the age of 35 or 40 and is not altered by menopause, and the thyroid becomes smaller with age but thyroid function tests are not significantly altered, despite a declining basal metabolic rate.

VULVA. The labia majora become flatter because of their loss of fat, and the labia minora also flatten and become less distinct. The introitus tends to gradually constrict, the skin becomes thin and there is a loss of pubic hair.

VAGINA. With advancing years the vagina shortens, narrows and loses its rugation. Decreased vascularity causes the mucosa to appear pale. In estrogen-deficient states, the mucosa is thin, having only a few cell layers, with superficial cells uncornified. The supportive tissue surrounding the vagina and uterus loses its elasticity and tone, producing a characteristic vaginal relaxation which leads to cystocele and rectocele. Uterine prolapse may also result, and urinary stress incontinence may appear. The thin vaginal mucosa is easily traumatized and bleeds easily, also it has less resistance to infections.

UTERUS. The uterus promptly atrophies following the reduction of estrogen, progressing from a premenstrual weight of 120 Gm. to 50 to 60 Gm. postmenopausally. In more advanced years the uterus may weigh only 25 or 30 Gm. The cervix also shrinks but not as much, and becomes pale. In women many years after menopause, it may be hard to distinguish the cervix from the surrounding vaginal mucosa. The uterine fundus may assume a midposition as the relaxed uterosacral ligaments fail to keep it in the usual anteflexed position. The endometrium becomes thin, with short glands and cuboidal epithelium, and the stroma becomes fibrotic.

OVARIES. The ovaries gradually decrease in size to 1 or 2 cm.; the normal postmenopausal ovary is not palpable. As atrophy progresses the quality of ova decreases, and there is more nondisjunction after age 40, resulting in increased Down's syndrome babies and spontaneous abortions. Follicles gradually disappear and the surface of the ovary becomes convoluted. Ovulation usually stops 1 or 2 years before menopause, although this varies. The time of transition in menstrual patterns is about 6 to 8 years preceding menopause, with a mixed pattern of short and long cycles. Thus declining ovarian function is quite gradual, with no objective criteria for the beginning of menopausal transition.

BREASTS. The glandular tissue of the breasts undergoes atrophy, as there is inadequate estrogen to stimulate duct growth or progesterone to support alveolar development. The supportive and fatty tissues also atrophy, and the loss of elasticity of Cooper's ligaments causes sagging and pendulousness. The nipples become smaller, flatter, and lose their erectile ability. Fibrocystic disease and adenosis diminish after menopause. There is also a greater proportion of fatty to glandular tissue in the breasts of older women, making breast examinations generally easier.[12]

Physical Symptomatology of Menopause

Decreasing estrogen levels are primarily responsible for the physical symptoms experienced by women going through menopause. The absolute amount of circulating estrogen is probably not as important as the rate of change and the interplay of other hormones, including progesterone deficiency and the presence of high levels of pituitary gonadotropins.

VASOMOTOR INSTABILITY. "Hot flushes" are the hallmark of menopause; they are the sensation of sudden overwhelming heat spreading from the waist or chest upward over the neck, face, and upper extremities. Women often feel they are suffocating and rush to a window for fresh air. They may become drenched in perspiration despite removing layers of clothes. The skin of the upper chest, neck, and face may also become flushed in appearance. There is considerable variation among women, for some never have hot flushes and others range from infrequent bouts to daily recurrences, causing severe discomfort. Rapid changes in the diameters of blood vessels causes hot flushes, and this is thought to be due to erratic swings of estrogen and progesterone or to high levels of FSH. Hot flushes can be provoked by situations that change body temperature, such as anger, sexual arousal, sadness, or getting under the bed-covers. In a large survey of 45- to 54-year-old women, 48.5 percent experienced hot flushes. Those women having regular menses reported that flushes were rare, while four out of five postmenopausal women were having hot flushes. The flushing continued throughout postmenopausal subgroups, tapering off in the group whose last menstrual flow was more than nine years previous.[13] Hot flushes thus are directly related to menopausal changes, as are other vasomotor symptoms, including cold hands and feet, numbness and tingling, and possibly headaches and heart palpitations.

MENSTRUAL IRREGULARITIES. Variations in menstrual cycles begin to occur some years before menopause, and this change differs with individual women. Cycles may alternate between being longer or shorter than usual, and flow may diminish. Heavy bleeding and longer periods happen frequently and are probably due to anovulatory cycles and unopposed estrogen effects on the endometrium as ovarian function wanes. There may also be some intermenstrual spotting. These last two conditions must be viewed with suspicion, however, because of the increased chance at this age of endometrial and cervical carcinoma. Any bleeding occurring six months or more after the last menses should be investigated.

ATROPHIC VAGINITIS. An increased susceptibility to infections due to the atrophy of the vaginal mucosa produces the typical symptoms of discharge, itching, and burning. Occasionally itching and burning may be felt in the absence of infection and be due simply to tissue changes. Postcoital discomfort and dyspareunia are frequent problems, and spotting

after douching or intercourse can also occur. Vaginal atrophy may progress to the point where intercourse is impossible, although this is uncommon in women who remain sexually active.

BACK PAIN. If significant osteoporosis is present, the postmenopausal woman may complain of back pain. Acute episodes are caused by compression fractures of the vertebrae, which usually heal spontaneously only to occur again. Increased kyphosis and lordosis can produce muscle strain. Pain caused by vertebral fractures may radiate on a segmental basis due to nerve root irritation. It has been established that most women lose bone substance after menopause. The presence of adequate estrogen during the reproductive years inhibits bone breakdown and maintains a balance between bone resorption and formation. A decrease in estrogen exacerbates resorption and there is a loss of bone substance, with a marked rise in serum phosphate and a slight but variable rise in serum calcium. Postmenopausal osteoporosis is rarely seen less than 10 years after physiologic menopause, but it can occur within 3 years after the surgical removal of the ovaries.[14]

MANAGEMENT OF COMMON MENOPAUSAL PROBLEMS

Many women seek care for the symptoms which they associate with menopause, most commonly hot flushes, nervousness, irritability, and a decrease in energy. Common knowledge has informed them that estrogen therapy relieves these symptoms and promotes a sense of well-being, and often women will specifically request "hormones" for the change of life. Estrogens have been widely used over the last 20 years to treat menopausal symptoms, and prophylactically to retard bone demineralization, prevent vaginal atrophic changes, and, it is hoped, retard the aging process. Their theoretical effects on skin tone and cardiovascular dynamics contributed to the promotion of estrogens for menopausal women. "Estrogen Forever" seemed to be the philosophy of many physicians and women until recent studies indicated that the use of exogenous estrogens was associated with the increased incidence of endometrial cancer and, possibly, other types of cancer. The current controversy over estrogen and cancer is discussed later in this chapter.

Whatever the presenting problem of the patient in her middle years, a careful history and physical examination appropriate to the symptoms reported is carried out. Obviously, a number of common menopausal symptoms can also be caused by disease, and the most likely causes in the differential diagnosis should be explored. In the absence of abnormal physical findings and laboratory studies, the history is a most important tool for establishing climacteric changes as the basis of the patient's symptoms.

Hot Flushes and Vasomotor Instability

Hot flushes usually occur in women who have noticed irregular menses or who have ceased to menstruate. They may last from a few seconds to an hour or more and can be very distressing, especially at night when they may interfere with sleep. Although almost half of the women going through menopause experience flushes, only about 20 percent seek medical assistance. Most women can accept and tolerate flushes as transient discomforts, with the understanding that they do decrease and eventually disappear. When women do seek help, it is important to determine the extent of the disruption caused by hot flushes and, if the history is not typical, to consider other causes such as infection or tumors. The night sweats, malaise, and fatigue which often go along with hot flushes raise the possibility of tuberculosis or other infectious processes. It would be reasonable to order a purified protein derivative test to rule out tuberculosis, and a complete blood count, sedimentation rate and urinalysis to rule out other infections.

A pelvic examination is usually done to rule out tumors or infections and to obtain a Pap smear. A maturation index for estrogen effects on the vaginal mucosa can be done, but adequate estrogen levels are common, even with vasomotor symptoms, because the relative values of hormones are more important in symptomatology than absolute estrogen levels. A breast examination should be carried out as routinely as a pelvic examination and Pap smear.

If the conclusion drawn from the examination is menopausal hot flushes or other vasomotor symptoms, the first step in therapy is education. Misconceptions and fears about

menopause are explored and correct information is shared. Often other concerns and other symptoms, such as nervousness or depression are present. Identifying the extent of the crisis that menopause poses for the particular woman helps the practitioner to determine whether emotional counseling is indicated. If the woman desires estrogen therapy, or if the assessment of severe, disruptive hot flushes is made by the practitioner, the dangers and advantages of exogenous estrogen need to be discussed with the patient. Attitudes vary among health providers on the use of estrogen, and each must make her or his own decision whether to include this medication in the therapeutic regimen.

Estrogen is generally contraindicated in patients with breast or reproductive malignancies, kidney disease, severe cardiac decompensation, or liver disease. Often it is not given to women with a history of endometriosis or fibroids because exacerbations may result. Women with certain characteristics are at higher risk for endometrial cancer, thus with these women estrogen should be avoided or used with great caution. These characteristics include obesity, hypertension, diabetes, infertility and oligoovulation, and they are usually found in some combination with each other.

The most commonly used estrogen preparations are: conjugated estrogen (Premarin, Conestron, Menotabs) 0.3 to 1.25 mg. daily; esterified estrogen (Amnestrogen, Evex, Menest) 0.3, 0.625, or 1.25 mg. daily; and diethylstilbestrol (a nonsteroidal estrogen) 0.2 to 0.5 mg. daily. The Federal Drug Administration recommendations for estrogen therapy during menopause include the use of the smallest dose which relieves symptoms; the administration of the drug in a cyclic manner, with about 1 week per month off the medication; the use of the drug for the shortest time possible; and the close monitoring of the patient, with examinations every 6 months.[15]

The side effects of estrogen use include gastrointestinal disturbances, fluid retention and weight gain, breast and pelvic discomfort due to engorgement, headache, vaginal discharge, and skin pigmentation. These symptoms usually result from an estrogen dosage which is too high for the individual or are an initial response to therapy which can be reduced by decreasing the dosage or which may resolve with continued use. The most potentially significant side effect is vaginal bleeding which often occurs as a withdrawal effect when estrogen is used cyclically. Particularly during the initial months of therapy, spotting or moderate bleeding, usually within 1 week when the medication is stopped, is not uncommon. Some experts advise using a progestational agent to promote controlled cyclic bleeding, although it is unlikely that a woman past 50 would want to continue to "menstruate" indefinitely. Alternate treatment could be the use of a mild tranquilizer or a progestational agent alone (i.e., megestrol acetate or Megace) which is often effective against menopausal symptoms. In the light of recent studies linking estrogen use with endometrial cancer, some gynecologists recommend an endometrial biopsy before starting estrogen therapy in order to rule out hyperplasia and repeat biopsies every 6 months, whether the woman is bleeding or not.[16]

Breakthrough bleeding during the time when estrogen is being taken is even more significant than withdrawal bleeding. A first episode may be managed by the discontinuation of estrogen and close observation for several weeks, but repeated episodes of heavy bleeding indicate the need for a thorough diagnostic work-up and, usually, referral to the physician for a D and C and a cervical biopsy. Likewise, if withdrawal bleeding following cyclic estrogen use is heavy, recurrent, or lasts more than 10 days, the woman needs referral for a D and C. Women with persistent breakthrough bleeding or heavy cyclic bleeding who have been found by D and C to have atypical adenomatous hyperplasia cannot continue with estrogen therapy as long as the uterus is intact. Hysterectomy may be the better choice for these women, particularly if they derive benefits from estrogen therapy and wish to continue using replacement hormones.[17]

Menstrual Irregularities

Many women accept changing menstrual patterns as natural for the menopausal transition and recognize that their periods may vary in frequency and may skip one or more months. Decreased flow with lighter and shorter periods rarely causes concern; it is the women with heavier and longer periods who seek help. Very heavy bleeding with periods or intermenstrual bleeding are not normal for women during the middle years, even though they are common. Declining ovarian function often

leads to failure of ovulation, and the prolonged estrogen effect so caused, unopposed by progesterone, produces endometrial hyperplasia. Eventually the overgrown endometrium breaks down and begins to bleed in a profuse uncontrolled manner. Another problem arises from a corpus luteum which does not regress properly, again due to aging ovaries. Progesterone effects are then prolonged but not sufficient to maintain the lush secretory endometrium; bleeding occurs erratically and extends over a longer time than usual, with gradually decreasing flow followed by some days of spotting. Under either condition, the endometrium is often not sloughed efficiently, and there are patchy areas of unsloughed tissue remaining into the next cycle which serve as sites of intermenstrual spotting.

Although many menstrual irregularities experienced by menopausal women are basically physiologic, the question of pathology is always present. Fibroids, uterine and endocervical polyps, adenomyosis, and cervical, uterine and ovarian cancer are more common in the over-40 age groups. Individual characteristics and history are important indicators for the health provider's approach to perimenopausal bleeding problems (see Chapter 4, Menstrual Problems).

Atrophic Vaginitis

There is considerable variation among postmenopausal women in the degree of their estrogen deficiency and in the resultant changes of the vulva and vagina. If the estrogen level is low enough, however, atrophic changes will occur, including thinning of mucosal surfaces, shrinking and loss of pliability of vulvo-vaginal tissues, decreased vaginal lubrication and the loss of the vagina's ability to expand during sexual excitement, painful uterine contractions with orgasms, and altered vaginal flora, with decreased resistance to infection and trauma. Women with adequate supplies of endogenous estrogen do not exhibit these changes.

Estrogen therapy can dramatically reverse atrophic changes, with the growth of the vaginal epithelium; an increase in the glycogen content of the cells which favors the formation of lactic acid and the return of normal vaginal flora; and the cornification and shedding of superficial epithelial layers, helping protect against infection. The ability of the vagina to undergo changes during sexual excitement and orgasm are increased, and painful orgasmic uterine contractions are often decreased. Itching and burning, secondary to bacterial effects on atrophic tissue, and dyspareunia due to vaginal dryness and tissue rigidity usually disappear. Some postmenopausal women who complain of burning on urination are also suffering the effects of estrogen deprivation; if their urinalysis is normal and atrophic changes are present, estrogen therapy generally helps dysuria secondary to local irritation of urethra and periurethral tissues.

The local application of estrogen cream or lotion to the vulva and vagina is often effective in relieving atrophic symptoms. A cream containing 0.625 mg. per Gm. is applied with a vaginal inserter in doses ranging from 2 to 4 Gm. of cream daily. Once the symptoms are relieved, the cream can be applied once or twice per week as needed. Vaginal estrogen creams are absorbed to some degree into general circulation, so the side effects of oral estrogens must be borne in mind. Any bleeding must be referred for thorough evaluation. Women taking oral estrogens will experience the same effects on vaginal and vulval atrophy, thus therapy can be either local or systemic. Precautions in the use of oral estrogen have been discussed previously.

Osteoporosis

Osteoporosis is a disorder in which not enough bone is present to maintain skeletal strength, so fractures occur with minimal stress. It occurs in 25 percent of postmenopausal women and is usually manifest symptomatically about 10 years after the cessation of menses. Men, however, rarely have osteoporosis until their 80s or 90s. Many factors are involved in bone loss, not all of which are well understood. The amount of bone increases during the childhood growth period, reaching a peak at about age 20. It remains at a plateau for the next 10 to 20 years, then begins to diminish. Women tend to lose bone faster than men, and this loss begins, on the average, a decade earlier in women. Such factors as exercise, which promotes a larger complement of bone; race, with blacks accumulating more bone then whites; and several dietary factors determine the amount of bone an individual develops during maturity.

Calcium deficiency has been associated with osteoporosis, for it is known that calcium intake decreases with age beginning at about age 20. Older people also have a reduced ability to absorb calcium from the intestines when it is present. Recent data have indicated that the ratio of calcium to phosphorus is the important factor. In adults, the dietary intake of phosphorus is at least 2 to 3 times that of calcium, regardless of milk consumption, because many of the foods commonly consumed are high in phosphorus with almost no calcium (bread, cereal, meat, potatoes). Very few foods contain a large amount of calcium and almost no phosphorus (sesame seeds, maple syrup, turnip greens, seaweed). Milk, cheese, lettuce, and greens contain slightly more calcium than phosphorus, but the ratio is essentially 1:1. This dietary intake of phosphorus creates a rise in serum inorganic phosphorus concentration, which stimulates parathyroid hormone release thus releasing calcium from bone to equalize the serum calcium-phosphorus balance. Over time, this will produce a phosphate-induced bone loss. The ratio of calcium to phosphorus rather than the absolute amount of either mineral is the most important factor; when calcium is proportionally low, then demineralization of bone occurs. The maintenance of a dietary ratio of 1:1 for calcium and phosphorus is recommended as a preventative for osteoporosis; since this is unlikely, due to American eating habits, supplementation with calcium beginning at age 25 is suggested. With early calcium supplementation, it may be possible for a person of age 70 to retain the bone mass, and therefore bone strength, of a 40-year-old.[18]

High protein diets with an increased intake of nitrogen are also thought to result in bone loss. High nitrogen diets create more acid for the kidneys to dispose of, buffered in part by calcium. Since calcium intake is not also increased, this is accomplished at the expense of bones. A negative calcium balance is produced which, if continued, can cause osteoporosis. Fluoride is also implicated as a cause of bone disease, with an increased incidence of osteoporosis and osteomalacia in those geographic areas where the level of fluoride in drinking water exceeds 7 ppm, unless the calcium content is also high. Fluoride and calcium together promote bone density, but fluoride alone removes calcium from bone in the process of mineral exchange. Vitamin D deficiency interferes with calcium utilization and can cause bone loss, but it is rare in the United States.[19]

The role of estrogen in bone loss involves its restraining action on bone breakdown because it maintains a homeostasis between bone formation and resorption. When estrogen levels drop with menopause, this stabilizing influence is often lost and there is an increased loss of bone substance, with a marked rise in serum phosphate and a variable slight rise in serum calcium. In postmenopausal osteoporosis, the mineral pool for rapid exchange is small, the turnover of bone-seeking material is subnormal, and bone formation is decreased, producing high bone resorption. Initially the weight-bearing vertebrae are most affected, from the eighth thoracic vertebra down. Later the entire spine becomes involved and various deformities may result, the most common being biconcavity due to the pressure of the tough intervertebral discs on the weakened vertebrae. Soon anterior wedge fractures follow—compression fractures that result in a loss of height. This can progress to the "dowager's hump" of thoracic kyphosis and a significant loss of height. Hip and wrist fractures suffered during falls are also frequent.

The diagnosis of osteoporosis is based upon history and laboratory and x-ray findings; there is no specific diagnostic test. The patient usually presents with lumbar or low thoracic back pain, or pain in the hip or wrist. Tenderness is usually localized and there may be a history of a mild injury, such as lifting a heavy object, missing a step, or falling on an extended arm. If there is pain and tenderness in other bones, especially with proximal muscle weakness, other causes are suggested including osteomalacia and myeloma. Other causes of bone pain to consider are osteoarthritis and metastatic cancer.

Measurement of height loss is a helpful aid in diagnosis, and can be done in two ways. The measurement of the crown of the head to the symphysis pubis should equal the distance from the symphysis to the heels. Also, the span of the outstretched arms from fingertip to fingertip should be equal to total height. This measurement is best done with the patient standing against the wall without shoes, heels together, knees straight, and head erect. The crown is marked on the wall and the height taken with a tape measure. Also with the patient standing against the wall, the arms are raised at right angles to the trunk and the elbows and hands held straight. Marks are made on the wall at the fingertips and this distance taken with tape measure. Any difference between height and arm span indicates how much height has been lost due to vertebral osteoporosis.

Conventional x-ray studies are often not helpful, for they are sensitive only to greater than 30 percent bone loss. However, they can be helpful in ruling out other bone lesions such as myeloma, osteoarthritis, and malignancy. X-ray examination of the hands can be useful to determine whether or not the cortices of the metacarpals are thin, which would indicate bone loss. If the cortical thickness were decreased, one could suspect that the spine was also demineralized, although the reliability of extrapolating data has been questioned. Measuring bone density of the spine or, more commonly, the radius by radiographic photodensitometry may be used if the necessary equipment is available. Photodensitometry is an accurate measure of early bone mineral loss but is not specific for osteoporosis because density can also be lost in osteomalacia, cancer, myeloma, and other conditions. With a history typical of osteoporosis and findings on examination, measuring cortical thickness or bone density can be useful adjuncts to making the diagnosis of osteoporosis.

Laboratory values expected in osteoporosis include serum calcium normal or slightly elevated, phosphorus elevated or normal, alkaline phosphatase normal and sedimentation rate normal. In osteomalacia and metastatic cancer, the alkaline phosphatase is elevated and in myeloma it is low. In osteomalacia, the calcium is decreased or normal and the phosphorus is low. The urine may be examined for Bence Jones proteins to rule out myeloma. The parathyroid hormone level in serum is normal in osteoporosis. Hyperthyroidism is a possible though uncommon cause of osteoporosis, but if suspected it can be either confirmed or ruled out with T_3 and T_4.[20]

Estrogens are the primary treatment for postmenopausal osteoporosis and are effective in preventing fractures and decreasing pain. Estrogen therapy does not restore lost bone, but does slow down bone resorption. The timing of the initiation of estrogen therapy seems to be important; if given within 3 years of estrogen deficiency, bone mineral loss may be prevented. A realistic goal for the patient with osteoporosis is to prevent accelerated bone loss. The treatment for established osteoporosis is the administration of conjugated estrogen 1.25 mg. daily, omitting the first 5 days of each month, or, alternately, ethynil estradiol 0.05 mg. daily or diethylstilbestrol 1 mg. daily, omitting the first 5 days of the month. Conjugated estrogen seems to have fewer side effects than either ethynil estradiol or diethylstilbestrol. Unless otherwise contraindicated, estrogen therapy is continued for the remainder of the woman's life.[21]

The question of prophylactic estrogen therapy presents a difficult challenge. It is well established that exogenous estrogen can prevent the development of osteoporosis and its resultant deformities, disability, and pain. However, only about one-fourth of postmenopausal women have insufficient endogenous estrogen and develop serious bone demineralization. The use of estrogen is not without its dangers, and the benefits must be carefully weighed against the risks. Perhaps the prevention of demineralization could be approached on a dietary basis, by supplementing calcium intake and reducing high levels of nitrogen. If prophylactic estrogen is elected, the dosage recommended is 0.625 mg. conjugated estrogen on a cyclic regimen. Activity is another important method of prevention, as immobilization is known to enhance bone loss. Maintaining regular activity schedules, walking daily, and exercises to strengthen back muscles can help prevent muscle atrophy and the demineralizing effects of inactivity.

THE ESTROGEN-CANCER CONTROVERSY

Studies published in the *New England Journal of Medicine* in 1975 and 1976 reported a significant increase of endometrial cancer in women taking replacement estrogen. The Food and Drug Administration is sufficiently concerned to plan a revision of package inserts for estrogens, restricting their use in the menopausal syndrome to the small minority of women with vasomotor symptoms that are serious and incapacitating. The implications of this step by the FDA would be to change radically the use of exogenous estrogens and to limit severely the conditions under which they would be prescribed.

The study by Dr. Donald C. Smith and his colleagues retrospectively compared 317 patients with endometrial adenocarcinoma against an equal number of patients with other gynecologic neoplasms, and it found that the risk of endometrial cancer was 4.5 times greater for users of estrogens.[22] Drs. Harry K. Ziel and William D. Finkle reported on 94 patients with endometrial carcinoma who were age-matched with two sets of controls from the same population, and who showed an average risk ratio of 7.6 varying from 5.6 to 13.9, depending upon the duration of conjugated estrogen use.[23] Dr. Thomas M. Mack and his colleagues compared 63 cases of endometrial cancer in a retirement community with four sets of controls of the same age and length of residency and found a 5.6 risk ratio for conjugated estrogen use.[24]

The obvious inference to be drawn from these studies is that exogenous estrogen can be a cause of endometrial carcinoma. Making this inference has been criticized, however, as unjustified by present evidence. A retrospective study showing an increased incidence of endometrial carcinoma cannot prove causality, and there are many variables in the association of exogenous estrogen and endometrial cancer. There is a greater opportunity for the discovery of cancer in a patient being followed regularly for estrogen therapy, particularly as episodes of unusual bleeding would lead to a prompt diagnostic biopsy or D and C. Since estrogens are used to treat perimenopausal bleeding, it is possible that cancer was already present at the initiation of therapy but not diagnosed until the response to estrogen was unsuccessful. The pathologists' interpretation of tissue slides is subject to some variation because it is difficult to differentiate frank adenocarcinoma from atypical adenomatous hyperplasia. Often Grade 0-1 adenocarcinoma is actually atypical adenomatous hyperplasia which does not progress to invasive cancer but returns to normal endometrial tissue when estrogen is discontinued. Differences in socioeconomic status between subjects and controls may also skew the data because endometrial cancer is more common in affluent, obese women. Other biases may also be operating in the selection of the groups studied.

Estrogen does cause cancer in experimental animals, and even if it does not transform healthy cells into cancerous cells in humans, it may hasten the growth of preexisting cancer cells. Whether or not there has been an increased incidence of endometrial cancer paralleling the widespread use of estrogen replacement is unclear. One report noted that endometrial cancer caused only 1.38 percent of all female cancer deaths in 1974 and that the disease had not increased in incidence, according to the National Cancer Surveys, from 1948 to 1971.[25] The California Tumor Registry reported a dramatic increase among affluent white women over 50 years of age in the San Francisco Bay area over the last 15 years—a 230 percent increase of endometrial cancer compared to 15 percent for all other gynecologic cancers.[26] Some believe that this increase may be an artifact caused by better detection, more complete reporting, improved diagnostic criteria, or skewed population surveys. In neither case was the use of estrogen considered. Fur-

thermore, the hysterectomy rate among these two samples needs to be taken into consideration.

Although additional studies are needed, there is a consensus that the existing evidence merits concern. Many physicians are taking a conservative approach to estrogen replacement therapy, and some are going so far as to require a pretreatment endometrial biopsy and repeat biopsies every 6 months while estrogen use continues. The use of progestogens for 5 to 7 days every month to encourage the shedding of the endometrium is increasingly advocated, with biopsy or D and C for unusual bleeding or spotting. There is some evidence that progestogen may have a protective effect against endometrial cancer. In counseling women on estrogen use, its benefits and risks must be fully explored.

Risks of Estrogen Therapy	Benefits of Estrogen Therapy
Salt and water retention	Reversal or prevention of vulvovaginal and breast atrophy
Slight increase in thrombophlebitis and embolism	Relief of hot flushes and vasomotor symptoms
Aggravation of fibrocystic breast disease, fibroids, migraine, endometriosis	Prevention or stabilizing of osteoporosis
Mastodynia	Amelioration of depression, irritability, or insomina (possible)
Nausea, vomiting, or stress incontinence with large doses	Relief of atrophic vaginitis
Hypertension (rare)	
Endometrial carcinoma (possible)	

The principles of therapy to minimize risk include the following:

1. Use the lowest effective dose possible.
2. Use for the shortest time possible to achieve therapeutic goals.
3. Give estrogen cyclically, with 5 to 7 days per month off the medication. Consider using progestogen during the cyclic off-week to promote withdrawal bleeding and to avoid endometrial hyperplasia.
4. Follow closely with return visits every 3 to 6 months, at which time do a pelvic and breast examination. Do Pap smears every 6 months. Check BP.
5. Educate the woman about reporting unusual bleeding at once, and refer for endometrial biopsy or D and C if this occurs.
6. Inform the woman of the possible risk of endometrial cancer and discuss pros and

cons of using estrogen in her particular instance. Cover the diagnostic sequence if she has abnormal bleeding and discuss when hysterectomy is indicated.

7. If the woman has had a hysterectomy, discuss other risks and follow all the above principles that apply. Cyclic therapy is still recommended.
8. The final decision is the woman's to make unless there are contraindicating factors. Obesity and nulliparity are the most important characteristics in increasing individual risk.

At least 40 percent of postmenopausal women maintain estrogen levels comparable with the early follicular phase of the menstrual cycle until late in life; thus, for many women the estrogen question may never arise.[27]

THE NEW OUTLOOK

Middle age is the way you would feel about summer if you knew there would never be another spring.

Clare Boothe Luce, *The Women*

Women in their middle years are questioning sexual stereotypes and confining social roles, as are women of all age groups. Although the change of life is certainly a point of demarcation, it increasingly represents an entry into a promising new era rather than an end of purpose and meaning. Many women do not view the cessation of fertility itself as a tragedy but are actually relieved that concerns about contraception and monthly menstrual cycles are now over. Freedom from the pervasive demands of childbearing and child rearing and their release from conventional roles permit many women to feel like individuals for the first time.

Moving into the "leisure years" can be a special bonus for the individual woman. But realizing her potential may not be easy; it is hard to break the habits of a lifetime and espouse new values. To be self-directed, women must be confidently self-centered—no little feat for someone whose life has involved sacrifice to others and 50 years of setting aside personal interests. Inner resources are more important than money in the utilization of leisure time; many women have followed beliefs and priorities which never allowed them to build up the self and the interests necessary to develop such resources.

Increasingly middle-aged women are transcending the limitations placed on them by "women's role" and "getting old." They are going to work and to college in unprecedented numbers and making very good workers and students. They are traveling to all parts of the world, experiencing other cultures and histories, providing valuable volunteer services, increasing their physical fitness, joining consumer and conservation causes, and becoming involved in the political process. Some middle-aged women who have always pursued personal goals are rising to positions of leadership and great influence in their fields. By communicating and sharing their feelings and experiences, by being in contact, women are breaking the unrecognized conspiracy which has kept them separated from each other and

hidden. In so doing, the self may be rediscovered.

Although the image of financially secure middle-aged housewife with abundant leisure time causes envy, the reality of older women's financial status is often dismal. Older single and widowed women are one of the country's most impoverished group, partly because of financial ignorance and partly due to inadequate Social Security benefits and pension plans. When older women work, it is usually for very low wages and on a temporary basis because their interrupted work pattern has developed neither years of experience nor seniority. For these women there is little job security, for they are often the last hired and the first fired. There are no "executive placement" agencies for mature women. Much needs to be done, both in the personal realm—in developing their knowledge of finances—and in the political sphere—in realizing employment opportunities and changing laws related to Social Security, taxes, and pension benefits.

Sexuality and Relations

Women in the middle adult years may face changes in their sexual relations, as the female's sexual capacity increases at a time when the male's is decreasing. Women between the ages of 40 and 50 often feel less inhibited, more willing to enjoy sex, and more physically responsive than ever before. After 50 this pattern begins to diminish, but high levels of sexual enjoyment often continue well into the 60s. The most important factor in a continued capacity for sexual enjoyment is the continuation of regular sexual intercourse over the years, which is associated with the lack of atrophic changes so influential in pelvic physiology. Although many relations mellow and are enriched with time, making sex more satisfying, others fall prey to the partners' changing biological and emotional rhythms, creating greater incompatibility. Women may seek to express their increased sexuality in other ways, or may simply suppress it and drift toward a neuter old age.

For middle-aged and older women, the problem of being without a partner is widespread. Because of their greater longevity, older women outnumber older men, and the social expectations of pairing become unrealistic. Relatively little is known about the sexual behavior of single middle-aged adults, but research does indicate that nearly all divorced females resume sexual activity, while only about 50 percent of widows do so.[28] Probably widows are more subtly inhibited from engaging in new relations with men through their continuing bonds with in-laws, or they may feel restricted by guilt and gratitude to their dead husbands. Single women in the middle years need to escape the bonds of convention to partake of a full social life, developing friendships and relations with each other, and not feeling constrained by rigid social codes. In becoming freely self-expressive, they keep all their options open for relations with men or with women in mutually comfortable arrangements. (See Chapter 2, Sexuality and Affectional Relationships, for a fuller discussion of sexuality and the middle-aged and older woman.)

Women in the middle years face many problems but also come to the threshold of a fascinating passage: a second identity upheaval with a new chance to grow and change, a time to redefine goals and find other meanings. Social forces wield great influences and must be confronted by those who are in a position to take them on—as indeed is happening—but for the individual, change begins within:

> We—women in our middle years—have a number of avenues open. We can stand still, passively accepting the end of our function as society has defined it for us, and drift early into old age. We can go backward, furiously clutching at lost youth. We can cop out, numbing ourselves with drugs and alcohol, or retreat into chronic bad health. Or we can choose to move forward—into bonus years of self-exploration, self-development, self-creation. Each of the choices is dictated, in the last analysis, by our own attitudes.[29]

NOTES

1. J. Harris, *The Prime of Ms. America: The American Woman at 40* (New York: G. P. Putnam's Sons, 1975), p. 23.
2. V. N. Prock, "The Mid-Stage Women." *American Journal of Nursing* 75,6 (June 1975): 1019-22.
3. B. Friedan, *The Feminine Mystique* (New York: W. W. Norton, 1963).
4. Harris, *The Prime of Ms. America*, p. 4.
5. B. Friedan, as quoted in Harris, *The Prime of Ms. America*, p. 67.
6. P. Weideger, *Menstruation and Menopause* (New York: Alfred A. Knopf, 1976), pp. 195-200.
7. N. Diekelmann, "Emotional Tasks of the Middle Adult." *American Journal of Nursing* 75,6 (June 1975): 997-1001, and I. M. Burnside, *Nursing and the Aged* (New York: McGraw Hill, Blakiston, 1976), pp. 57-68.
8. Weideger, *Menstruation and Menopause*, p. 202.
9. *A Clinical Guide to the Menopause and Postmenopause* (New York: Ayerst Laboratories, 1968), pp. 21-22.
10. Burnside, *Nursing and the Aged*, pp. 81-82 and 92-98.
11. *Ibid.*, pp. 82-91.
12. S. L. Romney, et al., eds., *Gynecology and Obstetrics: The Health Care of Women* (New York: McGraw Hill, Blakiston, 1975), pp. 170-72 and 610-14.
13. Weideger, *Menstruation and Menopause*, p. 202.
14. G. S. Gordan and C. Vaughan, "Postmenopausal Osteoporosis." *Primary Care* 1,4 (December 1974): 565-82.
15. R. W. Kistner, "Estrogen Controversy Updated." *The Female Patient* 1,9 (October 1976): 25-27.
16. "Cancer Controversy: Six Experts Advise on Estrogen Use." *Patient Care* 10,8 (April 15, 1976): 63-65.
17. "Hysterectomy—The Kindest/Unkindest Cut of All." *Patient Care* 10,19 (October 1, 1976): 56-90.
18. J. Jowsey, "Osteoporosis—Its Nature and the Role of Diet." *Postgraduate Medicine* 60,2 (August 1976): 75-79.
19. *Ibid.*
20. "The Postmenopausal Patient: Thwarting the Erosion of Osteoporosis." *Patient Care* 7,10 (May 15, 1973): 50-72, and G. S. Gordan, "Preventing Osteoporosis," *The Female Patient* 1,6 (July 1976): 45-49.
21. Gordan and Vaughn, "Postmenopausal Osteoporosis," pp. 565-82.
22. D. C. Smith, et al., "Association of Exogenous Estrogen and Endometrial Carcinoma." *New England Journal of Medicine* 293 (December 4, 1975): 1164-67.
23. H. K. Zeil and W. D. Finkle, "Increased Risk of Endometrial Carcinoma Among Users of Conjugated Estrogens." *New England Journal of Medicine* 293 (December 4, 1975): 1167-70.
24. T. M. Mack, et al., "Estrogens and Endometrial Cancer in a Retirement Community." *New England Journal of Medicine* 294 (June 3, 1976): 1262-67.
25. G. S. Gordan and B. G. Greenberg, "Exogenous Estrogens and Endometrial Cancer." *Postgraduate Medicine* 59,6 (June 1976): 66-77.
26. "The Estrogen-Cancer Flap: What You Need to Know." *Current Prescribing* (April 1976): 19-34.
27. Romney, et al., eds., *Gynecology and Obstetrics*, p. 612.
28. N. Diekelmann, *Primary Health Care of the Well Adult* (New York: McGraw Hill, Blakiston, 1977), pp. 127-37.
29. Harris, *The Prime of Ms. America*, pp. 243-44.

9

Vaginal Discharge and Itching

Vaginal secretions are a normal, regularly occurring experience for women during the years of active gonadal function, from about ages 11 to 45. There are many variations in the amount and character of vaginal secretions, which are influenced by physiology, emotional state, and pathological conditions. Women respond very differently to vaginal discharge and other vaginal symptoms, depending on a complex interplay of many factors such as attitudes and self-concept, interactions with others, and meanings associated with bodily and sexual functioning. Problems related to vaginal discharge and itching seen most frequently in primary care are of an infectious or irritative nature. While the managment of vaginitis is usually seen as a simple and straightforward process, the health provider must keep in mind the unity of psychobiological processes in assessing the cause and evaluating the outcome of treatment. Although infrequent, more serious diseases occasionally underlie symptoms of vaginitis.

PHYSIOLOGY AND HOMEOSTATIC CONDITIONS OF THE VAGINA

The *vagina* is a muscular tube, lined with mucous membranes, which can be thought of as a potential space. Most of the time its walls lie in approximation to each other so that on cross-section the cavity appears as a slit shaped like the letter H. The length of the vagina is 7.5 to 10 cm. along its anterior wall and 12.5 to 15 cm. along its posterior wall. The pelvic diaphragm and perineum support the vagina and surrounding tissue, with the *pubococcy-*

geal muscles as the principal supports of the lower portion of the vagina. The *bulbocavernosus* muscles partly encircle the vagina on each side and act as constrictors of the introitus (Figures 9-1 and 9-2). The *cervix* enters through the anterior vaginal wall, and the vagina enters onto the perineum between the *labia minora*. The greatest vaginal diameter at the introitus is anteroposterior, but some distance up the canal it becomes transverse. Above the pelvic floor, the vaginal walls dilate easily, particularly at the upper end of the vaginal vault, the *fornix*.

The mucous membrane lining the vagina is arranged in transverse folds called *rugae*, which branch outward from longitudinal ridges (rugous columns). These ridges extend along the midline of the anterior and posterior vaginal walls. The *squamous epithelium* of the mucosa undergoes cyclic changes which are under the control of ovarian hormones. The vaginal epithelium is stratified; its three layers are called basal, intermediate, and superficial. Estrogens cause an increase in the rate of cell division in the basal layer, thus stimulating growth, with the intermediate layer beginning with the development of granular cells containing more darkly staining nuclei than the basal cells. With continuing estrogen stimulation, the intermediate cells grow into the large, thin cells with small, densely staining nuclei that form the superficial layer of the mucosa. Since the intermediate and superficial layers resemble the corresponding layers of the skin, the terms *precornified* for intermediate cells and *cornified* for superficial cells are used. Progestogens oppose the estrogenic effects on the

219

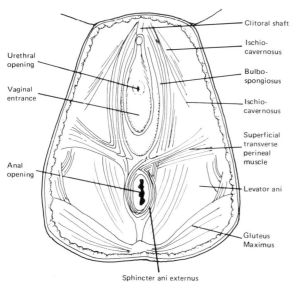

Figure 9-1. The muscles of the female perineum. M. J. Sherfey, *The Nature and Evolution of Female Sexuality* (New York: Random House, 1972), p. 62.

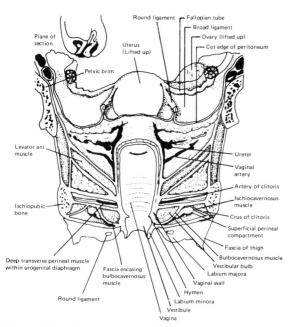

Figure 9-2. Ligamentous, fascial, and muscle support of the pelvic viscera.

vaginal epithelium, and the superficial and intermediate layers are shed with menstruation, leaving the basal layer to begin cyclic regeneration.

Papanicolaou (Pap) smears of the vaginal mucosa can identify cyclic changes of the vaginal epithelium, aiding in the identification of high and low estrogen states. These are reported as high to absent estrogen effects, percentage of cornified or precornified cells, or as a maturation index depending on the ratio of mature (fully cornified) cells on the smear to intermediate and basal cells. During the years of active estrogen secretion, a typical maturation index would be 0-40-60, meaning no basal cells, 40 percent intermediate, and 60 percent superficial cells. After menopause, this ratio would typically be 30-40-10.

Women with adequate estrogen, whether from endogenous or exogenous sources, will have vaginal secretions. *Cervical mucus* is the major source of normal vaginal secretions. There are also small amounts produced by the vaginal epithelium and the Bartholin's, sebaceous, sweat, and apocrine glands of the vulva, and also, though rarely, by the uterus and oviduct. The vaginal mucosa contains no glands and is not truly secretory, but copious lubrication from vaginal "sweating," a transudate from the congested vaginal venous plexus, occurs during sexual excitement (see Chapter 2, Sexuality and Affectional Relationships). Vaginal secretions are usually white or greyish and of semisolid consistency, due to the presence of clumps of superficial epithelial cells. The cervix secretes an alkaline, glary, mucoid substance which is most abundant and least viscous at the time of ovulation. A microscopic examination of vaginal fluid from the normal vagina of a mature woman during the intermenstrual phase shows a large number of exfoliated vaginal cells, occasional endometrial and cervical cells, and numerous bacteria, leukocytes, and histiocytes. The bacteria are largely of the *Lactobacillus* genus. Normal secretions of the vagina are acid, with a pH range from 3.8 to 4.2, and are usually not malodorous. The amount increases at the time of ovulation, several days before menstruation, and during sexual excitement.[1]

Microbiology of the Vagina

The concept of "normal vaginal flora" has been undergoing change in recent years. The biochemistry and microbiological relations in the vagina are more complex than previously believed, and although there is ample evidence of normal vaginal flora, the exact nature of this flora is unclear. The etiology of the disease states of the vagina is now recognized to involve more than merely the entry of pathogens into the vagina, combined with a decreased resistance due to pH changes or decreased glycogen in the vaginal mucosal cells.

It had been believed that an increase in estrogen caused an increase in glycogen in the cells of the vaginal epithelium and that cyclic variations in estrogen production, with resultant changes in cellular glycogen, influenced a woman's susceptibility to vaginal infections. *Döderlein's bacilli (Lactobacillus acidophilus)* were found to be the predominant organisms in the vagina when there were increased glycogen effects, and these bacilli acted upon the glycogen to produce *lactic acid*, contributing to a lower pH (Figure 9-3). Supposedly lactic acid suppressed the growth of pathogens such as enteric bacteria. However, quantities of vaginal glycogen in women in their reproductive and postmenopausal years measured through tissue biopsy showed no statistical differences during various phases of the reproductive and life cycles. Thus, cyclic vaginal glycogen does not appear to be a major factor in the changing microbiotic vaginal flora. The concept of a pathogenic flora causing vaginitis also needs modification because a large number of "pathogenic" bacteria have been recovered from asymptomatic pregnant women and from endocervical cultures of women prior to IUD insertion, without any subsequent disease. A difference has also been found in the number of "pathogenic" bacteria present in the genital tracts of women, according to social class and sexual activity. Women of lower social class and those with a higher number of male sexual contacts had a larger number of "pathogenic" bacteria, including such organisms as *Staphylococcus aureus* and *albus*, *Escherichia coli*, *Proteus vulgaris*, and the *Streptococcus*, *Micrococcus*, *Bacteroides*, *Mycoplasma*, *diphtheroides*, *Aerobacter*, and *Pseudomonas* genera.[2]

These organisms are capable of producing disease in the vagina, as elsewhere, yet are present in significant number in the genital tracts of asymptomatic women. The host-pathogen relation is based on a multitude of factors

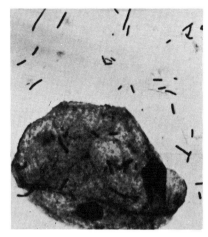

Figure 9-3. Lactobacilli in normal vaginal secretions. H. L. Gardner and H. R. Kaufman. *Benign Diseases of the Vulva and Vagina* (St. Louis: C. V. Mosby, 1969), p. 159.

encompassing genetic, physiological, emotional, social, and environmental conditions. For instance, people who are malnourished are more susceptible to infection, particularly those with protein-calorie malnutrition. In malnourished patients with infections there is a decreased leukocytosis and decreased bactericidal and glycolytic activity of the leukocytes. Malnourished infants have lower complement levels, and complement has been shown to interact in several ways with antigen-antibody response and other components of the immune system. Certain systemic illnesses cause a decreased resistance to infection because of the depression of the immune response or bactericidal functions of leukocytes. An inherited lack of certain components of complement is associated with defects of total complement levels or the presence of collagen disease such as lupus erythematosus and rheumatoid arthritis. It is well known through empirical observation that intense or prolonged stress is frequently associated with the onset of systemic disease or may precipitate acute minor illness of various types. Persons of a lower socioeconomic status have a higher incidence of disease which is probably associated with nutritional or stress factors, among others.

Thus, many factors must be taken into consideration in the diagnosis and treatment of vaginal infections. Although identifying the causative organism and prescribing the correct antimicrobial treatment are the core of the management of vaginitis, the health provider's awareness needs to extend beyond the "bug and drug" approach and to encompass the many other factors in the patient's life which may be contributing significantly to the presenting problem. When the host defense mechanisms are altered, whether locally or systemically, and whether due to nutritional, emotional, or physical factors, there is a greater susceptibility to infection and, no doubt, there are also differences in the rates of recovery and response to treatment.

Related Structures

Several other structures may be involved in vaginal itching and discharge. The symptoms of itching or burning may be related to the labia majora or minora, with edema, erythema, and excoriation. The paraurethral or Skene's glands on either side of the urethra may be inflamed or infected, and the urethral meatus may be edematous or irritated. In certain types of infections, there may be purulent discharge from the urethra or Skene's glands. Bartholin's glands, located just inside the lower vagina at about 5 o'clock and 7 o'clock, can develop cysts and abscesses of their ducts, usually due to gonorrheal infection. The cervix is frequently involved in infections and contributes significantly to increased vaginal discharge. The characteristics, cytology, and lesions of the cervix are discussed in detail in Chapter 14, Abnormal Pap Smears. In addition to the vulval structures, the perineum and skin of the inner thighs can be involved in vulvovaginal infections.

SYMPTOMS AND MEANINGS FOR WOMEN

Women have not been taught in our culture to be comfortable with their bodies. Although barriers preventing the full expression of sexuality exist for both sexes, women seem to have a particular problem with attitudes toward their physical selves. Men tend to get around the smutty image of sex more easily and manage to take some pride and direct pleasure in their sexual organs. To women, however, the vagina often remains an enigma. After all, who can see it? For many years the vagina may be unknown or dimly perceived as some mysterious part of the body, hardly to be spoken of or asked about. If caught in the proc-

ess of exploring the area or testing sensations, the message generally received by the girl is that "it" is dirty or she is "not nice."

To the woman fully socialized into a lower status and decreased self-worth on the basis of her sex, all unique attributes of femaleness signify her second-class existence. Without realizing why, she is hostile toward her female physical and physiological characteristics. Ironically, these become both her cross to bear and her equity in the world, as she is defined and simultaneously limited by a 50 percent chance expression of chromosomes. Her body must meet standards of perfection virtually unattainable by the average woman, and she constantly strives toward this impossible goal—to meet male imagery. Underneath it all she must resent this double bind: a woman's body is inferior and relegates her to lower status in society, yet it is for her body and its functions that she is most valued.

Women and men have mixed feelings about the functions of the female body, and the vagina is central in this ambivalence. Often vaginal secretions, as perfectly normal and healthy as saliva or tears, are thought of as unclean. Women are frequently chided about the "fish smell" of vaginal secretions and feel self-conscious about possible unpleasant vaginal odors. The cosmetic industry has shrewdly taken advantage of women's insecurities, creating a long list of products to cleanse, deodorize, and perfume the vagina and vulva. Some women have been led to believe that they must douche daily or insert suppositories frequently. Not only is this unnecessary, but it also upsets the normal vaginal flora and may predispose a woman to vaginal infections. Some vaginal sprays have been found to be chemically irritative, leading to inflammation and tissue destruction. Health providers have warned women against using such products, and governmental agencies have even banned a number of them from further sales.

The great lengths women are encouraged to go to in order to conceal menstrual discharge or even the mere suggestion that they might be menstruating reinforces the unacceptibility of their physiological processes.

Vaginal secretions do have a faint odor, which varies slightly during different phases of the menstrual cycle. It is not unpleasant. Infrequent bathing produces genital odors which are strong and sharp in both female and male;

seminal fluid has a particularly acrid scent. Even so, many people find these smells sexually exciting. Body odors in general have become so unacceptable in our society, however, that most of us have far to go in becoming comfortable with or enjoying this normal physical characteristic.

The increase in vaginal discharge and itching that accompany vaginal infections may be perceived by some women as signs of "dirtyness," and they are often quite concerned about how the professional will react toward them. Other women may have a better understanding, recognizing these as symptoms of a pathophysiological process. Almost all women are interested in the causes of vaginitis, and the practitioner has an important educational role in helping women to come to know and accept their bodies.

APPROACH TO DIAGNOSIS AND MANAGEMENT

Symptoms of discharge from the vagina and itching of the vulva are common reasons for women to seek care in ambulatory settings. A growing number of women have some knowledge about vaginal infections or have had previous experience with infections, so it is not unusual for a patient to say, "my vaginal infection is back," or, "I think I've got yeast again." Several symptoms may be present, together or alone, including an increased amount of discharge, changes in the character or color of the discharge, unpleasant odor, itching, burning, cramping, or dysuria. If itching is a symptom, it may range from mild to severe; in some instances it may be so unbearable that the labia, perineum, or thighs are raw and weeping from scratching.

The most common types of vaginitis are caused by infectious or irritative processes involving bacteria such as *Hemophilus vaginalis*, protozoa such as *Trichomonas vaginalis*, fungi such as *Candida albicans* (formerly called *Monilia*), parasites such as pinworms, contact allergans such as vaginal deodorant sprays or contraceptive creams and jellies, mechanical irritants including nylon underpants, pantyhose, and tight pants, foreign bodies, and pelvic congestion. Each of these irritants is associated with a fairly typical history and characteristic physical findings, although it is not unusual to have a mixed picture, making diagnosis diffi-

cult. Effective treatment is founded upon an accurate diagnosis, including the identification of the causative agent, the determination of contributing factors, ruling out serious pathology, and the selection of appropriate therapeutic modality, with attention to preventive measures.

The most important element in making the diagnosis is in some cases the history, in others the findings of the physical examination, and laboratory testing in still others. Since the health provider must piece together bits of information while proceeding through the diagnostic work-up, data will be described here in the usual sequence in which it is obtained in the clinical setting. Types of vaginal infections, their characteristics and treatment are summarized in Table 9-1.

The History

Questions in the history taken for vaginal discharge and itching include the following:

When did the symptoms begin? Recent onset signifies an acute condition; longstanding symptoms may be related to a chronic condition such as chronic cervicitis or polyps, endometrial polyps or hyperplasia, or other lesions of the upper or lower genital tract.

What is the character and color of the discharge? Thick, purulent discharge suggests bacterial or gonorrheal infection; curdy white or watery white discharge is characteristic of Candida; frothy green or yellowish discharge may be Trichomonas; serous or blood-tinged discharge suggests the presence of a foreign body or genital tract lesion; greyish-white, scant, cloudy discharge may be Hemophilus.

Has there been a change in the amount of discharge? The amount can vary greatly, as can the woman's perception of what is an increased vaginal discharge. In assessing the amount, ask whether the discharge stains underclothes to such a degree that the woman wears a pad or tampon. Remember that all women with adequate estrogen have vaginal discharge, and it can be normal to have some staining throughout the menstrual cycle. If the discharge soaks through underclothes onto pants or skirt, then it is considered copious. If the amount is more than usual for that particular woman, this can be significant. Or, if the discharge is much less than usual, it may imply decreased estrogen or some type of obstruction. Also bear in mind that pregnancy, oral contraceptives, and cer-

Table 9-1
Common Types of Vaginitis: Characteristics and Treatment

Type of Vaginitis	Erythema/ Itching	Discharge	Wet Prep	KOH	Culture	Treatment
Candida albicans (formerly Monilia)	Vulva, labia, perineum, thighs Mild to severe	Mild to moderate Curdy white	May show hyphae or spores Many lactobacilli	May show hyphae or spores	Nickerson's grows brown or black colonies	Nystatin vaginal suppositories
Trichomonas vaginalis	Severe vulval itching, ± erythema Petechiae of cervix and vagina	Copious Yellow-green frothy	Tricho-monads Few lactobacilli Many WBCs	Negative	None	Trichofuron suppositories Flagyl orally
Hemophilus vaginalis	Mild or absent	Mild to moderate Homo-geneous grey, foul	Clue cells Small rods ± WBC Few lactobacilli	Negative	Blood agar ± colonies	Sulfa vaginal cream Ampicillin orally
Nonspecific	Mild to moderate	Varied	Many WBC Few lactobacilli	Negative	Blood agar ± colonies	Sulfa vaginal cream
Allergic or irritative	Mild to severe	Varied	Unremarkable	Negative	No growth	Remove source of allergy or irritation Topical steroid if severe inflammation
Foreign body	Mild or absent	Serous, purulent, fetid	Many WBC	Negative	+ specific organism if 2° infection	Remove foreign body Treat 2° infection with specific antibiotic

tain ovarian tumors produce increased estrogen states and can produce increased vaginal discharge.

Does the discharge have a bad odor? A foreign body in the vagina, Hemophilus, and Trichomonas usually have a foul-smelling discharge. The woman may be overly fastidious, however, and perceive the discharge as malodorous when it is inoffensive to the examiner. Or, generally poor body hygiene can produce unpleasant genital odors which could be confused with the odor of the discharge.

Are there any associated symptoms? Dysuria could be due to a local irritation of the meatus secondary to vaginitis, to secondary urethritis, or to cystitis. Some women may associate abdominal cramping with their vaginal discharge, or a sense of pelvic fullness. This would raise suspicions of endometritis or salpingitis, cystitis, or pelvic congestion. Irregular bleeding or dysmenorrhea could be symptomatic of organic pelvic disease or a psychogenic disorder.

Is there itching? How severe? Intense itching of the vulvar area is reportedly associated with Trichomonas, although any infection causing erythema and irritation of the labia and vulva could produce itching, if severe enough. Uncontrollable scratching, particularly during the night, suggests pinworms. Itching involving the upper mons area, as well as the vulva, and associated with pinpoint spots of blood on the underpants suggests pediculosis pubis (crabs).

What type of contraception is used? Oral contraceptives increase cervical secretions and may produce changes in the vaginal climate which encourage the growth of Candida. There also appears to be an increased susceptibility to gonorrheal infections in women on oral contraceptives if they are exposed to the disease. The use of vaginal spermicidal foam, cream, or jelly can cause irritative or allergic vaginitis in sensitive individuals, as can the rubber used in diaphragms or condoms. An IUD may cause endometritis or cervicitis related to increased vaginal discharge.

Have you been on antibiotic therapy? The long-term use of broad-spectrum antibiotics produces changes in the vaginal flora which may trigger candidal infections. Antibiotics reduce the amount of *Döderlein's bacilli* in the vagina, and alter the vaginal environment in such a way that resistance to pathogens is impaired.

Have you had any previous vaginal infections? What was the treatment? Recurrent vaginitis, particularly Candida, raises the suspicion of diabetes. Reinfection with Trichomonas indicates the "ping-pong" syndrome between male and female in which the organism is passed back and forth. Other types of infection, including gonorrhea, herpes, and Candida, are passed between partners and recurrences imply an untreated partner or an inadequate course of therapy for the patient. Also, recurrent vaginitis can be due to emotional factors, with the vagina as the target organ for stress-induced physiologic changes. If earlier treatment was successful and the symptoms now are the same, this provides a cue for diagnosis; if unsuccessful, the previous diagnosis was probably wrong, or the course of treatment too short, or the patient's compliance poor.

Do you douche or wear tight-fitting pants, pantyhose, or nylon underclothes? Frequent douching, especially with a highly astringent or concentrated solution, can cause the irritation of vaginal tissue. Douching more often than once every week or two, even with a mild solution, can upset the vaginal environment and predispose a woman to infections. Nylon panties do not conduct air and moisture as do cotton panties, and thus, can cause an accumulation of perspiration and secretions in the vaginal-perineal area, leading to chafing and irritation. Tight-fitting clothing also traps moisture and causes mechanical irritation.

Do you use sprays, powder, perfume, antiseptic soaps, deodorants, or ointments in the perineal area? Many of these chemicals can produce vaginal or perineal irritations and allergic reactions in sensitive women. Occasionally, colored or perfumed toilet tissue or bits of toilet paper in labial folds or the vagina can be the cause of irritation and discharge.

Are you presently under any unusual emotional stress? Particularly in recurrent vaginitis, causes of conflict need exploration. It is estimated that upward of half of all gynecological problems have psychosomatic components, and vaginal infections are no exception. The effects of stress upon host resistance to pathogens must be kept in mind as a significant factor in recurrent vaginitis.

Is there a family history of diabetes? Occasionally diabetes can present as candidal vulvovaginitis, because the increased cellular glycogen alters the usual vaginal environment. Repeated candidal vaginitis indicates the need for further exploration for diabetes as a possible cause.

Depending upon the cues obtained from these initial questions, further exploration of past medical history, family history, menstrual history, or sociopsychological conditions may be necessary. Since a pelvic examination will be done as part of the physical, inquire whether it is time for the woman's annual Pap smear and, if so, this health maintenance procedure can be done at the same time. If a Pap smear is desired, a breast examination should also be included.

Physical Examination

The pelvic examination proceeds in an orderly sequence, and important data are gathered at each step. It is important that the woman's bladder be empty, because a distended bladder interferes with palpation of the uterus, tubes, and ovaries. If dysuria was one of the symptoms elicited during the history, a clean-catch midstream urine specimen should be obtained. Both a speculum examination, with a collection of specimens for smear or culture, and a bimanual examination are included.

INSPECTION OF THE VULVA.   With the patient in the lithotomy position, the vulva is inspected carefully. Erythema and swelling may be present, involving the perineum, labia minora and majora, and the inner thighs or buttocks. This may range from mild to severe with excoriation, involving all or only portions of one of these structures. Bright red, shiny, very inflamed labia and vulva suggest Candida; although quite extensive erythema and swelling can occur with other types of infection. If the vulva is inflamed, a smear should be made of this area and potassium hydroxide (KOH) applied. Vulvar eruptions and lesions may be present; common types being condylomata accuminata (venereal warts) which appear as pale, irregular clusters of raised lesions; and herpes vaginalis which are vesicles filled with clear fluid in various stages of eruption, some having central ulcerations. Herpes are small lesions that appear in clusters (see Chapter 11, Venereal Disease). The chancre of syphilis may be present, as may areas of pale discoloration or of an unusual mottled appearance. Any lesion which is suspicious or cannot be identified should be biopsied.

The appearance of the urethra, Skene's glands, and Bartholin's glands should be noted. An everted, edematous meatus suggests urethritis, and swelling on either side of the urethra may be caused by the inflammation of Skene's glands. The urethra should be "milked," whether there are signs of inflammation or not. This is done by the examiner placing one gloved finger in the vagina, palm up, with the finger against the anterior vaginal wall, milking outward and upward. Pressure is thus exerted against the urethra, and purulent discharge may appear at the meatus, signifying gonorrheal infection. When using this technique, a few drops of purulent discharge may also be noted coming from the ducts of Skene's glands if they are also involved in the gonorrheal infection. Culture any purulent discharge for gonorrhea. Next, the condition of Bartholin's glands is assessed, again with one intravaginal finger, this time palm down, as the labial tissue is gently palpated at 5 o'clock and 7 o'clock between the intravaginal finger and the thumb pressing externally on the labia. If a mass is felt, it is a cyst or an abscess of Bar-

tholin's ducts. The mass may be as small as a pea or large enough to be seen as a distinct labial swelling before palpation. Small Bartholin's cysts often resolve spontaneously and can be treated with sitz baths; large, infected ones often need incision and drainage and antibiotic therapy.

INSPECTION OF THE VAGINA.   A speculum examination of the vagina is undertaken next. Preferably a warm, dry, sterile speculum is used if the examining table is equipped with a speculum warmer. Usually there is adequate vaginal secretion to permit comfortable speculum insertion if the proper technique is used. However, if a warmer is not available, a sterile speculum may be warmed with a small amount of warm tap water which also serves to lubricate the speculum. A cold speculum should not be used unless it is absolutely necessary for a sterile procedure, such as IUD insertion, and when a cold speculum must be used, the woman should be informed about the unpleasant sensations. Lubricant jellies must not be used when vaginal smears, cultures, or Pap smears are to be taken because they interfere with the specimens and can change the characteristics of the cells obtained.

With the speculum in place, observe the appearance of the vaginal discharge and the walls of the vagina. The nature of the discharge provides an important cue to diagnosis if the typical characteristics of the different infections are present. Rarely does vaginal discharge conform to classic textbook descriptions, however, and all sorts of variations and mixed pictures are commonly seen. Some health providers claim that they can identify the type of vaginitis by the characteristics of the discharge, and in some cases this is possible, but confirmatory smears provide additional evidence which is of the utmost importance. The classical discharges for common vaginal infections are the following:

Candida has a cottage cheese, lumpy, curdy, thick, white discharge which adheres to the vaginal walls, cervix, or labia. In severe cases there is often a bright erythema of the vulva, and the vaginal walls and cervix may appear uniformly bright red and edematous. No erythema may be present, however, and the discharge may be thin, white, and watery. Usually vulval itching is more of a symptom than is increased vaginal discharge. Look also for onychia and paronychia, oral thrush, or intertrigo of the groin, thighs, and buttocks as additional cues that the infection is candidal. Take vaginal smears from patches of the white discharge in the vagina and from inflamed labia or perineum and apply KOH. A wet prep with normal saline solution should also be done. Details of techniques for taking vaginal smears and cultures, what to look for, and how to interpret them are described on pp. 228 to 232.

Trichomonas has a yellowish-green, frothy or bubbly discharge which is often very copious and has a strong, foul odor. The cervix and upper vagina may have several "strawberry spots" which consist of tiny hemorrhages or petechiae. If Trichomonas is severe, there can be acute inflammation of the vaginal wall and cervix with edema and erythema. The vulva may be swollen, with multiple superficial erosions which are found most commonly on the labia majora and the fourchette and have irregular edges and a necrotic base. Unrelenting itching, burning, dysuria, and dyspareunia often accompany severe infections. Trichomonas vaginitis can be moderate to mild also, with numerous variations in the severity of the above signs and symptoms. The discharge can be thin and relatively scant, whitish-yellow, and without the typical frothiness and foul odor. Not infrequently, routine Pap smears will report the presence of trichomonads in asymptomatic women. No treatment is necessary in this case, unless symptoms appear or the Pap smear also reports that inflammation is present in the cervical cells. For some women, a small number of trichomonads seem to be part of their normal vaginal flora. In the symptomatic woman, a wet prep of vaginal discharge is done, and if there is any question about the diagnosis, another smear is done with KOH.

Hemophilus has a greyish, homogeneous, turbid, foul-smelling discharge that is usually scant in amount. Various degrees of vaginal and cervical inflammation may be present, but it is not as dramatic as in severe candidal and trichomonal infections. Itching is not a major symptom unless the discharge is copious enough to drain continuously onto the perineum, causing some maceration and mechanical irritation. Hemophilus vaginitis is usually diagnosed by the typical appearances of certain cells on wet prep.

Nonspecific vaginitis is the term often applied to difficult to diagnose or mixed picture infections that are assumed to be bacterial in nature. Such infections can be caused by *Escherichia coli*, *Proteus*, staphylococci, streptococci, or bacterial mixtures. If Hemophilus can be confirmed by cellular characteristics on wet prep, it is a preferable diagnosis to nonspecific vaginitis.

Foreign body discharge has a blood-streaked, serosanguineous, or purulent appearance and ranges from thin to thick and usually has a fetid odor. The foreign body should be observable by speculum examination, often high in the posterior fornix. Common foreign bodies found in the vagina are tampons, condoms, and diaphragms in adult women, and such things as buttons, clips, bobby pins, beans, and seeds in young girls. The object is removed, and if there is a secondary infection with local inflammation and purulent discharge, it should be cultured.

Occasionally the practitioner may be surprised to see clumps of hair in the vagina, seemingly protruding from folds in the vaginal wall. This does not signify a "hairy vagina," because the hair has been introduced during intercourse, as penile thrusting pulls off tufts of the woman's labial hair. It can easily be removed by grasping it with the sponge forceps.

Allergic or irritative vaginitis does not have a typical type of discharge, although it most probably would not be any of the types described above. An increase in the usual type of vaginal secretions, or itching and burning of the vulva are more common. Here the diagnosis is primarily made by exclusion: if no Candida, Trichomonas, Hemophilus, or other bacterial infection seemed present and the history was positive for the use of an allergen or irritant, the diagnosis is apparent. A rash of considerable extent in the vulval area is possible, especially in women with known skin allergies or a positive allergic history. Little upper vaginal and cervical inflammation would be expected, unless the woman was douching with a strong solution or was allergic to the rubber used in condoms and diaphragms. Confirmation of the diagnosis could be made by the disappearance of symptoms after removing the suspected offending agent.

Gonorrhea typically causes a purulent discharge exuding from the cervical os, and the urethra and Skene's glands may be involved as previously described. The vagina may have varying amounts of yellow purulent discharge. There are other signs helpful in diagnosing gonorrhea, and these as well as treatment are discussed fully in Chapter 11, Venereal Disease.

INSPECTION OF THE CERVIX. The appearance of the cervix often gives cues in the diagnosis of vaginitis for it may or may not be involved in the pathophysiologic process. Note the character of the secretions coating the cervix, recalling that curdy white patches imply Candida. The type of secretions exuding from the cervical os is important. Normally the endocervical glands produce a clear mucus which varies in viscosity according to the phase of the menstrual cycle. Under increased estrogen influence, as during pregnancy and while taking oral contraceptives, this mucus can be quite copious. However, an increased secretion of clear or mucoid material from the cervix can also be a sign of cervicitis. This is confirmed by noting an enlarged, edematous, pale, and shiny cervix which is often tender upon palpation. Copious amounts of thin, watery discharge collecting in the vaginal vault and draining from the cervix raises suspicions of fallopian tube carcinoma, particularly in the postmenopausal woman. If the discharge from the cervical os is yellow and purulent, a gonorrhea culture is a must because this type of discharge is one of the classic signs of gonorrhea.

The appearance of the cervix itself can be pathognomonic, if, for example, it were to have the strawberry spots of Trichomonas. Extensive eversion of the endocervical mucosa accompanies hyperestrogen states, and the overgrowth and hypersecretion of the cervical glands produce large amounts of mucoid or clear discharge. Friability of this everted (ectropion) tissue implies an inflammatory process of the cervix. Pap smears of cervical eversions are helpful in establishing the diagnosis and ruling out carcinoma in situ. Any suspicious lesions of the cervix should be biopsied. For a further discussion of cervical conditions, see Chapter 14, Abnormal Pap Smears.

BIMANUAL EXAMINATION. After a speculum examination and the collection of the appropriate specimens, a bimanual pelvic examination is performed. The upper vaginal vault and fornix, as well as the uterosacral ligaments, are palpated for nodules. The cervix is felt for size, shape, irregularities, and tenderness. The parous cervix often has irregularities of the os and small nodules around the os. Larger masses that distort the contour of the cervix should be referred to the physician. If the cervix is tender when moved, this is suggestive of gonorrheal infection. The uterus is palpated for size, shape, consistency, and tenderness. Normally, vaginal infections are just that: infections confined to the vagina. The bimanual examination of the cervix and uterus is usually negative. If the uterus is tender, suspect endometritis. If it is enlarged, suspect pregnancy or a submucous fibroid, depending upon the woman's age and history and on the consistency of the uterus. In palpation of the adnexa, check carefully for tubular masses, enlarged ovaries, and fullness of the lower quadrants. The degree of discomfort caused by an adnexal examination is also important. Normally there will be mild discomfort with wincing or grimacing when the ovaries are squeezed, just because of the sensitivity of these organs. Some women who are tense will have increased discomfort, with tightening of the abdominal muscles and may perhaps scoot upward on the examining table. However, significant salpingitis, oophoritis, or endometritis will produce what is known as the "chandelier sign" when the uterus and adnexae are palpated: the woman will exhibit severe discomfort, jump sharply, or jerk away (reach for the chandelier), and not allow firm palpation due to the exquisite pain it causes. Severe pain or palpable masses or enlargement in the adnexa may indicate tubal or ovarian infection and possible pelvic inflammatory disease, the most common cause of which is gonorrhea. Relatively painless masses of the adnexae suggest tumors and need immediate referral.

With most types of vaginitis, the bimanual examination will be negative. The next step in the diagnosis is examination of smears of the vaginal discharge and other laboratory testing, if indicated.

Laboratory Tests

Often the diagnosis of vaginitis is based upon laboratory tests that identify the specific causative organisms. Even in the absence of known vaginal pathogens, however, smears provide useful information which gives additional circumstantial evidence to help the practitioner

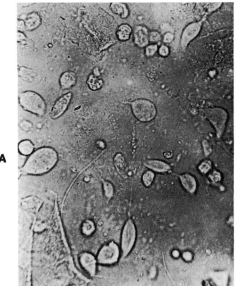 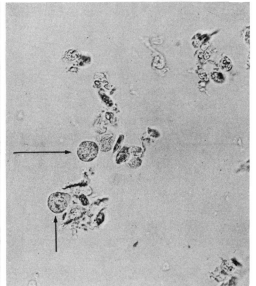

Figure 9-4. Trichomonas on microscopic examination. (A) Numerous trichomonads in wet prep. (B) Balled-up trichomonads in urinary sediment. Gardner and Kaufman, *Benign Diseases of the Vulva and Vagina*, p. 182.

to arrive at a diagnosis. Collecting good vaginal samples is a matter of some acumen, and the proper preparation of samples is crucial to obtaining meaningful results. In some clinical settings, smears are sent to the laboratory to be read by technicians; in others, the health provider not only takes and prepares the slides, but also reads them. Cultures are frequently collected by the provider and sent to the laboratory for incubation and interpretation. However, bacteriological kits are available for several cultures including Candida, gonorrhea, and general bacterial media. Interpreting the growth of colonies requires considerable bacteriological knowledge, but in isolated settings where no clinical laboratory is readily available, acquiring the necessary knowledge to read cultures in the office or clinic can be very helpful.

WET PREP. The wet prep or wet smear is a standard vaginal test useful in detecting Trichomonas, Candida, and Hemophilus. The sample is obtaind on speculum examination, taken from a pool of vaginal secretions with a Q-tip or Pap stick. If the secretions in the vagina are scant, a few drops of saline can be added to the vagina with a pipette, the speculum opened and closed several times for adequate lavage, and then some solution aspirated with the pipette. If curdy, white plaques are seen on the cervix or vaginal wall, a specimen should be obtained from these. The specimen

is placed on a slide and a drop of saline added, a cover slide placed over the specimen, and the slide read as soon as possible. The reason for speed is that trichomonads are most easily identified when still motile, and will die rapidly if not kept warm. To avoid this, one approach is to collect the vaginal specimen with a Q-tip and place the tip of the applicator in a test tube with a few drops of saline in the end. The patient or an assistant holds the test tube during the remainder of the examination to keep the solution warm and the trichomonads motile. At the end of the examination, the specimen is transferred onto a slide and prepared for microscopy.

Under high magnification, the slide is examined for its cellular and microbiological components. The one-celled flagellate trichomonads are easily seen as they dart back and forth. Any vibrating cells may overlie a trichomonad; move the focus back and forth to try to see the protozoa. Trichomonads are somewhat larger in size than white blood cells and they have a single nucleus within the cell membrane. Usually oval in shape, they may alter their external shape as they elongate or contract to swim about or wrap around epithelial cells (Figure 9-4).

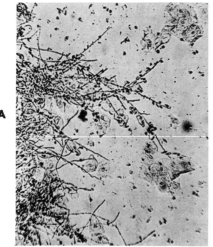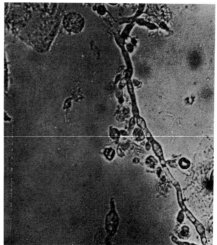

Figure 9-5. Candida on microscopic examination. A, low power; B, high power. Gardner and Kaufman, *Benign Diseases of the Vulva and Vagina*, p. 159.

Occasionally, the spores or hyphae of *Candida albicans* (formerly called *Monilia*) can be seen on wet prep. Spores are somewhat larger than white blood cells (Figure 9-5). They are very difficult to identify, however, and are often hidden by the epithelial cells and the debris usually present in generous amounts in wet preps. If no trichomonads are seen and the health provider suspects Candida, there are two cues which can be helpful, even though buds or hyphae cannot be identified. Relatively few white blood cells present in the vaginal discharge argues against bacterial and trichomonal infections, suggesting Candida by the process of elimination. And the presence of a large number of lactobacilli (*Döderlein's bacillii*) suggests that the vaginal infection is due to Candida because most other vaginal pathogens compete with and destroy lactobacilli while Candida can coexist with the normal vaginal inhabitant.

The epithelial cells have a characteristic appearance in Hemophilus infections. Usually the cell outline is not clear, and the cell itself has a granulated or stippled effect due to adhering bacilli. Such stippled or studded epithelial cells are called "clue cells." At times the organism may be seen: fine Gram-negative bacilli with rounded ends in short chains, often in a formation resembling a school of fish. The number of white blood cells present in Hemophilus infections varies considerably, but

usually it is less than with other bacterial infections. Many of the leukocytes may be filled with the small rods and clearly seen under high magnification (Figure 9-6).

Other cellular components of vaginal secretions will be seen on wet prep, and the health provider needs to be familiar with their appearance. Epithelial cells from the vaginal mucosa are usually quite abundant; these are large, irregularly shaped, nucleated cells which usually have a distinct cell outline. It is from these cells that the maturation or cornification index is determined. White blood cells, with their multiple nuclei, grainy appearance, and generally round, regular shape, are almost always present in small amounts. Occasionally the smaller, round, discoid red blood cells, distinct for their lack of nuclei, are seen in vaginal secretions. An occasional red blood cell is normal even in the absence of menses or other bleeding; a large number indicates bleeding from some source. Cellular debris can be of various shapes and sizes and is present in small to large amounts. Occasionally crystalline forms are seen and hair, which appears enormous in comparison to the other cells. Mucous threads, cotton fibers, and sperm are also frequently seen in vaginal discharge.

POTASSIUM HYDROXIDE (KOH). Whenever Candida is considered as a possible cause of vaginitis, a KOH slide should be done specifically for this organism. The KOH lyses other cells found in vaginal secretions, leaving the Candida intact. The specimen is obtained in the same manner as for wet prep, with a Q-tip

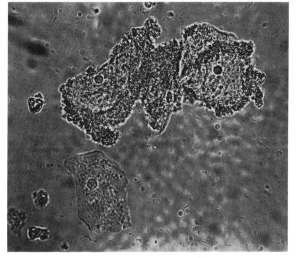
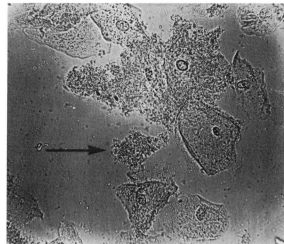

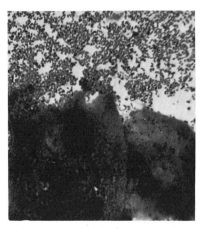
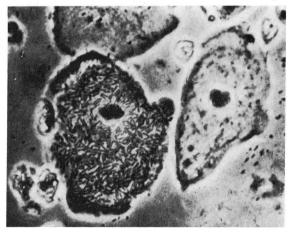

or a Pap stick. It is very important to take a sample from white curds or patches if they can be seen on the cervix or vaginal wall, for these are colonies of Candida. If, however, the discharge is not typical, it is better to take the sample from erythematous areas of the labia or vulva. The Candida on the mucosa is suspected to be responsible for the erythema; thus it is likely that a sample from this area would contain the organism. Place the sample on the slide and apply one drop of 10 to 20 percent KOH, then cover it with a cover slide. The slide can be warmed to hasten the action of the KOH by passing it quickly back and forth over the flame of an alcohol burner. Some believe that the KOH solution should bubble slightly, but not too actively as this destroys the Candida too. Or, the provider can simply wait for the lysing action to take place without heating the slide.

Figure 9-6. Hemophilus and clue cells on microscopic examination. (Top, left to right) Clue cells with normal epithelial cell in lower left. Arrow indicates clumps of *H. vaginalis* floating free in fluid. (Bottom, left to right) Hemophilus from vaginal secretions, Gram-stained smear. False clue cell, incident to adherence of larger bacilli to surface of an epithelial cell. Gardner and Kaufman, *Benign Diseases of the Vulva and Vagina,* pp. 200-202.

Examine the slide under high magnification, looking for spores and hyphae of Candida. It is very difficult to obtain a good specimen of Candida from vaginal discharge, and probably the majority of slides so prepared will be disappointing because no organisms can be seen. If even a few hyphae are seen, they can substantiate the diagnosis. Although skilled laboratory technicians can identify spores readily, the provider may have great difficulty because there are so many objects, ranging from bubbles to debris, which can resemble the round or oval buds. To increase the success rate in finding Candida in KOH, add a drop of Lugol's solution when fixing the slide to color the organisms and make them more visible (see Figure 9-6).

Occasionally other cells in the vaginal secretion will not be completely lysed by KOH and can be seen on the slide. However, their appearance is often altered. Overheating the KOH solution can produce crystals of varying sizes.

CULTURES. Cultures of vaginal discharge are of varying usefulness and may or may not be used by the health provider. The most important culture is for gonorrhea, although there is a high incidence of false negatives. The sample is taken from the cervical os (or urethra, Skene's glands, and rectum) and inoculated on *Thayer-Martin*(TM) culture plates or in *Transgrow* bottles. Details of diagnostic tests for gonorrhea are discussed in Chapter 11, Venereal Disease. *Nickerson's* medium is used to identify organisms of the *Candida* genus. Single vial culture tubes are streaked with a sample of vaginal discharge, obtained from a pool of vaginal secretion with a sterile applicator. The culture is incubated for 1 to 2 weeks, and is positive if brown and black colonies grow on the medium. Since not all *Candida* is *Candida albicans*, the cause of vaginal infections, it is possible to have a false positive. Also, the long incubation time does not make Candida culture a practical office diagnostic tool for making treatment decisions during the visit. For recurrent infections without clear-cut diagnosis, however, it can be an important adjunct to identifying the underlying cause. *Casman's blood agar* or *thioglycollate medium* is used for culturing Hemophilus, but the success of growing this organism varies extremely. A specimen of vaginal discharge is obtained with a sterile applicator, and the medium streaked. Incubation must be in a reduced oxygen atmosphere. A positive culture shows the growth of typical colonies[3] (Figure 9-7).

GRAM STAIN. Certain bacterial pathogens can be further identified by their Gram-staining qualities, such as the Gram-negative rod Hemophilus. A thin smear of vaginal secretions is placed on a slide, air dried for 1 or 2 minutes, then fixed by holding it above a gas flame for 15 seconds. The smear is covered with crystal violet for 10 seconds, then washed with tap water. Gram's iodine is next applied for 10 seconds, then the slide washed again in tap water. With the slide held at a slight angle, an acetone-alcohol solution is poured over the slide until no more blue color washes away (5 to 10 seconds). The slide is washed again with tap water, and safranin is applied to it for 10 seconds. The slide is then washed off with water, and allowed to air dry. Excess moisture is evaporated by holding the slide over a gas flame. For microscopic examination, the oil immersion technique is used.

Gram-positive bacteria are colored blue because they retained the blue stain after their exposure to acetone-alcohol. Gram-negative bacteria are colored red, having lost the blue stain when exposed to acetone-alcohol, and then staining red when safranin was applied. Gram stain is not useful in identifying gonococci in vaginal or cervical secretions because the numerous other cells and organisms confuse the picture.

URINALYSIS. Whenever dysuria is a symptom accompanying vaginitis, a clean-catch midstream urine specimen should be obtained for microscopic examination and possible culture. Not infrequently a urinary tract infection can be present as a primary or secondary source of infection, and the same organism is often involved when urinary tract infection and vaginitis occur together. Chemical and microscopic examination of urine, as well as diagnosis and treatment of urinary tract infection, are discussed in Chapter 10, Urinary Problems.

Diagnosis of Vaginitis

Data from the history, physical examination, and laboratory tests are put together to determine the type of vaginitis. At times the diagnosis is quite clear, but at other times no causative agent can be identified. The key points in the diagnosis of the most common types of vaginitis are as follows:

Candida albicans has a typical cottage cheese, curdy, thick, white discharge with placques adhering to the cervix and vaginal walls. Usually, itching is more of a problem than increased discharge. The labia, perineum, and other vulval structures are often bright red and swollen, very sensitive, and painful during intercourse. The wet prep has few white blood

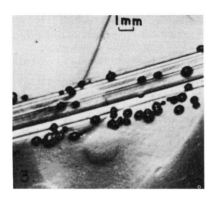 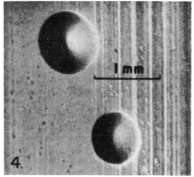

Figure 9-7. Positive culture for Hemophilus. Gardner and Kaufman, *Benign Diseases of the Vulva and Vagina*, p. 203.

cells, normal appearing epithelial cells, and a large number of lactobacilli. If the health provider is in luck, the KOH or wet prep will show hyphae and spores.

Trichomonas vaginalis has a yellow-green, frothy, foul-smelling discharge which is often copious. Itching may be severe, there may or may not be vulval irritation, and the cervix and upper vagina have small hemorrhagic spots. Wet prep reveals motile trichomonads. There often is an increase in the amount of white blood cells, and a decrease in lactobacilli.

Hemophilus vaginalis produces a grey, homogeneous, foul-smelling discharge of varying amount. Vulval erythema is usually not present. On wet prep the epithelial cells appear studded or stippled, with less distinct cell outlines. There is an increased amount of white blood cells, although this is quite variable, and the leukocytes may be filled with rods. Lactobacilli are decreased in amount.

Nonspecific vaginitis is diagnosed by the exclusion of the above types. The discharge shows an increased number of white blood cells, normal appearing epithelial cells, and decreased lactobacilli. Physical findings are usually minimal or equivocal.

Allergic or irritative vaginitis is characterized by the absence of specific vaginal pathogens. Erythema and edema of the vulva, buttocks, or thighs are common, and vaginal discharge may or may not be increased. The patient's history is most important here and typically would reveal exposure to some allergenic or irritative subtance.

Foreign body vaginitis presents as a serous or purulent blood-tinged discharge of increased amount and fetid odor. Speculum examination reveals the lost object usually high in the posterior fornix of the vagina.

Gonorrhea typically has the appearance of a purulent discharge exuding from the cervical os. On bimanual examination the cervix is tender when moved, and the uterus and adnexae are also frequently very tender when palpated. A purulent discharge from the meatus or Skene's ducts, after milking the urethra, is also highly suggestive of gonorrhea. On wet prep there is an increase in the number of white blood cells, but the gonococcus is almost impossible to see in vaginal discharge because so many other organisms closely resemble it. Positive gonorrhea culture confirms the diagnosis.

Psychogenic vaginitis is a diagnosis to be made with caution because so many factors can be involved in causation and the identification of specific pathogens presents some difficulties in technique and test reliability. Vaginitis with a pathogenic or physical cause can have emotional components, of course, which must be taken into consideration. A conclusion that the vaginitis is psychogenic would be justifiable in the case of repeated subjective symptoms with no physical findings. If there were any signs suggestive of a particular type of pathogenic infection, the health provider would have to make sure that the course of treatment had been adequate and the patient's compliance good. Usually, sensitive questioning will reveal historical data which substantiate the presence of stresses in the woman's life that can be related to her vaginal symptomatology.[4]

The Treatment of Vaginitis

Therapeutic agents for the treatment of most types of vaginitis are very specific, underlining the importance of arriving at an accurate diagnosis. When a pathogen is causing the vaginal itching and discharge, specific medications are prescribed to halt the infectious process. When the problem appears to be allergic, irritative, mechanical, or emotional in nature, local symptomatic treatment is given, with the elimination of the source of the symptoms if it can be identified. The usual treatment for the most common types of vaginitis is as follows:

CANDIDA ALBICANS. Nystatin (Mycostatin, Nilstat) vaginal suppositories, two tablets inserted high into the vagina at bedtime for 2 to 3 weeks, or one tablet *per* vagina twice a day for 2 to 3 weeks. Instruct the woman to remain recumbent for about 30 minutes after inserting the tablets to allow some absorption. Also inform her that there will be some yellow drainage from the vagina due to the tablets, and if she is concerned about this she might want to wear a perineal pad. Tampons should not be used because they will absorb the medication. Although the symptoms will diminish in a few days, stress the importance of completing the full course of treatment for optimal eradication of the pathogenic organism. The treatment should continue during menses, and it is advisable to avoid intercourse during the course of therapy. If avoiding intercourse for 2 weeks is unreasonable to the woman, it is advisable to use a condom to prevent the introduction of any new organisms. Some providers prefer to have the woman give herself a cleansing acid douche (one teaspoon white vinegar in one quart water, or Massengil douche powder) before each insertion of the vaginal tablets; others do not think douching is indicated.

Chlordantoin (Sporostacin) vaginal cream twice a day for 14 days; or twice a day for 4 to 5 days, then once nightly for 15 to 20 days total is an alternate medication. Other medications include Candicidin (Candeptin, Vanobid) vaginal tablets twice a day for 14 days, or Miconazole nitrate cream (Monistat) at bedtime for 2 weeks. The same instructions as those described above would be provided.

If there is extensive erythema and swelling of the vulva or labia, causing the woman discomfort, the local application of a topical antifungal agent combined with a corticosteroid antiinflammatory agent is very helpful. Most combinations also contain a topical antibiotic, which is useful in mixed infections. Examples of such combination creams which contain anticandidal medication are Myclog, Nystaform, Fungizone, Nilstat, Monistat, and Kenalog. These creams are to be rubbed onto the affected areas 2 to 4 times daily. Sitz baths several times daily are also helpful in reducing inflammation and promoting comfort.

TRICHOMONAS VAGINALIS. Treatment with vaginal preparations is indicated in mild cases of Trichomonas; in more severe cases, oral treatment or combined oral-vaginal treatment is necessary.

Metronidazole (Flagyl) 500 mg. vaginal inserts, placed high in the vaginal vault, one each evening at bedtime for 10 days, is used in mild cases. Diiodohydroxyquin (Floraquin) 100 mg. tablets, two per vagina at bedtime for 2 to 3 weeks is an alternate therapy; as is the use of Trichofuron (furazolidone and nifuroxime mixture) suppositories one twice a day vaginally for 1 week, then one at bedtime for 2 to 3 weeks. Trichofuron also contains an agent effective against Candida and is considered safe for use during pregnancy. Therapy should continue during menses, and the same instructions as those for anticandidal vaginal inserts should be given.

Oral Flagyl 250 mg. three times a day for 10 days has been a standard treatment for severe Trichomonas infections. A single dose of 2 Gm. (eight 250 mg. tablets) is now recommended. Since Trichomonas is functionally a venereal disease in that it is transferred between sexual partners and since the organism lives in the genital tracts of both sexes, it is recommended that the male partner also be treated. Men usually are asymptomatic, harboring the trichomonads in the urethra or prostate, and ejecting them upon ejaculation. Occasionally Trichomonas may cause urethritis in the male. A single dose of 2 Gm. is also recommended for the man. In particularly severe infections in women, both oral and vaginal Flagyl can be used. When oral Flagyl is prescribed, the patient must be advised not to drink alcoholic beverages, due to the very unpleasant side effects of nausea, abdominal distress, vomiting, headache, and a modification in the taste of the drink. Often patients report a sharp, metallic, and unpleasant taste when taking Flagyl. Gastrointestinal symptoms, headache, stomatitis, and moderate leukopenia are common side effects even in the absence of alcohol consumption. Flagyl is contraindicated in patients with a history of blood dyscrasias, those with central nervous system disease, and during pregnancy.

Although Flagyl is highly effective against Trichomonas infections, particularly when used orally, it has become the subject of some controversy. Recent studies have indicated that metronidazole (Flagyl) causes mutation in bacteria in controlled testing.[5] Drugs which can produce mutations in the rapidly reproducing bacteria are suspected to be carcinogenic.[6] Although causing cancer in humans is far removed from creating mutations in bacteria, because of the dosage levels and a myriad of host-environment factors, some health providers are avoiding the use of Flagyl unless other therapies prove ineffective. One approach is to use Trichofuron vaginal suppositories for at least two courses of treatment, then to resort to oral Flagyl only if the infection clearly persists. A single dosage is recommended, however, Flagyl 2 Gm. (eight 250 mg. tablets) at one time.[7]

HEMOPHILUS VAGINALIS. There are different opinions as to the preferred mode of treatment for Hemophilus vaginitis. Some health providers prefer antibiotic vaginal creams; others argue that systemic antibiotics are indicated for any significant bacterial infection regardless of which system it involves. A severe infection would sway the provider toward the systemic route, as would a history of recalcitrant vaginitis treated several times by the vaginal method.

Sulfa vaginal cream is the standard treatment for Hemophilus and nonspecific vaginitis. Sultrin, AVC, or Triple Sulfa creams are inserted high in the vagina, one applicator full daily for 6 to 14 days. Other medications include Floraquin tablets or a combination tablet such as Baculin (diiodohydroxyquin, phenylmercuric acetate, sodium lauryl sulfate, and papain) or Lycinate (diiodohydroxyquin, sodium lauryl sulfate, and dioctyl sodium sulfosuccinate) twice a day per vagina for 2 weeks. If systemic treatment is given, the antibiotic of choice would be ampicillin (Amcil, Polycil-

In case of sulfa allergy, Furacin vaginal suppositories one twice a day for 10 days can be used. If the woman is allergic to penicillin and systemic therapy is to be used, *Tetracycline* 250 mg. four times a day for 10 days is an acceptable substitute.

NONSPECIFIC VAGINITIS. Sulfa vaginal cream is the usual treatment for nonspecific vaginitis thought to be of bacterial origin. See the discussion under Hemophilus vaginalis for the names of preparations and directions for their use. Generally, oral antibiotics are not used to treat nonspecific vaginitis.

ALLERGIC OR IRRITATIVE VAGINITIS. The identification and removal of the allergen or irritative substance or process is the basic treatment for this type of vaginitis. The health provider can advise the woman to avoid the use of vaginal sprays and deodorants, perfumes or powders applied to the perineal area, antiseptic soaps, nylon underpants, pantyhose, tight-fitting pants, and douching. Another area to explore is a recent change of sexual partner, for the introduction of new flora into the vagina may cause transient symptoms even if no specific infection can be identified. In this case, the symptoms should improve after the woman's body has had time to adapt to the new vaginal environment. Rarely are individuals truly allergic to each other's genital secretions—an extremely difficult problem to solve.

If there is considerable vulval irritation, with itching and burning, local relief of these symptoms should be part of the therapy. Sitz baths several times daily promote comfort and reduce inflammation. Hydrocortisone cream (Corte-Dome, Heb-Cort) or triamcinolone cream (Aristocort, Kenacort) .5 to 1 percent can be applied to irritated vulval tissues three or four times a day to alleviate the local inflammatory reaction.

When a foreign body is the cause of irritative vaginitis, removal of the object is usually adequate to alleviate the symptoms in a few days. If an infected area has developed around the foreign body, however, the purulent discharge or indurated tissue should be cultured on a general medium. Specific antibiotic therapy is then given, depending upon the pathogen identified. Needless to say, in this situation a sensitivity test should routinely be ordered with the culture.

RECURRENT VAGINAL INFECTIONS. Recurrent vaginitis, regardless of the cause, presents special problems in management. The health provider must try to determine whether the recurrences are due to reinfection, improperly used medications, inadequate absorption of medications, or foci of organisms in sheltered sites. If the woman does not complete the entire course of treatment, whether vaginal or oral, probably the organisms have not been completely eradicated, and another course of therapy with special emphasis on completion is in order. Sometimes a second course is necessary even when medications are properly used. Perhaps an extremely heavy vaginal discharge with much mucus and cellular debris has interfered with the absorption of vaginal medication, or perhaps the woman has used tampons or douched shortly after inserting the tablets or cream. Reinforce the necessity of not using tampons. Then instruct the patient to douch *before* inserting the vaginal medication, explaining carefully why this is necessary.

Skene's glands, Bartholin's glands, the urethra, bladder, or rectum can harbor the infecting organism and serve as sources of reinfection. If Candida is involved in such recurrences, oral nystatin can be used effectively to rid the bowel of Candida when it is a focus of infection. In cases of chronic infection where one of the other sites is responsible, it is best to refer the patient to a gynecologist.

Consider the sexual partner as a source of reinfection, particularly in Trichomonas vaginitis. However, testing of male urethral secretions, urine, prepuce, and bowels might also be considered for candidal and bacterial infections.

Recurrent Candida in the woman taking oral contraceptives is a very difficult problem to solve satisfactorily. Because of the effects of oral contraceptives on the vaginal environment, it may be necessary to discontinue their use in order to end the candidal infection. The woman should be assisted to select another method of birth control.

Women with repeated Candida infections should also be tested for diabetes with a 2-hour postprandial blood sugar test. Occasionally diabetes may present as a severe candidal vulvovaginitis.

Preventive measures are especially important for women with recurrent vaginitis. Good general body hygiene is a beginning, with adequate washing of the perineal area and buttocks during bath and shower, done frequently enough to prevent the accumulation of smegma and perspiration. Proper technique in wiping the vulva after voiding and the anus after bowel movements can help prevent contamination from drawing rectal organisms across the vaginal orifice. Wiping should always be in a front-to-back motion, and the toilet tissue dropped without drawing it forward. Stress the importance of not wearing clothing which fits tightly onto the perineum, for this can also transfer rectal organisms to the vulva. All sorts of chemicals should be avoided by the woman prone to vaginitis, as these irritate the skin and mucosa and alter the vaginal environment. Douching should be avoided or kept to a minimum because the regular introduction of a douche solution or even plain water into the vagina interferes with the natural flora and may aggravate any inflammation. If douching is part of the therapeutic regimen, the woman must be carefully instructed to use the proper technique (Table 9-2). Reinfection with *E. coli* or *Proteus* after these preventive measures have been used for some time can be due to sexual practices. Ask whether alternating vaginal and rectal intercourse is part of the couple's sexual repertory; if so, explain the mechanism of transfer of organisms and suggest that a new condom be used each time the mode of intercourse is changed.

PSYCHOGENIC VAGINITIS. A significant part of the therapy for psychogenic vaginitis is the process through which the conclusion is reached that this indeed is the cause. The woman should be involved and the health provider's knowledge shared at every step of the way. Most people know when they are under unusual stress and can accept the concept of psychophysiologically caused symptoms if they are allowed to reason along with the provider and follow the logic of the diagnosis. As one cause after another is eliminated, the woman comes to see that her emotional conflicts are finding outlets through vaginal symptomatology and to understand that this is not unusual. Once the diagnosis is established, treatment options include simple counseling, psychotherapy, or psychotropic medication,

Table 9-2
The Dos and Don'ts of Douching

To douch means to wash out the vagina, usually with a stream of water or cleansing solution.

In treating vaginal infections or irritations, a douche usually is used only as an addition to medications. Although some women regard douching as a form of cleanliness, it is seldom necessary for women with normal vaginal secretions to douche unless they are irritated or offended by the secretions.

During pregnancy, douching is not advised unless prescribed by the physician. He will then provide special instructions.

General rules

1. Follow doctor's instructions for making the prescribed douching solution.
2. The solution should be lukewarm (not hot). Test it on your arm.
3. A douche bag, rather than a douche syringe, should be used to get a steady stream of flow without too much force.
4. Don't rush the douching process. It should take several minutes for a thorough cleansing.
5. The douche bag and nozzle should be kept clean and used only by you.

What you need

1. A douche bag (preferably two-quart size). Portable types that fold can be used while traveling.
2. An ample length of rubber tubing to ensure that the nozzle will reach the vagina when the bag is hanging.
3. A hook not more than two feet above the bathtub level. You can also hook the douche bag on the top of a straight-backed chair.
4. A clasp on the tubing which you can reach to regulate the flow.
5. A hard-rubber douche nozzle (which curves slightly and has several holes around the sides at the end of the tubing). An enema attachment is *not* suitable for douching.

Proper technique

1. Prepare the solution and fill the douche bag, suspending it from the hook.
2. When douching, it is best to recline at a 45° angle rather than to sit upright. In a sitting position the water flows in and out of the vagina without really reaching or cleansing the entire vaginal passage.
3. The most effective position is to recline along the slanting portion of your bathtub (feet towards the drain). Raise your knees slightly and spread them apart.

In a shower enclosure, sit against a wall at an angle so that you can recline with your knees raised and spread apart. If you must douche while sitting on a toilet, lean back as far as you can so that you are not sitting upright. Use a stool if possible to raise your legs off the floor. This will permit you to recline further.

4. When inserting the nozzle into the vagina, guide it gently in the natural path of the canal (slightly downward and slanting) until it goes in as far as it can.
5. The vaginal canal has many folds and creases, like a deflated rubber balloon. To reach and cleanse these surfaces it is necessary to fill the vagina with fluid (and hold it there) just as you would the air in a balloon. As the water flows in, press the lips of the vulva together around the nozzle with thumb and forefinger of one hand.
6. When there is a sense of fullness and pressure over the bladder area, shut off the flow by pinching the tubing with fingers of the other hand or by snapping the clasp shut.
7. Hold the fluid in with the vagina lips pressed together for as long as it takes to count to 15.
8. Let the fluid gush out.
9. Release more water into the vagina so that it fills up, hold the water in for a while, then let it gush out.
10. Repeat this procedure until all of the douche solution has been used.
11. Dry the entire area thoroughly after the douche. If your doctor has prescribed a surface cream or vaginal medication for a particular disorder, you are now prepared to use it. The inside of the vaginal area is cleansed and the medication can penetrate.

From *Patient Care* (September 15, 1974) p. 70.

depending upon the nature and extent of the emotional disturbance. Chapter 15, Nervousness and Fatigue, covers the management of psychosomatic problems by the nurse practitioner.

Vaginitis in Prepubertal Girls

Vulvovaginitis occurs fairly frequently in children because their immature epithelium is thin and easily traumatized or infected. The most common causes are foreign bodies, non-specific, intestinal parasites, poor hygiene, Candida, and urinary tract infections. If the problem involves increased vaginal discharge, it is necessary to collect vaginal samples for microscopy and culture and to examine the vaginal vault. A vaginal examination can be done without trauma if the proper techniques are used. To test for pinworms, give the girl's mother a microscope slide and transparent adhesive tape, instructing her to press the adhesive side of the tape to the child's perineal area after the child has been asleep for a while. Then apply the tape to the slide, adhesive side down, and bring it in for microscopy. Pinworms deposit their ova outside the rectum during the night, and ova should stick to the tape and be seen on microscope examination. Particularly if vulval itching is most severe at night, pinworms are suspect. Treat with Povan, with the dosage adjusted according to the child's weight.

Candidal vulvovaginitis in children can be treated with nystatin cream locally, or with nystatin liquid both orally and instilled vaginally with an eyedropper four times a day for 10 days. Older girls can be treated with intravaginal nystatin cream or suppositories broken in half. The local or intravaginal application of sulfa cream is used for nonspecific vaginitis.

Good hygiene and sitz baths may be enough by themselves to correct vulvovaginitis in girls. Systemic antibiotics are not recommended because of sensitization problems and the promotion of candidal vaginitis. A persistent infection may be helped by applying estrogenic cream to the vulva and vagina nightly for 2 weeks because this will promote reepithelialization and encourage a resistance to infections. Continued use of estrogens is contraindicated. If a urinary tract infection is present, it should be treated appropriately.

Any nonspecific vaginitis or purulent vaginal discharge should be cultured for gonorrhea. Female children as young as 18 to 24 months have been found to have gonorrheal infections. The disease can be contracted from contact with warm moist discharges on bedding when infected persons share beds with children; or sex play may also be the source.[8]

Vaginitis is a common problem for women of all ages and is usually a self-limiting and minor disease. Its discomforts are considerable, however, both physically and emotionally. The management of vaginitis deserves the health provider's careful and thoughtful attention. Causes, contributing factors, therapy, and prevention should be discussed with the woman, so that she can learn more about her body and take the initiative in keeping herself healthy. Atrophic vaginitis, a special problem of older and postmenopausal women, is covered in detail in Chapter 8, Menopause.

NOTES

1. D. W. Beacham and W. D. Beacham, *Synopsis of Gynecology* (St. Louis: C. V. Mosby, 1972), pp. 1-12 and 169-85.
2. S. L. Romney, et al., eds., *Gynecology and Obstetrics: The Health Care of Women* (New York: McGraw Hill, Blakiston, 1975), pp. 439-42.
3. "Best Tests for the Office Lab and How to Do Them: Bacteriology." *Patient Care* 6,12 (June 30, 1972): 54-56.
4. H. L. Gardner and R. H. Kaufman, *Benign Diseases of the Vulva and Vagina* (St. Louis: C. V. Mosby, 1969), pp. 149-215 and 287-97.
5. "Is Flagyl Dangerous?" *The Medical Letter* 17 (1975): 53-54, and C. E. Voogd, et al., "The Mutagenic Action of Nitromidazoles: Part I: Metronidazole, Nimorozole, Dimetridazole and Ronidazole." *Mutation Research* 26 (1974): 483-90, and M. S. Legator and T. H. Conner, "Detection of Mutagenic Activity of Metronidazole and Niridazole in Body Fluids of Humans and Mice." *Science* 188 (1975): 1118-19.
6. J. McCann, et al., "Detection of Carcinogens As Mutagens: Bacterial Tester Strains with R Factor Plasmids." *Proceedings of the National Academy of Science, U.S.A.* 72 (1975): 979-83.
7. J. R. Dykers, "Single-Dose Metronidazole for Trichomonas Vaginitis." *New England Journal of Medicine* 293 (1975): 23-24.
8. "When Vaginitis Keeps Coming Back." *Patient Care* 8,16 (September 15, 1974): 44-77.

10

URINARY PROBLEMS

Dysuria—painful or difficult urination—is a symptom experienced by women in most age groups at some time in their lives. Often dysuria is associated with urinary tract infection (UTI): about 50 percent of the time in women and 75 percent of the time in men. Although very little is known about the natural history of urinary tract infections, surveys of large populations of normal persons have uncovered a considerable amount of such infections in women. The incidence of UTIs increases steadily throughout life from about 1 percent in school-age girls to a peak of 10 to 12 percent in women in their 70s.[1] All dysuria does not signify UTI, and some other causes in women include trauma, obstruction, irritation, and unrelated concomitant infection.

Another very common symptom experienced by women is urinary incontinence. Inadvertent loss of urine is a problem found in all age groups, although it is more common among women in the late reproductive and menopausal years. It is estimated that 14 percent of women in the United States have urinary incontinence, with some expert opinion holding that all women will have had urinary leakage at some time during their lives. There are different types of incontinence, and it is of the utmost importance to identify the specific type for the individual woman. Surgery is helpful only in certain types and is contraindicated in others.[2]

PHYSIOLOGY AND HOMEOSTATIC CONDITIONS OF THE URINARY TRACT

The urinary tract consists of the right and left kidneys, the right and left ureters, the bladder, and the urethra (Figure 10-1). The *kidneys* are bean-shaped structures situated on the posterior abdominal wall near the point at which the last rib joins the vertebral column. The outer layer of the kidney is the *cortex*, and the inner portion is the *medulla*, which is divided into cone-shaped pyramids. *Calyces*, a number of short, broad tubes, project into the kidney substance on one end and drain into a large cavity called the *renal pelvis* on the other. The *ureter* is contiguous with the renal pelvis and is a muscular tube which carries urine to the bladder, partly by pressure and gravity and partly by the peristaltic contractions of the walls of the ureter. The formation of *urine* and the regulation of the body's internal environment by the kidney are a composite of four processes: 1) the filtration of the blood through the renal corpuscle, 2) the selective reabsorption of materials, by the renal tubule, which are required in maintaining the body's internal environment, 3) the excretion and secretion by the tubules of certain substances from the blood into the tubular lumen, and 4) the conservation of base for the body by the exchange of hydrogen ions for sodium ions.

The *bladder* is a hollow muscular bag, located in the pelvic cavity behind the pubic bone, which varies in size and shape depending upon how much urine it contains. When empty, the bladder resembles a deflated balloon. When slightly distended, it is spherical in shape, and as its contents increase it becomes pear-shaped and can rise to a considerable height in the abdominal cavity. The bladder is lined with *transitional epithelium* and has a three-layer smooth muscle coat, the *detrusor muscle*. At the base of the bladder the smooth muscle coat passes around the urethral opening in a series of loops, forming the *inter-*

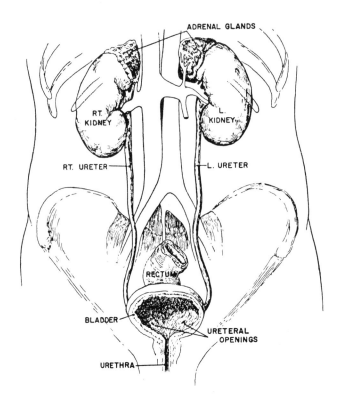

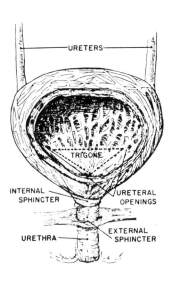

Figure 10-1. Urinary tract structures.

nal sphincter. When the bladder is empty, this sphincter is normally in a state of contraction. There are three openings in the posterior wall of the bladder arranged in a triangle, forming the *trigone*. The two ureters open into the posterior part and form the base of the triangle; the urethral opening is in the midline below and anterior to the openings of the ureters, forming the vertex of the triangle. Parasympathetic fibers from the sacral spinal segments innervate the detrusor muscle and the internal sphincter, and their stimulation causes the contraction of the detrusor and the relaxation of the internal sphincter. Sympathetic fibers from the lumbar segment via the hypogastric nerves relax the detrusor and increase the tone of the internal sphincter. The *external sphincter* surrounds the urethra a short distance below the internal sphincter and is composed of striated muscles innervated by the pudendal nerves. These spinal somatic nerves place the regulation of this sphincter under voluntary control. Sensory fibers accompany both the sympathetic and parasympathetic paths.

The *urethra* is a short tube which conveys urine from the bladder to the external opening of the urinary tract, the *meatus*. The urethral walls are composed of mucous membrane and a muscular layer, and in the nonurinating state the anterior and posterior walls lie against each other. The posterior wall of the urethra is united firmly with the anterior wall of the vagina. The urinary meatus opens into the vestibule of the vulva, appearing as a small slit. In women, the urethra is only 1 to 1½ inches long.

Mechanism of Voiding

Voiding (micturition) is the emptying of the urinary bladder; it is a reflex act subject to voluntary control. When 200 to 300 ml. of urine has accumulated in the bladder, the stretch receptors in the wall of the detrusor muscle are stimulated by distention. Sensory impulses are transmitted to the central nervous system and the sensation of a full bladder is appreciated, with the desire to void. Subsequently, there is a reflex relaxation of the detrusor muscle of the bladder neck, with the descent and rotation of this region. The base of the bladder and the urethra flatten, and the urethra shortens as part of this action. The detrusor muscle of the bladder wall begins rhythmic contractions, and when the pressure within the bladder exceeds the intraurethral pressure, the urethra will open, beginning at its proximal end, and urine will enter. As urine passes along the urethra, more contractions of the bladder wall occur, and there is a relaxation of the external sphincter of the urethra. Intraabdominal pressure from straining often is exerted to aid in the passage of urine and the complete emptying of the bladder.

Although the external sphincter cannot be made to relax voluntarily, its contraction is under voluntary control. Thus urination can be delayed by an act of will. Voiding can also be caused voluntarily before the bladder wall is distended enough to produce the stimulation of the stretch receptors. This is done through impulses arising in the cortex due to conscious effort, which then descend down the spinal cord and, in a reflex manner, throw into action the micturition center in the cord, removing the inhibition of the normal reflex response to distention. Thus voluntary control, the ability to start or delay voiding, is accomplished through the removal of an inhibition or the creation of an inhibition of the normal reflex response to distention. If the bladder is not emptied when the urge is noticed, it will of course continue to distend. Voiding can be voluntarily controlled until about 700 ml. of urine has accumulated, at which point pain will be felt and there is an urgent need to empty the bladder.

Pelvic Support and Urethrovesical Angle

Disorders of pelvic support and insult to the urethrovesical angle, usually resulting from pregnancies and gynecological instrumentation, cause many problems for women. Considering the phylogenetic heritage of Homo sapiens, it is remarkable that there is not a higher incidence of such disorders. With a pelvis originally designed for quadrupedal ambulation, humans had to undergo numerous evolutionary changes to accommodate their bipedal preference. Additionally, humans evolved along the lines of other primates toward a long gestation of the single fetus, born relatively mature, in order to achieve maximum brain development. It appears that these two evolutionary paths now at times clash, because the pelvic changes necessary for the conversion from quadrupedal to bipedal gait can make childbirth hazardous for mother and infant.

The funnelling and lengthening of the pelvic outlet, the 45-degree angle of the pelvis to the vertebral column, and the development of both a pelvic muscular diaphragm and a urogenital diaphragm were the major adaptations of the human pelvis to the bipedal gait (Figure 10-2; see also Figures 9-1 and 9-2). These strong multi-layer muscular slings support the pelvic viscera, being perforated by the urethra, vagina, and rectum. The oblique angle at which the urethra and vagina enter through the pelvic diaphragm, and the ligamentous supports of the uterus add to the effectiveness of the support mechanisms. The enlargement of the vagina, widening of the levators, partial disruption of the urogenital diaphragm, or damage or stretching of the uterine ligaments which occur with pregnancy weaken this support system, however, and predispose women to herniation (uterine prolapse) and may damage the urethrovesical angle.

Urine will be excreted whenever the intravesical pressure exceeds the intraurethral pressure, whether voluntary when voiding or involuntary due to stress incontinence, bladder spasm, or neurological disease. Injury or trauma to pelvic tissues resulting in an alter-

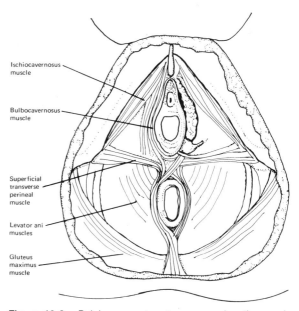

Figure 10-2. Pelvic support system, muscular sling, and urogenital diaphragm.

ation in the urethrovesical angle is usually the cause of stress incontinence, the loss of urine when coughing, sneezing, laughing, lifting or otherwise increasing intraabdominal pressure (Figure 10-3). Urge incontinence, on the other hand, is often caused by the irritation or stimulation of the bladder, secondary to infection, inflammation, or neurologic deficits. In the normal continent female, the posterior urethrovesical angle is generally between 90 and 110 degrees. When this angle is flattened in excess of 110 degrees, the woman often experiences stress incontinence. In urge incontinence, in which there is an involuntary loss of urine shortly after the sensation of a full bladder and before the woman can reach the toilet, the urethrovesical angle is normal.

The changed urethrovesical relation in stress incontinence closely resembles the processes in the first stages of voiding in normal women: the posterior urethrovesical angle is flattened to greater than 110 degrees, the bladder neck descends and funnels, and there is some backward and downward rotation of the urethral axis. When the bladder is in the anatomic position for the first stage of voiding all the time, any increase in downward thrust (by coughing or laughing) is enough to force urine to escape from the urethra.[3] A short or patulous urethra is not related per se to incontinence; what is of primary importance is the strength, tone, and elasticity of the pelvic support tissues. Trauma and stretching due to childbearing, atrophic changes after menopause, and the effects of aging are the common causes of lack of tone and elasticity. While a cystocele, the ballooning out of the bladder into the vaginal vault due to a weakness in the muscular wall, may also result from trauma or atrophic changes, it alone does not cause incontinence. As long as the posterior urethrovesical angle is maintained, which is possible even with a large cystocele, continence is preserved. Not infrequently, however, stress incontinence and a cystocele do occur together when both the normal urethrovesical angle has been lost and there is a ballooning defect in the wall of the bladder.

Composition of Urine

Urine is composed of water, dissolved substances, and cellular components. It can provide a broad range of easily available information about certain body processes, and

urinalysis is essential in the diagnosis of urinary problems. Some of the principal characteristics and constituents of urine are listed in Table 10-1.

In healthy persons, the urine contains a small number of cells and other formed elements from the whole length of the genitourinary tract. These elements may include casts and epithelial cells from the nephron; epithelial cells from the renal pelves, ureters, bladder, and urethra; mucus threads; and erythrocytes and leukocytes which have passed through intact blood vessel walls (diapedesis) from various parts of the urinary tract. Many crystals may appear both in acid and alkaline urine, and their presence has relatively little clinical significance except in certain special circumstances. Ammonium urate, triple phosphate, calcium carbonate, and calcium phosphate crystals appear in alkaline urine; uric acid, sodium urate, and calcium oxalate crystals appear in acid urine. Calcium oxalate crystals may be significant if found persistently in patients with renal stones. Some drugs such as sulfa can produce crystals, and metabolic or systemic diseases may cause, for example, cystine or other amino acid crystals.

Microorganisms and the Urinary Tract

Generally microorganisms gain access to the urinary tract via the urethra. Given the woman's anatomy, the likelihood of the ascent of microorganisms up the urethra seems great due to the urethral meatus's proximity to the vaginal introitus. Vaginal secretions, the introduction of tampons, sexual intercourse and other methods of sexual stimulation, and the close contact of clothing or perineal pads all have the potential of bringing pathogenic organisms very near the meatus. Additionally, the rectum is only inches from the introitus and meatus and can be another source of microorganisms by which these areas can be contaminated. Even given these many factors, relatively few women have persistent problems with urinary tract infection.

Apparently, the average woman has a defense mechanism that usually prevents the growth of pathogenic bacteria on the vaginal introitus. If weekly vaginal cultures were done on women who never had UTIs, Gram-negative bacteria, the most common urinary tract pathogens, would rarely be found. Some women seem to have no biological suscepti-

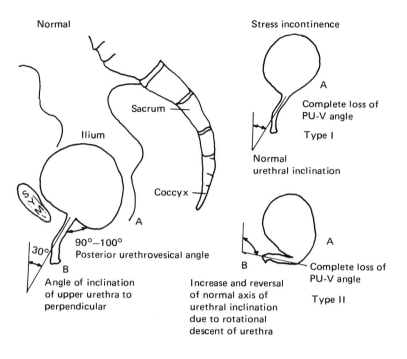

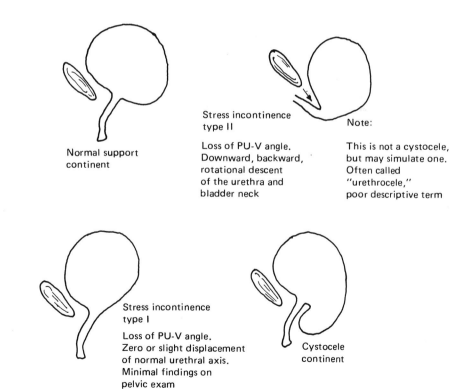

Figure 10-3. Urethrovesical angle and urinary continence. Stress incontinence contrasted with cystocele.

Table 10-1
Principal Characteristics and Constituents of Urine

Characteristics
specific gravity	1.003-1.030
pH	4.6-8.0 (average 6.0)
volume	600-2500 ml/24 hours (average 1200)
color	straw to yellow; clear to hazy

Chemical constituents   Gm. per 24 hours
urea	33.0
uric acid	0.6
creatinine	1.0-1.6
sulfate	2.0
phosphate	1.7
chlorine	7.0
ammonia	0.7
potassium	2.5
sodium	6.0
calcium	0.2
magnesium	0.2
protein	0-0.1 (qualitative 0)
glucose	0-0.3 (qualitative 0)
ketones	(qualitative 0)
hemoglobin	0
cystine	0

Cellular constituents   *Amounts in urine*

red blood cells (RBC) Up to 1 million excreted daily in normal healthy adult; average rate 150,000 to 300,000 daily. Normally not seen in centrifuged urine, but 1-2 RBC per high power field is considered normal in women and men.

white blood cells (WBC) Up to 2 million excreted daily in normal healthy adult. In centrifuged urine, 1-2 WBC in men and 1-5 WBC in women and children per high power field is normal. More than 5 WBC per high power field constitutes pyuria.

epithelial cells Often present in small numbers and are of little significance in either men or women. Large numbers indicate a "contaminated" specimen in which correct technique was not used in collection.

casts These cylindrical molds formed in the lumina of renal tubules or collecting ducts are normally not present. An occasional hyaline (proteinaceous) cast per high power field is considered normal especially if urine is concentrated or acidic. Hyaline casts may also be seen following fever or extreme exercise. All other casts indicate intrinsic renal disease.

crystals Urinary sediments may precipitate and form crystals of different chemical composition. Crystalluria may be entirely asymptomatic or associated with the formation of calculi.

microorganisms A clean-catch midstream urine sample should not contain microorganisms (but if allowed to stand at room temperature for several hours it is an excellent culture medium). Presence of organisms generally indicates infection. Common pathogens include coliform bacteria, *Candida albicans*, and *Trichomonas*.

artifacts Commonly oil particles, dandruff, hair, fabric fragments, talc, starch, cellulose.

bility to UTI; their bodies effectively destroy any pathogens finding their way to the vaginal introitus or urethra. In other women, however, weekly vaginal cultures would show that they intermittently carry Gram-negative bacteria in the vaginal introitus. These are the 10 to 15 percent of women in the United States who have recurrent UTIs. The pathogen causing a succeeding UTI can be predicted from the results of the preceding vaginal culture in these women.[4] Recurrent UTIs are now believed to be due mainly to new infections rather than flare-ups of some locus of chronic infection within the urinary system. The kidney is rarely the residual locus; infection is by urethral ascent.

Some health providers believe that women with unusually short urethras become infected more easily from vaginal secretions. This concept is questioned by others, however, who consider the complex host-pathogen relation to be the core of the problem, not anatomic variation. If this is the case, then the ability of host defenses to overcome the pathogenicity of the organism, as influenced by physiologic, emotional, social, and environmental factors, would determine a woman's susceptibility to infection (see also Chapter 9). For years it has been known that the bowel is the source of many of the pathogenic bacteria responsible for UTIs in girls and women, but before the onset of infection, these bacteria must establish themselves in the vaginal vestibule and colonize extensively. Here the many other factors influencing susceptibility come into play.

Fecal soiling is an obvious factor, so good hygienic practices would reduce the exposure of the vaginal vestibule to pathogens. The effectiveness of the antibacterial characteristics of the urethral and bladder mucosa, and the body's mobilization of defense forces to fight infection are of primary importance. The elimination of bacteria by urination also plays a significant role. Inability to empty the bladder completely leaves a residuum of urine, kept at body temperature, which provides an excellent culture medium for bacterial growth. Impaired emptying of the bladder can occur in several ways: neurogenic conditions in which there is a decreased perception of the need to void or in which reflex bladder contraction to expel urine is impaired; vesicoureteral reflux in which urine backs into the ureters during void-

ing and dribbles down into the bladder afterwards; and urethrovesical reflux, in which increased pressure on the bladder, such as sneezing, forces urine into the upper urethra, and the urine subsequently reenters the bladder, bringing bacteria with it. Regardless of the mechanism, urine remains in the bladder and serves as a medium for bacterial growth.

The bacteria most often involved in UTIs are *Escherichia coli*, *Aerobacter aerogenes*, *Klebsiella pneumoniae*, *Proteus vulgaris*, *Pseudomonas aeruginosa*, and *Steptococcus faecalis (enterococcus)*.

Sexual Trauma and Dysuria

Not infrequently a pattern emerges for some women in which dysuria follows sexual intercourse by 36 to 72 hours. Urinalysis and culture may reveal the presence of pathogenic bacteria, but at times these tests are negative. Remember that the urethra is anchored to the anterior vaginal wall and can receive considerable trauma during very active or prolonged intercourse. Particularly in women who have never had children, the perineum is high and the introitus tight, with undisturbed tone of the muscles of the pelvic sling. These conditions bring the penile shaft in close contact with the anterior vaginal wall, and frequent, strong thrusts just under the urethra and against the base of the bladder can lead to tissue trauma, capillary rupture, edema, and inflammation. Typically, no infection can be found in this situation, although the symptoms of urgency, frequency, and dysuria are present. Cystoscopic examination of such patients has shown that the mucous membrane in the area of the trigone is greyish and granular in appearance, like cake frosting. Women with symptoms of dysuria and bladder irritability, but with uninfected urine, are thus felt to have "trigonitis," a noninfectious inflammatory process. Generally antibiotics are not indicated, although some practitioners do feel these changes in bladder mucosa are anatomic residua of previous bacterial infections. This syndrome is also called "honeymoon cystitis," as it frequently occurs when the sexual pattern changes from little or no activity to rigorous and frequent activity.[5] Changes in sexual patterns could also introduce new pathogens or alter the local vulval environment in such a way that an infection would be triggered. Infectious processes must always be ruled out, as discussed later in this chapter.

SYMPTOMS AND MEANINGS FOR WOMEN

Acute dysuria is a symptom for which few people have much tolerance. It is painful and disconcerting, for a process which normally causes no discomfort and affords relief of bladder fullness rather suddenly causes a burning, pulling, shooting type of pain. To make matters worse, frequency also occurs and the woman must void more often while she desires to void less. Urgency sends the woman scurrying for the toilet, hoping desperately she reaches it before urine begins to leak. Usual activities are impossible with acute dysuria, and although the severity of the symptoms varies a great deal, even mild dysuria interferes with a woman's ability to function and concentrate. It is a condition for which treatment is generally sought shortly after the onset of the symptoms.

Urinary symptoms are often frightening, especially if the urine is bloody or purulent. Public awareness of the consequences of kidney disease is quite high, and women know death is a result of kidney failure, or that kidney dialysis could be needed for the rest of one's life. Spectacular medical feats such as kidney transplants are played up in the popular media, so the public has learned that damage to the kidneys can cause a desperate situation. Unless the woman is medically sophisticated, she may fear her symptoms signal kidney damage. Conversely, women with repeated urinary infections who have seen their symptoms disappear with simple treatment may not give enough attention to recurrences. They may think of urinary infections as benign conditions, overlooking the fact that bladder infections can ascend and can indeed cause kidney damage.

To some women, these urinary symptoms signify that their bodies are not functioning properly. It is a good feeling to know that body functions are normal, and that the body can be depended on to do its work smoothly. This is particularly true when the woman is under emotional stress and needs considerable psychic energy to cope with interpersonal or situational problems. "All I needed was something like this" is a typical remark in such situations, signifying frustration at having now to divert effort and energy to righting the body

malfunction. Ironically, women are more prone to infections when under stress, for stress significantly affects the body's defense systems.

Repeated infections may lead to a perception of the body as unreliable. Particularly if the woman has been taught preventive measures and has practiced them, she may develop the attitude that "something is really wrong with me." Self-esteem may be lowered, frustration raised, and a sense of helplessness fostered. Embarrassment is often part of the picture when incontinence is experienced. Some women avoid almost all social occasions because they can never be sure that they can keep dry. The ammonia odor from constant urine leakage may be very distressing also.

Urinary problems are related to sexuality in several ways. One common association of problems is between voiding and childbirth. Many women experience their first urinary difficulties in the postpartum period, with retention and infection being common problems. Bladder and kidney infections also are common during pregnancy and pose a threat to its safe outcome. Trauma to tissues following labor and delivery can leave residual damage, and a woman may notice leakage of urine with increased abdominal pressure following pregnancy. Thus an expression of female sexuality leads to a damaged body, causing inconvenience and discomfort to the woman. Trigonitis or "honeymoon cystitis" is even more directly connected with sex. For the woman susceptible to this condition, a very discouraging situation may develop in which almost every act of intercourse is followed by dysuria. While infection may or may not be present, the unpleasant or painful symptoms of bladder irritability are; this certainly must reduce a woman's motivation for sex. The woman also perceives her body as defective. Sexuality, supposedly one of our great pleasures, brings pain which most women are spared. Even if a woman has an intellectual understanding of the causes and mechanisms of her problem, some degree of alienation from her body probably occurs.

APPROACH TO DIAGNOSIS AND TREATMENT

When a woman presents with dysuria, the health provider will probably think first of UTI, and will be right 50 percent of the time.

It is necessary to consider other causes, however, and carefully work up these patients so that the appropriate treatment can be given. initial UTIs are usually caused by *Escherichia coli* or other enteric bacilli, and are easily treated with sulfonomides. Subsequent infections require a careful determination of the causative organism because upward of 90 percent of them are reinfections that could be due to resistant strains which have developed after antimicrobial therapy. Scars in the cortex of the kidney associated with the dilatation of the underlying calix constitute the pathology of chronic pyelonephritis, and bacterial infection is a major source of such scarring. Many factors affect the progression of urinary tract disease, and there is not necessarily a correlation between UTI or acute pyelonephritis and chronic pyelonephritis. The presence of an anatomical defect of the urinary system or another disease state such as diabetes are key factors in the development of serious kidney disease.

Infection, inflammation, and obstruction produce dysuria and other urinary symptoms. The first two are by far the most common causes in women. The history, a physical examination, and laboratory testing provide the data for diagnosing the cause and planning the treatment.

The History

The following history is obtained when the patient presents with urinary symptoms.

What symptoms are you having? Frequency, urgency, and nocturia are common when there is an inflammation of the urinary tract. Severe infection produces a constant desire to urinate even though there may be only a few drops of urine in the bladder. When bladder capacity is diminished by disease or the bladder cannot be emptied completely, frequency and nocturia occur. Dysuria and burning pain in the urethra on voiding is associated with infection and inflammation. Flank and back pain signifies renal disease, as does fever. Incontinence can be due to anatomic defects, stress, the urgency of an infection or neurogenic disease, or the dribbling of an overdistended flaccid bladder.

When did the symptoms begin? A recent onset indicates an acute process which is severe enough to motivate the patient to seek attention quickly. Onset days, weeks, or months earlier implies a chronic process with less pronounced interference with functions.

Has there recently been any activity which could irritate the urethral area? A long jolting ride by auto, motorcycle, or bicycle could traumatize the urethra and produce dysuria. Changes in sexual patterns, with increased activity or a new partner, can cause local inflammation. Vaginal tampons, chemicals applied to the vulva, condoms or diaphragms could cause irritation in women sensitive to these materials.

Does pain or burning occur before, during, or after urination? Pain at onset of voiding may signal urethritis, postvoiding pain is more typical of trigonitis or an irritation of the internal vesical sphincter area. A urethral stone may also cause these symptoms, but they are very rare in women (except for stones in urethral diverticula).

Is dysuria intermittent or constant? Intermittent discomfort on voiding, occurring for a short period of time on one day then disappearing for days or months, suggests a neurogenic (spastic) bladder. Sometimes the patient can associate her symptoms with events which place her under stress. Hesitancy and a diminished stream may also be part of this syndrome, as the spasm of the sphincters causes urethral resistance to the urine stream. Round-the-clock dysuria and frequency signify lower tract inflammation or infection.

Is there blood in the urine, and if so does it appear at the beginning, end, or all through voiding? Hematuria is a significant sign and may be due to infection, trauma, stones, glomerular disease, neoplasms, vascular accidents, or anomalies. When blood appears only during the initial voiding, its most likely source is the anterior urethra. When it appears toward the end of voiding, it is probably from the posterior urethra, vesicle neck, or trigone. Blood mixed throughout voiding can be from the kidney, ureters, or bladder.

Have you had fever, chills, nausea, or vomiting? Lower tract infection (bladder, trigone, urethra) is rarely accompanied by fever. These symptoms indicate pyelonephritis, or unrelated concomitant infection such as flu or tuboovarian or gallbladder infections. In acute pyelonephritis, there is typically a fever of 102 to 105 degrees F., chills, nausea, and vomiting, flank pain, and prostration. However, absence of these symptoms does not rule out pyelonephritis.

Is there increased vaginal discharge or itching? Vaginitis frequently can cause urethritis, or the organisms may have ascended to also involve the bladder. Obtain vaginal smears and evaluate for vaginitis as described in Chapter 9.

Is there flank or back pain? Dull, aching pain in the flanks or costovertebral angle, often extending along the rib margin toward the umbilicus, is typical of renal disease. Some people may describe this as back pain and be unable to localize it well.

Is there abdominal pain? Severe, colicky pain of abrupt onset which radiates from the costovertebral angle across the abdomen and into the vulva and inner thigh is typical for ureteral stones. Some mild lower abdominal discomfort may accompany cystitis and moderate bladder distention but could also be due to other pelvic and abdominal causes. Significant bladder distention produces severe generalized abdominal pain.

Do you void large or small amounts? Do you leak urine? Frequent voiding of small amounts implies diminished bladder capacity, or the woman may be voiding so often that very little urine can accumulate. If she voids larger amounts but has dysuria, bladder capacity is not diminished and the urethra or trigone is probably involved. Frequent voiding of larger amounts, however, is probably related to increased fluid intake (which many women deliberately do at the onset of symptoms) and may lead to a dilute urine specimen. In this case, bacterial and cellular counts have significance at lower numbers.

If the leaking of urine is a symptom, find out if it occurs with stress only, dribbles constantly, occurs with urgency, occurs only at night, and so forth. Constant dribbling signifies a flaccid bladder, with overdistention, which will need to be emptied. Some leakage with urgency is common in urethritis and cystitis. Leakage with stress can be due to anatomic defects following childbirth or gynecological instrumentation trauma; neurogenic problems can also cause various types of leakage.

Have you ever had a UTI before? What was the treatment? It is important, though sometimes difficult, to ascertain if the woman has had any previous UTIs. Some women can definitely reply in the affirmative and give the exact dates and treatment. Others may be more vague and must be quizzed about their symptoms. It is possible that previous UTIs might have gone undetected, and the practitioner should be suspicious if the patient recalls typ-

ical symptoms or unexplained fever. Asymptomatic infections also can occur. Whenever possible, find out how many UTIs the woman has had, the length of time between them, the antibiotic treatment, and when the last episode occurred. Recurrences due to a persistence of the same organism tend to occur earlier than a reinfection with a new microbe. About 90 percent of recurrent UTIs is due to new infection.

Have you recently completed a pregnancy or had a gynecological procedure? Dysuria may be related to trauma following childbirth or gynecological instrumentation. This is particularly important to note when one of the symptoms is incontinence. While infection may be the cause, inflammation alone can also produce dysuria. The time elapsed since the trauma is significant because inflammation would not be expected to persist as long as infection.

Is there a past history of kidney or bladder problems? Although the answer to this question will probably be elicited when asking about previous UTIs, it is important to establish the presence of known renal disease. A positive answer will necessitate consultation.

A further exploration of past medical history, family history, menstrual and reproductive history, or sociopsychological conditions may be needed, depending upon the patient's responses to these initial questions. Be certain to ask about drug allergies, especially to sulfas and penicillin.

Physical Examination

Generally the physical examination for urinary problems is short and provides limited information. Some health providers may not examine at all, but rely on the history and laboratory tests. In most cases, however, an abdominal and back examination should be done as a minimum. The presence of bacteria in the urine does not differentiate their sources within the urinary tract, and certain physical findings can be helpful in making this determination. The examination must be correlated to the history, of course, and additional parts must be examined, depending upon the historical cues.

TEMPERATURE. Particularly with a history of fever, chills, nausea or vomiting, the patient's temperature should be taken to ascertain if there is fever. If malaise is reported, it too could indicate fever. Even in the absence of a positive history, taking the patient's temperature is a good screening test and provides helpful information suggestive of upper versus lower tract involvement.

PALPATION OF ABDOMEN.   This procedure is useful in determining if there is suprapubic tenderness and seeking cues to the presence of abdominal masses. A distended bladder appears as a lower abdominal, midline, cystic mass. At times the poles of the kidneys may be felt on abdominal examination, but enlargements or masses in this area would be more significant. Except for some mild suprapubic tenderness which might or might not be present in cystitis, the abdominal examination is usually negative in an uncomplicated UTI.

PERCUSSION OF THE BACK.   For cues to renal involvement, the percussion of the costovertebral angle is important. The kidneys lie close to the peritoneal cavity wall at this point and are extremely sensitive to jolting when infected. Even light tapping at the costovertebral angle will cause sharp, shooting pain when there is significant renal infection. As some patients are surprised by sudden pounding on their back, it is best to explain what is to be done, then to percuss the entire spine before percussing the costovertebral angle. Otherwise, what is essentially a surprise reaction or a response to external sensation can be mistaken for costovertebral angle tenderness.

PELVIC EXAMINATION.   If the history indicates, a pelvic examination may be done. If there is dysuria or hematuria only at the initiation of voiding or if the urine stream is diminished or the bladder cannot be emptied completely, urethritis or obstruction of the urethra is likely. On inspection of the vulva, the meatus is examined for erythema, patulousness, polyp, and induration. The urethra should be milked and any discharge from the meatus or Skene's glands should be cultured. (see Chapter 9). Gonococcal urethritis is common, and these findings are highly suggestive.

Vaginal and cervical inspection with the collection of specimens is done when the history indicates a possible vaginitis (see Chapter 9). A bimanual examination can be done to rule out pelvic tumors, tuboovarian disease, preg-

nancy, and pelvic relaxation. The woman is examined for a cystocele by having her strain downward as if moving her bowels, while the examiner observes for the typical ballooning outward of the anterior vaginal wall through the introitus. Rectocele is the ballooning out of the posterior vaginal wall, and it can also be discovered during this procedure. Often these ballooning defects in the vaginal wall can be felt on bimanual examination, as can uterine prolapse.

Laboratory Tests

The most important information in diagnosing urinary tract infections comes from the microscopic examination and culture of the urine. The collection of the specimen must be done properly if findings are to be reliable. Specimens may be collected in the clinical area, or the patient may be sent to the laboratory for both collection and analysis. In some settings, the nurse practitioner does the urinalysis in the clinical area; in others the urine is sent to the lab with a request for stat urinalysis.

URINALYSIS.   A one- or two-specimen approach is used depending upon whether the practitioner suspects urethritis or higher infections. The patient is instructed to collect specimens after cleansing to avoid the contamination of the sample. The genital area is washed with gauze or cotton pads which can be soaked with water, benzalkonium chloride (Zephiran), povidone-iodine (Betadine), or other antiseptic solution. A front-to-back motion should be used, with separate pads for each labia and over the vulva. If antiseptics are used, the cleansing is repeated with water to rinse. Be certain that the labia are spread for cleansing of the vulva. A sterile container is used to collect the urine. If two specimens are required, the woman is given two containers. She catches the initial voiding in one, then catches midstream voiding in the other, while keeping the labia separated. If a single midstream specimen is desired, the patient begins voiding and then catches urine in the container. It is preferable if the urine can be tested immediately, but if that is not possible it should be stored in a refrigerator at 4 to 6 degrees C. right away. Bacteria proliferate rapidly in urine at room temperature, and the specimen will be unreliable if allowed to stand for 30 minutes. Plating for culture must thus be done before 30 minutes for a specimen kept at room temperature, or within 24 hours if it is refrigerated.

Catheterization is generally avoided because it introduces organisms from the urethra into the bladder. This procedure may be necessary, however, if the patient is unable to void or if the specimen would be contaminated by voiding, such as with heavy vaginal bleeding. Suprapubic aspiration is most accurate for obtaining an uncontaminated specimen, using a 10 cc. syringe and 1½-inch, 22-gauge needle. This procedure is not commonly used, however, because of the danger of bowel perforation.

Microscopic examination of urinary sediment is done to identify cellular and formed components of urine. In a clean, conical centrifuge tube place about 15 ml. of urine. With a balancing tube with 15 ml. of water in place, spin the urine for 5 minutes at 1500 or 2000 r.p.m. in the centrifuge. Remove the urine tube, invert it quickly and allow the supernatent urine to escape. Then stand the tube upright, and a small amount of urine with the solid sediment will be in the conical tip of the tube. The sediment and remaining urine need to be mixed, either with a small glass pipette or by agitating the tube. A drop of the well-mixed specimen is placed on a clean glass slide (either with pipette or by pouring) with a cover slide placed over it, and examined microscopically while it is still wet.

Subdued light is used because hyaline casts and other partially transparent solid elements can be obscured by bright light. Use low power first and higher magnification later, if necessary. Because many of the formed elements are somewhat refractile, the fine focus of the microscope should be varied continuously while examining the urine. A drop of methylene blue added to the sediment helps to delineate the formed elements. If the urine is very dilute, it may cause the lysis or distortion of formed elements; cross-reference to specific gravity confirms a dilute specimen.[6]

The entire cover glass area is examined under low power in the search for casts (Figure 10-4). These cylindrical molds formed in the lumina of renal tubules, or collecting ducts, can be proteinaceous, epithelial, or red or white blood cell in composition. An occasional hyaline cast is considered normal; more than a few or other types indicate renal disease. Red blood cells (RBCs) appear as biconcave discs without nuclei, but they may also be globular, crenated, or shrunken (Figure 10-5). They are best seen under high power and appear quite pale. One or two RBCs per high-power field is considered normal in the urine of women; a greater number indicates hematuria. Bleeding without proteinuria, casts, or other evidence of kidney disease usually originates from the lower urinary tract. Red blood cells are lysed by hypotonic or alkaline urine, so if urine appears bloody but no RBCs are seen, measure the pH and specific gravity. A dipstick testing for hemoglobin can be done. While hematuria is additional evidence of UTI, it also occurs with calculus, neoplasm, stricture, acute fever, strenuous exercise, collagen diseases, and numerous other systemic diseases and conditions. White blood cells (WBCs) are larger than red blood cells, have a grainy appearance, and have one or more nuclei. Leukocytes from the kidney are commonly larger and more degenerated than those from the bladder. They are also called "pus cells," and their presence in large numbers indicates pyuria. In women, one to five per high-power field is considered normal; above five indicates infection. Also, if the cells appear in clumps, it is suggestive of UTI. The quantity of WBCs in the urine is not necessarily related to the severity of the infection, and the absence of pyuria does not exclude the possibility of infection because pyuria is frequently intermittent. It has been found that at least 20 percent and possibly as many as 50 percent of patients with UTIs do not have pyuria.[7] If the specimen is cloudy and it is difficult to identify the cells, 2 percent acetic acid can be used to dissolve phosphates and clear the specimen. White blood cells are smaller than epithelial cells, although it may be hard to differentiate them from degenerated or distorted epithelial cells. White cells may be better identified by using a Sternheimer-Malbin stain (crystal violet and safranin). If more than five WBC are seen per high-power field, it is routine procedure to culture the urine also. Finding WBCs in the urine is not by itself diagnostic of urinary tract infection because white cells may appear in any inflammatory process in the renal parenchyma, such as Bright's disease, lupus erythematosus, and others. White blood cell casts are strongly suggestive of upper urinary tract disease.

Epithelial cells commonly appear in urine sediment, and their significance is variable.

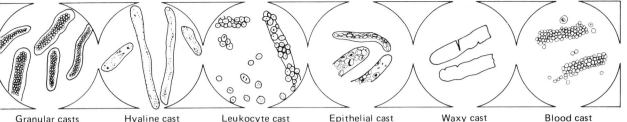

Granular casts   Hyaline cast   Leukocyte cast   Epithelial cast   Waxy cast   Blood cast
fine and coarse

Figure 10-4. Casts found in urine.

Squamous epithelial cells from the urethra and the vagina appear large and flat, with a small nucleus. They may also be rolled or cigar-shaped. Some squamous epithelial cells will be in any voided specimen and are of little significance unless WBCs are also present. A large number of them may indicate a contaminated specimen that was not properly collected. Smaller tubular or transitional epithelial cells may be seen, and a few of them appear in normal urine. A large number of these indicates a sloughing process in the bladder, ureters, or kidneys. It is difficult to identify accurately the origin of urinary tract lesions from the morphology of epithelial cells because of cell degeneration.

Crystals are easily seen as discrete structures quite different in appearance from cells and casts (Figure 10-6). The presence of crystals in the urine has little clinical significance except in certain special circumstances. Alkaline and acid urine each have characteristic crystals. Calcium oxalate crystals are associated with the formation of urinary calculi; cystine crystals with familial cystinosis; tyrosine and leucine crystals with liver disease. Special types of light are necessary to see certain crystals. Other *artifacts* may be seen in the urine, and the health provider needs to be able to identify them in order to differentiate them from cells and casts (Figure 10-7).

Bacteria are normally not present in healthy urine. If bacteria are seen under high power, then there are probably over a million organisms per ml., providing the urine specimen was properly collected and examined right away. If a laboratory count of bacteria is done, it may be reported as a "full field" of bacteria. To aid decision-making about antimicrobial treatment, a Gram stain can be done (see Chapter 9). Coliform bacteria are responsible for virtually all first UTIs and 50 to 60 percent of chronic, recurrent infections. *Escherichia coli, Aerobacter, Klebsiella, Proteus,* and *Pseudomonas* are Gram-negative rods; *enterococcus (Streptococcus faecalis)* is a Gram-positive coccus.

Urine should also be examined for pH, protein, and glucose; the dipstick test is a convenient method. *Proteinuria* is suggestive of pyelonephritis or renal disease, *glycosuria* signals the need for further testing to rule out diabetes, and *alkaline pH* is often seen in Proteus infections. If its *specific gravity* is less than 1.008, the urine specimen is dilute, and lower cellular and bacterial counts are significant.

Figure 10-5. Bacteria in urine. Cells found in urine.

ELLS FOUND IN URINE

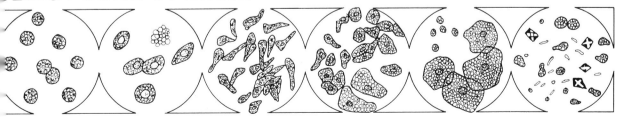

RBC and WBC   Renal epithelium   Caudate cells of Renal Pelvis   Urethral and bladder epithelium   Vaginal epithelium   Yeast and bacteria

CRYSTALS FOUND IN ACID URINE 400 X

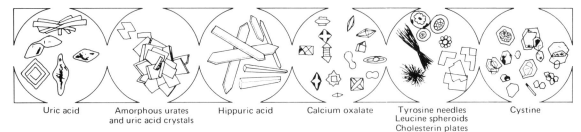

Uric acid   Amorphous urates and uric acid crystals   Hippuric acid   Calcium oxalate   Tyrosine needles Leucine spheroids Cholesterin plates   Cystine

CRYSTALS FOUND IN ALKALINE URINE 400 X

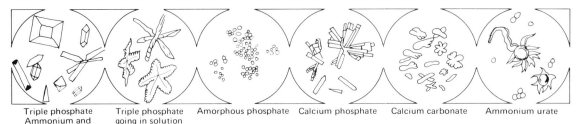

Triple phosphate Ammonium and magnesium   Triple phosphate going in solution   Amorphous phosphate   Calcium phosphate   Calcium carbonate   Ammonium urate

SULFA CRYSTALS

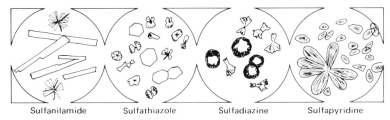

Sulfanilamide   Sulfathiazole   Sulfadiazine   Sulfapyridine

Figure 10-6. Crystals found in urine.

CULTURE. Urine specimens should be cultured when the patient is symptomatic or when routine urinalysis reveals more than 5 WBC per high-power field. Some health providers think it is not necessary to culture first UTIs, as 90 percent of first infections are due to *Escherichia coli*. There is mixed opinion whether routine sensitivity tests should be done when cultures are ordered. The high concentration of antimicrobial agents in the urinary tract (a normal result of the elimination of the drug) is believed to augment its effectiveness. It is prudent to order cultures, so that the organism will be identified, in case of treatment failure. In chronic UTIs or recurrent infections, both cultures and sensitivity tests are indicated because the organism is likely to be a resistant strain of coliform or a different type of pathogen.

Generally the urine specimen is sent to the laboratory for plating on culture media, but in some circumstances the health provider may have to plate and incubate cultures. Using the same size plating loops and constant, controlled plating procedures gives more reliable results. There are a number of bacteriological kits available for office use to aid in the identification of Gram-positive, Gram-negative, and beta-hemolytic organisms. The interpretation of cultures and sensitivity tests requires special knowledge, especially if the particular organism is to be identified.

For clean voided specimens, a microscopic colony count of greater than 100,000 bacteria per ml. of urine is diagnostic of infection, although a smaller colony count may be significant. A count of less than 10,000 bacteria per ml. generally excludes infection, unless the urine is dilute. In specimens obtained by catheterization, a count of 10,000 indicates infection. If counts are between 10,000 and 100,000

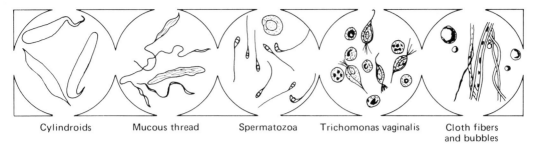

Cylindroids   Mucous thread   Spermatozoa   Trichomonas vaginalis   Cloth fibers and bubbles

Figure 10-7. Artifacts found in urine.

per ml. of urine, clinical judgment assumes primary importance. Symptomatic patients probably have an infection and should be treated. Asymptomatic patients with two consecutive clean-voided specimens with the same organism, with counts in this range are also considered to be infected.[8]

SENSITIVITY. The identification of specific antimicrobial agents to which a particular infecting organism is sensitive can be the key to successful therapy. In most first or second infections in women, sensitivity tests are not ordered due to the known high susceptibility of *Escherichia coli* to sulfonamides. In third infections and thereafter, sensitivity tests are essential because the likelihood of infection by resistant organisms increases greatly with each reinfection. Urine samples for culture and sensitivity tests must be obtained before the initiation of treatment. Sensitivity tests are generally performed by the clinical lab and may be reported in qualitative or quantitative terms.

The older, qualitative, method lists various antimicrobial drugs and labels each one "S" when the organism is sensitive, and "R" when it is resistant. Some labs report "I" for intermediate response, or they may include them in the resistant category. These sensitivity determinations are based primarily on the achievable antimicrobic concentrations in the serum when standard drug dosages are used. Drug concentrations achievable differ for blood, urine, bile, and other body fluids, with urine often having a higher concentration because many drugs are excreted via the urinary system.

The newer, quantitative, method uses a microdilution procedure, with demonstrated accuracy and reliability, and determines the minimum inhibitory concentration (MIC) for organisms against various antimicrobial agents. The MIC is the lowest concentration for an antimicrobic agent that will inhibit the in-vitro growth of an infectious organism, reported in mcg. per ml. The achievable levels of the antimicrobic in-vivo in the blood or urine (sometimes other body fluids) under the standard therapeutic dose is also given. To select the appropriate antimicrobic drug for use, the achievable in-vivo concentration at the site of the infection (blood, urine, and so forth) should be a minimum of 2 to 4 times the MIC. For urinary infections, an antibiotic concentration of at least two times the MIC is considered sufficient. This quantitative method of determining the sensitivity of an organism to a drug provides more precise information than does the qualitative method on which to base drug therapy and allows greater flexibility in therapeutic decision making.[9] Figure 10-8 illustrates the MIC quantitative sensitivity report. Figure 10-9 illustrates a positive urinalysis report and a standard qualitative sensitivity report.

Diagnosis of Common Urinary Tract Infections

Although there will of course be variations among individual patients, the following combinations of symptoms, physical findings, and laboratory results are typical of the most common types of UTIs:

URETHRITIS. There is persistent dysuria, frequency, and urgency which is present around-the-clock (24-hour dysuria), often with hematuria on initial voiding. There usually is no fever, malaise, or systemic symptoms, and no nausea and vomiting. The abdomen is negative on physical examination and there is no costovertebral angle tenderness. Urinalysis of first-voided specimen shows WBCs and bacteria, but the bladder specimen (midstream) is negative. Urine culture is positive. Urinalysis is negative for WBC casts and protein.

ANTIMICROBIAL SUSCEPTIBILITY REPORT
MINIMAL INHIBITORY CONCENTRATION (MIC)

Patient _____   Date _____

Doctor _____   Source site(s) _____

IMPORTANT: The achievable antibiotic concentration at the site(s) of infection should be 2-4 times the MIC, unless infection is confined to urine where maximum antibiotic concentrations of at least 2 times the MIC is sufficient. The concentration of antibiotics inactivated by penicillinase should be at least *10 times* the MIC for treatment of Staph. aureus.

ORGANISM	1.					
	2.					
	3.					
	MIC. mcg/ml			ACHIEVABLE PEAK BLOOD LEVELS	ACHIEVABLE URINE LEVELS	THERAPEUTIC ADULT DOSE
	1	2	3	mcg/ml	mcg/ml	
Clindamycin				2-4 6-10	> 20 > 60	PO 150-300 mgm q6h IV 300-600 mgm q6h
Erythromycin				1-2 10-20		PO 250-500 mgm q6h IV 300 mgm q4-6h
Methicillin				1-5 20-40		PO 0.25-0.50 gm q4-6h** IV 1.0-2.0 gm q4h
Penicillin G				2-3 6-8 20-40	> 300	PO 600,000 U q6h IM 900,000-1.2 mill. U IV 3.0 mill. U q4h
Ampicillin	2			1-3 2-6 10-25	> 50 > 20 > 100	PO 0.25-0.5 gm q6h IM 0.25-0.5 gm q6h IV 1.0-1.5 gm q6h
Cephalothin	8			3-18 9-24 30-85	> 300 > 1000 > 1000	PO 0.25-0.5 gm q6h* IM 0.5-1.0 gm q4-6h IV 1.0-2.0 gm q6h
Gentamicin	0.5			5-15	> 25	IM/IV 3-5.0 mgm/kg/day
Tetracycline	2			2-8 10-20	> 200 > 200	PO 0.5-1.0 gm q6h IV 0.5 gm q6-12h
Carbenicillin				100-450	> 1000 > 2000	PO 764 mg q6h IV 4 gm q4h
Chloramphenicol				10-12 20-30	> 100 > 200	PO 1 gm q6h IV 1 gm q6h
Kanamycin				12-32	> 100	IM/IV 7.5-15 mgm/kg/day
Colistin	4			4-10	> 40	IM 1.5 mgm/kg
Nitrofurantoin	16				> 100-300	PO 50-100 mgm/q6h
Trimeth/Sulfa	.5/9.5			1-2/40-60	> 100	160 mgm/800 mgm q12h

COMMENTS: *Cephalexin or Cephradine
             **Oxacillin

Tobramycin	0.5				Same as Gentamycin

Date reported _____   Tech _____

Figure 10-8.   MIC quantitative sensitivity report.

Form A (Left):

☑ ROUTINE ☐ PRE-OP 4/5/76
☐ STAT ☐ PATIENT WAITING

PHYSICIAN	ROOM
Connell	710
NURSE/CLERK	BED
	WARD

☒ ROUTINE URINALYSIS

COLOR	Yel
CLARITY	Clear
SP. GRAVITY	1·010
REACTION (pH)	6·5
SUGAR	
KETONES	
PROTEIN	
OCCULT BLOOD	

DATE REQUESTED

MICROSCOPIC

WBC/HDF	many, clumps
RBC/HDF	1-2
EPITH CELLS	few round
BACTERIA	many (rods)

CASTS/LDF

A. HYALINE
B. FINE GRANULAR
C. COARSE GRANULAR
D. OTHER

CRYSTALS

| BILE |
| PREGNANCY TEST |
| OCCULT BLOOD — FECES |
| GROSS |
| GUAIAC |
| OVA AND PARASITES |

REMARKS:

TECHNOLOGIST

URINALYSIS – PREGNANCY – FECES
COMMUNITY HOSPITAL
FRED H. DRAPER, M.D.
3325 CHANATE ROAD
SANTA ROSA, CALIFORNIA 95402
PHONE: (707) 544-3340

Form B (Right):

☐ ROUTINE ☐ PRE-OP
☐ STAT ☐ PATIENT WAITING

PHYSICIAN	ROOM
Crooks	
NURSE/CLERK	BED

SOURCE

☐ BLOOD ☐ STOOL
☐ CSF ☐ THROAT
☐ GENITAL ☑ URINE
☐ SPUTUM ☐ WOUND
☐ OTHER

| AFB SMEAR |
| FUNGUS |
| GRAM STAIN |

REMARKS:

CULTURE RESULTS:
100,000/ml E. coli
100,000/ml alpha
strep. not group

ANTIBIOTIC SUSCEPTIBILITY

1	2		1	2	
	S	CHLORAMPHENICOL		R	STEREPTOMYCIN
	S	ERYTHROMYCIN	S	R	TETRACYCLINE
	S	CLINDAMYCIN	S		CARBENICILLIN
	S	METHICILLIN	S	R	COLISTIN
	S	AMPLICILLIN	S	R	GENTAMICIN
S	S	CEPHALOSPORIN	R	R	SULFISOXAZOLE
S	S	KANAMICIN	S		NALADIXIC ACID
S	R	PENICILLIN	S		NITROFURANTOIN
R	S				

TECHNOLOGIST

MICROBIOLOGY

COMMUNITY HOSPITAL
DRS. THOMAS, CLARY, DRAPER, LEISSRING, De MEO
3325 CHANATE ROAD
SANTA ROSA, CALIFORNIA 95402
PHONE: (707) 544-3340

Figure 10-9. (A) Positive urinalysis report. (B) Qualitative sensitivity report (Sensitive-Resistant Macro Method).

ACUTE CYSTITIS. There is twenty-four hour dysuria, often with hematuria toward the end of voiding. The bladder specimen (midstream) is positive for WBCs and bacteria. There are no WBC casts or protein, and the urine culture is positive. The patient usually has no systemic symptoms, fever, malaise, nausea, or vomiting. The abdominal examination is generally neg-ative, except for some supra-pubic tenderness, and there is no costovertebral angle tenderness.

TRIGONITIS. There is 24-hour dysuria and essentially the same symptoms as in urethritis and acute cystitis. Usually there is no hematuria. Often the history includes sexual intercourse 36 to 72 hours before. Urinalysis is negative for WBCs, RBCs, bacteria, WBC casts, and protein. There are no systemic symptoms of infection, the abdominal examination is negative, and there is no costovertebral angle tenderness. Urine culture is negative. Definitive diagnosis is made by cystoscopy, with characteristic appearance of the trigone (see p. 240). There can be a superimposed infection complicating trigonitis.

ACUTE PYELONEPHRITIS.   Typically the patient presents with fever, malaise, nausea, and vomiting and complains of back or flank pain. Symptoms of bladder irritability (urgency, frequency) and inflammation of the lower tract (dysuria) may or may not be present. Hematuria may or may not occur, but when it does it tends to be throughout voiding. Midstream voiding shows, on urinalysis, WBCs and bacteria in great concentrations, with WBC casts also frequently present. Pyuria can, however, be absent or intermittent. Protein may or may not be seen. Urine culture is positive. On examination, there may be some midabdominal tenderness, but costovertebral tenderness is more typical. The costovertebral angle may be exquisitely tender, so that light tapping elicits a marked pain response. This tenderness is more often unilateral but can be bilateral.

CHRONIC CYSTITIS.   Often the patient is asymptomatic or has minor symptomatology of bladder irritation and inflammation. The history reveals repeated UTIs. Systemic symptoms are absent. Urinalysis shows WBCs and bacteria, and the culture is positive. The physical examination may be unremarkable, or some structural defect may be found, such as a cystocele or uterine prolapse. Such infections are often found on routine urinalyses and called asymptomatic bacteriuria.

CHRONIC PYELONEPHRITIS.   This UTI may be manifest as chronic renal insufficiency or it may be discovered when investigating for other disease. Usually there is no dysuria or symptoms of bladder irritation or inflammation and no typical systemic symptoms of infection. Proteinuria and WBC casts (as well as other types of casts) are often present, though they may be present intermittently. Other typical UTI findings (WBCs, RBCs, bacteria in urine, positive urine culture, costovertebral angle tenderness) may or may not be present. If there is pyuria without bacteriuria and the urine culture is negative, suspect *renal tuberculosis*. Usually with this condition there is bilateral costovertebral angle tenderness.

NEUROGENIC BLADDER.   Intermittent dysuria or intermittent discomfort not directly related to voiding, often associated with stressful situations, implies a spastic bladder. Urinalysis and culture are negative. If incontinence is a symptom, it might be related to anatomic deficits or neurologic disorders of the bladder. A relaxed rectal sphincter suggests a neurologic problem; a cystocele often accompanies the loss of the posterior urethrovesical angle, secondary to trauma. Infection may be superimposed on any of these conditions.

Figure 10-10 summarizes the characteristics of common urinary tract infections.

Treatment of Urinary Tract Infections

Symptomatic women with a positive urinalysis (pyuria, bacteriuria, hematuria) are treated with antimicrobial agents. Immediate therapy may be necessary before the culture results are available, and decisions about medication are determined by whether this is a first UTI, by the results of previous cultures, the knowledge of antimicrobial sensitivities of common urinary pathogens, a history of recent or previous UTIs, and other salient points in the history. The most commonly used drugs which are effective against Gram-negative bacteria include *sulfonamides, ampicillin, tetracycline, nitrofurantoin, carbenicillin, nalidixic acid,* and *cephalexin.* If a Gram stain was done, it can confirm the presence of Gram-negative organisms. Gram-positive organisms (staphylococci and enterococci) occasionally cause UTIs and are sensitive to *penicillin G* and *V, penicillinase-resistant penicillin,* and *cephalosporins.*

First UTIs, generally caused by *Escherichia coli,* respond well to most of the above agents for Gram-negative bacteria. Since sulfonamides are inexpensive and have a relatively low toxicity, they are the agents of choice for first infections. Gantrisin and Gantanol are the two most frequently used sulfonamides. If the patient is allergic to sulfa, tetracycline or ampicillin are equally acceptable as therapeutic

	Urinary Sx: Dysuria Urgency Frequency	Systemic Sx: Fever Malaise N + V	Hematuria	Urinalysis					CVA tender-ness	Urine culture
				RBC	WBC	Bact-eria	WBC casts	Protein		
Urethritis	24 hour	0	initial voiding	+	+	+	0	0	0	+
Acute cystitis	24 hour	0	end of voiding	+	+	+	0	0	0	+
Chronic cystitis	mild ±	0	±	±	+	+	0	0	0	+
Trigonitis	24 hour	0	0	0	0	0	0	0	0	0
Acute pyelonephritis	±	+	throughout voiding	+	+	+	+	±	+	+
Chronic pyelonephritis	0	0	±	±	±	±	±	±	±	±

Figure 10-10. Characteristics of common urinary tract infections.

agents. The treatment should last for 10 days to 2 weeks, and ideally the patient and her urine should be rechecked in 2 or 3 days. Bacteria clear from the urine rapidly with effective treatment, thus an examination of urinary sediment or Gram stain should no longer show bacteria. White blood cells persist several days longer and may still be present. A reculture of urine done at this time should be sterile. If bacteria persist, there is treatment failure; obtain sensitivity tests and treat with an appropriate medication for 10 days to 2 weeks. Recheck again in 2 or 3 days to be sure that the second drug is effective. The treatment is the same whether the problem is urethritis, cystitis, or pyelonephritis.

With a repeat infection, the interval between infections is important. Recurrences due to the reemergence of a partially suppressed organism tend to occur sooner than reinfections with different organisms. It is advisable, however, to treat the repeat infection with a different agent from the one used in the previous infection, particularly if a sulfonamide was used. Sulfonamides are usually ineffective after the first few courses because the stool flora tend to develop resistant strains. Cultures and sensitivity tests are critical here to select the proper medication. The course of therapy is again 10 days to 2 weeks, with a recheck in 2 or 3 days.

Highly recurrent and closely spaced infections require suppressive therapy for 1 to 3 months following the eradication of the infection. After the urine has been cleared of bacteria using the antimicrobial agent indicated by the culture and sensitivity reports, *methenamine mandelate* is given with an agent to acidify the urine to a pH of 5.0 to 6.0. After a few months, suppressive therapy should be discontinued to see if the patient will remain infection-free. If infection recurs, it must be treated, and the suppressive therapy is repeated. Methenamine salts work only in the urine and not in the kidney, thus they are of use only for bladder prophylaxis. Nitrofurantoin is a good antimicrobial agent to use in highly recurrent infections if the organism is susceptible to it, because it remains effective after many courses of treatment as it does not appear in measurable quantities in the patient's stool.

ANTIMICROBIAL AGENTS. Dosages, particular information, and the toxic effects of the most commonly used oral antimicrobial agents for UTIs are as follows:

Sulfisoxazole (Gantrisin)—initially 2 to 4 Gm., then 1 Gm. four times a day for 10 to 14 days. Avoid this drug if the patient is allergic to sulfa. It is the most widely used, safe, and economic oral agent. Hypersensitivity reactions affecting the skin and mucous membranes occur most frequently (urticaria, purpura); other effects include nausea, vomiting, headache, dizziness, mild or serious blood dyscrasias, crystalluria, serum sickness, toxic nephrosis, and other rare toxic effects.

Sulfamethoxazole (Gantanol)—initially 2 Gm., then 1 Gm. twice a day for 10 to 14 days. Avoid if the patient is allergic to sulfa. This is a slowly excreted sulfonamide, requiring lower doses, and it has the same toxic effects as sulfisoxazole.

Ampicillin, 250 to 500 mg. every 6 hours for 10 to 14 days. Avoid, if the patient has a penicillin allergy. This drug is well absorbed from the gastrointestinal tract and is acid resistant. It is a broad-spectrum antibiotic with comparatively few adverse reactions. Toxic effects include rash, fever, serum sickness, stomatitis, nausea, vomiting, diarrhea, anaphylaxis, reversible blood dyscrasias, and elevated transaminases.

Tetracycline, 250 to 500 mg. four times a day or every 6 hours for 10 to 14 days. It is a broad-spectrum antibacterial agent, with relatively low toxicity. It forms insoluble complexes with calcium, magnesium, iron, and aluminum salts, thus it should not be taken with food, milk and milk products, cathartics and antacids which have these salts. It is teratogenic if taken early in pregnancy, and causes discoloration of teeth in infants if taken later. Toxic effects include skin eruptions, stomatitis, anorexia, nausea, vomiting, flatulence and diarrhea, anaphylaxis, hepatotoxicity, and delayed coagulation.

Nitrofurantoin (Furadantin, Macrodantin), 50 to 100 mg. four times a day for 10 to 14 days. It attains therapeutic concentrations only in urine and is absorbed rapidly from the gastrointestinal tract; its effectiveness is reduced when it is taken with antacids. A high urine pH reduces the activity of this drug. The toxic effects are nausea and vomiting, skin eruptions, polyneuropathy, allergic pneumonitis, and hemolytic anemia. Bacterial resistance to this drug develops slowly and to a limited degree.

Nalidixic acid (Negram), 1 Gm. four times a day for 1 to 2 weeks. It is a drug with a narrow antibacterial spectrum and is particularly useful against *Proteus* since many strains of this genus are resistant to other agents. Generally a culture and sensitivity test is needed before this drug is used. Some organisms rapidly become resistant to nalidixic acid. The toxic effects include nausea, vomiting, rash, urticaria, diarrhea, fever, gastrointestinal bleeding, and photosensitivity.

Cephalexin, 250 to 500 mg. four times a day for 10 to 14 days. This drug is effective against some Gram-negative and -positive organisms, but sensitivity testing should be done before prescription. It is acid stable and food does not interfere with its absorption. Adverse reactions include diarrhea, pyrosis, nausea, vomiting, abdominal pain, rare rashes, neutropenia, serum sickness, and others.

Methenamine mandelate (Mandelamine), 1 Gm. four times a day with acidifying agents such as ascorbic acid 500 to 1000 mg. two to four times a day and methionine 2 to 3 Gm. four times a day. This drug is a urinary antiseptic that acts by liberating formaldehyde in an acid medium. It is not to be used as the only therapeutic agent for UTIs, but it is useful for prophylaxis in recurrent infections. It can be given for a long time, without having the bacteria develop a resistance to it. The drug has a low toxicity, but it may cause gastric irritation, rash, nausea, and acute urinary tract inflammation when administered in large doses.

INSTRUCTIONS TO THE PATIENT. The symptoms should disappear in 48 to 72 hours, but the full course of medications must nevertheless be taken. The infection may only be partially suppressed and recur in a few days or weeks if medications are not completed. If the symptoms are not much improved within 2 or 3 days, the medication is not effective and retesting is necessary, as is a change of medication. It is important for the patient to drink large quantities of fluids and to empty her bladder frequently. This helps to prevent crystal formation in the urine (particularly with sulfonamides), keep the kidneys well hydrated, and prevents the concentration and stagnation of urine in the bladder. If the drug is one which should not be taken with meals, milk, antacids, or other substances, explain this to the patient.

FOLLOW-UP. The response to treatment should be assessed in 2 or 3 days. The culture results (and sensitivity reports, if they were ordered) are available, and the choice of a drug can be verified. Telephone contact with the patient may be enough if the antimicrobial is correct and if the patient reports improvement of her symptoms. If not, the patient should be seen right away to retest her urine and change the drug. Another appointment is made for 2 weeks later, following the course of treatment, to repeat the urinalysis and culture. The urine should be cultured again at monthly intervals for 3 months, then every 3 months for the next 9 months, then twice a year for the next year. If there are no further infections in this 2-year period, the patient's UTI is considered cured. If further infections do occur, the entire process starts over with each infection. Additional diagnostic testing is indicated after the woman's third episode of UTI, although some may wish to do this after one episode of pyelonephritis.

FURTHER UROLOGICAL TESTING. Women with recurrent urinary infections need further urological studies. The health provider can order a screening IVP (intravenous pyelogram), excretory (voiding) urogram, and renal function tests such as BUN (blood urea nitrogen), creatinine, P.S.P. excretion and clearance tests. If these tests are normal, referral to a urologist can be delayed while preventive measures and suppressive treatment are tried. Major structural abnormalities and renal damage must have been ruled out. Any abnormalities in these tests indicate the need for referral, however, for additional studies such as a cystourethrogram, cystoscopy, and urethral calibration. After a thorough urological study has proven normal, it is unusual for urological lesions to occur at a later time. Thus repeated IVPs, voiding urograms and cystoscopy need not be done again unless there is a clear indication of their need.[10]

Preventive Measures

Women who are prone to repeated UTIs can benefit greatly from learning preventive measures. Using the proper technique in wiping the vulva after voiding and bowel movements is essential so that bacteria from the rectum is not carried toward the urethra. The importance of the front-to-back motion is to be stressed. The highly susceptible woman should not take tub baths, for bacteria from the skin or rectum are washed into the water and can work their way into the urethra. She should shower, or wash herself while standing in a tub bath. Good bladder habits must be developed, including emptying the bladder regularly and often so that the urine does not stagnate, giving bacteria time to multiply. Many women hold urine for long periods of time, take little fluid, and avoid getting up to urinate at night. Al-

though urinating often is inconvenient, it is very helpful in avoiding recurrent UTIs. Fluid intake must be increased in susceptible women, keeping urine dilute and flushing urine out of the bladder frequently.

Particular precautions need to be taken with sexual intercourse. Showering before intercourse reduces the number of bacteria in the genital area that can be carried to the urethra during intercourse. Emptying the bladder both before and after intercourse also removes a potential source of organisms. Applying povidone-iodine (Betadine) to the urethral meatus before intercourse and after voiding further diminishes organisms in this area. If UTI is clearly related to intercourse, occurring after nearly every occasion, it may be necessary to give the woman a single dose of 250 mg. penicillin V one-half hour before intercourse. Or, a maintenance dose of 50 to 100 mg. nitrofurantoin at bedtime can prevent recurrences once the UTI has been eliminated. This should be combined with an agent for acidification of the urine (ascorbic acid, methionine).

MANAGEMENT OF INCONTINENCE

An accurate diagnosis of the type of incontinence is of the utmost importance, because the management of stress and urge incontinences (see pp. 241 to 242) differs substantially. In pure stress incontinence, the diagnosis is easy and is usually made from the history alone: leakage is clearly associated with coughing, laughing, lifting, straining, or any activity which increases intraabdominal pressure, and the problem is continuous. In urge incontinence, urine cannot be controlled once the need to void has been felt, and this problem may be intermittent. A past history of UTIs and symptoms of dysuria are associated with urge incontinence. A neurogenic bladder, whether spastic or atonic, causes leakage unassociated with any activity. Spontaneous unexpected leakage and a history of bed-wetting alert the health provider to possible neurologic deficits. Fistulas may also be a cause, usually with a history of trauma or instrumentation.

The physical examination may provide cues to the proper diagnosis. In classical *stress incontinence*, the woman is examined with a full bladder and the region of the vesicle neck and urethra during coughing or straining can be seen to provide poor pelvic support. Loss of urine also occurs in this situation. If continance can be demonstrated by supporting the vesicle neck with the fingers intravaginally, then the diagnosis of a flattened urethrovesical angle causing stress incontinence is reinforced. Some women have stress incontinence without the characteristic pelvic findings of a cystocele and relaxation, and these can be diagnosed by a chain cystourethrogram. A posterior urethrovesical angle of greater than 90 to 110 degrees confirms the diagnosis. (See Figure 10-3). Referral to a urologist is necessary for this procedure. This condition may be corrected surgically, and the degree of distress from the symptoms would be the major indication of whether or not surgery is justified. The Marshall-Marchetti procedure is major surgery, though the risks are relatively low. The woman must evaluate the degree of distress she experiences versus the risks and discomforts of anesthesia, surgery, hospitalization, and recovery. Chances of success are best with the first operation.

In urge incontinence, there are no particular pelvic changes unless there is concomitant pelvic relaxation. This condition does not bear directly on the cause of urge incontinence, and the correction of a cystocele will have little effect on urinary leakage. The bladder and urinary tract must be studied to identify the cause. Infection is a frequent cause of urge incontinence and should be treated with the appropriate antiomicrobial agent. Recurrent infections require referral for cystoscopy, excretory urogram, and cystourethrograms. Chronic irritative processes such as trigonitis are often involved. This type of incontinence is not helped by surgical repair, but a mixed picture of urge and stress incontinence might be partially improved by correcting the pelvic relaxation and posterior urethrovesical angle. With a mixed-picture incontinence, the woman should be informed of the limits of surgery and the two different causes of her problems.

A pelvic examination is rarely helpful in diagnosing a neurogenic bladder, although marked distention is felt as a large cystic mass in the hypogastrium, signifying flaccidity. A spastic bladder may appear as a small, firm, tender mass anterior to the uterus, and the relaxation of the rectal sphincter may be present. If a neurogenic bladder is suspected, referral for a cystometrogram is indicated. Incontinence associated with a neurogenic lesion is not amenable to surgical correction; in fact, urge incontinence and a neurogenic bladder without stress incontinence are considered contraindications to surgery.

Medical Management

Many factors affecting incontinence can be improved with other types of therapy. In stress incontinence, isometric excercises described by Kegal (contraction of rectal and perineal muscles) may improve muscle tone to the point of significant relief from incontinence. Loss of weight in obese patients can be helpful, as can the control of a chronic cough due to smoking or pulmonary disease. In postmenopausal women with atrophic pelvic changes, the use of estrogen vaginal creams may increase the tone and vascularity of tissues to relieve both urgency and stress leakage. Any estrogen therapy must be used with caution. When bacterial infection is associated with urge incontinence, the correction of this condition can afford a great relief of symptoms. Chronic infections should be carefully managed to give long-term relief. The use of anticholinergic drugs may be valuable in some mixed urge and stress incontinence, especially if there is a neurogenic component. Stress incontinence may also be relieved by using a vaginal tampon or a pessary to provide support for the vesicle neck. Some neuromuscular conditions have been improved by the use of electric stimulation of the perineal area.

There is one situation in which asymptomatic pelvic relaxation does require surgical repair. This is when a cystocele exists and there is persistent residual urine, with recurrent urinary tract infection. This reservoir of urine provides a focus for infection, and until the cystocele is corrected, repeated infections will occur, with continuing damage to the urinary tract. In this situation, surgical repair should be done even though there are no symptoms of incontinence.[11]

NOTES

1. P. P. Kelalis, "Recurrent Urinary Infections." *Update International* (June 1974): 417-21.
2. T. J. Williams, "Urinary Incontinence in the Female." *Primary Care* 2,4 (December 1975): 555-70.
3. S. L. Romney, et al., *Gynecology & Obstetrics: The Health Care of Women* (New York: McGraw-Hill, Blakiston, 1975), pp. 895-98 and 907-11.

4. "Tight Focus on Urinary Tract Infections." *Patient Care* 9,8 (April 15, 1975): 21-59.
5. Romney, et al., *Gynecology and Obstetrics*, p. 915.
6. R. M. Kark, et al., *A Primer of Unrinalysis*, ed. 2. (New York: Harper & Row, 1973), pp. 60-64.
7. "Tight Focus," p. 22.
8. C. M. Kunin, *Detection, Prevention and Management of Urinary Tract Infections* (Philadelphia: Lea & Febiger, 1972), pp. 1-25.
9. *Quantitative Antimicrobic Susceptibility Testing Manual*, ed. 2. (Palo Alto, Calif.: Micro-Media Systems, 1976).
10. Kunin, *Detection, Prevention and Management*, p. 182.
11. Williams, *Urinary Incontinence*, pp. 561-67.

SUGGESTED READINGS

"Dysuria: UTI May Not Be the Cause." *Patient Care* 8,3 (February 1, 1974): 134-48.
M. Wintrobe, et al., eds., *Harrison's Principles of Internal Medicine* (New York: McGraw-Hill, Blakiston, 1970), pp. 269-72.
Urine Under the Microscope, ROCOM Reference Series (Nutley, New Jersey: ROCOM Press, Division of Hoffman-LaRoche, Inc., 1973).
"Urology: Three New Aids to UTI Workup." *Patient Care* 9,2 (January 15, 1975): 128-30.

11

Venereal Disease

Named after Venus, the Roman goddess of love, venereal diseases (VD) are those infectious diseases associated with sexual intercourse or the genital area. The mons veneris of the woman, or "mound of love," has represented both pleasure and danger for untold ages and the Old Testament included rules for the man with "unclean issue." Used in its broadest sense, venereal disease includes gonorrhea, syphilis, herpes genitalis, condylomata, pediculosis pubis (crab lice), and vaginal infections such as Trichomonas and Candida, as well as the much more uncommon granuloma inguinale, lymphogranuloma venereum (lymphopathia) and chancroid. This chapter will cover the first five common venereal diseases which are frequently encountered in health care settings. Trichomonas and Candida are included in Chapter 9, Vaginal Discharge and Itching. The remaining uncommon venereal infections are seen mainly in tropical and subtropical countries and may be reviewed in appropriate medical texts.

DEMOGRAPHY, DETECTION, AND PREVENTION

The actual incidence of gonorrhea and syphilis in the United States is difficult to determine due to underreporting and the existence of many undiagnosed cases. In 1972 there were an estimated 2.5 million cases of gonorrhea and 85,000 cases of syphilis, with a new case of gonorrhea occurring every 15 seconds.[1] For years all states have required that syphilis and gonorrhea be reported to the boards of health, but probably only one out of nine cases is ac-

tually reported. Reporting of the several other sexually transmitted diseases is not required; thus there is little data on their incidence. Crabs are often self-treated with over-the-counter preparations, and the assistance of health providers is infrequently sought. Genital herpes is generally believed to be on the increase and probably is more often encountered in private practice than is gonorrhea.

Much discussion centers on the "VD pandemic" which the greater sexual freedom, increased leisure and mobility, the intermingling of persons from different cultural and economic backgrounds, decreased social control by established conservative institutions, and the increased sexualization of mass media have helped to promote. Whether or not there actually is an increase in the amount of sexual activity or in the exchange of partners, an increase in total population, with earlier maturation and expanded longevity, does create a longer sexual life span. The population at risk for VD is thus increased. Predictors of the populations most likely to contract VD, such as socioeconomic status, race, color, geographic location, are not accurate; the incidence of VD is widespread among any group that has sexual mobility. Three persons of either sex are all that is required for sexual mobility, and any sexual contact holds the potential for transmitting VD.

Sexual contact is almost always necessary to contract gonorrhea or syphilis. The idea that infections can come from toilet seats is very farfetched when the characteristics of the organisms are considered. Both the gonococcus and the spirochete require a special environment for growth and die rapidly outside the human body; thus,

> You might contract VD from the proverbial toilet seat, if you happen to have a toilet that was kept at the invariant temperature of 98.6 F and flushed with lukewarm blood plasma. . . .[2]

As this type of toilet apparatus is highly unlikely, some type of sexual contact must be considered the mode of transmission for VD, with two rare exceptions: First, gonorrhea may be contracted by contact with moist sheets or bedclothing of an infected person, but the contact must be almost immediately after the drainage of infected secretions. In this way it is possible for children who sleep with infected parents to contract gonorrhea. Because the gonococcus cannot penetrate intact skin and needs access to mucosal surfaces, the likelihood of exposed children developing gonorrhea is still quite small. Second, syphilis can be spread by contact with infected blood or lesions, and the spirochete can penetrate the skin as well as mucous membranes. Contaminated blood used for transfusions was a source of the disease prior to widespread serological testing. Infected needles, causing accidental pricking or shared among drug users, can spread the disease. Contact with skin lesions, such as chancres on the mouth or fingers, or condylomata lata, or the skin rash of secondary syphilis, are other possible modes of transmission. However, infection from such sources is undoubtedly very uncommon. Congenital syphilis transferred from the infected mother to her unborn child is another method of transmission. Although the predominant mode of transmission is sexual, it must be borne in mind that genital intercourse is not the only way VD is spread. Kissing, oral-genital and rectal intercourse, and manual stimulation also can transfer both gonorrhea and syphilis.

The detection of venereal disease is a continuing problem in health care. There may be an absence of symptoms after VD is contracted, or the symptoms may be so vague and mild that they do not cause alarm. Men generally have more readily recognized symptoms than do women because of the difference in the structures of each sex's genital organs. The penile discharge and dysuria caused by gonorrhea and the chancre of syphilis on the glans or shaft are obvious causes of concern for which treatment is usually sought. Women, for whom some vaginal discharge is normal, may not notice slight changes following gonorrhea infection. Since the urethra is often not involved in women, no urinary symptoms alert them to possible danger. The chancre of syphilis is usually on the cervix, hidden high in the vaginal vault. It is estimated that about 60 percent of the women with gonorrhea are asymptomatic. There is a much lower percentage of asymptomatic men, possibly between 12 and 15 percent, but among the male sex partners of infected persons this percentage is much higher.[3]

Most gonorrhea is detected when symptomatic persons seek treatment and refer their contacts. The lack of a simple, accurate, screening blood test for gonorrhea is a major deterrent to widespread testing to detect the disease in asymptomatic cases. Particularly for women, gonorrhea (GC) cultures are necessary for diagnosis, and these must be obtained during a pelvic examination. Although there is an increased use of routine GC cultures, particularly among higher risk groups seen at family-planning clinics and among younger, sexually active women, it must be assumed that a significant number of cases of gonorrhea in women are going undiagnosed. The situation for syphilis is different because there are available simple, inexpensive, and fast screening blood tests which are widely used. In the United States, 45 states require premarital blood tests for syphilis, 42 require serological testing for syphilis for pregnant women before or after delivery, and about one-half of the hospitals in the country perform routine syphilis testing on patients admitted for hospital care.[4] This routine testing reveals numerous asymptomatic cases which would not have come to medical attention for years, if ever. Also, syphilis is often detected during the work-up for other diseases because its reputation as "the great mimicker" causes health providers to frequently consider syphilis among the diagnoses to be ruled out. The continued incidence of new cases indicates that syphilis is still being spread, despite routine testing. Because the symptoms of primary and secondary syphilis resolve spontaneously, treatment may not be sought, and the disease may be transmitted many times over before serological testing makes the diagnosis. The numerous barriers to case-finding, including underreporting and reluctance to name contacts, contribute to the continued spread of both syphilis and gonorrhea.

Prevention of VD is a much-harped-upon theme in primary health care and public health, but little headway seems to have been made among the population as a whole. Partly this is due to changed methods of contraception, with less reliance on the condom among the teenage and young adult age groups in which most new cases of VD are found. The change of attitude toward VD, particularly gonorrhea, from public avoidance of the whole subject to today's rather jaded nonchalance, probably also contributes to inertia with regard to prevention. The condom is the only contraceptive device which is prophylactic for VD, although the diaphragm may have some effect in preventing cervical infections. The effects of oral contraceptives on cervical and vaginal physiology are believed to increase significantly the woman's susceptibility to gonorrhea, perhaps to nearly 100 percent incidence, following exposure. Women with an IUD in place are considered at increased risk for fulminant gonococcal salpingitis and pelvic inflammatory disease.[5]

Probably the only way to prevent VD is for two virgins to begin their sexual life together and stay together forever—remaining always sexually faithful. To prevent the spread of VD among the rest of the population, it would be necessary to have an "annual VD treatment day," with everyone receiving penicillin shots (a double dose, including the specific penicillin regimens for syphilis and gonorrhea), including the supposed celibate. Both of these measures are, of course, totally impossible to carry out, so VD will continue to spread and constitute a significant health problem. The VD pandemic spreads across socioeconomic groups and age lines to the extent that if present trends are not changed, the probability that those now in their preteens will contract VD before age 25 will be 50 percent.[6]

MEANINGS FOR WOMEN

The shame, secrecy, and fear which have surrounded venereal diseases for centuries are still operant today to some degree. Venereal disease, as is sex, is more out in the open now, but misinformation and confusion about both are still common. The use of the "fear approach" in many VD pamphlets directed at various age groups stresses the dangers of such terrifying consequences as blindness, sterility, insanity, and death. This reflects an underlying moralistic approach persisting from puritanical and Victorian traditions; VD suggests immoral, promiscuous behavior by persons of low character. Fear of retribution (legal or disease-caused suffering) has not been known to constitute an effective deterrent, either to crime or sex. Similar to the oversell on the consequences of marijuana use, an exaggerated approach to VD control promotes a casual attitude among the young, who experience both marijuana and VD without suffering the dire consequences that were predicted. That there are serious consequences of both syphilis and gonorrhea is undeniable, and health providers are well aware of them. But there is no point in adopting a moralistic or punitive approach to patients; a realistic, factual, and dispassionate discussion, aimed at helping individuals or groups understand their risk of contracting VD, the usual course of the disease, the high rate of effectiveness of the treatment, and the common dangers of untreated or inadequately treated VD seems to be a more reasonable approach.

Both men and women who engage in more liberal sexual behavior must simply accept the risk of contracting VD with any given sexual partner. Even those who believe they are selective, who have limited sexual contacts, or who think they know their sexual partner well are at risk. For those who change sexual partners frequently or have occasional casual sexual encounters, there must be a high index of suspicion about any signs and symptoms possibly indicating VD. Even in situations where VD is an inherent risk, people often are angry and upset when their VD is actually diagnosed. The anger is directed at the presumedly irresponsible sexual partner who should have informed the patient or should have avoided intercourse until he or she was cured of the disease. The prevalence of asymptomatic infections often is a surprise. Individuals vary in their responsibility about informing their contacts; some cooperate fully and others resist taking any action, either out of shame or a desire for vengeance.

Couples in marital or committed relations face additional problems when VD is diagnosed. When the toilet-seat theory is debunked, sexual activity in one or the other partner must be faced. Anger, guilt, recriminations, accusations, and other emotions may threaten the relations; physical abuse may be the woman's lot in some situations. The health provider may need to provide counseling or to refer couples to a psychologist so that they may deal with the implications of VD for their relations. The many differences in how couples conceptualize their relations are crucial here; these may range from the old double standard in which men are expected to have outside sexual activities—thus VD is not unexpected nor disastrous for the relation—to the romantic idealism of undying exclusive love in which this evidence of infidelity is a crisis of major proportion, to the progressive contract in which each partner has some degree of sexual freedom and VD is an inevitable if unfortunate risk.

Women are often concerned about the implications of gonorrhea for their future fertility. It is difficult to answer their questions, because the residual effects of the disease are highly individual and are not necessarily related to the extensiveness of the infection. Residual effects may be absent if treatment is early and adequate, but the functional capacity of the fallopian tubes following gonorrheal infections is difficult to predict. Even mild infections which had appropriate treatment can produce enough alteration in tubal physiology that infertility, ectopic pregnancy, or chronic disease process may result.

APPROACH TO MANAGEMENT

The health provider must maintain a high index of suspicion for VD and be particularly alert to symptoms or data from the history which might be suggestive of these infections. Some patients will present with the problem of possible or known exposure to VD, helping focus the work-up from the beginning. Others will describe symptoms which could indicate VD or could be due to other types of vaginal or pelvic problems. Symptoms of vaginal discharge, dysuria, and lower abdominal pain should always trigger the thought of gonorrhea in the differential diagnosis; painless sores on the genitals or mouth raise suspicions of syphilis, and exquisitely painful genital lesions suggest herpes. However, other causes for such symptoms are frequent, and a thorough exploration, including a history, a physical examination, and laboratory testing, is necessary to arrive at an accurate diagnosis.

The routine screening of asymptomatic patients for both gonorrhea and syphilis is advisable to the extent that it is practicable and economically feasible in the given setting. Obtaining cervical GC cultures when women are seen for contraception, prenatal care, or routine Pap smears is a growing practice among primary health care providers. The VDRL is a routine procedure as part of a prenatal panel, hospital admissions work-up, premarital panel, and any thorough work-up for complete health assessment or diagnostic purposes. Adding to this a GC culture and VDRL for all pelvic complaints would increase the rate of detection.

The History

What are the presenting symptoms or reasons for seeking care? Cues to possible VD are often obtained in the motives for seeking care and the initial symptoms the patient describes. Known or suspected exposure to VD often sends asymptomatic women to the office. Ascertain whether the exposure could be to gonorrhea or syphilis or both and when the exposure might have occurred. Explore any other symptoms, as below. If the following are not mentioned spontaneously by the patient, they should be brought up by the practitioner.

Is there any vaginal discharge, itching, burning, or pain? Have the woman describe the discharge, its color, amount, and odor, the time of its onset, and changes since it has been present. Some vaginal discharge is normal so a change in amount or character from what is usual for the individual is of importance. Although there are typical discharges for the various types of vaginitis, in clinical practice it is rare to see the classic types. Of significance to VD is a yellow, purulent discharge; this is uncommon, however, even when gonorrhea is present. A large amount of vaginal discharge would actually be more indicative of some other type of vaginitis, such as Candida or Trichomonas. Itching or burning of the vulva or labia indicates drainage of the discharge onto this area, causing irritation and inflammation; it is more common in Candida or Trichomonas than in gonorrhea. Actual pain, especially if it is severe, alerts the health provider to herpes or an infected lesion such as a Bartholin's cyst or a sebaceous cyst.

Is there dysuria? Pain, burning, blood, or pus

in the urine and urgency and freqency indicate urethral or bladder involvement. Urethritis could be due to gonorrhea or to other pathogens; urinary tract infection must be ruled out. A urinalysis, with a culture if it is indicated, is essential if there are any urinary symptoms. Dysuria, some burning or discomfort with urination, or some urgency are common with localized urethritis which could be due to gonorrhea. A GC culture of the urethra should be obtained with such symptoms.

Is there abdominal pain or cramping? The suspicion of upper reproductive tract involvement is raised with these symptoms. Abdominal pain is very difficult to evaluate objectively, but its characteristics should be explored, including the time of the original onset, associated factors, what provokes or precipitates the pain, the character and radiation of the pain, what relieves the pain, any medications or treatment, any previous similar episodes, and the relation of the pain to the menstrual cycle. The onset of pain during the first 7 days of the menstrual cycle is particularly suggestive of gonococcal salpingitis, while in nongonococcal infections the onset of pain occurs throughout the menstrual cycle.[7] The many causes of lower abdominal pain must be considered, ranging from tumors to functional processes, and an appropriate work-up must be undertaken if abdominal pain is a significant symptom. Chapter 12, Lower Abdominal Pain, covers this problem in greater depth.

Has there been any fever, nausea, or vomiting? Fever in association with lower abdominal pain and abdominal findings of tenderness or rigidity are suggestive of salpingitis or pelvic inflammatory disease. Nausea or vomiting may indicate systemic infection or a reaction to pelvic involvement and pain. Explore other possible causes of fever such as upper respiratory or gastrointestinal infections. Ask whether the woman took her temperature with a thermometer, and if so how high it was. Frequently people will say they had a fever because they "felt hot" but did not take their temperature. Ask if they had shaking chills in this instance, being careful to differentiate real chills from a feeling of chilliness, which is quite common among women.

Have there been any menstrual changes? One of the subtle signs of gonorrhea involving the upper reproductive tract is some change in menstruation—usually an increased flow with more cramping than usual, although there may be decreased flow. Skipping a period could also point to possible gonorrhea. Any menstrual irregularities indicate that pregnancy must be ruled out.

What type of contraception (if any) is used? Oral contraceptives increase a woman's susceptibility to gonorrhea if she is exposed. Women with IUDs are not more susceptible to gonorrhea, but if they do contract the disease they are 2 to 2½ times more likely to develop pelvic inflammatory disease than are women without IUDs.[8] The use of a diaphragm or contraceptive jellies, creams, or foams might provide some measure of protection from gonorrhea because these preparations often contain bactericidal substances. However, this in no way implies that the use of these contraceptives prevents gonorrhea.

Has there been a recent change of sexual partners? The risk of exposure to VD could be increased if there is a new sexual partner, although of course a regular partner could transfer an infection acquired from someone else. Because of the difference in bacterial and viral flora with a new partner, the incidence of other types of vaginitis and of herpes is also increased. Particularly for first infections with herpes, this information is an important component of the history.

Is there painful or uncomfortable intercourse? Dyspareunia of recent onset in a woman previously having comfortable intercourse can mean pelvic infection if the pain occurs on thrusting or deep penetration. If vaginal entry causes the pain and there is a burning type of pain with intercourse, not associated with deep penetration, a vulval inflammation caused by a vaginal discharge is more likely.

Have there been any sores, bumps, or lesions on the genitals or any type of skin rash? Women may develop the chancre of syphilis on the labia, vulva, or perianal skin, although it is more commonly found on the cervix. If there has been or currently is a genital lesion, have the woman describe it. A single, painless ulcer signifies syphilis; multiple small vesicles which progress to ulcers accompanied by marked pain and varying amounts of swelling are typical of herpes. A single subcutaneous lump or swelling which is tender and may or may not drain purulent material is suggestive of a Bartholin's infection which could be gonococcal or due to some other bacteria. Itchy, small bumps distributed through the pubic hair may indicate crab lice or scabies. A collection of fleshy, white, wartlike bumps around the labia and rectum could be condylomata acuminata (venereal warts) or condylomata lata (due to secondary syphilis). Skin rashes on other parts of the body alert the practitioner to the rash of secondary syphilis; fine, small, red bumps, occasionally pussy, are particularly suspect if they are found on palms and soles. A disseminated gonococcal infection causes red, pussy, necrotic, discrete lesions, usually on the extremities.

Is it possible that you could have been exposed to gonorrhea or other VD? If the woman has not raised this possibility, the nurse practitioner should bring it up in the exploration of positive answers to the preceding questions. In addition to perhaps providing another cue to the nature of the problem, the woman's response to this question may indicate that she has difficulties in her relation with her partner or with the implications of the diagnosis of VD. The extent of the crisis which the possibility of VD creates provides an early indication of whether emotional therapy will be needed as an adjunct to physical treatment.

If there is a known exposure, ascertain if the woman's partner was treated and, if so, was it before or after she was exposed. Try to determine what type of VD is involved.

Have you ever had VD before? What type? How was it treated? These questions can provide information about possible treatment failures, inadequate treatment, or residua of previous infections which could affect the woman's current symptoms. If the patient did have a previous VD, were her partners treated also? The type of treatment given, such as a single treatment with penicillin versus a series of shots, helps to suggest whether the disease being treated was gonorrhea or syphilis. A history of positive blood tests points to syphilis.

With patients who are not known to the health provider or agency, a brief past medical history, including major illnesses, hospitalizations, operations, and current medication used, as well as a family history of significant illnesses, is helpful to eliminate other considerations in the diagnosis and treatment. It is essential to determine any specific allergy to penicillin, as well as other medications, before planning therapy.

Physical Examination

If dysuria was a symptom elicited during the history, a clean-catch midstream urine specimen should be obtained. The examination for suspected VD includes an abdominal examination, a speculum and bimanual pelvic examination, with the collection of cultures and smears as indicated, an inspection of the skin, and blood testing.

ABDOMINAL EXAMINATION. Both superficial and deep palpation of the abdomen is carried out to determine the presence of masses and tenderness, especially in either lower quadrant. Abdominal rigidity and pronounced guarding may indicate peritonitis, secondary to gonorrheal or other bacterial pelvic infections. A lower-quadrant mass may be a tubal ovarian abscess, pyosalpinx or hydrosalpinx, ectopic pregnancy, or ovarian tumor. Suprapubic tenderness could signify cystitis or endometritis. Decreased bowel sounds support the diagnosis of peritonitis. Liver, kidney, and spleen should also be palpated to determine if there is any enlargement or tenderness. The presence of enlarged or suppurative lymph nodes in the groin indicates the need for consultation to determine the presence of chancroid, lymphogranuloma venereum, or granuloma inguinale; adenopathy may also mean a chancre or herpes.

INSPECTION OF THE VULVA. The labia, perineum, anus, and surrounding tissue are examined for lesions. Single or multiple *chancres* may erupt at the site of contact in any of these areas and may appear as a punched-out ulcer crater with indurated edges (Figure 11-1). It is uncommon for the chancre to be painful when it is touched unless it is secondarily infected. Chancres are usually singular and may be accompanied by hard, nonfluctuant, painless, enlarged inguinal lymph nodes (satellite bubos). *Herpes* lesions appear as tiny fluid-filled vesicles, usually multiple and in clusters, which may be in various stages of eruption including shallow ulcers which tend to coalesce. An erythematous areola around these lesions, with edema, may be seen, and the surrounding area is usually exquisitely tender to the touch. A clear, watery discharge may be present, and there may be inguinal lymphadenopathy. An *erythematous vulva* with discharge present at the introitus could mean vaginitis due to Candida, Trichomonas, or Hemophilis. *Condylo-*

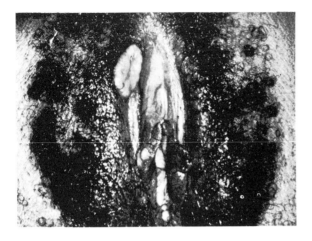

Figure 11-1. Chancre of primary syphilis on labium majus.

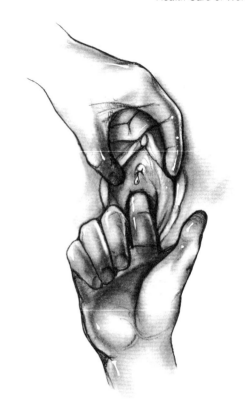

Figure 11-2. Gonorrheal discharge upon milking the urethra.

mata acuminata appear as pale, irregular clusters of fleshy, raised lesions, usually on the labia, perineum, or perianal skin. The *condylomata lata* of secondary syphilis are broadbased outgrowths in the same areas which are more flat and pale and tend to ulcerate and produce a highly contagious, foul discharge (see Figures 11-3 and 11-5 pp. 273 and 278).

INSPECTION OF BARTHOLIN'S GLANDS, SKENE'S GLANDS, AND THE URETHRA. A swollen, indurated area in the lower portion of the labia, usually unilateral, indicates a cyst or abscess of Bartholin's glands which could be due to gonorrheal infection. Palpation of these glands in the absence of an obvious swelling can reveal smaller lesions. Erythema, swelling, or discharge from the urinary meatus or from Skene's glands indicates an infection which could be gonorrheal. The urethra should be milked whether or not these signs are present, and any purulent discharge obtained from the urethra or Skene's ducts is highly suggestive of gonorrhea. A GC culture should be done on any discharge from these three structures. (See Chapter 9, Vaginal Discharge and Itching, for a description of the procedure for milking the urethra and palpating Bartholin's glands, and Figure 11-2).

INSPECTION OF THE VAGINA AND CERVIX. With speculum in place, the vaginal mucosa is examined for its appearance, discharge, and lesions. An erythematous mucosa, with considerable discharge present in the vault, is more suggestive of Candida or Trichomonas infection. Primary vaginal chancres are rare, but if they are present they appear as a light, whitish lesion or a soft, irregularly shaped sore which is flush with the adjacent mucosa. Cervical chancres are the most common site of spirochete invasion, but they are usually discovered by accident. It is often difficult to distinguish a chancre from other cervical lesions; syphilis should be suspected, however, when a cervical lesion is isolated from the os by an area of normal epithelium or when lesions do not respond to the usual treatment methods. Chancres usually disappear spontaneously within 3 to 5 weeks, complicating both the discovery and evaluation of the response to treatment. A discharge from the cervical os must be carefully evaluated. A yellow, purulent discharge is typical of gonorrheal cervicitis but is not commonly seen. Clear, mucoid or white discharge from the os is normal, but despite the appearance of the discharge a cervical culture is essential in the diagnosis of gonorrhea.

Any vaginal and cervical cultures indicated must be taken using an unlubricated speculum because most lubricant jellies contain bactericidal preparations, and the gonococcus, a fastidious organism, can be easily inhibited. Warm water or simply a warmed speculum is adequate. It is recommended that rectal cultures be taken to increase the yield of positive GC cultures.

BIMANUAL EXAMINATION. The cervix is palpated to discover if it is tender when moved, an indication of cervicitis or salpingitis. Palpation to determine the size and shape of the uterus may help to rule out pregnancy or uterine lesions. If the uterus is tender when compressed it indicates a possible endometritis, but a careful evaluation of the severity of the pain elicited is necessary. The adnexae are examined to discover any fullness, masses, or tenderness. Salpingitis may appear as a feeling of fullness, usually bilateral, but with no definable mass. Considerable tenderness should be elicited in an active infection. An adnexal mass may be a tubal ovarian abscess and should also be exquisitely tender. Other causes of adnexal masses, such as tubal pregnancy and ovarian tumors, must be kept in mind. In acute infections such as pelvic inflammatory disease, the adnexae are very difficult to evaluate due to pain and guarding of the abdominal muscles. Typical acute pelvic inflammatory disease appears as exquisitely tender bilateral adnexal masses which usually cannot be clearly delineated due to the pain; movement of the cervix also elicits pain. Chronic pelvic inflammatory disease is manifested by bilateral, usually irregular and fairly fixed adnexal masses which are also tender but not as pronounced as in an acute infection.

Ovarian cysts or tumors are more typically unilateral and nontender. An ectopic pregnancy is unilateral; its tenderness varies depending upon whether or not the tube has ruptured and on the extent of the distention. In a ruptured tubal pregnancy, there is marked pelvic tenderness, rigidity of the lower abdomen, and tenderness of the cervix when it is moved (see also Chapter 9, Vaginal Discharge and Itching, and Chapter 12, Lower Abdominal Pain). A rectovaginal examination is done to confirm the pelvic findings and to evaluate the adnexal masses further.

SKIN. When a venereal disease is suspected, the patient's skin should be examined, and she should be specifically asked about skin lesions. The rash of secondary syphilis is usually maculopapular and generalized, although lesions may also be papulosquamous and pustular (never vesicular or bulbous) and localized. Lesions on the palms and the soles of the feet are particularly suggestive. There is usually no itching associated with syphilitic skin rash. Disseminated gonorrhea is most often manifested by an arthritis-dermatitis syndrome, in which the skin lesions appear as isolated hemorrhagic, pustular or necrotic papules usually on the hands, arms, or legs. If these are seen, the patient should be questioned and examined for polyarthritis of the wrists, ankles, knees, hands, and feet.

PHARYNX. Particularly if a history of oral-genital intercourse is obtained, or if there are symptoms of sore throat, the pharynx should be examined and cultured for gonorrhea. Gonococcal pharyngitis appears as a beefy red posterior pharynx with purulent exudate from the tonsils if the tonsillar bed is involved. Because several species of the *Neisseria* genus other than gonococcus are common inhabitants of the oropharynx, the diagnosis of gonorrhea must be confirmed by sugar-fermentation tests.

GONORRHEA

Neisseria gonorrhoeae is an intracellular Gram-negative diplococcus which has flattened adjacent sides and resembles a pair of coffee beans. The organism can invade any mucosal surface in the body, but most commonly it invades the urethra in men and the endocervix, urethra, Skene's and Bartholin's ducts or glands in women. About 60 percent of all infected women will have rectal gonorrhea, whether by rectal coitus or from the drainage of infected vaginal secretions. Those who engage in oral-genital intercourse may develop gonococcal pharyngitis. Direct physical contact, usually sexual, is the method by which infection is spread in most cases, although indirect spread by instruments or linens is possible. The gonococcus is a delicate organism and is readily killed by drying, heat, and washing with an antiseptic solution; thus indirect spread is rare.

From 3 to 21 days after exposure, the gonococcus produces an endotoxin which causes redness and swelling at the site of contact. A purulent exudate often develops, with the potential for abscess formation. The disease process may remain localized or may spread by direct tissue extension, bloodstream invasion, or both. The most common method of spread is by direct extension through the endocervical canal to the endometrial cavity, fallopian tubes, and peritoneal cavity. This process is facilitated at the time of menstruation, when the endocervical canal becomes dilated, the mucous plug disintegrates, and the necrotic tissue and serum in the menstrual discharge encourages the growth of the organisms. Endometrial infection is usually transient, unless a recent delivery or surgical procedure has rendered the uterine cavity less resistant to infection. The organism spreads through the uterine opening of the fallopian tube, which is patent during menstruation, invading the mucosa of the tube and producing an exudate which often drains into the peritoneal cavity. Various degrees of pelvic peritonitis then result. If the disease progresses, the tubes may become thickened, edematous, and hyperemic, leading to their occlusion and inability to drain and producing abscess formation.

The key factors in the progression of gonorrheal infection are the virulence of the organism, the innate tissue resistance of the host, and the availability and adequacy of treatment. If the disease remains localized, the most common findings are urethritis, periurethral abscess, Bartholin's abscess, and cervicitis. A purulent, yellow discharge with signs of inflammation is classic, and the cervix is by far the most commonly involved structure. The vulva and vagina are not usually invaded unless the patient's resistance is lowered by a coexistent disease or debilitation, or there is little or no estrogen, as in prepubertal girls or postmenopausal women.

Most women who have gonorrhea, with estimates ranging from 60 to 90 percent, are either asymptomatic or have minor symptoms which are overlooked. A small number may complain of vaginal discharge, dysuria, or frequency. Bartholinitis is not common, and most Bartholin's abscesses are due to other organisms. Changes in menstruation may be a symptom, but are caused by so many other factors that women often disregard this symptom believing it to have no significance. Most gonorrhea is diagnosed by culture results or by a

history of contact with an infected sexual partner. Unless this happens, the disease may remain in a subclinical status, with the woman essentially a carrier who is capable of spreading the disease to her sexual partners. Or, the infection may progress to pelvic inflammatory disease (discussed in the next section).

A disseminated gonococcal infection is usually seen as the arthritis-dermatitis syndrome, occurring twice as often in women as in men and with 25 percent of all cases occurring during pregnancy or in the immediate postpartum period. The onset of symptoms is often during or immediately after a woman's menses, with sudden chills, high fever, and migratory polyarthralgia; or symptoms occur subacutely as joint stiffness, swelling, or tenderness. Usually two or more joints are involved, with tenosynovitis in over 75 percent of all cases. Skin lesions of the extremities, usually tender and sparse, often accompany the arthritis. Meningitis and endocarditis are rare but severe complications of gonococcal septicemia.

Diagnostic Tests

Cultures for gonorrhea are essential for confirming the diagnosis in women. If only a single site is to be cultured, the cervix should be selected because about 85 percent of infected patients will harbor organisms here. A culture of the rectum will increase the yield of confirmed gonococcal infections by 3 to 5 percent.[9] A routine culture of the urethra is rarely productive, without coexisting cervical disease; rarely is the urethra alone found to be positive. Discharge from the urethra, or ducts of Skene's or Bartholin's glands should, of course, be cultured. To obtain a good cervical culture, first carefully remove the mucous plug and discharge. Gently massage the cervix repeatedly between the blades of a bivalve speculum lubricated only with warm water. Insert a sterile cotton-tipped applicator well into the endocervical canal, allowing enough time for the swab to absorb any organisms present. Or, a small platinum loop can be used to collect the specimen. Streak the tip of the swab directly onto the culture medium and place it immediately in a candle jar or CO_2 incubator. Although the gonococcus is an aerobic organism, many strains require an atmosphere of 2 to 10 percent CO_2 to initiate growth and must be incubated at 35 to 36°C. A specific medium, the Thayer-Martin (TM) plate, which encourages the selective growth of the gonococcus and inhibits the growth of the usual vaginal and rectal contaminants has been developed. Plated and incubated properly, it yields about 85 to 90 percent accuracy in growing the gonococcus. If laboratory facilities are not readily available, a holding medium such as Transgrow or Clinicult can be used for up to 48 hours, then the specimen must be plated. The Transgrow bottle must be kept upright to prevent the escape of CO_2, and the swab must be kept away from the layer of water to avoid lysing the gonococci.

Rectal specimens must be carefully obtained in order to avoid as much contamination as possible. Taking a specimen from the anal crypts following a direct inspection with an anoscope or proctoscope is recommended. A TM plate is used for rectal and pharyngeal cultures also and should be appropriately labeled.

A Gram stain of cervical secretions is generally not recommended for women because of the several other vaginal organisms which resemble *Neisseria gonorrhoeae*, including the *Mimmina* group and other *Neisseria (N. sicca, N. subflava)* as well as staphylococci and streptococci. In men, the diagnosis of gonorrhea is confirmed by the presence of Gram-negative intracellular diplococci on a urethral smear; in women, cultures are always necessary to make the diagnosis. Treatment is instituted with a positive history of exposure, without awaiting culture results, and in the absence of any signs or symptoms.

Treatment and Follow-Up

The treatment of choice in uncomplicated cases of gonorrhea in both women and men is aqueous procaine penicillin G 4.8 million units IM, half in each buttock. It should be preceded within 30 minutes by 1 Gm. probenecid taken orally to elevate the serum levels of penicillin by decreasing its excretion in the urine. If oral therapy is preferred, use 3.5 Gm. ampicillin with 1 Gm. probenecid simultaneously. Long-acting penicillins, such as benzathine penicillin G, alone or in combination with short-acting forms, should not be used to treat gonorrhea because they do not produce the high blood levels required. A relative resistance has developed in some strains of gonorrhea to penicillin, and larger doses are now required for treatment than were needed a decade ago.

In cases of penicillin or probenecid sensitivity, oral tetracycline HCL 1.5 Gm. initially, followed by 0.5 Gm. four times a day for 4 days, is recommended for a total dose of 9.5 Gm. Because a number of substances prevent the absorption of tetracycline, advise the patient to take it with water on an empty stomach. The newer tetracyclines, doxycycline (Vibramycin) and minocycline (Minocin, Vectrin) are not noticeably affected by milk or foods.

If an injectable drug is desired for penicillin-sensitive patients, use spectinomycin HCL (Trobicin) 2 Gm. in a single IM injection. If the initial treatment with penicillin has failed, as evidenced by a positive second culture without the patient's being reexposed to gonorrhea, then spectinomycin is the preferred agent.

Pharyngeal gonorrhea may be more difficult to treat than anogenital; if 4.8 million units of aqueous procaine penicillin G with 1 Gm. probenecid fails to eradicate the infection, use tetracycline in the dosage described above. Ampicillin and spectinomycin in the doses described are ineffective against pharyngeal gonorrhea.

A VDRL should be done when gonorrhea is diagnosed, because incubating syphilis is present in 3 to 10 percent of all patients with gonorrhea. Treatment with 4.8 million units of penicillin IM will abort incubating syphilis, but ampicillin, tetracycline, and spectinomycin will not. If the VDRL is negative at this time and the patient is without clinical signs of syphilis, follow-up serological testing is not necessary if the treatment is by parenteral penicillin. If a drug other than penicillin is used, a follow-up VDRL should be done in 3 months to detect untreated syphilis.[10]

The woman should return for a second culture of the cervix and rectum 7 to 14 days following treatment. Informing her that cures on the first treatment are becoming increasingly difficult to obtain can reinforce the need for a follow-up visit. The woman's sexual partners also need treatment, whether symptomatic or not, and she must be advised to so inform them. Public health officials should be notified and communicable disease reports filled out.

PELVIC INFLAMMATORY DISEASE (PID)

Upper reproductive tract gonorrheal infection can involve the tubes, uterus, ovaries, and pelvic peritoneum; it is generally called salpingitis or pelvic inflammatory disease (PID) and may be acute or subacute. Pelvic inflammatory disease is the most common complication of gonorrhea, occurring in 10 to 17 percent of women who have this disease; it is directly or indirectly involved in almost one-fifth of all gynecological problems.[11] Acute PID presents with bilateral, sharp, cramping pain in the lower quadrants and adnexal tenderness during a pelvic examination. The history may reveal a purulent vaginal discharge which cleared up, irregular bleeding, a longer, heavier menstrual period, or a recent abortion or D and C. An elevated temperature of 102°F and nausea or vomiting indicate peritoneal involvement or abscess formation; a pelvic examination typically reveals an adnexal mass, abdominal rigidity, and extreme tenderness. An elevated sedimentation rate and white blood count support the diagnosis of an acute infection.

Subacute PID is less dramatic, with great variation in its severity and the extent of its symptoms. Chronic lower abdominal pain, dyspareunia, low-grade fever, menstrual irregularities, and urinary symptoms may be present. An examination may reveal adnexal masses, varying degrees of adnexal tenderness or fullness, and some pain when the cervix is moved. The findings may be minimal, however, and symptoms may be vague. In seeking objective data for the confirmation of PID, it must be remembered that only 40 percent of the patients who have gonococcal PID are febrile, about 60 percent have elevated white blood counts, and about 70 percent have elevated sedimentation rates.[12] In acute PID, with a hot abdomen, the diagnostic considerations must include ectopic pregnancy, septic abortion, appendicitis, urethral stones, ruptured diverticula, and other causes of an acute abdomen. Subacute PID suggests the possibility of urinary tract infection, ruptured ovarian cysts, appendicitis, endometriosis, and other uterine or tubal problems.

Cervical and rectal cultures for gonorrhea are necessary to establish the diagnosis. About 50 percent of the patients who have acute PID do have gonorrheal infections; other invading organisms causing a PID include bacteroides, *Streptococcus, Staphylococcus, Escherichia coli, Mycobacterium* tuberculosis, or even a fungus or parasite. Cervical cultures for causes of a nongonococcal PID are not generally done because reliable results can not be obtained. If

an examination reveals that fullness is present in the cul-de-sac, the patient should be referred for a culdocentesis; gonococci and other bacteria can often be aspirated to confirm the diagnosis.

Treatment and Follow-Up

The treatment for PID which can be managed on an outpatient basis includes: Aqueous procaine penicillin G 4.8 million units, half in each buttock, with 1 Gm. probenecid just before injection, followed with 0.5 Gm. oral ampicillin four times a day for 10 days. Or, ampicillin 3.5 Gm. orally together with 1 Gm. probenecid, followed with oral ampicillin 0.5 Gm. four times a day for 10 days. For penicillin-sensitive patients, use oral tetracycline HCL 1.5 Gm. as a loading dose, followed by 0.5 Gm. four times a day for 10 days. If the patient is pregnant, acutely ill, has findings suggestive of pelvic abscess, or fails to respond to treatment, she should be referred to the physician for possible hospitalization.

Follow-up syphilis screening and the treatment of sexual partners is the same as previously described for lower-tract gonorrhea. The residual effects of gonococcal PID are difficult to predict, but even with a first attack the potential for tubal scarring and adhesions, with subsequent infertility, exists. There is no immunity against reinfection, and successive attacks certainly increase the probability of permanently altered tubal function. Some inflammation may also be a residuum of PID, causing what some view as a chronic disease process. Others think that chronicity is not a feature of PID, and that symptoms are caused by reinfections rather than flare-ups.[13] Adhesions and scarring in the lower abdominal cavity, secondary to pelvic peritonitis are, however, probably a source of continuing discomfort and lower abdominal pain associated with "chronic PID."

SYPHILIS

Treponema pallidum is a spiral-shaped bacterium which is thin, translucent, and motile and has 6 to 14 regularly spaced corkscrewlike spirals. It belongs to a family of other spirochetes, some of which cause disease in humans and some of which do not. Humans are the only natural host of *T. pallidum*, although other mammals can be infected; rabbits have been used since 1912 to grow Nichol's strain of the organism, which is used for studies and to prepare specific antibody tests for syphilis. T. *pallidum* can invade mucosal surfaces and intact skin, and it is usually transmitted by sexual contact between moist mucous membranes. The organism is extremely fragile and is easily destroyed by heat, drying, soap, water, and chemicals. In addition to sexual contact, syphilis may be spread by contact with infectious lesions, blood transfusions if improper screening occurs, sharing of needles among drug addicts, and as congenital syphilis transmitted from an infected mother to the fetus in utero.

After invading the mucosa, T. *pallidum* spreads throughout the body via the blood within 24 hours, remaining without signs or symptoms for 10 to 60 days, the incubation period. Usually a chancre erupts within 2 to 3 weeks of exposure at the site of contact, ranging in size from a few mm. to approximately 2 cm., with varying appearances but usually having erosion or ulceration. While genital lesions are most frequent, chancres may also occur on the lips, mucosa of the mouth, tongue, nipple, or fingers. The lesion is usually painless and resolves spontaneously in 2 to 9 weeks. The only other sign may be painless, hard, nonfluctuant, enlarged inguinal lymph nodes. This is the primary stage of syphilis.

Symptoms of secondary syphilis usually begin 2 months after exposure, but may occur before the chancre disappears or many months later. A local or generalized, usually symmetrical, skin rash is the most common manifestation. Other reactions include a flulike syndrome of malaise, headache, fever, and anorexia; patchy alopecia, condylomata lata, (Figure 11-3) iritis, and mucous patches in the mouth. Secondary symptoms and signs usually last 2 to 6 weeks and disappear spontaneously, but may range from a few days to a year before resolving.

Syphilis then goes into a latent stage with no clinical manifestations, and an extremely wide range of outcomes. Some people may never have other effects, some may have benign later lesions, and still others progress to very destructive cardiovascular or neurosyphilis. The diagnosis in the latent stage is made by reactive serological tests after other possibilities have been ruled out. Latent syphilis is arbitrarily divided into two stages:

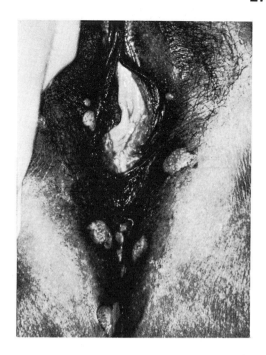

Figure 11-3. Condylomata lata of secondary syphilis.

early latent, which begins when secondary symptoms disappear and ends 1 to 4 years after the infection was contracted (up to 1 year is most significant for infectiousness), and late latent, which begins when it is decided that early latent ends. These stages are part of a continuum, and the person remains latent unless there are relapses of secondary symptoms or the disease progresses to late symptomatic stages.

Late or tertiary syphilis may occur 5, 10, or 30 years after the infection, or it may never develop. Benign lesions include gummas and nodular or ulcerative skin lesions. Destructive lesions can involve any body organ, causing inflammation, induration, necrosis and tissue destruction, scarring, and hyperpigmentation. The most common manifestations include saccular aneurysms (cardiovascular syphilis); neurosyphilis, causing central nervous system damage (blindness, psychosis); and parenchymal neurosyphilis, causing the paresis of tabes dorsalis.

Diagnostic Tests

The *darkfield examination* of exudate from a suspected chancre or rash can establish the diagnosis of primary or secondary syphilis. Using a compound microscope with a darkfield condenser, a drop of exudate placed on a slide is viewed under the oil immersion lens. The spirochete cannot be seen under direct light because it is translucent and cannot be stained with the usual dyes. The darkfield reflects light through the organism rather than directly on it, and if positive the spirochete can be seen undulating back and forth. If the patient has applied alcohol, Merthiolate, systemic or local antibiotics, or other local preparations, the surface spirochetes will have been destroyed. If findings are negative from a suspicious lesion, repeat the darkfield examination daily for 3 consecutive days; if still negative, follow-up with serological tests.

Serological tests are used to detect, confirm, and follow syphilis. Results will vary according to the stage of the disease. For the first week or so after the appearance of the chancre, serological tests (STS) will be negative as the antibody titer has not had time to rise sufficiently. The STS usually becomes positive 1 to 3 weeks after the chancre appears (4 to 6 weeks after the initial infection), and usually rises rapidly to high titer levels during secondary syphilis. If primary syphilis is treated, STS titers will almost always descend to nonreactive levels within 6 months. In secondary syphilis, blood titers are generally very high and remain so for several months after treatment, but in most cases they will become nonreactive within 2 years. In latent stages, titers often are low before treatment and change little afterward; people treated in these stages often remain seropositive for life.[14]

Serological tests for syphilis (STS) are based upon the presence of an antibody-like substance (called reagin) which is present in the serum shortly after the onset of the disease. The addition of a lipoidal antigen made from an extract of beef heart causes a reaction in syphilitic serum, resulting in precipitation (called flocculation) or in complement fixation. Complement is a lytic substance in normal serum that combines with antigen-antibody complex, producing lysis when the antigen is an intact cell. These nontreponemal antigen tests are not absolutely specific or sensitive for syphilis, but they are economical and practical, and their findings are highly indicative. The results of these tests are read qualitatively as reactive, weakly reactive, or nonreactive. If any reactivity is obtained, a quantitative test should be performed in which the serum is diluted geometrically until there is no longer a reaction. The *VDRL* (Venereal Disease Research Laboratory) reports reactivity at 2+, 3+, 4+, and so on; the *Kolmer, Kahn, Kline* or *Mazzini* serological tests report reactivity at dilutions of 1:1, 1:2, 1:4, 1:8, 1:16, 1:32, 1:64, and so forth until weakly reactive and nonreactive. A titer of 1:8 or below may indicate a false positive or the presence of syphilis. A second titer should be obtained, and a specific treponemal antigen test done. Titers of 1:32 or higher signify the presence of syphilis, and more specific testing is usually not necessary. Titers can be affected by antibiotic treatment, and there is an estimated 1 in 4000 biological false positives. False positives have also been reported with lupus, mononucleosis, hepatitis, malaria, rheumatic fever, pneumonia, and measles. It is also possible that false positives may be due to cancer, narcotics addiction, and pregnancy.

Treponemal tests detect the specific treponemal antibody and are more expensive and time-consuming than nontreponemal tests, thus are generally used to confirm the presence of syphilis when the latter are positive. The *treponema pallidum immobilization* test (TPI) uses a live virulent strain of the organism as an antigen. When combined with the patient's serum, the test spirochete becomes immobilized if specific treponemal antibodies are present. A more recent test currently used by most laboratories is the *fluorescent treponema antibody-absorption test (FTA-ABS)*, considered to be the most sensitive test to diagnose all stages of syphilis. Immunofluorescent techniques allow the identification of specific *T. pallidum* antibody after antibodies common for other treponemes are absorbed from the specimen. False positive reactions are rare. These test results are reported as reactive, weakly reactive, and nonreactive; there are positive reactions with these tests later in the disease than with other testing methods and the reactions remain positive long after treatment in many cases.

A *spinal tap* to rule out neurosyphilis is indicated if the disease is diagnosed after the secondary stage. Dosages for treatment of neurosyphilis are considerably higher, and the risk of serious complications is great if the disease is not properly treated. Many physicians perform spinal taps routinely 2 years after treatment, regardless of the stage in which syphilis was diagnosed, or on any patient whose titer remains positive 12 months after treatment.

Treatment and Follow-Up

The recommended treatment schedules for syphilis issued by the United States Public Health Service Center for Disease Control in Atlanta, Georgia in 1976 include the following:

Benzathine penicillin G 2.4 million units IM, half in each buttock; or

Aqueous procaine penicillin G 600,000 units IM daily for 8 days for a total of 4.8 million units; or if the patient is penicillin-sensitive

Tetracycline HCL 0.5 Gm. orally four times a day for 15 days; or erythromycin 0.5 Gm. orally four times a day for 15 days. These dosages are for primary, secondary, and latent syphilis of less than one year's duration.

For syphilis of more than one-year's duration, including latent syphilis of indeterminate duration, cardiovascular, late benign, and neurosyphilis:

Benzathine penicillin G 7.2 million units total, 2.4 million units IM weekly for 3 successive weeks; or aqueous procaine penicillin G 9 million units total, 600,000 units IM daily for 15 days. If the patient is sensitive to penicillin use tetracycline HCL 0.5 Gm. or erythromycin 0.5 Gm. orally four times a day for 30 days. However, there are no published clinical data which adequately document the effectiveness of drugs other than penicillin for syphilis of more than one year's duration.[15]

Patients with early syphilis should have repeated quantitative nontreponemal tests 3, 6, and 12 months after treatment. With syphilis of more than one year's duration, a repeat STS should be done 24 months after treatment. Neurosyphilis requires retesting yearly for at least 3 years. Retreatment of any patient should be considered when clinical signs or symptoms persist or recur, when there is a sustained fourfold increase in STS titer, or when an initially high STS titer fails to show a fourfold decrease within one year. Reinfection is always possible after treatment for early syphilis, but probably some immunity develops if the treatment is later. For patients treated with drugs other than penicillin, a spinal tap should be done at the last follow-up visit. The patient's sexual contacts should be elicited and treated, and a communicable disease report should be made to the public health department for epidemiological investigation.

Syphilis During Pregnancy

Congenital syphilis is transmitted by an infected mother to the fetus in utero, and despite antibiotics and prenatal care there were 1,932 infected infants born in 1972.[16] The treatment of the mother prior to the sixteenth week of pregnancy usually prevents congenital syphilis, presumably because the spirochete cannot cross the placental barrier before this time. Treatment later in pregnancy will eradicate the infection but may not prevent damage to the fetus, which could include uneven spacing of teeth, osteochondritis of the long bones, hydrarthrosis of the joints, blindness, deafness, and facial scars from infected nasal discharge after birth. Higher rates of abortion, stillbirth, and neonatal death are associated with syphilis in pregnancy. Women with a positive STS should have confirmatory treponemal tests, and if the tests are positive or equivocal they should be treated at once. The treatment of choice for pregnant women with primary, secondary, and latent syphilis with normal spinal fluid is benzathine penicillin G 2.4 million units IM. If a spinal tap is positive or not done, the larger doses for neurosyphilis are given. A pregnant woman with a penicillin allergy presents a difficult treatment situation, and consultation should be sought. Because a woman with a nonreactive VRDL in the first trimester may be incubating syphilis, and because the infection can be contracted after testing, a repeat STS in the third trimester is indicated for high risk women.

HERPES GENITALIS

Genital herpesvirus infections have been steadily increasing over the last several years, and it is the second most common venereal disease (after gonorrhea) among women seen in VD clinics.[17] Herpes simplex virus type 2 is believed to be responsible for most genital lesions, and herpes type 1 for most lesions occurring above the waist; however, there is some crossover, with about 14 percent of the patients seen in private practice having herpes type 1 infections involving the genitals. The herpes virus can be transmitted by sexual contact, and it is apparent that many infections are subclinical or asymptomatic, in the range of 45 percent. Persons with prior extragenital herpes type 1 infections (fever blisters, cold sores) may have some degree of protection from type 2 infections through their formation of heterologous antibodies, which could account for their having only mild or asymptomatic primary type 2 infections.

Primary herpetic genital infections are usually more severe than recurrent ones and are most often seen in teenagers and young adults. Within 3 to 7 days of exposure there may be constitutional symptoms of fever, malaise, or anorexia, with mild paresthesia and burning or tingling in the genital area preceding the eruption of lesions. The labia minora or majora, perianal skin, vestibule, or vaginal or cervical mucosa may be involved in primary herpes (Figure 11-4). Vesicles appear early but rupture quickly to form shallow, painful ulcers that may cover extensive areas of the vulva and perianal skin. Erythema and induration are often present, and the vulvovaginal ulcers tend to coalesce and become covered with a grey-yellow exudate. Lesions on the buttocks and perineum are more typically vesicular, while those on the cervix vary from diffuse inflammation to multiple tiny superficial ulcers or occasionally a single large necrotic ulcer. With the appearance of the lesions there is severe vulvar pain and exquisite tenderness, a watery discharge, and often inguinal lymphadenopathy. Severe dysuria or retention is occasionally seen, probably due to herpes lesions in the urethra and bladder.[18] The primary lesions persist from 3 to 6 weeks, then heal spontaneously with no residual scarring or ulceration.

Recurrent herpes is a milder infection involving the same sites which can be affected by primary herpes. One to 5 mm. lesions with an erythematous base develop in localized patches, progress from vesicular to ulcerative stage in 1 or 2 days, and resolve completely in 7 to 10 days. Not all women with primary herpes infections will have recurrences; the cause of recurrences is unknown, but they are precipitated by temperature elevation, emotional disturbances, premenstrual tension, and systemic disease. The herpesvirus is probably harbored in the dorsal nerve root ganglia that receive sensory fibers from genital tissues, and migrates down the nerve fibers to the areas of eruption when the infection recurs. There are few immediate complications of herpes infections, which resolve completely unless they become secondarily infected. The severe pain and the recurrence of infections are the most important parts of the woman's experience as they cause a disruption in her usual activities and signify to her the malfunctioning of her body. Herpes does have serious implications for pregnancy, and it has a suggestive relation to cervical carcinoma, as discussed below.

Diagnostic Tests

The simplest method of confirming the diagnosis of herpes genitalis is with the *Tzanck test*. One of the genital lesions is ruptured and scrapings taken from the base of the ulcer are placed on a slide and fixed with absolute or methyl alcohol for 10 minutes and stained with Giemsa's or Wright's solutions. Typical findings microscopically are giant multinucleated cells or acidophilic intranuclear inclusion bodies. *Virologic cultures* also can be used to confirm herpes if they are available. Specimens are taken with cotton-tipped applicators from the base of ulcerated lesions, placed in special virologic culture medium (Eagle's medium with 5 percent calves' serum), and taken quickly to the laboratory. The virus grows on special culture media, producing typical plaques. *Blood testing* may also be done to detect a rise in the serum titer of antibody against herpes simplex virus type 2. In common practice, however, the diagnosis is usually based upon the clinical appearance of the lesions, with typical symptoms and history.

Treatment

There is no curative treatment of herpes, and therapy is aimed at symptom relief primarily. The topical application of steroid creams, antihistamines such as Benadryl, alcohol, ether, camphor, or dilute Betadine solution have been used with varying results. Sitz baths, compresses of Burow's solution or boric acid solution, and analgesics may provide some pain relief. Viscous lidocaine (Xylocaine) 2 percent applied to lesions every 3 or 4 hours exerts a local anesthetic pain-relieving effect. Idoxuridine (Stoxil), an antiviral agent used topically to treat herpes type 1 infections of the eyelids, conjunctiva, and cornea, has been used for genital herpes with some reports of relief. Herpes genitalis is not, however, an FDA-approved indication for idoxuridine.

Photoinactivation of the virus with a tricyclic dye (neutral red or proflavine dihydrochloride) reduces pain almost immediately and possibly shortens the attack, but this treatment is now controversial due to concern about its carcinogenicity. After the vesicles are denuded, the dye solution is applied to the lesions for several minutes, followed by exposure to white fluorescent or incandescent light for 15 minutes. Patients are then advised to repeat the light exposure 4 hours later, or 3 or 4 times during the next 24 hours. In severe infections, the dye/light procedure can be repeated every 3 or 4 days. When the herpesvirus incorporates these dyes, it becomes extremely sensitive to light, which inactivates it. In vitro tests showed, however, that although replication of the virus was inhibited by this technique, sufficient genetic information remained to cause cell transformation. These transformed cells also had a loss of contact inhibition, a property associated with malignant potential.[19] In an untreated infection, defective virus particles are produced along with normal infective virions, and these defective particles are themselves suspected of being carcinogenic. Thus a prolonged herpes infection could produce a large number of potentially dangerous defective virus particles, while inactivating the virus with photodynamic therapy might also leave behind virus particles capable of cell transformation. In the case of severe, debilitating herpes genitalis the relief of pain and the shortening of the disease process might be worth the risk to the woman. As data are inconclusive, with fully informed consent on the patient's part, some physicians proceed with photodynamic inactivation.[20]

Herpes During Pregnancy

If a genital herpes infection occurs prior to the twentieth week of pregnancy, the result is spontaneous abortion in about half of these gestations. If the infection occurs after the twentieth week, there is a significantly increased risk of prematurity. After 32 weeks, there is a 60 percent risk of neonatal herpes if the infant is delivered vaginally or by cesarean section more than 4 hours after the rupture of the membranes. Herpes in the newborn infant is a serious disease which is frequently fatal or leaves the infant with severe brain damage. In addition, several congenital anomalies have been associated with maternal herpetic infection, including microcephaly, intracranial calcifications, microophthalmia, retinal dyspla-

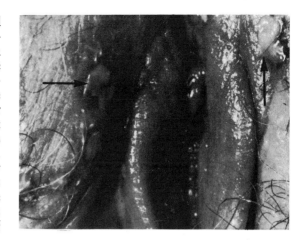

Figure 11-4. Herpes genitalis of the labia.

sia, chorioretinitis, diffuse brain damage, and mental retardation. Neonatal herpes may be disseminated, localized, or asymptomatic at birth, and although the prognosis for each is not well known, it presently appears that about one-half of all infected infants either die or have serious neurologic or ocular complications.[21]

Herpes infections during pregnancy are thought to be transmitted to the fetus through direct contact with infected maternal tissues during vaginal delivery, ascending infection following the rupture of the membranes, and via the maternal bloodstream through the placenta to the fetal circulation. Cesarean section is often recommended for the woman with genital herpes lesions in the third trimester, but some physicians prefer to do amniotic fluid analysis for herpesvirus before operating. If the virus can be demonstrated to be present in the amniotic fluid, the fetus is already infected and cesarean section is pointless. Also, if more than 4 hours have elapsed since the rupture of the membranes, the incidence of ascendant infection increases significantly and cesarean section is usually not done. If herpes during pregnancy does not occur near term, vaginal delivery would probably be safe 1 or 2 weeks after a recurrent infection, but in a primary infection viral particles continue to be shed for 2 or 3 months.

Herpes and Cancer

Three areas of research seem to link herpesvirus type 2 with cervical cancer, although the

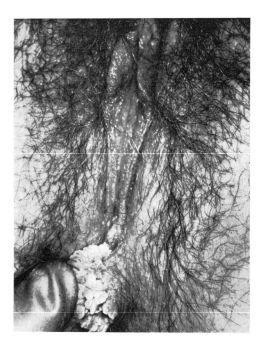

Figure 11-5. Condylomata acuminata of the perineum and lower labia.

evidence is still circumstantial. A number of serologic studies have shown that 80 to 100 percent of the patients who have invasive cervical cancer have antibodies to herpes type 2.[22] Significantly more women with cervical dysplasia and carcinoma in situ, compared to controls, also have these antibodies. The second area, epidemiological studies, has shown a relation between high herpes antibody titers and both early onset of sexual relations and multiple sexual partners. High titers are also correlated with cervical cancer, and cancer is correlated with early sexual relations and multiple partners. In the third area of research, viral nucleic acids and proteins have been recovered from patients with carcinoma in situ and invasive carcinoma. The herpesvirus is also used to transform cells in culture, and has been seen to be virulent in vitro.

The cervix of the young woman after puberty, and during and shortly after the first pregnancy, is thought to be particularly susceptible to potentially carcinogenic insult. The enormous amount of cell activity taking place in the squamous metaplasia which is typical of these events, and the relatively lower immunocompetence of the younger person or the

modification of immune responses during pregnancy may set up conditions where there are susceptible host cells and less effective immune defenses. If the young woman is sexually active during these times, the set of conditions possibly leading to cancer 15 to 20 years later may be initiated.[23]

CONDYLOMATA ACUMINATA

Venereal warts are wart papillomata of the genitalia believed to be caused by the epidermatrophic virus responsible for the common wart. Condylomata appear as pale, irregular clusters of raised fleshy lesions on the labia, perineum, or perianal skin. They appear first as small, discrete papillary structures which often spread and enlarge, coalescing to form cauliflowerlike masses with broad bases (Figure 11–5). The warts are usually painless unless they become secondarily infected or are irritated by friction. Associated vaginal infections such as Candida or Trichomonas may be present, contributing to the irritation. If large or extensive enough, condylomata can make intercourse painful or interfere with vaginal delivery. Venereal warts are sexually transmitted, although individual susceptibility varies. They are persistent once developed and require frequent retreatment to effect their clearing. There probably is an increasing incidence of venereal warts, as is the case with herpes genitalis, and it is a common problem encountered in primary care.

Treatment

Concurrent vaginal infections should be treated as indicated. For small lesions, the application of 20 percent podophyllin in tincture of benzoin is usually effective. The solution is applied with a cotton-tipped applicator, or the wooden stick portion can be broken and the irregular ends used to soak small amounts of the solution and apply it precisely to the warts. Podophyllin causes a blanching of the warts within a few hours and sloughing in 2 to 4 days. The patient must be instructed to wash off the podophyllin with soap and water 4 to 6 hours after its application, or the chemicals may burn the surrounding and underlying skin. Repeated applications about 1 week apart may be needed until all the lesions have been removed. Trichloroacetic acid is also effective in eradicating isolated lesions. Warts over 2 cm.

diameter can be removed by cryocautery, using liquid nitrogen with an applicator or gun. The wart should be frozen until completely white; repeated freezings may also be needed. Extensive venereal warts should be referred for surgical excision or removal with an electric cutting loop.

PEDICULOSIS PUBIS

Crab lice are insects that infect the hair-bearing area of the genitals, though the eyebrows, axillary hair, and hairs on the back of the head may also be infested. The main symptom is pubic itching, which can be quite severe. The patient may notice tiny red specks of blood on her underclothing. The lice can be seen by a close examination of pubic hair, appearing as red, dark brown, or grayish dots, 1 to 2 mm. in size, at the base of pubic hairs attached to the skin. Feeling the pubic hairs helps detect the presence of eggs, or nits, which attach themselves to the hairs and make them feel bumpy or irregular. A magnifying glass facilitates seeing the parasites and eggs, and if placed on a slide they can also be examined under the microscope. If skin lesions are present they are minute, inflamed maculopapules, often with crusts. Scratching may cause excoriation and lichenification. The transfer of crab lice is primarily by direct contact, such as person-to-person, bed linen-to-person, or toilet-seat-to-person. The louse is relatively hardy and can survive apart from the host for 1 week to 10 days in the active form and about a month as ova.

Treatment

Gamma benzene hexachloride (Kwell) 1 percent is the standard treatment for pubic lice as for all other lice and scabies infestations. It is effective for eggs as well as lice. Kwell lotion or shampoo is applied to the pubic, perineal, axillary hair after moistening with water, worked into a lather, and allowed to remain for 5 minutes. It is then rinsed thoroughly, repeated in 24 hours, and again in 4 or 5 days if necessary. Linens and clothing are washed in hot water; woolens are dry cleaned. Stressing the importance of washing bedding, linens, and clothes can prevent reinfection.

Venereal diseases are basically no different from other communicable diseases transferred by direct human contact or close proximity, except in their site of invasion and selection of target organs. The outcomes of these infections range from mild and annoying to serious and life-threatening. The eradication or control of all types of communicable infections is a goal of health care, but it is essential for the public to assume major responsibility if control is to be achieved. Responsibility does not imply any particular brand of morality; instead it means the individual's obligation to be informed, to exhibit concern for other persons, and to take action rationally in a situation of risk. Health providers have the additional responsibility of making available the knowledge which enables the individual to act responsibly, a task which is most effectively accomplished through a nonjudgmental approach.

NOTES

1. B. M. Morton, *VD: A Guide for Nurses and Counselors* (Boston: Little, Brown, 1976), pp. 3–4.
2. E. Z. Friedenberg, a review of Theodore Rosebury's *Microbes and Morals: The Strange Story of Venereal Diseases* (Viking, 1971) in *New York Review of Books* 30 December 1971.
3. "Are Your VD Regimens Adequate?" *Current Prescribing* (May 1976): 71-79.
4. W. J. Brown, et al., *Syphilis and Other Venereal Diseases* (Cambridge: Harvard University Press, 1973), pp. 42-44.
5. S. L. Romney, et al., eds., *Gynecology and Obstetrics: The Health Care of Women* (McGraw-Hill, Blakiston, 1975), p. 569.
6. E. C. Pierson and W. V. D'Antonio, *Female and Male: Dimensions of Human Sexuality* (Philadelphia: J. B. Lippincott, 1974), pp. 110-24.
7. "Gonorrhea Infection: Discussing Complications." *Contemporary OB/GYN* 5 (May 1975): 36-48.
8. *Ibid.*
9. "Are Your VD Regimens Adequate?," pp. 71-79.
10. "Update: Keeping Up with Gonorrhea Guidelines." *Patient Care* IX 2 (January 15, 1975): 72-87.
11. M. A. Krupp and M. J. Chatton, *Current Medical Diagnosis and Treatment.* (Los Altos, Calif.: Lange Medical Publications, 1974), pp. 421-22.
12. "Gonorrhea Infection," pp. 36-48.
13. "Cooling Down Pelvic Inflammation." *Patient Care* VIII, 21 (December 1, 1974): 90-99.
14. Brown, *Syphilis*, p. 28.
15. "Syphilis: Recommended Treatment Schedules, 1976." *American Family Physician* (September 1976): 119-21.
16. Morton, *VD: A Guide*, p. 25.
17. A. W. Chow, "Genital Infection with Type 2 Herpes Simplex Virus." *Postgraduate Medicine* 58,2 (August 1975): 66-70.
18. "Symposium Herpesvirus Infection of the Genital Tract." *Contemporary OB/GYN* 6 (July 1975): 116-40.

19. F. Rapp, J. L. Li, and M. Jerkofsky, "Transformation of Mammalian Cells by DNA-Containing Viruses Following Photodynamic Inactivation." *Virology* 55 (1973): 339.

20. "Symposium," pp. 132–5.

21. A. J. Nahmias, W. E. Josey, and Z.M. Naib, "Significance of Herpes Simplex Virus Infection During Pregnancy." *Clinical Obstetrics and Gynecology* 15,4 (December 1972): 929-38.

22. "Managing the Rising Risk of Herpes Genitalis." *Patient Care* VIII, 19 (November 1, 1974): 140-53.

23. "Symposium," pp. 124-26.

12

Lower Abdominal Pain

The presenting problem of lower abdominal pain is a common one in primary ambulatory care. It is estimated that functional pelvic pain, not associated with any organic cause, occurs in 5 to 25 percent of all gynecological patients.[1] Lower abdominal pain is a difficult symptom to evaluate because of the many organs which could be the site of painful stimuli and because of the subjective nature of pain. Many physiologic functions of the bowels and female reproductive organs may occasionally be accompanied by varying degrees of discomfort. Structural stresses on muscles, bones, joints, and ligaments due to the accommodation of the human to bipedal ambulation and the many daily demands placed upon these parts of the anatomy contribute their share to aches and pains. Discomfort in its varying degrees and pain in its many shades provoke highly individual responses to their implications and a wide range in patients' level of tolerance. Objective attempts to confirm the severity of the pain are notoriously unreliable because patients' responses to palpation and percussion are influenced by anxiety, fear, dislike of being examined, tension, attitudes toward their bodies, attitudes toward health care, their relation with the provider, events immediately preceding the examination, and a multitude of other things, as well as the actual pain elicited.

Although functional problems constitute a significant proportion of complaints related to lower abdominal pain, many organic causes may also be involved, ranging from infections to malignant neoplasms. Because this symptom may herald serious disease, women with lower abdominal pain require a careful and thorough diagnostic work-up. Even the patient with a long history of psychogenic pain can develop pathology. A determination of the cause of lower abdominal pain, as much as can reasonably be established, is thus an important goal for both health provider and patient. When no pathology can be identified, an explanation of the likely physiological processes underlying the pain stimuli may be an important therapeutic tool in assisting the woman to live with her discomforts. If pathology is found, the decision of the health provider to treat the problem or to refer the patient to a doctor depends upon the nature of the disease and the individual provider's ability to provide the care needed.

MEANINGS FOR WOMEN

Pain associated with the reproductive organs has many implications for feminine identity. Pain is a warning, a sign of danger within the body, a sign that something is wrong. When pain is located in the lower abdominal area, women generally associate it with the uterus, tubes, and ovaries because their pelvic location is common knowledge. Many women are not aware of the other organs and structures which could be involved, and the similarity of painful sensations arising from lower abdominal and pelvic structures further complicates the picture. The pain experience crosses over any boundaries which may have been created through the person's psychic organization between the body and the mind. Psychic energy may be discharged through such mechanisms as conversion, displacement, symbolization, and guilt expressed through pain. Thus pain may be experienced unconsciously as punishment, a symbol of rejection, an expression of trauma, or a plea for help.

Often pain is experienced as a threat to the self-concept or body image, which produces an emotional reaction that profoundly affects the pain response. The phenomenon of pain helps the organism to maintain its integrity, and threats to this integrity have emotional implications. The person will fantasize about the cause and meaning of her pain and may use defenses against implied threats. Whether physical or emotional, pain has a paralyzing effect upon the person's ability to function and can disable personalities of great strength. It may be easier for a person to tolerate physical suffering than the mental anguish of facing underlying emotional conflicts. Bodily pain, once experienced, opens the way for its substitution for mental pain; thus it may be used to symbolize anger, fear, sexual desire, or guilt. There is also a psychological type of anticipatory pain which includes the associated ideas, expectations, and fears that accompany the sensory perceptions initiated by painful impulses. This type of pain may become indistinguishable from the original pain.

Sociocultural factors also affect pain response according to the specific meanings and values assigned to pain. Cultural norms are a major conditioning influence in the formation of individual patterns of reaction to pain. There are moral and religious meanings attached to pain, prescribed reaction patterns, and positive or negative values, depending upon whether the particular experience of pain is seen as having an affirmative or detrimental effect upon the welfare of the group. Pain in certain parts of the body is often more culturally acceptable and brings more sympathy than pain in other parts.

Pain defies definition for it is a personal and subjective experience, a sensation of hurt. Its expression may be minimal or dramatic, involving physiological, verbal, vocal, facial, body movement, and physical contact behavior. The pain experience encompasses all the person's sensations, feelings, and behavioral responses, and it has three phases: anticipation, presence, and aftermath. Essentially the definition of pain must be whatever the person experiencing it says it is and must exist whenever she says it does.[2]

PHYSIOLOGICAL CONSIDERATIONS

It is not usual to think of pain as a normal concomitant of living, but this sensation is often a part of the daily experiences of otherwise healthy persons. There are thousands of explainable or elusive pains occurring among all age groups which tend to disappear as rapidly as they come, or which persist just below the threshold of real discomfort. For instance, there is the sudden hard pain over an eye, in the temporal region, or in the ear or jaw which lasts only a moment; the fleeting precordial discomfort which raises the specter of heart disease; the breath-taking catch in the side or lower abdomen; the persistent ache or sharp darting pain in a muscular area of the arm, leg, neck, or back; the meandering abdominal pains with intestinal rumbling; the dull lower abdominal ache with sensations of fullness and pressure; the brief discomfort at the movement of a joint. These are all normal pains, due to transitory conditions in the organ or structure, a part or a result of the physiological functions taking place.

These normal pains may be brought up during the history if they are elicited by a health questionnaire, in the review of systems, or when presented as a complaint by a worried patient. Emotional states which result from coping with stress, fear, conflict, anxiety, or depression, predispose some persons to exaggerate or focus more attention on minor aches and pains. Or, periodic recurrence of a pain may prompt the person to seek care primarily for reassurance that the pain is not pathological. Many pains will always remain unexplained, but it is hoped that the characteristics of pain which signify organic illness can be identified or ruled out—if not on one visit, then by observation over time.

The lower abdomen contains numerous organs and structures which are potential sites for both physiological and pathological pain. The bowel is a leading source of pain, with the *cecum* and *appendix* in the right lower quadrant, a portion of the *ascending colon* just above these, and the *descending* and *sigmoid colon* in the left lower quadrant. The *rectum*, *anus*, and *perianal area* can also be involved. Attached to all this bowel is the *mesentery*, itself supplied with vessels and nerves and subject to painful stimuli. The *ilium* of the small intestine also occupies the lower abdomen, with many loops and twists.

The female reproductive organs are frequent sites of pelvic and lower abdominal pain. The *uterus* is related to pain in the suprapubic and deep midline portions, the *fallopian tubes* and *ovaries* to pain in the right and left adnexae; and the location of pain in their several supportive ligaments, particularly the *round* and *broad ligaments*, extending to the pelvic peritoneum is variously perceived. *Vaginal, labial,* and *perineal* pain tends to be perceived more superficially, although this pain may be referred.

Genitourinary structures located in the lower abdomen include the *bladder*, just anterior to the uterus in the pelvis, which often gives rise to suprapubic pain; the *ureters*, which descend from the kidneys through the left and right lower quadrants to join the bladder; and the *urethra*, which may cause deep pelvic or superficial sensations. In rare persons, a *kidney* may be misplaced into the pelvis; but the kidneys are usually upper abdominal organs.

In addition, there is the *muscular abdominal wall* of the lower quadrants and pelvic sling; the parietal and visceral *peritoneum*; the *bones* of the pelvis, sacrum and coccyx; and the many *blood vessels, lymphatics,* and *nerves* supplying all these organs and structures (Figure 12-1).

Pain Receptors and Pathways

Pain receptors in the skin and deep structures are fine, freely branching nerve endings which form an intricate network. The cutaneous areas supplied by peripheral branches of each neuron are several square millimeters in size, with an overlap between neurons so that every spot of skin is within the domain of 2 to 4 sensory neurons. This network permits extremely accurate sensing of the location of pain stimuli on the skin. Free nerve endings are also found in other specialized sensory receptors in the skin, such as Krause's end-bulbs, ruffinian plumes, and pacinian corpuscles; these receptors probably account for the sensation of the extremes of heat, cold, and pressure being felt as pain. The skin is also sensitive to painful stimuli arising from pricking, cutting, and burning.

In contrast to the closely distributed and overlapping nerve endings in the skin, the vis-

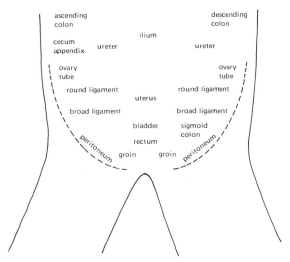

Figure 12-1. Structures of the lower abdomen.

cera and deep skeletal structures have relatively sparsely occurring sensory endings. The locus of pain in these structures is poorly perceived, and its borders are not clearly delineated. It is perceived as being deep—that is, not close to the skin—and it is usually dull, aching, or burning in quality. Visceral pain is produced by inflammation, distention or spasm, and traction upon mesenteric attachments. Pains from viscera and deep skeletal structures have common sensory pathways and are essentially the same in character and behavior.

Sensory nerve fibers from lower abdominal structures course through somatic and visceral nerves, where they mix with motor fibers and are transmitted into the posterior horn of the spinal cord at levels from L1 through T9. The secondary sensory neurons cross to the opposite side of the spinal cord within 1 or 2 segments, combining to form the lateral spinothalamic tract, which terminates in the posterolateral nucleus of the thalamus. From there the third sensory neuron conveys the impulse to the cortex, at which point there is a conscious awareness of the pain stimulus. The threshold for the perception of pain is defined as the lowest intensity of stimulus which can be recognized as pain, and it is approximately the same constitutionally in all persons. The inflammation of peripheral nerve endings lowers the pain threshold; local anesthetics, peripheral and central nervous system (CNS) lesions, analgesics, distraction, and suggestion raise the pain threshold. The concept that some persons have a "lower pain threshold" is misleading; rather, their reaction to a painful stimulus is excessive or exaggerated compared to the average person's response.

The most important characteristics of deep pain (visceral, deep skeletal) are its imprecise segmental localization beneath the surface of the body and the frequent occurrence of referred pain to particular areas. Centrally, the deep tissues supplied by a given cord segment have only a general representation. Impulses received in the brain from a viscus or a deep somatic tissue would create similar sensory impressions, and would be localized over a general sphere without precise margins. The pain is recognized and perceived as having its locus roughly in any or all structures innervated by cord segments subserving the structure affected. The pain also appears to be projected toward the body surfaces supplied by these segments, naturally enough, as these superficial areas habitually provide sensory impressions due to their much finer innervation. Referred pain is an integral part of the phenomenon of visceral pain. In most cases, the location of referred pain is perceived in the parts of the body which are supplied by the cord segment of the viscera involved. Because of the uneven inhibitory effects on large and small afferent pain fibers within any given segment of the cord, however, visceral pain sometimes overflows to excite areas completely unrelated to the known innervation of the viscus. One example of this phenomenon is the appearance of anginal pain in the jaw. An unusually intense pain tends to spread beyond the cord segment serving the involved viscera. Also, pain may extend outside normal boundaries when abnormalities exist in structures innervated through nearby cord segments. For example, patients with gallbladder disease often have epigastric pain with a myocardial infarction. Why pain radiates to a previously diseased area is not understood. Because of the possibility of a summation effect of stimuli, visceral pains overflowing into neighboring cord segments tend to wander into higher rather than lower segments.[3] Figure 12-2 shows skin areas to which pain in various organs is referred.

The sensory stimulus of pain has several characteristics which are not shared by the other sensory stimuli. Pain does not appear to be subject to negative adaptation or extinction, while most other stimuli will become ineffective if applied continuously, or else an increase in intensity is necessary to produce excitation. Pain usually persists as long as the stimulus continues and may even outlast the stimulus by establishing a central excitatory state. It is accompanied by a strong negative feeling tone or affect which is perceived almost universally as unpleasant. When severe enough, it supercedes all other drives or needs and can become an obsessional focus of attention. Unlike other sensory stimuli, pain often causes involuntary spasms in the skeletal muscles that are supplied by the same or adjacent segments of the spinal cord. In chronically painful states, the affected part is unusually sensitive to all stimuli, even those normally not considered painful or unpleasant. The pain elicited is unnatural, outlasts the stimulus, radiates, and is modified by emotional states, fatigue, certain activities, and other conditions.

Functional Causes of Lower Abdominal Pain

MITTELSCHMERZ.   Cyclic lower abdominal pain occurs in many women in association with ovulation. The mechanism of this pain is thought to be related to the increased intrafollicular pressure prior to rupture, or to the release of small amounts of follicular fluid or blood into the peritoneal cavity, causing a localized chemical peritonitis. The discomfort usually comes on fairly rapidly, lasts from a few hours to a day, and affects the right lower quadrant more often than the left. It may be sharp initially but is generally dull and constant, with a sense of fullness or pressure. Straining or coughing tends to accentuate the pain; pressure applied over the lower quadrant affords some relief. This pain is rarely severe or incapacitating and resolves spontaneously. Its most characteristic aspects are its occurrence in midcycle, about halfway between menses, its short duration and relatively mild intensity, and an associated light pinkish vaginal discharge of 1 to 2 days' duration. Not all women experience mittelschmerz, and of those who do, it is not invariably a monthly phenomenon. Some women note alternating quadrant pain, others have pain predominantly in the same quadrant. The light pink discharge, called mittelstaining, occurs variously among women and in the same woman. Right-sided mittelschmerz has been confused with appendici-

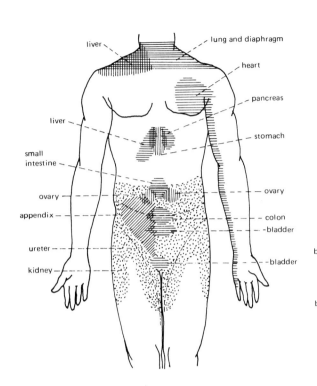

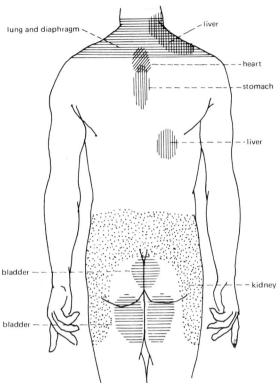

Figure 12-2. Skin areas of referred pain from various organs.

tis because both cause localized peritonitis, giving rise to signs and symptoms which they share.

PELVIC CONGESTION AND DYSMENORRHEA. Premenstrually, many women experience a type of pelvic and lower abdominal discomfort which is dull and aching in character, with associated sensations of fullness, bloating, pressure, and achiness in the perineum, upper thighs, and lower back. Termed pelvic congestion, this discomfort is also cyclic and occurs 7 to 10 days before a menstrual period. There is often a complex of associated symptoms including constipation, diarrhea, gas, cramping, headache, irritability, or depression. The symptoms are worse just prior to the onset of menses, and they gradually subside after the flow starts. Pelvic congestion tends to be a regular occurrence among women subject to it, and discomfort usually is more severe in the later reproductive years.

Dysmenorrhea, painful menstruation, is an obvious cause of pelvic and lower abdominal pain. While the diagnosis is easy to make, the etiology is difficult to establish unless there is some demonstrable pelvic abnormality such as uterine fibroids, cervical stenosis, endometriosis, or a chronic pelvic inflammatory disease. Primary or functional dysmenorrhea has no identifiable organic cause. The pain ranges from mild to severe and incapacitating, and the pattern and character differ, depending upon whether the woman experiences spasmodic or congestive primary dysmenorrhea. Premenstrual syndromes and dysmenorrhea are discussed more fully in Chapter 4, Menstrual Problems.

GAS, CONSTIPATION, AND DIARRHEA. The distention and spasm of a hollow viscus account for innumerable episodes of lower abdominal pain. Virtually everyone has experienced the sharp, shooting pain of momentarily trapped flatus; sometimes intense enough to take away the breath. Typically this type of pain comes on suddenly, reaches maximum intensity rapidly, and decreases or disappears after a short time. People readily recognize the grumblings and rumblings of the bowel which accompany gas and often can feel the movement of gas bubbles across the abdomen. A change in position, belching, or passing flatus usually relieves gas pains. Constipation may be associated with gas, and there is frequently a sensation of fullness and pressure in the lower abdomen and pelvis. Cramping, colicky pain which rises quickly to a high pitch then subsides, only to occur again shortly, is typical of bowel spasm accompanying both constipation and diarrhea. A bowel movement relieves the pain, at least temporarily. Severe diarrhea can cause very intense pain, perceived as deep and widespread within the lower abdomen. Bowel spasm can cause people to double over with pain, or thrash about desperately in purposeless movement. Not uncommonly, a constant lower grade ache may persist between severe spasm, probably in part due to bowel inflammation or edema associated with the cause of the diarrhea.

The gastrointestinal system is highly responsive to emotional influences, as evidenced by the frequency of gastritis, ulcers, functional diarrhea and constipation, and spastic colitis. Usually persons with functional bowel problems are eventually properly diagnosed and come to recognize the emotional components of their regularly occurring discomfort, although they may undergo numerous tests and occasional surgery in the process. Informed of their "irritable bowel syndrome," they often seek ways to avoid triggering the colicky, cramping pain by altering their diet, taking medication, or dealing in some way with the underlying tensions and stresses.

DEEP SKELETAL MUSCLE AND LIGAMENT STRAIN. The muscles and ligaments of the sacral and lumbar spine, the pelvic bones, the ligaments of the uterus and ovaries, and the muscles of the pelvic sling and lower abdominal wall are all subject to strains and minor traumas having to do with activity and positional changes. Pain originating from these structures is very similar to visceral pain, and often the person cannot distinguish the real source. The sharp, sudden one-sided lower abdominal pain women not infrequently experience upon running some distance probably is

related to a strain of the uterine or ovarian ligaments, or to traction on their supporting mesentery. A strain of the right lower rectus muscle may produce constant dull aching right lower quadrant pain, making the person wonder about appendicitis. Other signs and symptoms of organic disease, however, are missing in these functional muscle and ligament aches and pains.

APPROACH TO DIAGNOSIS AND MANAGEMENT

Acute, severe abdominal pain presents as an emergency and usually is not seen in office or ambulatory settings. The focus here is on less severe lower abdominal pain for which office treatment rather than emergency room or hospital care would be sought. As the severity of the pain experienced by the patient does not necessarily correspond to the seriousness of the cause, the nurse practitioner must keep in mind the full range of conditions responsible for lower abdominal pain—the functional and benign as well as the pathological and dangerous. Initial questions to keep in mind are: Is it urgent, emergent, or routine? What system is it in? And, is it medical or surgical?

The History

Obtaining an accurate history for lower abdominal pain is often difficult, but must be pursued rigorously because information critical to an accurate diagnosis is gathered from the patient's description of the characteristics and circumstances of the pain. The full significance of the pain is usually not revealed by any one characteristic or circumstance but by a combination of data which helps to determine its anatomic site and its mechanism. The following are the classic questions asked in the exploration of pain, with special applicability here to the lower abdomen in women.

WHERE IS THE PAIN LOCATED? The exact locating of visceral and deep somatic pain is difficult, but certain typical sites are known. Appendicitis usually begins as periumbilical pain which several hours later becomes localized in the right lower quadrant. Unilateral lower quadrant or adnexal pain accompanies the torsion of an ovarian cyst, an ectopic pregnancy, mittelschmerz, ureteral stone, or tumors or cysts of the ovary. Diverticulitis most characteristically causes left lower quadrant pain, as does a diverticular abscess. Colonic obstruction or ischemia may cause mid-lower abdominal pain. Cystitis is more typically suprapubic; pain from uterine tumors or congestion may be midabdominal or in the low back due to rectal encroachment. Salpingitis or pelvic inflammatory disease (PID) tends to be bilateral and frequently involves the entire lower abdomen in painful sensations. Pain in the groin or labia is often related to ureteral colic or an incarcerated hernia. Figure 12-2 indicates additional areas where abdominal pain may be felt.

DID THE PAIN COME ON SUDDENLY OR GRADUALLY? The mode of onset of the pain suggests the mechanism underlying it. Pain which comes on suddenly and reaches maximal intensity almost at once or shortly thereafter suggests perforation, rupture, embolus, or ureteral colic. Appendicitis may come on very acutely. Pain having a gradual onset developing over days or weeks, for which the exact time of onset cannot be clearly identified is often due to low mechanical bowel obstruction, urinary tract infection, ectopic pregnancy before rupture, PID, uterine or ovarian tumors, pelvic congestion, endometriosis, and, sometimes, appendicitis.

HOW LONG DOES THE PAIN LAST AND IS IT CONSTANT OR DOES IT COME AND GO? The duration and rhythm or pattern of the pain provide cues about the nature of the problem. Inquire specifically if the pain lasts seconds, minutes, or hours, or all day or night, and if it always lasts about the same amount of time. Does the pain occur intermittently several times a day or is it constant once it has begun? Does it occur every day? If not, how many times a week or a month does it occur? Does it have a cycle of recurrence? Cyclic pain occurring about once a month is usually tied to the menstrual cycle, as in such instances as premenstrual congestion and mittelschmerz. The pain of bowel distention or spasm usually is intermittent but recurrent, whereas ureteral colic is constant once it starts but varies in intensity. The pain of appendicitis and peritonitis is constant.

WHAT IS THE QUALITY OF THE PAIN? DESCRIBE ITS CHARACTER. The choice of words the pa-

tient uses to describe pain is influenced by many factors, such as vocabulary and educational level, previous experiences with health providers, medical knowledge and sophistication, and what the patient imagines to be taking place in her body. "Cramping" denotes an intermittent, short-term, poorly localized pain which is usually indicative of irritation, congestion, inflammation, or obstruction. "Aching" suggests a continuous, dull and poorly localized, usually not incapacitating pain that may be steady for some time and may fluctuate in intensity. This type of pain suggests congestion, swelling, muscle spasm, or strain. "Pulling" may be used to describe the deep dull ache of mesenteric traction and adhesions. Pain identified as "burning" is accompanied by sensations of hotness and often indicates mucosal irritation of the bowel, bladder, or urethra, although it can also be due to muscle contraction. "Sharp" pain rising in waves to a peak then subsiding is typical of colic. There may be pain-free intervals, or the intense pain may give way to a dull ache, only to be followed soon again by another wave of sharp pain. Colicky pain occurs with the mechanical obstruction of bowels, the more distal the obstruction the longer the pain-free interval. It can also be due to ureteral stones, neoplasm, inflammatory diseases such as diverticulitis and regional ileitis, spastic colitis, and thrombosis. "Feeling bloated" is a term used to describe a distention caused by gas in the colon or by premenstrual congestion. Gas pains can be either sharp or dull but are usually of short duration. Another type of sharp, transitory pain is caused by a disease of the nerve roots or ganglia, or by a strain or tear in somatic tissue such as a muscle or ligament. "Throbbing" pain usually indicates that an arterial pulsation is giving rise to painful stimuli; it is frequently seen with infections, or inflammations, or the spasm of an artery.

WHAT BRINGS ON THE PAIN? WHAT MAKES IT WORSE? WHAT MAKES IT BETTER? These factors are often of greater diagnostic value than the character of the pain, which may be described differently by individual patients. Lower abdominal pain which follows eating, particularly certain types of foods, is due to some condition of the bowel. If accompanied by gas, bloating, or diarrhea the relation is even more obvious. This pain may be caused by gastrocntcritis, an inflammatory bowel disease, obstruction, functional bowel problems, or parasites. If the problem is made worse by foods high in roughage, irritable colon and diverticulitis are suspect. When expulsion of flatus, a bowel movement, or an enema relieves lower abdominal pain, the distal half of the colon is likely to be involved. These problems can be either functional or organic. In cases of inflammation or peritonitis, however, emptying the bowels or bladder causes a sudden change in intraabdominal pressure and may aggravate the pain. Pain that is increased by a cough, a sneeze, and strain can be radicular in origin, can arise in ligamentous structures or may be due to inflammation and peritonitis. If the movement of certain parts of the body or if certain postures relieve the pain, it is usually centered in bones, muscles, or ligaments. Lower abdominal pain which increases with deep breathing can be due to peritonitis, abscess or inflammation, or distention from obstruction. Urination is often painful in peritonitis, pelvic abscess near the bladder, appendicitis which irritates the right ureter, and urinary tract infections. Vomiting can accompany any type of severe abdominal pain. It tends to occur early (within a few hours) in appendicitis, late with lower bowel obstruction, and variously in gastroenteritis. Pain which occurs after physical effort is often vascular in origin. Postural changes or activity can cause pain when there are adhesions or peritoneal bands. Pain caused by a jolting ride may be due to the incarceration of a renal calculus or to diverticulitis.

WHEN WAS YOUR LAST MENSTRUAL PERIOD? Is THE PAIN RELATED TO THE MENSTRUAL CYCLE? If the woman has skipped one or two menstrual periods, suspect ectopic pregnancy as the cause of lower abdominal pain. When pain begins about a week after the last menstrual period, gonorrheal or bacterial salpingitis may be the cause. Premenstrual congestion and dysmenorrhea are obviously connected with the menstrual cycle. Mittelschmerz occurs midcycle and may be intermittent, skipping some months and alternating sides. Pelvic pain due to a chronic PID may be exacerbated by menstruation.

DOES INTERCOURSE AGGRAVATE THE PAIN? Pain on intromission may be due to inflammatory conditions of the vagina or labia or to other vulval or vaginal conditions. It can also be psychogenic, such as in vaginismus. Pain on deep penetration is of more significance to lower abdominal pathology, although it also can be functional. Pelvic congestion, endometriosis of the uterosacral ligaments or cul-de-sac, severe uterine retroversion, broad ligament tear, PID, and ovarian tumors are some organic causes of deep pelvic pain with intercourse. Any cause of peritonitis would also cause painful intercourse, such as appendicitis and mittelschmerz. A functional problem can result when the woman is nonorgasmic, and the vasocongestion which develops in pelvic structures following sexual arousal is not relieved by the muscle contractions of orgasm. This causes an aching type of chronic pelvic pain (see Chapter 2, Sexuality and Affectional Relationships).

HOW SEVERE IS THE PAIN? The severity of the pain is not a very reliable indicator of how serious the problem may be. Patients differ greatly in their tolerance of pain and their ability to communicate its intensity. Some indicators can be helpful, although not invariably accurate, in detecting organic problems, including whether the patient can continue her usual activities when the pain is present, if she has to lie down or stop her activities, if the pain prevents her from falling asleep or awakens her from sleep, and what type of medicine provides pain relief. Pain relieved by aspirin probably is not severe, as opposed to that requiring narcotics or opiates. The position assumed when the pain is present also gives cues about the underlying mechanism. The characteristic postures for extremes of abdominal pain include writhing, restlessness, thrashing about, moving constantly with colic in a hollow viscus as with ureteral stones or bowel spasm, and lying very still, supine, as with peritonitis.

HAVE YOU HAD ANY PREVIOUS ILLNESSES, HOSPITALIZATIONS, OR OPERATIONS? The patient's past history is important to ascertain the presence of an illness which could be related to her lower abdominal pain, or to rule out certain possibilities. If the woman has had an appendectomy, appendicitis must be left out of the differential diagnosis. Hysterectomy, salpingectomy, or oophorectomy rule out some diagnostic categories but suggest others. The history of any abdominal surgery must be carefully explored in order to determine what was done, why it was done, and the patient's perceptions about it. Adhesions and abdominal bands are common following abdominal procedures. A history of gonorrheal PID or treatment for GC is significant and should be routinely asked about when exploring lower abdominal pain. The woman's pregnancy history and any problems with labor or delivery provide additional cues. It is also important to ask specifically about drug use, both for relief of the pain and the treatment of other unrelated conditions. Many medications cause gastrointestinal symptoms as a side effect, whether medically prescribed drugs, over-the-counter self-medication, or illegal street drugs.

HAVE THERE BEEN ANY RECENT CHANGES, STRESSES, OR CONFLICTS? The bowel is often a sounding board for emotions, and any stressful situation can be translated into gastrointestinal symptoms. People also become concerned about the possible significance of the pain they are experiencing, and emotional reactions surrounding this symptom often act to aggravate it. It is a rare person who cannot report some type of stress in his or her life, however, or who does not become distressed about a continuing or recurring pain. Depending upon the practitioner's familiarity with the patient and impressions based upon the patient's mannerisms and presentation of her symptoms, the exploration of stresses may be delayed or emphasized immediately.

The Physical Examination

VITAL SIGNS. Temperature, pulse, respiration, and blood pressure may provide important information in evaluating lower abdominal pain. An elevated temperature indicates an infectious or inflammatory process. Rapid pulse and respirations may accompany fever or may indicate anxiety states. Hypertension raises the suspicion of vascular disorders or it may be an incidental finding.

ABDOMINAL EXAMINATION. With the patient supine, the abdomen is inspected for scars, contour, symmetry, peristalsis, or pulsations. Auscultation is done next so that the bowel sounds will not be disturbed by palpation. The frequency and character of bowel sounds are noted. Increased bowel sounds occur with diarrhea and early intestinal obstruction. High-pitched tinkling sounds suggest intestinal fluid and air under tension in a dilated bowel. There are rushes of these sounds coinciding with cramping or pain with an intestinal obstruction. Functional bowel spasm is also associated with increased bowel sounds. Decreased and then absent bowel sounds occur with peritonitis and paralytic ileus. Bruits may occur over the renal arteries, abdominal aorta, or femoral arteries. These suggest partial arterial obstruction or turbulent flow, as in an aneurysm.

Percussion of the four quadrants may be done for the proportions and distribution of tympany and dullness. Tympany usually predominates due to gas in the bowel. The liver is percussed to determine its size. Any masses or lumps found by palpation are also percussed, if the spleen is felt it should be percussed to help determine its size. Light palpation is carried out to identify muscular resistance and to ascertain any tenderness of superficial organs or masses. Deep palpation is used to delineate abdominal organs and masses. If masses are felt, note their location, size, shape, consistency, tenderness, pulsations, and mobility. If tenderness is present, note its location, whether increased by deep palpation or by rebound, and its approximate severity. Any abdominal wall ridigity and guarding are also noted. Rebound tenderness, rigidity, and guarding suggest peritoneal irritation. The size and consistency of any enlarged organs, including the liver, spleen, kidneys, or uterus are described.

Abdominal tenderness is often difficult to assess accurately. Structures and organs in the abdomen are sensitive, and deep palpation normally elicits some discomfort. Distracting the patient by talking or asking questions not directly related to the abdominal examination may help to reduce any reflex guarding and reactions to normal discomfort. When the patient is suspected of overreacting, the stethoscope may be used, supposedly to listen but actually to press down quite firmly as in palpation, while distracting the patient. If there is a marked difference in discomfort with this technique as compared to actual palpation with the hands, anticipation and overreaction by the patient is most likely. Some apparent masses or thickenings felt in an abdominal examination are not abnormal and should not be confused with organomegaly or pathology. The abdominal aorta may be felt in thin people as a midline, pulsating mass. It usually is not wider than 4 to 5 cm., and it transmits pulsation forward. A prominent pulsation with lateral expansion suggests aneurysm. Stool present in the ascending or descending colon can also feel like a mass, particularly if it is hard and large in amount. This usually feels like a tubular-shaped mass which molds and changes shape as the examiner feels it. The most typical location is the left lower quadrant. Reexamination a day later, or after an enema or bowel movement, should reveal that the mass has disappeared. The enlarged uterus during pregnancy is a cystic-feeling midline mass with regular contours. Occasionally the rectus muscle may be confused with a possible mass, as the examiner's fingers slide over the edge of the contracted muscle sheath.

Patients with very obese abdomens, thick abdominal musculature, abdominal distention, and truly severe pain are almost impossible to examine successfully. Greater reliance must be placed upon their history and on diagnostic tests in these instances, unless the severe pain is typical and therefore diagnostic of certain conditions. With significant pain, the amount of information which can be obtained from the examination is proportional to the gentleness of the examiner.

PELVIC AND RECTAL EXAMINATION. With lower abdominal pain, a pelvic and rectal examination is essential since the abdominal examination is often negative or equivocal. The pelvic examination follows the usual routine, with a speculum examination and the collection of specimens, as indicated. The inspection of the vulva, vagina, and cervix is done, and any abnormalities are noted. A bimanual examination is most revealing, however, when there is lower abdominal pathology. Palpation of the affected side first is recommended, because pain elicited by the examination may lead to guarding and so may reduce the chance of the practitioner's accurately feeling the adnexa during continued palpation. Gentleness is critical, and assisting the woman to breath deeply may also help her to relax. Search carefully for tenderness, masses, thickening, and fullness. Tenderness when the cervix is moved, with bilateral adnexal fullness or masses, suggests PID. Uterine tenderness may indicate endometritis; if it is associated with nodular uterosacral ligaments or fullness in the cul-de-sac suspect endometriosis. With cervical congestion, slight uterine enlargement, and a unilateral tender adnexal mass, an ectopic pregnancy is likely, particularly if the woman is experiencing amenorrhea or menstrual irregularity. When pregnancy is unlikely, an irregularly shaped or enlarged uterus which is mildly tender during the examination could indicate the presence of fibroids.

The size, shape, consistency, tenderness, and mobility of definite masses in the adnexae must be described. It is difficult to determine whether an adnexal mass is ovarian or tubular or a pedunculated uterine fibroid. Most masses indicate the need for an immediate consultation or referral to the physician, unless the characteristics of the mass and the patient's history and symptoms clearly point to a functional ovarian cyst. Table 12-1 summarizes the characteristic of lower abdominal masses. In general, however, mobile cystic masses are most likely ovarian in origin. Nonmobile cystic masses adherent to other pelvic structures or to the lateral pelvic walls may be an ovarian neoplasm, an inflammatory mass such as a tuboovarian abscess, or an endometrioma. A solid mobile mass could be a solid ovarian tumor, a pedunculated fibroid, a benign bowel neoplasm, or an unruptured ectopic pregnancy. A solid nonmobile mass suggests a malignant ovarian tumor, a bowel neoplasm, inflammatory mass, or retroperitoneal neoplasm.

The identification of other pelvic organs is important when a mass is present. If a normal uterus and both ovaries can be palpated along with a mass, it is extraovarian in nature. A solid mass adjacent to or fixed to the uterus, when both ovaries feel normal, probably is a fibroid. Masses adherent to the uterus could also be due to inflammatory disease, malignancy, or endometriosis. Masses in the cul-de-sac could be an enlarged ovary, a tuboovarian abscess, an ectopic pregnancy, a retroflexed uterus, fibroid, a diverticular or appendiceal abscess, a displaced kidney, or retroperitoneal neoplasms. Fullness in the cul-de-sac suggests the presence of blood or pus.

The rectovaginal examination provides additional information about pelvic findings and permits a deeper exploration of the lower abdomen. It is particularly helpful in feeling the

Table 12-1
Lower Abdominal Masses

Condition	Location	Size	Consistency	Mobility	Shape	Tenderness	Pain	Fever	N/V/D	Other Associated Factors
OVARY										
Functional cyst (follicular, corpus luteum)	Adnexa usually unilateral	5-6 cm.	Cystic	Mobile	Round to ovoid	None to slight	None to dull, aching	No	No	Delayed menses; spontaneous resorption in 6-12 weeks
Benign neoplastic (cystadenoma, cystic teratoma)	Adnexa, usually unilateral	6-12 cm.	Cystic	Mobile unless large	Round to ovoid	None	None or vague fullness, aching	No	No	Disturbed menses ±
Malignant (cystadenocarcinoma, adenocarcinoma)	Adnexa, usually unilateral	5-25 cm.	Cystic or solid	Mobile early, fixed or frozen late	Varies	None	None or vague fullness, aching	No	No	Disturbed menses ±
Endometrioma (chocolate cyst)	Adnexa, usually unilateral; cul-de-sac	>10 cm.	Cystic	Usually fixed	Irregular	±	±	No	No	Nodules on uterosacral ligaments; fixed retroflexed uterus; cul-de-sac nodules
Granulosa-theca cell tumor	Adnexa usually unilateral	Few mm. to 20 cm.	Solid	Mobile	Round to ovoid	None	None unless large	No	No	Precocious puberty; postmenopausal vaginal bleeding, breast hypertrophy; premenopausal menometrorrhagia
FALLOPIAN TUBES										
Tuboovarian abscess	Adnexa, bilateral; cul-de-sac	Varies	Solid	Fixed	Poorly defined	++++	Severe constant	Yes	N/V	Elevated WBC, ESR; History of VD or PID ±; Movement of cervix painful

Table 12-1
Lower Abdominal Masses (Continued)

Condition	Location	Size	Consistency	Mobility	Shape	Tenderness	Pain	Fever	N/V/D	Other Associated Factors
Pyosalpinx	Adnexa bilateral, cul-de-sac	Varies	Solid	Fixed	Retort	+++	Varies	±	±	Elevated WBC, ESR ±; History of VD or PID ±; Movement of cervix painful
Parovarian cyst	Adnexa, usually unilateral	5-8 cm.	Cystic	Mobile	Round to ovoid	None	None or vague, aching	No	No	Ovary separately palpable
Ectopic pregnancy	Adnexa, unilateral; cul-de-sac	5-6 cm.	Solid	Mobile	Ovoid	++ to ++++	Mild to severe	No	N/V	Menstrual irregularities; signs, Sx of pregnancy; peritonitis if ruptured
UTERUS										
Fibroid pedunculated	Midline; Adnexa or cul-de-sac	Varies	Firm and rubbery	— Mobile	Irregular	No	None or vague aching	No	No	Uterus enlarged, nodular, irregular contour; pressure; irregular menses
Adenomyosis	Midline	2-3 mo. gestation	Firm to hard	Mobile uterus	Uterus globular	+++	Cramps	No	No	Abnormal bleeding, dysmenorrhea; multipara age 40-50
Endometrial carcinoma	Midline	Often normal	Firm	Mobile uterus	Usual	None	None usually	No	No	Abnormal bleeding
Endometritis	Midline	Often normal	Firm	Mobile uterus	Usual	+++	Cramps, Aching	±	±	Hx of VD, vaginal discharge; menstrual changes
BOWEL/OTHER										
Dilated cecum (feces, gas)	LLQ Midline	Varies; Changes	Varies	Moves around	Tubular	None to mild	Sharp colicky	No	No	Hyperperistalsis, ↑ bowel sounds, diarrhea, constipation

	Location	Size	Consistency	Mobility	Borders					Comments
Diverticular abscess	LLQ; left adnexa	Varies	Soft, fluctuant to firm	Fixed	Poorly defined	++	Mild to severe	±	±	Minimal Sx to bloody diarrhea, peritonitis, cramping
Appendiceal abscess	RLQ; right adnexa; cul-de-sac	Varies	Firm	Fixed	Poorly defined	+++	++	±	N/V	Rebound, peritonitis, ↓ bowel sounds, ↑ WBC with shift to the left
Ectopic kidney	Cul-de-sac	6-7 cm.	Solid	Mobile	Round	None to mild	No	No	No	IVP shows displaced kidney
Retroperitoneal abscess	Cul-de-sac	Varies	Firm	Fixed	Poorly defined	++	++	±	±	Hx of VD or PID

uterosacral ligaments for nodules and the rectovaginal septum and in evaluating the posterior uterine surface and the cul-de-sac. Rectal lesions and adnexal masses can also be better evaluated in a rectovaginal examination.

OTHER EXAMINATIONS FOR APPENDICITIS. With right lower quadrant pain and tenderness, two additional tests can be done to detect peritonitis caused by an inflamed or ruptured appendix. The appendix may be found in a pelvic, iliac, or ascending colon location (as well as occasionally on the left side). For an extrapelvic (ascending) appendix, the *iliopsoas sign* is elicited, in which the patient is asked to raise the right leg against the resistance of the examiner's hand while lying supine. Pain is elicited if the inflamed extrapelvic appendix has caused irritation of the lateral iliopsoas muscle. The *obturator sign* reveals an intrapelvic (iliac, pelvic) appendicitis. The supine patient is asked to flex her right thigh to 90 degrees; the examiner then immobilizes the ankle with one hand, and pulls the knee, first laterally for external, then medially for internal rotation. Pain elicited by this rotation indicates an inflamed obturator internus muscle due to irritation from an inflamed intrapelvic appendix.

Diagnostic Measures

A complete blood count is often ordered in cases of lower abdominal pain or masses in order to assist in establishing the diagnosis. An elevated white blood cell count, with immature forms of leukocytes in the peripheral blood smear, is indicative of infection and is particularly helpful in diagnosing appendicitis, PID, a tuboovarian abscess, and a diverticular abscess. However, leukocytosis greater than 20,000 cu. mm. can occur with the perforation of a viscus, intestinal infarction, and other infections. The absence of leukocytosis cannot rule out PID, appendicitis, or diverticular abscess because they have all been known to occur with a normal white blood cell count and with no shift to the left. A decreased red blood cell count, hematocrit, and hemoglobin indicates anemia, possibly secondary to blood loss. Changes will not occur until several hours after the onset of bleeding. An erythrocyte sedimentation rate is often helpful in verifying the presence of an inflammatory process such as PID, although it is not invariably elevated

and if normal does not rule out these conditions.

Urinalysis is an important test to determine if lower abdominal pain is of renal or urinary origin, such as urinary tract infection or ureteral stones. A pregnancy test should be done if pregnancy is suspected among the diagnoses to be ruled out. The most useful x-ray tests for lower abdominal pain or mass include 1) a flat plate x-ray examination of the abdomen to discover any calcifications characteristic of an ovarian teratoma or a uterine myoma, or the air-fluid levels in an abscess cavity; 2) a barium enema for detecting diverticular abscess, diverticulitis, or colonic obstruction; and 3) an intravenous pyelogram, particularly when pelvic malignancy is a consideration, but which may also detect a misplaced pelvic kidney presenting as a cul-de-sac mass. In all cases of left lower quadrant masses of undetermined cause, a barium enema is recommended.

The patient should be referred for culdocentesis when there is fullness in the cul-de-sac. The aspiration of nonclotting blood in the cul-de-sac confirms the presence of intraabdominal bleeding, and when it is associated with a unilateral mass, an ectopic pregnancy or a bleeding corpus luteum is strongly suggested. Pus in the aspirate indicates pelvic or intraabdominal infection. Ultrasound scanning of the abdomen and pelvis can help to identify the mass by identifying various features of ovarian neoplasms; or if an extrauterine gestational sac is found it indicates an ectopic pregnancy. A laparoscopic examination may be indicated when the possible causes of the pain include ectopic pregnancy or a persistent corpus luteum cyst, and a decision must be made about the necessity for surgery. This examination is also useful when a pelvic mass is suspected but cannot be clearly felt in a bimanual examination. It is not indicated when there is a definite significant mass. In cases of persistent adnexal or cul-de-sac masses of significant size, surgery is usually necessary for definitive diagnosis and treatment.

COMMON CAUSES OF LOWER ABDOMINAL PAIN
Infectious Conditions

PELVIC INFLAMMATORY DISEASE. Salpingitis, tuboovarian abscess, and pelvic peritonitis may result from gonorrheal or other bacterial infections. The classic syndrome consists of exposure to gonorrhea with local infection of the cervix which spreads during the next menstrual period through the uterus to the tubes and ovaries. The onset of bilateral lower abdominal pain occurs about one week after menses, with the presence of other signs of infection such as fever, leukocytosis, elevated sedimentation rate, malaise, and, possibly, vomiting. On examination both adnexae are exquisitely tender, with fullness or bilateral masses that are fixed and poorly defined. Movement of the cervix elicits pain, and a cervical culture reveals gonorrhea. There are numerous variations in the signs and symptoms of PID, which are covered more fully in Chapter 11, Venereal Disease.

APPENDICITIS. The obstruction of the appendix with infection, edema, infarction, and rupture is a common cause of acute abdominal pain, but it can present in a subacute manner. The attack usually begins with epigastric or periumbilical pain and vomiting. Within 2 to 12 hours the pain shifts to the right lower quadrant, is constant, and is aggravated by coughing, straining, or walking. Anorexia, malaise, and slight fever are present, usually with constipation but occasionally with diarrhea. An examination reveals a progressive right lower quadrant tenderness which can often be localized to a single point of maximal tenderness. A spasm in the overlying abdominal muscle and rebound tenderness usually are found. Rectal tenderness is common and may be more definite than abdominal tenderness with a pelvic appendix. A positive iliopsoas or obturator sign is strongly suggestive of appendicitis. Peristalsis is diminished or absent. Moderate fever and leukocytosis of 10,000 to 20,000 per cu. mm. are typical. There are variations with age, obesity, location of appendix, and progression of the inflammation. A consultation with a physician is indicated as appendicitis is treated surgically.

GASTROENTERITIS. Acute gastroenteritis is commonly confused with appendicitis. Vomiting and diarrhea are more common with acute gastroenteritis than with appendicitis and more pronounced. Fever and leukocytosis may rise sharply and appear out of proportion to the relatively minimal abdominal findings. Pain and tenderness are difficult to locate spe-cifically because they are shifting and indefinite. Hyperactive peristalsis is typical of gastroenteritis. Localized abdominal muscle spasm and rebound are usually absent. Gastroenteritis usually runs a short course, and a period of observation over several hours in which there is no progression of abdominal signs characteristic of appendicitis often establishes the diagnosis.

Other conditions which may be confused with appendicitis are mesenteric adenitis, Meckel's diverticulitis, regional enteritis, ureteral colic, acute salpingitis, mittelschmerz, ruptured ectopic pregnancy, and twisted ovarian cyst.

DIVERTICULITIS. The inflammation of diverticula of the colon causes intermittent cramping left lower quadrant pain most characteristically, but the pain may be steady and severe and last for days. Constipation is usual, but diarrhea may occur, or the two may alternate. In more severe inflammation there may be signs of peritoneal irritation, chills, fever, ileus, partial or complete obstruction, and abscess formation. An examination reveals left lower quadrant tenderness and the presence of a fixed, tender mass if an abscess has formed. Blood may be present in the diarrhea and leukocytosis may occur. A barium enema x-ray study reveals diverticula and colonic spasm, thickening or narrowing of the colon or the presence of a mass, when it is abscessed. Acute diverticulitis is treated with antibiotic therapy, preferably ampicillin; then the underlying diverticular disease is treated with a high residue diet, bulk additives such as Metamucil, stool softeners such as Colace, and anticholinergics such as Donnatal or Pro-Banthine. The formation of abscesses may require surgical resection.

URINARY TRACT INFECTION. Burning pain during urination, with urgency, frequency, and hematuria usually make the diagnosis of a urinary tract infection evident. Occasionally, however, there may be vague suprapubic lower abdominal pain and tenderness without the typical symptoms described above. Upper tract involvement usually presents more striking symptoms with costovertebral and abdominal pain, malaise, vomiting, chills, and fever. A urinalysis is indicated as a routine part of the work-up for lower abdominal pain because the symptomatology may be vague, and it is important to rule out urinary problems (see Chapter 10, Urinary Problems).

Endometriosis and Adenomyosis

The presence and proliferation of endometrial tissue in sites outside the endometrial cavity cause *endometriosis,* a benign disease of widely varying character, and *adenomyosis,* also a benign disease, which is due to the invasion of the myometrium of the uterus by endometrial glands and stroma. While there are morphologic similarities in these two diseases, the histogenesis, clinical picture, and natural history are different. Endometriosis and adenomyosis are not commonly found together. Because the symptoms may be minimal and may resemble those of other pelvic diseases or may occur in conjunction with other pathology, the diagnosis of these two diseases is often made following surgery for some other condition. These diseases probably occur more frequently than they are suspected, and they account for a considerable amount of discomfort and disability among women.

Endometriosis presents most commonly as pelvic pain, often taking the form of acquired dysmenorrhea, beginning in the late 20s to early 30s, and progressing in severity. The pain is usually dull, aching, or cramping in the lower abdomen or back, occurring with menstruation and diminishing gradually after the onset of the flow. The pain is not always related to menstruation, however, and some women experience a vague aching, cramping, or bearing down sensation in the pelvis, lower abdomen, or back. This may be constant or intermittent and it may show no variation with menses. The pain is due to irritation of the peritoneum, distention of tissue, or traction from adhesions.

The cause of endometriosis is thought to be the transplantation of endometrial fragments, via retrograde tubal flow of menstrual discharge, or via lymphatic or venous spread to sites most commonly involving the ovary, pelvic peritoneum, cul-de-sac, rectovaginal septum, and the uterosacral ligaments. The transformation of pelvic peritoneum or celomic epithelium into endometrial epithelium and stroma due to hormonal influences, inflammation, or some inductive substance in menstrual discharge is another theory about the cause of endometriosis. The sites of ectopic

endometrium less often found include the round ligaments, tubes, the peritoneal surfaces of the uterus and the bladder, and the rectosigmoid colon. These misplaced pieces of endometrial tissue respond to the hormones of the menstrual cycle, with proliferation, secretion, and bleeding, which leads to the irritation of surrounding tissue, scarring, and fibrosis, with dense adhesions and the formation of blood-filled cysts. In the ovary, the lesion may form an endometrioma, a cyst rarely larger than 10 cm. in diameter, filled with blood and blood pigment which looks like chocolate syrup, the "chocolate cyst of the ovary." Other symptoms caused by endometriosis are dyspareunia and painful defecation when lesions are present in the cul-de-sac, and occasionally rectal bleeding with bowel lesions.

In a pelvic examination, multiple tender nodules may be palpable along the uterosacral ligaments or in the rectovaginal septum of the posterior fornix or in the cul-de-sac. These nodules enlarge and become more tender during menstruation. The uterus may be fixed in a retroflexed position due to adhesions, and pain is elicited when attempts are made to move it. There may be a thickening and nodularity of both adnexae, suggestive of pelvic inflammatory disease, and the ovary may be irregularly enlarged, fixed, closely adherent to the uterus, and tender when an endometrial cyst is present. Fullness in the cul-de-sac may be due to the collection of blood from ruptured cysts and bleeding of the endometrial implants in the pelvic cavity.

Endometriosis is a pathologic finding in about 20 percent of all gynecological operations but is significant in only about one-third of these cases.[4] It may cause no symptoms or it may be progressively disabling. The diagnosis is established by observing the lesion, often by laparoscopy or laparotomy. There are no laboratory studies particularly helpful for this diagnosis. When the symptoms are enough to warrant treatment, factors including the woman's age and desire for future children are key in decision-making. The treatment choices are observation and symptom palliation, surgery, and hormone therapy. If the symptoms are mild to moderate in young women, education about the disease process and reassurance that it is not serious often enables them to cope with the discomfort without further measures. A mild analgesic may be needed for dysmenorrhea. In some cases the disease may become inactive, and it has been noted that endometriosis may improve or disappear with pregnancy. However, the concept that pregnancy is curative appears unfounded, as the persistence of disease after pregnancy is more common than permanent regression, and in some cases there is active growth of lesions during pregnancy.

Hormone therapy is recommended for women whose symptoms are not relieved by reassurance and a mild analgesic and who either desire a subsequent pregnancy or are not candidates for surgery whether by their own choice or because it is contraindicated. Estrogens, androgens, and progestins have all been used with reported relief of symptoms in about 80 percent of cases. The drugs commonly recommended are Enovid 2.5 mg. daily for 1 week, 5 mg. daily for 2 weeks, with an additional increase, if it is needed for symptom relief or breakthrough bleeding, up to 20 mg. daily; Norlestrin 2.5 mg. daily, increased by 1 tablet for breakthrough bleeding; and Depo-Provera 100 mg. IM every 2 weeks for 4 doses, then every 4 weeks, adding Delestrogen 30 mg. IM for breakthrough bleeding.[5] Treatment is often continued for 6 to 9 months, with the usual estrogen side effects. Analgesics with codeine may also be needed.

Surgery is often necessary when the symptoms are severe, incapacitating, or acute. Decisions about the extensiveness of the surgery depend upon the woman's age and her desire for children, and on the nature and location of the lesions found. Procedures can range from resecting the lesions, freeing adhesions, and suspending the uterus, to the removal of the uterus, tubes, and ovaries along with as many lesions with adjacent fibrosis and adhesions as can be safely resected.

Adenomyosis usually occurs in multiparous women in the fifth decade, the average age being 45. The basal stromal cells of the endometrium burrow into the myometrium and are followed by glandular cells. The myometrium responds with hypertrophy and hyperplasia, becoming very firm or hard. Scattered throughout the muscle are small cystic areas which often contain blood and may develop into larger pseudoencapsulated cysts called adenomyomas. Eventually as this invasive endometrial tissue responds to cyclic hormonal changes, the uterus becomes firmer, the corpus broadens, and the enlarged uterus assumes an erect, rigid posture, often causing pressure on the bladder. This enlargement is slow and symmetrical, with the uterus gradually becoming globular and increasing 2 to 3 times in size, but rarely exceeding the size of a 3-month's gestation.

The most typical symptoms of adenomyosis are abnormal uterine bleeding and acquired dysmenorrhea. In her late 30s and early 40s the woman begins having heavier and more frequent menses, often with flooding through tampons and pads and causing anemia. Dark scant pre- and postmenstrual staining is often present. Dysmenorrhea becomes progressively worse as the hypertrophic rigid uterus can no longer yield to increased pressure from bleeding into the myometrium. While these symptoms occur together in 25 percent of the cases, each more frequently occurs separately: abnormal bleeding in over 60 percent and dysmenorrhea in about 27 percent of the women who have adenomyosis. The majority of these patients have another pathologic process in the uterus, the most common being fibroids, which occur 50 percent of the time. Endometrial carcinoma not infrequently occurs in conjunction with adenomyosis, but primary malignant change in adenomyotic lesions is very rare.

The incidence of adenomyosis in surgical specimens has been reported at about 60 percent, although only about half of these patients were symptomatic. When symptomatic, the only treatment is hysterectomy which completely corrects the problem. Adenomyosis is a disease easily obscured by other conditions which also cause abnormal bleeding and dysmenorrhea, such as uterine fibroids, endometrial hyperplasia, and polyps. It must be kept in mind, however, after the exclusion of other conditions as the underlying cause of the woman's symptoms.[6]

Pelvic Masses

Most pelvic masses are silent and are discovered incidentally during an examination, either routine screening examinations or as part of the work-up for other illnesses. When the mass does cause symptoms, these are usually vague, lower abdominal discomfort, aching, a feeling of fullness or pressure, or perhaps pain associated with intercourse, menstruation, or defecation. Acute, intense abdominal pain can be caused when a mass twists on its pedicle, as with ovarian cysts or pedunculated fibroids, or if there is infarction or bleeding into a cyst, or if a cyst ruptures, causing chemical peritonitis. Pelvic masses are potentially serious and almost always call for rapid referral to or consultation with a physician by the health provider. Table 12-1 summarizes the characteristics of many common lower abdominal masses (see pp. 291 to 293).

FUNCTIONAL OVARIAN CYSTS.   Cysts derived from the graafian follicle or corpus luteum are the most frequent causes of ovarian enlargement. Usually asymptomatic, these cysts occur in women between the ages of 20 and 40, are mobile, sharply demarcated, mildly tender, cystic, and round to ovoid in shape. Follicle cysts are frequently bilateral and multiple, usually no more than 4 cm. in diameter, and are due to the failure of an incompletely developed follicle to reabsorb. Occasionally there may be menstrual irregularities. Most resolve spontaneously within 60 days without treatment. Corpus luteum cysts are caused by an increase in secretion by the corpus luteum after ovulation, are 4 to 6 cm. in diameter, may cause local pain and tenderness and amenorrhea or delayed menstruation, and are usually unilateral. These cysts are also mobile, sharply demarcated, round to ovoid, somewhat tender and cystic, and they resolve within 60 days.

The most important consideration is to differentiate functional cysts from neoplasms. Symptoms and physical findings must be carefully weighed. Because functional cysts only persist a few days or weeks, it is common practice to follow women closely, reexamining them during a different phase of the menstrual cycle after an interval of 1 to 3 months. If the woman is taking oral contraceptives, the mass is greater than 8 to 10 cm., or if the woman is postmenopausal there should be no delay in treatment because functional cysts are unlikely. If the mass persists for more than 6 to 12 weeks, exploratory laparotomy is also indicated. Combination oral contraceptives are frequently used for 1 or 2 cycles to hasten the involution of functional cysts. If the cysts are gonadotropin-dependent, the inhibitory effects of contraceptive steroids on the pituitary and hormone secretion should shorten their life span, with resolution by 6 weeks.

MOBILE CYSTIC MASSES.   Adnexal masses which are mobile, cystic in consistency, clearly demarcated, round to ovoid, and generally nontender are evaluated according to their size, the woman's age, and her history and symptoms. Any mass in a very young or a very old woman is presumed abnormal, and there is no time for observation. An immediate surgical consultation is indicated. In women between the ages of 20 and 40, small mobile cystic masses may be functional cysts as described above. Masses greater than 8 to 10 cm. in diameter raise the suspicion of neoplasms and could be benign, such as cystadenoma or cystic teratoma, or malignant such as cystadenocarcinoma or adenocarcinoma. Parovarian cysts are usually smaller than these neoplasms, being about 5 to 8 cm. in diameter. The endometrioma, while cystic, is usually fixed, and other signs of endometriosis are present.

MOBILE SOLID MASSES.   Solid masses are not functional but are caused by some pathological problem or abnormality in the pelvis. Benign neoplasms which are felt as solid adnexal masses are ovarian fibromas, pedunculated uterine fibroids, or other, rarer, types of tumors. Cystadenocarcinomas and adenocarcinomas may also be solid as well as cystic. Other malignant solid tumors are undifferentiated ovarian carcinomas and metastatic cancers. Functioning tumors of the ovary, of which the more common is the granulosa-theca cell tumor, are solid and range in size from a few millimeters to 15 cm. or more. This tumor produces estrogen and is responsible for precocious puberty in girls and for the evidence of estrogen elaboration in postmenopausal women, such as vaginal bleeding and hypertrophic breast changes. In the menstruating woman, menometrorrhagia may be the only symptom. While most granulosa-theca cell tumors are benign, there may be malignancy in from 1 and 20 percent of them, usually associated with ascites. An ectopic pregnancy also is felt as a solid, mobile, unilateral adnexal mass, 5 to 6 cm. in diameter, usually quite tender, and with signs of acute peritonitis if ruptured. Amenorrhea or abnormal bleeding and other signs of pregnancy assist in differentiating an ectopic pregnancy from other conditions.

FIXED SOLID MASSES.   Adnexal masses which are heavy, solid, fixed, and not well defined arouse suspicions of malignancy. Indeed, advanced cystadenocarcinomas and adenocarcinomas, as well as undifferentiated ovarian carcinoma, usually feel solid or hard, are irregular and poorly delineated, and frozen to the surrounding structures or to the pelvic wall. These tumors are often not tender, and there are few, if any, other symptoms, except perhaps some vague pelvic fullness or aching. Infectious processes causing abscesses are responsible for solid fixed adnexal masses. These masses are usually readily identifiable because of their associated symptoms of pain, tenderness, fever, leukocytosis, and nausea or vomiting. Tuboovarian abscess, pyosalpinx or hydrosalpinx, diverticular abscess, and appendiceal abscess are some of the causes.

ENLARGED OR IRREGULAR UTERUS. A palpable midline or suprapubic mass often is an enlarged uterus, although a distended bladder, neoplasm of the bladder, bowel, or ovary, and fecal material in the bowel must be considered. Uterine enlargement may be due to pregnancy, pyometra, hematometra, adenomyosis, fibroid, or malignant neoplasm. Fibroid tumors (leiomyoma) are common and may be felt as firm, rubbery nodules on the uterus, or their presence will simply be felt as an enlarged uterus if they are submucous. Uterine size is expressed in terms of the number of weeks of gestation to which it is comparable. There may be associated vague pelvic pressure or aching and menstrual irregularities. With endometritis and pyometra, signs of infection are present, and the uterus is usually quite tender. Endometrial carcinoma typically presents with abnormal bleeding and few other signs and symptoms. With a midline mass the size of 20-week's gestation or larger, it is important to listen for fetal heart tones and to palpate for fetal parts; the most common cause of a suprapubic midline mass is a pregnant uterus.

CUL-DE-SAC MASSES. Most pelvic masses can at times be found in the cul-de-sac, where again it is important to determine the characteristics of the mass and the signs and symptoms reported by the patient. Common cul-de-sac masses are tuboovarian, appendiceal, and retroperitoneal abscesses, with their usual symptoms of pain, tenderness, and fever. Ectopic pregnancies and endometriomas often occupy the cul-de-sac. Pedunculated fibroids, ovarian cysts and tumors, and parovarian cysts may be found. It is important to be certain that the mass is not simply a retroflexed uterus or

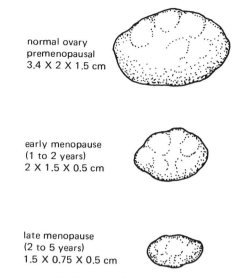

normal ovary
premenopausal
3.4 X 2 X 1.5 cm

early menopause
(1 to 2 years)
2 X 1.5 X 0.5 cm

late menopause
(2 to 5 years)
1.5 X 0.75 X 0.5 cm

Figure 12-3. Contrast in size between premenopausal and postmenopausal ovary.

fecal material in a redundant sigmoid colon which feels like a doughy nodular mass stretched across the anterior cul-de-sac. On rare occasions, an ectopic kidney may be felt as a mass in this location. Bowel or retroperitoneal neoplasms are also possible.

Masses in menopausal women aged 40 or older must be treated with a high index of suspicion because ovarian cancer and endometrial cancer are much more common in this age group. There is no indication for observation to see if the mass regresses, particularly if it is larger than 5 cm., adherent, and has both solid and cystic areas. It must be remembered that what is a normal-sized ovary in the premenopausal woman is an ovarian tumor in the woman more than 2 years postmenopausal. There are no functional cysts in this age group, and there is a striking difference in size between the premenopausal and postmenopausal ovary (Figure 12-3). Immediate consultation or surgical referral is indicated, for the presence or absence of a tumor must be substantiated.[7]

Psychogenic Pain

The experience of pain in the lower abdomen or pelvic areas may be part of a complex process involving a physical conversion of intrapsychic or interpersonal conflicts. Energy generated by unresolved conflicts seeks discharge; if the underlying problems cannot be confronted directly or in some cases even recognized because they are too threatening, a wide variety of expressions may be found, ranging from affective disorders, such as anxiety and depression, to the development of somatic symptoms. Stress sets into motion a series of common physiologic responses mediated by the sympathetic nervous system, producing the well-known symptoms of rapid heartbeat, sweating, cold clammy moist hands, the urge to void or defecate, dilation of the pupils, tremor, and a sinking feeling in the pit of the stomach. When stress becomes more chronic, common symptoms include headache, neck and shoulder pain, diarrhea, and abdominal pain.

The lower abdominal and pelvic areas are prime targets for emotionally triggered pain in women because of their association with sexual and reproductive functions, both of which are highly charged emotionally. The frequent occurrence of minor functional pains in this area of the anatomy may provide nervous pathways for the activation of pain impulses or for their exaggeration. Repeated focus or fixation on painful sensations originating from pelvic structures, and the characteristics of visceral and deep somatic pain, with its imprecise location and similar character, contribute to a syndrome of chronic pelvic pain without objective findings. There are structural bases for psychogenic pain, and the pain felt is very real to the woman, although an organic cause cannot be identified. To tell the woman the pain "is all in her head" is very different from saying that it has an emotional or psychological origin. The experience of pain must be recognized, not dismissed, before the treatment for psychogenic pain can be effective. The management of such pain basically has three phases: diagnostic evaluation to rule out organic disorders, assisting the woman to recognize and accept the emotional origins and components of the pain, and helping her to find an appropriate mode of therapy for dealing with the underlying problems.

To evaluate pelvic pain for possible organic bases, a careful history is taken as described in this chapter. Emphasis may be placed upon social, emotional, interpersonal, and occupational history if psychogenic problems are suspected. Cues to stress or conflict should be noted. It is often helpful to discuss with the patient the several differential diagnoses to be kept in mind as the work-up is planned, including that of psychogenic pain. Alerting the patient early that her symptoms could possibly be the result of stress, tension, or conflicts often initiates a process of thinking or reasoning this through which makes acceptance easier. When the patient feels involved in decision-making about problems affecting her body, and when she has contributed to the discussion and been responded to by the nurse practitioner in an easy exchange since the beginning, she may feel that she and the practitioner arrived at the conclusions together. This personal involvement can be an important learning experience, providing insight into both emotional and physical functioning. Because the woman follows the health provider's reasoning at each step of the diagnostic process, there are no surprises or shocks to create alienation and disbelief. When organic pathology has been ruled out and the conclusion is functional pain aggravated by emotional factors or psychogenic pain, the woman will not feel betrayed or discredited. It is her diagnosis as much as the practitioner's.

Although there are no hard and fast rules about differentiating organic from psychogenic pain, the general guideline presented in Table 12-2 are useful.

In some cases of psychogenic pain, going through the diagnostic work-up as a process of learning about the self and gaining insight may be enough to bring about an eventual resolution of the symptom. The woman may be able to deal with the causes of conflict or stress more directly, making decisions about changes or reordering the priorities in her situation in ways which relieve the need for the discharge of psychic energy in physical symptoms. Or, she may be able to accept counseling or psychotherapy for herself, and others who are directly involved in her situation, to deal with the underlying problems. The health provider may be able to conduct family therapy, either alone or jointly, or may need to refer the patient to a qualified therapist.

Some women cannot accept a psychogenic basis for their lower abdominal or pelvic pain, despite repeated examinations and tests which are negative for pathology. These women often refuse counseling or psychotherapy and seek medical care from another physician or health facility. The secondary gain derived from their symptoms or the deep-seated emotional disturbances underlying their pain are too significant to alter effectively. Some of these women

Table 12-2
Guidelines for Differentiating Organic from Psychogenic Pain

	Organic Pain	Psychogenic Pain
Time of onset	Any time, follows pattern typical for disease; may prevent falling asleep or awaken patient	Usually begins well after waking, following buildup of stresses; usually does not awaken from sleep
Character of pain	Sharp, cramping, intermittent	Dull, vague, continuous
Radiation	Follows definite neural pathways	Bizarre pattern; does not conform to neural pathways
Localization	May be located consistent with pathologic processes	Variable, shifting, generalized
Progress	Becomes either better or worse in a relatively short time	Remains essentially the same for weeks, months, or years
Precipitating factors	Often can be associated with definite factor; reproduced by palpation	Often triggered by interpersonal factors, stresses, conflicts; palpation usually does not reproduce
Physical examination and diagnostic tests	Positive physical findings or results from diagnostic tests to confirm organic disease	Negative physical examination and diagnostic tests

will end up with abdominal surgery, often with a hysterectomy, but without relief of the pain. It is a tragedy of hiding from the self and is ultimately self-destructive.

The use of medication in psychogenic pain must be carefully thought through. Narcotics and mood altering drugs can lead to physical or emotional addiction, and this is not an uncommon occurrence among women with chronic pelvic complaints. Certainly any use of such drugs should be short-term and pending definitive diagnosis. When depression or anxiety is found as an underlying cause, specific approaches to treatment are used which may include drugs. These problems are covered in Chapter 15, Nervousness and Fatigue.

Lower abdominal pain is a symptom which demands a thoughtful, thorough, and sensitive investigation by the health provider. While a significant proportion of such pain has an emotional basis, there is also a large number of potentially serious pathological processes and diseases which could be responsible. Psychogenic pain is a diagnosis made only by exclusion.

NOTES

1. M. A. Krupp and M. J. Chatton, *Current Medical Diagnosis & Treatment* (Los Altos, Calif.: Lange Medical Publications, 1976), p. 440.
2. M. McCaffery, *Nursing Management of the Patient with Pain* (Philadelphia: J. B. Lippincott, 1972), p. 8.
3. M. M. Wintrobe, et al., eds., *Harrison's Principles of Internal Medicine*, 6th ed. (New York: McGraw-Hill, Blakiston, 1970), 1:43-51.
4. J. A. Merrill, "Endometriosis." In S. L. Romney, et al., eds., *Gynecology and Obstetrics: The Health Care of Women* (New York: McGraw-Hill, Blakiston, 1975), pp. 883-94.
5. Krupp and Chatton, *Current Medical Diagnosis & Treatment*, p. 429.
6. C. W. Bird and T. W. McElin, "Adenomyosis of the Uterus." *Contemporary OB/GYN* 5, 6 (June 1975): 75-80.
7. H. R. K. Barber, "Diagnosing and Managing the Unilateral Mass." *Contemporary OB/GYN* 7, 1 (January 1976): 99-102.

13

Breast Masses

The female breast is a part of the body which has acquired a significance in our society out of all proportion to its actual functional value. In keeping with the typical American preoccupation with size, above average development of the mammary gland has been regarded by males with adulation, awe, and a kind of adolescent locker-room sexuality. Women have come to base at least some portion of their self-valuation, particularly their sense of their sexual self, on the size and appearance of their breasts. A disease which threatens to damage or distort the breast thus carries significance for a woman's perception of her body image and worth, in addition to the possible disability or death from the disease process itself.

Attitudes toward the breast are now changing as part of women's struggle toward recognition as full human beings rather than objects of sex, reproduction, or domestic servility. The change is gradual, however, with various degrees of persistence of older values among individuals. Loss or damage to any part of the body is very traumatic and affects our sense of wholeness. Breast masses are fraught with practical and symbolic dangers and are inevitably accompanied by strong emotional responses. Sensitivity to the woman's fears, the emotional repercussions of breast disease, and an honest and open approach on the part of the health provider are essential in the management of breast masses.

ANATOMY AND PHYSIOLOGY OF THE BREAST

The mammary gland is a specialized type of sweat gland whose purpose is to produce milk for feeding the young. Its development and functioning are intricately tied to the ebb and flow of hormones within the female body. Skin and superficial fascia surround the mammary gland on its external side, and deep fascia and the muscles of the chest wall surround it internally. The two muscles under the breast, the *pectoralis major* and *pectoralis minor*, lie over the ribs and control much of the mobility of the arm. Fibrous tissue, called *Cooper's ligaments*, extends from the deep fascia through the breast and fuses with the superficial fascia. A layer of fat of varying depth lies under the skin. The glandular tissue of the breast consists of 20 or more *lobes*, made of *lobules* which are clusters of many small *alveoli*. The alveoli are enmeshed in fatty and fibrous tissue and are the source of milk production. A system of *ducts* connects the alveoli and the lobes, and the 20 excretory ducts from the lobes merge into the *lactiferous sinus* as they enter the nipple. The external opening of this sinus has several tiny holes through which milk is secreted (Figure 13-1).

The blood supply of the breast is mainly from perforating branches of the internal mammary artery and axillary artery, with venous return via the internal mammary, axillary, and intercostal veins. Lymphatic drainage from the lateral side of the breast is through the axillary nodes, and from the medial side it is through the internal mammary chain. The infraclavicular nodes also provide some lymphatic drainage.

Breast growth is primarily under the influence of estrogen and progesterone, although to some degree human (pituitary) growth hormone, prolactin, insulin, cortisol, and thyroxine are also involved. After puberty, hormones effect constant change in the breast, with a rapid turnover of cells. During each hormone cycle the alveoli increase in size and there is ductal proliferation, causing premenstrual increases in breast size, engorgement, and tenderness. These changes regress with the decrease in hormones and menstruation, only to begin again with the next cycle.

During pregnancy there is rapid mammary growth due to an exaggeration in cyclic changes. Ductal proliferation and an increase in the number and size of alveoli are more extensive, and this increased amount of glandular tissue displaces connective tissue stroma. After delivery, additional prolactin release is stimulated, which initiates milk production. Intermittent suckling is required to maintain prolactin levels and lactation.

Variations of the Breast

Female breasts differ greatly in their size, shape, and other characteristics. It is normal for one breast to be somewhat larger than the other, though in some women there may be severe asymmetry. Amastia, the absence of breast development on one or both sides, is usually associated with maldevelopment of the pectoralis muscles and may be hereditary. Accessory breast tissue occurs in 1 to 2 percent of women, most commonly additional or supernumerary nipples which occur along the milk lines extending from the neck down the chest to the groin. Occasionally accessory glandular tissue occurs in the axilla, and this tissue is subject to neoplastic growth and hormonal influences.

Usually the breasts are reasonably symmetrical, similarly shaped with the nipples parallel in the same plane. The skin is smooth without discoloration or irregularities. The areola is darker and more deeply pigmented in women who have been pregnant, and small tubercles of Montgomery may be present. Nipples may be erect, flat, or inverted, but whatever their original status the nipples tend to remain that way. Any changes may be due to a neoplasm. Usually there is no discharge from the nipples except during pregnancy and lactation, but in a very small number of women premenstrual discharge may be normal. The administration or withdrawal of exogenous sex steroids, such as oral contraceptives, can cause nipple discharge or inappropriate lactation, as can certain other drugs, including phenothiazines, tricyclic tranquilizers, reserpine, and methyldopa.

As women get older, the glandular tissue of

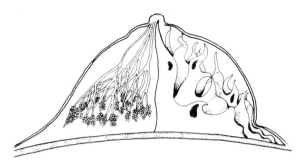

Figure 13-1. Anatomy of the normal breast with ductal and alveolar structures on left and fascial structures on right.

their breasts is gradually replaced by fatty tissue. There may be atrophic changes, depending upon the extent of body fat. The thickening of the inframammary ridge at the lower edge of the breast, which is a normal occurrence, becomes more pronounced with age. Only after menopause, during pregnancy, and while taking oral contraceptives are the breasts in a relatively quiescent phase as far as monthly cyclic changes are concerned. Pregnancy and possibly lactation are thought to confer some protection against breast cancer, although the mechanism by which this is accomplished is not understood. Estrogens in oral contraceptives cause breast changes of the proliferative type, but despite this tissue growth, use of oral contraceptives seems to be associated with a decreased incidence of some types of benign breast disease.[1] No causal relation between oral contraceptives and breast cancer has been demonstrated (see Chapter 4, Contraception). Both pregnancy and oral contraceptives provide a fairly continuous supply of estrogen and progesterone (or synthetic progestins) together, unlike the monthly rise and fall of these hormones in varying proportion during the menstrual cycle.

Women's breasts differ in the smoothness or lumpiness of their glandular tissue. Nulliparous breasts are dense and firm, and after pregnancy the tissue is usually softer and looser. Fine granular bumps, pea-sized or smaller, occurring in clusters widely dispersed throughout the breast are normal glandular tissue. Some women have larger lumps in irregular patterns due to cystic breast disease, making breast evaluation quite difficult. Lumpiness and soreness to the touch increase premenstrually and during menses, and are least noticeable the week following the menstrual period. Differentiation among lumps is discussed in the section on physical examination.

MEANINGS OF BREAST MASSES

The vast majority of breast masses are discovered by the woman herself, an event which creates in her an immediate state of panic and arouses her primitive fears. Perhaps the exception is the woman with longstanding breast disease, previously diagnosed as cystic or some other benign condition. For these women, however, the question of malignant changes is always present. It is much harder to identify a dangerous lump among many cystic ones than in smooth, regular breast tissue. In a small number of cases, breast masses are discovered by the nurse practitioner, physician, or other examiner including the woman's sexual partner. Whether it is a definite, distinct mass or some suspicious thickening or irregularity, the chilling fear following her discovery pervades the woman's consciousness and centers her attention on this alien growth within her breast. Continual feeling and pressing may cause increasing tenderness, only adding to her concern.

Mass Does Not Necessarily Equal Cancer

To most women today, finding a mass in the breast immediately flashes one terrifying thought—cancer! Cancer has become the dread disease of the 20th century, the plague of our times. The emotional reaction to cancer probably stems from certain characteristics of the disease and from outdated information about its treatment and prognosis. Cardiovascular disease, for example, kills more people than cancer but is not viewed with the same dread and terror. One reason cancer is so terrifying is that it is not well understood, and its causes, which are only now beginning to be identified, are multiple and complex. The term cancer actually covers over 100 different types of invasive diseases, each having some common and many particular characteristics. What cancers have in common contributes to their frightfulness: some agent (probably environmental) produces a change in the segment of DNA (deoxyribonucleic acid) in a given cell that controls the growth and reproduction of that cell. The altered or mutated cell replicates in kind, producing daughter cells with DNA informa-

tion that tells them to continue reproducing. This is in distinct contrast to the life cycle of the normal cell, which in the adult only reproduces at set intervals for the purpose of replacing other cells which have died. The malignant cells never stop reproducing and can outgrow the blood supply to their region, leading to necrosis. Another frightening characteristic of cancer is its ability to spread. Malignant cells can break off from the original tumor mass and travel via lymphatics or blood to distinct sites, setting up new tumors or metastases. Or they can invade local surrounding tissue, replacing it with malignant cells. These cancer cells have no useful function for the body or the organs they invade; they do not supply energy or contribute to the functions of the organ. In fact, they use up nutrients more rapidly than normal surrounding tissue does because of their more rapid rate of reproduction and their higher metabolic rate. Eventually the invaded organ becomes unable to function, as more and more of its tissue is taken over by the cancer. The changes caused by cancer in the structure and function of invaded organs leads to the pain and other symptoms of dysfunction typical of the disease.

The diagnosis of cancer has been viewed as equal to the pronouncement of death. This attitude developed because until recently there was very little that medicine could do to treat cancer, and the progression of the disease involved extensive suffering, disability, and fairly rapid death. Treatment was mainly surgical, often involving extremely mutilating procedures which were themselves disabling, but survival rates were poor because of metastasis. The disease was so lethal, so shrouded in mystery, and seemed so invulnerable to the tools of medical science that its mere mention struck terror in the hearts of most people and, for many years, cancer was not discussed.

Avoidance and Denial

Women with breast masses, fearing cancer, feel the primordial life threat triggering the organism's drive for survival, but the enemy is within and cannot be seen and attacked. This situation often leads to immobilization, in which the threat is so overwhelming or so nebulous that constructive actions cannot be undertaken. Instead, the psychological defenses of avoidance or denial are used, permitting the woman to escape from facing the threat.

These processes have a significant role in delaying treatment, as the woman may wait a considerable period of time before seeking help. With cancer, time is critical; the earlier cancer is discovered and the smaller the tumor, the better the chances for cure and long-term survival.

Women also fear the mutilation they associate with the treatment of breast cancer. Removal of a breast has so many implications for their self-concept, their worth and value in the eyes of society and men, and in their perception of sexuality that women may delay seeking care because of these fears. There is also the stigma of cancer, with the fear of isolation which occurs when other people withdraw and disengage from the doomed victim. These many factors combine to produce a profound fear that in its cumulative effect is much greater than realistic fears of pain, disability, and limitations which might result from surgical or other treatment.

In 1975 breast cancer was brought into a new focus by publicity in the mass media. Betty Ford, wife of the President, and Happy Rockefeller, wife of the former Vice-President, both had surgery for breast cancer. Their treatment was widely covered in the national news media, and their openness about the disease spurred many women into a new way of thinking. The American Cancer Society stepped up its campaign on behalf of early detection, breast self-examination, and the treatability of cancer. Late-night television shows and radio talk shows featured women who had undergone mastectomy. Rose Kushner, a medical journalist, published *Breast Cancer: A Personal History & an Investigative Report*,[2] in which she described her own experience with breast cancer. The book is a compilation of current information on the disease and an excellent source for both professional and lay persons. Women's groups attacked the sexism associated with breast amputation and encouraged women and men to view the disease and its treatment in the proper perspective rather than to consider it as devastating for their sexual relation. As a result, attitudes are changing toward breast cancer and its aftereffects. There is a climate of openness, hopefulness, and increasing involvement by women and their partners in all phases of treatment. The professional community must also change in order to accommodate the new attitudes of consumers and also to integrate new developments in the management of breast cancer.

MANAGEMENT OF BREAST MASSES

Problems related to the breasts may present as pain, lumps, or thickening, nipple discharge, changes in size or shape, or skin rashes of the nipple or areola. Any of these could be benign, minor problems or could signal a malignant neoplasm. Differentiating innocuous problems from potentially lethal ones becomes the task of the health provider—a difficult and often complex process. A woman's medical history can increase the index of suspicion by identifying her risk factors, but it is of less importance in the diagnosis than physical examination. While there are typical physical findings both for some types of breast cancer and for benign disease, they are unevenly present and are subject to numerous subtle variations. Diagnostic aids such as mammography and cytology are often crucial in establishing the nature of the lesion. There is currently much interest in predictive oncology and early cancer detection through screening, but these are areas which cause considerable controversy. Once breast cancer is diagnosed, management, involving surgery, radiation and chemotherapy, has progressed to the point of some precision and offers more options than were previously available. Although there are several large cancer research and treatment centers in the United States, family physicians and gynecologists continue to manage the majority of cancer patients, usually in consultation with local oncologists.

The History

Depending upon the presenting symptom, various combinations of the following questions are included in the history.

How long has the lump or thickening been present? Has it undergone any changes? If a lump has been present for 10 years or so and has not changed significantly, it is very unlikely that it is a serious condition. Women with a long history of multiple lumps and bumps usually report an established diagnosis of fibrocystic disease. If one area has changed recently, however, if a lump has become more pronounced or enlarged rapidly, the change is significant. The presence of a "dominant lump" in generally lumpy breasts must be approached in the same way as a new lump in smooth breasts because women with fibrocystic disease do develop breast cancer also. In fact, fibrocystic disease makes it harder to detect breast cancer early, as the numerous cystic masses and thickened fibrous tissue can conceal small malignancies. In a women with previously regular, smooth breast tissue, the appearance of a lump within a short time span must be viewed with great suspicion. A rapid increase in size does not always indicate a malignancy, however, because different types of tumors have different growth rates and some benign conditions are associated with a rapid increase in size.

Is the lump painful or tender? Breast cancer was previously believed to present typically as a painless, nontender lump, but new data have shown that unilateral breast pain is the second most common complaint in breast cancer patients, the presence of a lump being first.[3] The character of the pain associated with breast cancer is most often described as stinging, burning, pulling, or drawing, and it is confined to a localized area of the breast. Any type of breast tumor can cause pain when nerves are displaced or nerve endings are involved. Fibrocystic disease is associated with varying degrees of pain—at times enough to be almost disabling—which may or may not be cyclic. It is important to eliminate other extraneous causes of breast pain such as oral manipulation during sex, which can cause localized pain. Changes in activity, with the increased use of one arm, or repetitive activity involving one arm, can cause one-sided breast pain. Sometimes certain types of bras, particularly the underwire bra, have wire parts that can shift around and jab the breast. The woman may have thought she felt something in her breast, and continual poking and squeezing over a period of time can cause localized tenderness and pain. Mental stress could also be an indirect cause of pain.

Is the pain or tenderness cyclic? For many women, the cyclic changes involving enlargement and congestion in glands and ducts in the breasts produce regularly occurring pain, usually premenstrually. This may be more pronounced some months, leading to concern. Cyclic pain does occur with fibrocystic disease, with the use of oral contraceptives and, much less commonly, with cancer. With a negative examination, the woman with moderate cyclic breast pain can be reassured and educated about hormonal effects on the breasts. If pain is burning or stinging or if it persists and is of concern, a second examination in 1 or 2 months and mammography are indicated.

Has there been any nipple discharge? In the presence of a breast mass, any nipple discharge must be examined, no matter what its color. The incidence of cancer in women over age 50 with a lump and nipple discharge is at least 50 percent. Bloody or blood-tinged discharge is always significant, whether or not a lump is present. A Pap smear and a biopsy are both indicated. A spontaneous discharge, not associated with breast manipulation or drug use, must always be viewed with suspicion, and a guiuac test for occult blood as well as cytologic studies should be done. Women taking oral contraceptives or using other drugs which may alter hormone balance, such as phenothiazines, digitalis, diuretics and steroids, not infrequently have a clear nipple discharge. Vigorous stripping during examination or manipulation during sex can produce some clear discharge in most instances.

Is there any eczema or rash on the nipple? It is important to find out where the dermatitis began, if it is a symptom. Paget's disease starts with a small focus, usually covered with a crust, on the apex of the nipple. It then spreads outward to involve the areola. Eczema or other dermatitis usually begins on the areola or surrounding breast tissue and may subsequently spread to the nipple, but it very rarely begins on the nipple unless it is associated with breast feeding.

Has there been any trauma to the breast? Injuries to the breast are not thought to be related to the development of cancer although as environmental factors injuries may contribute to a set of conditions which might support cancer growth. To be causally related to breast cancer, the injury would have to have happened some 20 to 30 years before the lump was felt. What commonly happens is that after striking or bumping her breast on something, the woman feels the injured area and finds a lump that in reality was there for some time. Or, a lump found after an injury could be due to local edema from bleeding and trauma to the tissues. Such lumps should resolve in a short time; if they do not, the woman should be examined.

FAMILY AND PAST MEDICAL HISTORY.   There is an increased risk of breast cancer if the woman's mother, sister, or maternal grandmother, aunts, or first cousins had breast cancer before menopause. If her mother or sister had breast cancer after menopause, there is no significantly increased risk. When the woman herself has previously had breast cancer, she is at an increased risk of developing cancer in the remaining breast. Other factors associated with a higher incidence of breast cancer include early menarche, with menses for 30 years or more, no children or first pregnancy after age 35, infertility, or late or no beginning of sexual activity.[4] (See also the sections on Predictive Oncology and Early Detection and High Risk Profile).

Physical Examination

The physical examination of the breasts is extremely important because it serves as the major basis for clinical decisions on management. The examination must be approached systematically and both breasts examined thoroughly, regardless of when the lesion is identified. Inspection and palpation are utilized, and the complete examination includes axillary and supraclavicular palpation in addition to the breasts proper. It takes about 10 to 15 minutes to do a thorough breast examination, with the woman first sitting and then supine. The nurse practitioner needs access to the examining table from both sides because she or he cannot adequately palpate a breast when reaching across the patient. A good light is essential for showing the shadows and subtle variations in skin color and texture that often provide important information. Whether the examination begins sitting or lying is according to individual preference. The woman should be completely undressed to the waist to facilitate visualization.

EXAMINATION IN THE SITTING POSITION. With the woman sitting erect, arms at her side, inspect the breasts for size and symmetry. Some difference in size between them is normal, but the contours should be regular and similar bilaterally. Note any alterations in contour, indentation of the inframammary fold, or distortion of the edge of the areola which causes asymmetry. Breast cancers often involve fascial structures causing fibrosis and contraction producing skin retraction with its typical appearance of *dimpling* or *tethering*. This sign is almost pathognomonic of carcinoma.[5] Often, dimpling is seen better with the woman's arms raised. An inverted or flattened nipple, if of recent origin, is also usually associated with cancer, although one or two other lesions will produce this sign. The color and appearance of the skin is important to note because cancer can cause edema of the skin due to lymphatic blockage. Edema is manifested in thickened skin with enlarged pores which has the appearance of an orange peel and so is, appropriately, called peau d'orange. Edema with erythema and the presence of dilated blood vessels in a localized area of the breast can be associated with inflammatory carcinoma or with breast infections. Observe the appearance of the nipple and areola, as the presence of dermatitis with erythema, rough thickening, crusting, erosion, or ulceration could signal Paget's disease. The presence of peau d'orange or inflammation with a malignant lesion is considered a grave sign, indicating advanced or fulminant cancer.

Have the woman raise her arms above her head or rest her hands on her head, which is less tiring, and again inspect the breasts for symmetry. This position may reveal previously unnoticed dimpling. Fibrosis associated with cancer may also cause nipple deviation, in which one nipple deviates from a parallel axis in the direction of the cancer. Lifting the breasts or compressing them slightly will also accentuate dimpling. Have the woman point to the exact spot which concerns her before beginning palpation because this helps to locate the possible lesion and assures that the provider will carefully examine the area. Then, with the woman's arms raised, palpate by covering all the breast tissue, following a clockwise or counterclockwise pattern. Lift the breast with the fingertips and inspect the lower and lateral portions to determine if there are any changes in the color or texture of the skin. Pulling upward on the breast tissue near the clavicle may demonstrate nipple foreshortening or skin dimpling. Palpate the tail of the breast as it enters the lower axilla by gently compressing the tissue between thumb and fingers. The nipple can also be palpated in this position to check for small, centrally located lumps or duct thickening, and the nipple can be stripped softly for discharge. Some practitioners prefer to strip the nipple and collect specimens in the supine position.

After both breasts have been palpated with the woman's arms raised, have the woman press her hands against her hips. This flexion of the pectoral muscles may reveal dimpling or irregularities of contour previously not visible. Some health providers recommend palpating both breasts again in this position. Particularly if the breasts are large or pendulous, have the woman extend her arms and lean forward as her hands are supported by the examiner. The weight of the breasts carries them away from the chest wall, and subtle skin changes may be noted.

With the woman sitting relaxed, arms at her side, the examiner supports one arm while *palpation of the axilla* is carried out. The right hand is used for the left axilla and vice versa so that the fingers may reach upward and deeply into the axillary hollow. Push firmly upward and milk the axillary contents downward, even if vigorous palpation causes some discomfort. The presence of enlarged lymph nodes raises the index of suspicion, although this could be due to infections of the skin of the arms, hands, or breast. In rare cases, the first sign of breast cancer is an enlarged axillary node which has been invaded and can be found even before a breast mass can be palpated. The supraclavicular area should also be palpated because infraclavicular nodes drain a portion of the breast. This palpation is more easily accomplished if the woman turns her head toward the side being palpated and raises the same shoulder, allowing the examiner's fingers to reach more deeply into the fossa. Any enlarged nodes felt here are highly significant because they are caused by an invasion of the lymphatics by the carcinoma.

EXAMINATION IN THE SUPINE POSITION. After examining both breasts, axillae, and supraclavicular areas in the sitting position, have the woman lie supine with one arm behind her head (or abducted to 75 degrees). Placing a folded sheet or small pillow under her shoulder causes the breast to spread more evenly over the chest wall. Skin appearance and the symmetry of the woman's breasts are again noted. Techniques for palpation differ among providers, but the goal is to compress the breast tissue between the fingers and chest wall and to cover all tissue thoroughly. The pads of three or four fingers are used, compressing tissue in a rotary motion and proceeding in a clockwise motion starting at the periphery and moving inward. One or both hands may be used as breast tissue is systematically covered. Or, the palpation may proceed from top to bottom of the breast on one side, moving from periphery to the center, and repeated for the other side. The most important thing is to cover completely all breast tissue, including the tail of the breast which extends up toward the axilla. These maneuvers are repeated with the woman's arm at her side or rotated across her chest wall. This change in arm position changes the position of the breast and allows palpation when a different portion of her breast is over the woman's ribs.

Palpate around the nipple and areola for small masses or duct thickening. The nipple should be gently stripped for discharge. Watch the nipple closely to notice whether the discharge comes from a single or several ducts. If only a single duct is involved, there will be material exuding from one or several milk sinus openings just on one area of the nipple. The involvement of several ducts produces discharge from many more milk sinus openings. Multiple-duct discharge, whether clear or grumous, is most common with duct ectasia and papillomatosis. It often is caused by oral manipulation or poor nipple hygiene. Single duct discharge, whether bloody or clear, usually is caused by large-duct papillomas or intraductal carcinomas. If a mass is also present, any nipple discharge must be examined cytologically and for blood. In the absence of a mass, any discharge which is bloody or blood-tinged should be examined, and the woman should be referred for biopsy. Spontaneous discharge is also significant, even if it is clear. If nipple stripping is carried out gently enough during the examination, then any discharge produced could be important and must be examined cytologically.

If a mass is found in a breast, its size, shape, firmness, tenderness, fixation, and the degree of ease with which the margins can be identified must be characterized. Vague clinical findings in which there is no definite mass but a thickening or fullness that is somewhat more pronounced than in other areas, present the most difficult problem. Such vague differences are variously called fibronodular, ropy, granular, or indurated. In this situation, if other signs such as dimpling, asymmetry, and nipple discharge are present they can serve to confirm the practitioner's suspicions (Figure 13-2).

DIFFERENTIATING BREAST MASSES. When a definite mass is felt, there are certain characteristics which may help the provider to differentiate benign conditions from malignancies. However, definitive diagnosis depends upon a biopsy or the aspiration of cysts when a clear-cut mass is present. Carcinoma of the breast is usually a single mass, although it may coexist with other nodular or cystic lesions. Borders are generally irregular or stellate, and the consistency of the mass is firm or hard. There is no clear delineation from the surrounding tissues, and the mass may be fixed to the skin or underlying tissues. The mass may be either tender or nontender, and often signs of retraction such as dimpling or nipple inversion are present. Malignancies tend to grow constantly, and depending upon particular doubling time can increase in size very rapidly. Breast cancers occur most commonly in women age 30 to 80, but can occur in quite young women between 20 and 30 years old.

A fibroadenoma, a benign neoplasm, is usually a single mass, although fibroadenomas can be multiple. They are round, discoid, or lobular in shape, and range in consistency from soft to firm, although they are more commonly firm. Their borders are well delineated, and the lesion is very mobile and often described as slippery or wiggling as it moves under the fingers.

Usually fibroadenomas are nontender. They grow very quickly and constantly and are most common among younger women age 15 to 20, though they occur in women up to the age of 55.

Altered physiology with a long follicular or luteal phase is responsible for fibrocystic disease, in which continued ductal enlargement gives way to cystic structures which become filled with liquid under pressure. The cysts produced can become very tense and painful, and they feel like a tumor. There is also increased epithelial growth in the ducts and chronic inflammation, with an increase of fibrous tissue between the breast lobules. These changes lead to a firm, nodular feeling as multiple small or large cysts become surrounded by dense, fibrous tissue. Typically, women with fibrocystic disease have bumpy and nodular breasts, with continual fluctuation in any given area. The nodules are affected by hormones and tend to enlarge and decrease during the menstrual cycle. There is no symmetrical pattern to the lumps, which are round in shape and soft to firm in consistency. Usually both breasts are affected, with multiple nodules on both sides and no dominant nodule. Larger cysts are well delineated, mobile, and tender. Women age 30 to 55 are more likely to have fibrocystic disease and it usually regresses after menopause (Table 13-1).

When masses or other tissue abnormalities are found, the characteristics noted above are described, the size is given in centimeters, and

Table 13-1
Differentiating Breast Masses

	Fibrocystic Disease	Fibroadenoma	Cancer
Usual age	30-55, regresses after menopause	15-20+, occur up to 55	30-80, peak incidence 42-48
Number	Usually multiple, may be single	Usually single, may be multiple	Usually single, but may coexist with other lesions
Shape	Round	Round, discoid or lobular	Irregular or stellate
Consistency	Soft to firm; bumpy nodular breasts	Usually firm, may be soft	Firm or hard
Delimitation	Usually well delineated	Well-delineated, clear margins	Not clearly delineated from surrounding tissue
Mobility	Mobile	Very mobile, slippery	May be fixed to skin or underlying tissue
Tenderness	Often tender	Usually nontender	Usually nontender, but not always
Retraction signs	Absent	Absent	Often present

PAGET'S DISEASE

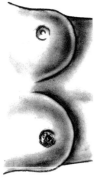

A form of breast cancer, Paget's disease progresses slowly from a smooth redness to rough thickening to erosion or ulceration of the nipple and areola. In any dermatitis of nipple and areola, cancer must be suspected.

NIPPLE DISCHARGE

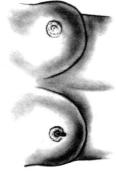

There are many causes of nipple discharge, most of them non-malignant. Note the color of the discharge and if possible identify its source.

SUPERNUMERARY BREASTS

One or more extra breasts may be located along the "milk line," most commonly in the axillae or below the normal breasts. A supernumerary breast usually consists of a small nipple and areola and may be mistaken for a mole. Less commonly glandu-

NIPPLE INVERSION

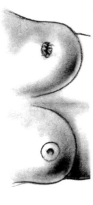

Simple nipple inversion is a common variant of normal and is usually of long standing. It may be unilateral or bilateral. The nipple can usually be pulled out of the sulcus in which it lies. Flattening, broadening and true retraction are absent. The recent development of inversion in a previously erect nipple, however, is highly suspicious of malignancy.

NIPPLE FLATTENING OR RETRACTION

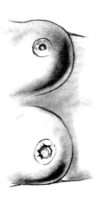

The fibrosis associated with a cancer behind the nipple pulls the nipple inward and may broaden and flatten it.

NIPPLE DEVIATION OR POINTING

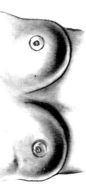

The fibrosis associated with cancer may deviate the axis in which the nipple points. The nipple deviates toward the cancer.

EDEMA OF NIPPLE AND AREOLA

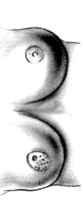

The pig skin or orange peel appearance produced by lymphatic

SKIN DIMPLING

Dimpling of the skin suggests an underlying malignancy. Look for this sign at rest, during special positioning, and on moving or compressing the breasts.

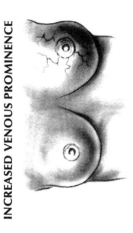

A breast cancer frequently causes fibrosis or scar tissue formation. Contraction of this fibrotic tissue produces *retraction signs*, including dimpling of the skin, alteration in breast contours and flattening or deviation of the nipple.

Dimpling

Flattening of nipple

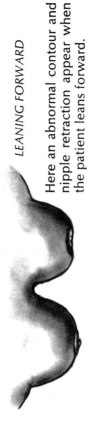

ABNORMAL CONTOURS

LEANING FORWARD

Here an abnormal contour and nipple retraction appear when the patient leans forward.

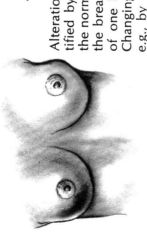

ARMS OVER HEAD

Alterations in contour are identified by careful inspection of the normally convex surfaces of the breasts and by comparison of one breast with the other. Changing the patient's position, e.g., by elevation of her arms, also helps.

IN ADDITION, *VASCULAR SIGNS* MAY BE NOTED. THESE INCLUDE:

INCREASED VENOUS PROMINENCE

An increased prominence of the venous pattern.

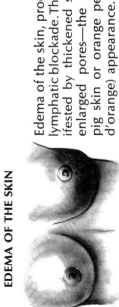

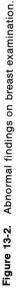

EDEMA OF THE SKIN

Edema of the skin, produced by lymphatic blockade. This is manifested by thickened skin with enlarged pores—the so-called pig skin or orange peel (peau d'orange) appearance.

Figure 13-2. Abnormal findings on breast examination.

their location in the breast is given according to the quadrant in which the mass is found, as for example, in the upper outer quadrant. Or, the breast may be divided according to the hours of the clock and the mass reported, for example, at 11 o'clock. The location of smaller nodules is also clarified by noting whether they are on the periphery of the breast or near the areola.

Diagnostic Aids

MAMMOGRAPHY. A radiological examination of the breasts is of great diagnostic value and can be used to identify the presence of a breast cancer as long as 2 years prior to the clinical appearance of signs and symptoms. Although false negative and false positive readings occur, the accuracy of the identification of breast lesions by mammography is 90 percent when their results are read by an experienced radiologist. Mammography aids in evaluating breasts with vague clinical findings, with ill-defined or questionable masses, multiple masses or nodules, nipple discharge or erosion, nipple or skin retraction, skin changes, or pain. In women with definite masses who will undergo biopsy, preoperative mammography provides information about the status of the mass, aids in the determination of the site most useful for biopsy and permits a survey of the opposite breast (5 to 8 percent of breast cancers occur subsequently in the opposite breast and 1 percent occur concurrently). Mammography is especially useful for screening women at high risk of developing breast cancer, such as those with a strong family history, with one breast removed for cancer, or with other predictive factors. Women with very large breasts or lumpy, nodular breasts due to fibrocystic disease are difficult to evaluate by physical examination, and mammography is the most accurate method for evaluating their breasts for significant masses.

There are two types of mammography commonly used, low dose x-ray mammography and xeromammography (xerography). Low dose x-ray mammograms are soft tissue x-ray studies using new techniques and lower doses than conventional x-ray studies. They look for differences in the density of breast tissues, and thus are more accurate in breasts of older women in which most of the glandular tissue has been replaced by fat. There is little difference in density between normal glandular tissue in the young breast and carcinoma, while in the older woman's breast the fatty tissue appears lighter than carcinoma. Also, cancer and cysts have the same density. However, there are characteristics of various types of lesions which aid the radiologist in identification. Cysts have a smooth border and clear margins, while cancer has tendrils with starburst margins. Large obvious calcifications within a mass occur in fibroadenomas, not in cancers, while calcifications in cancer are like small talcum powder granules. The presence of fibrocystic disease makes the interpretation of mammography more difficult.

Xeromammography uses a somewhat different technique in which x-ray images passing through the breast are received on a selenium-coated plate; these images are photoelectrically recorded on paper. A small x-ray dose is required, and the same rate of accuracy is obtained as with low dose x-rays. Xerography is easier to read than low dose x-ray methods, and provides the same information. It would be used for the same indications, the choice of methods depending upon what is available in a given locale (Figure 13-3).

Various other methods are currently under investigation, but their usefulness as diagnostic adjuncts has not yet been proven. Thermography identifies heat patterns in the breast, with cancer appearing as a "hot spot" because of its increased metabolism. It is an accurate technique in large cancers but often fails to identify small or deep cancers. Thus thermography is not yet helpful in the detection of small, early cancer. Ultrasonography, isotope scanning, and angiography are also being explored for their usefulness in early breast cancer detection.

BIOPSY. The definitive diagnosis of breast masses depends upon the pathologic examination of tissues removed by surgical biopsy. The safest course for the nurse practitioner is to refer all women who have suspicious masses

Figure 13-3. Mammographic appearance of breast lesions. A. Benign cyst. B. Benign fibroadenoma in patient who noted increasing size of the breast before feeling a mass. C. Benign calcifying adenoma that had clinical appearance of cancer. D. Moderately invasive carcinoma. E. Typical stellate image of carcinoma. *Patient Care*, (April 1, 1975):80 and C. D. Haagensen, *Diseases of the Breast*, ed. 2 (Philadelphia: W. B. Saunders. 1971), p. 136.

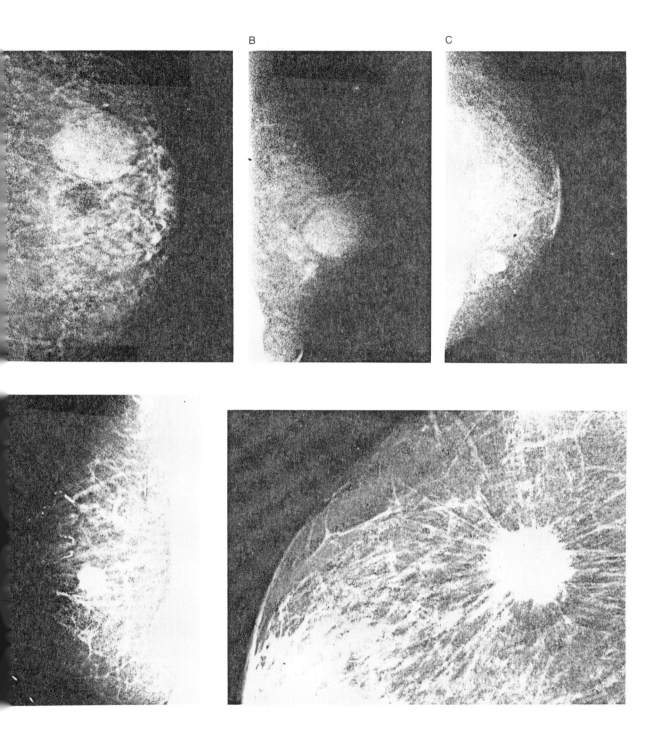

found in a physical examination or by mammography to a physician. Cystic masses may often be aspirated (see below), but if the fluid is blood-tinged or the mass persists after aspiration, a biopsy is indicated. A growing number of family practice physicians and surgeons are doing office biopsies for small breast masses with no skin changes or node involvement. A marked change is occurring in physicians' approach to the surgical management of breast masses, no doubt in part due to the furor over the "one-stage" versus the "two-stage" procedure. Evidence is accumulating that there is no increased risk to survival if biopsy and surgery for breast cancer are separated by a few weeks. In fact, there are several good reasons for separating biopsy from mastectomy. For one thing a frozen-section diagnosis is less accurate than a permanent section, which takes several days. Although the incidence is very small, the removal of the breast for a benign lesion is an incredible mistake. Combined surgical procedures do not allow for staging the cancer preoperatively, (see pp. 320 to 321) a step cancer specialists consider essential to the proper management of this disease. If there is metastatic disease, the very rationale for mastectomy—preventing the spread of the tumor from the breast—is negated. Preoperative preparation for a biopsy is quite different from preparation for major surgery such as mastectomy, and scheduling these procedures separately allows for proper planning. For biopsies done under light anesthesia, chest films are often not mandatory. Going right from light to deep inhalation anesthesia for the mastectomy could mean that some condition of the lungs which contraindicates inhalation anesthesia might be missed. A more thorough surgical work-up would no doubt be undertaken when a woman diagnosed as having breast cancer by biopsy was to be admitted for a mastectomy.

The psychological benefits for the woman and her family are enormous when diagnostic biopsy is separated from mastectomy. To be wheeled into an operating room, to be put to sleep without knowing whether or not a breast would be removed, to awaken to a groggy state of half-consciousness in the recovery room, and only then to discover whether she still has two breasts or only one, is an excruciating mental anguish for a woman. Absorbing the meaning of breast cancer, and rallying the resources necessary to cope with it, demands all the positive forces a person can muster. People are able to cope better with crises and problems if they can anticipate and prepare for them, and there is less disruption in the family if its planning for the woman's operation can be based on a realistic understanding of the extent of the problem. Women who have undergone the one-stage biopsy-mastectomy procedure attest eloquently to its devastating effect, to feeling dehumanized, excluded from decision-making, mutilated, frightened, and shocked to the depth of their beings.

Some surgeons think that a two-stage procedure is impossible in certain situations because occasionally a carcinoma cannot be left when diagnosed by frozen section, but there is controversy about this point. Another theory holds that the cancer might be seeded during the operation and have more time to spread if the biopsy and mastectomy are performed separately. Many oncologists do not believe that this theory is valid, however, and think that there is no danger of seeding if the proper technique is used in the biopsy. There is also evidence that the patient's immune system attacks and destroys circulating cancer cells, and that these cells are found in the peripheral circulation of patients with cancer who have not had a surgical procedure.[6]

The economic advantages to the health care system in outpatient biopsies of breast masses should also be considered. Costly hospital operating rooms would not be utilized for a minor procedure, and the two inpatient days needed to prepare for and recover from anesthesia would be eliminated. Those eight women out of ten who have breast masses which turn out to be benign would also be spared the surgeon's and anesthetist's fees for the hospital biopsy.

NEEDLE ASPIRATION OF CYSTS. When breast masses have the characteristics of a cyst, aspiration with a needle and syringe can help to distinguish benign cysts of fibrocystic disease from solid tumors which might be malignant. If any signs of malignancy such as dimpling or fixation are present, aspiration should not be attempted. To aspirate a cyst with a needle, anesthetize an area over the mass with a wheal in the skin from a local anesthetic. Then introduce a 20-gauge needle attached to a syringe into the mass. If the mass is cystic, fluid will be returned immediately, often under pressure. Cystic fluid is usually clear to turbid green or dark brown, and is almost always thin. Cytological study is not recommended, and the color is unimportant unless the fluid is blood-tinged. Bloody fluid increases the suspicion of cancer. A cyst should disappear completely after aspiration, and generally it does not recur. If a small residual amount of fluid is left, however, it can encourage the cyst to refill. Most cysts yield 3 to 10 cc. of fluid, but can have as little as 0.5 cc. or as much as 125 cc. fluid. Those with less than 5 cc. have a lower incidence of recurrence because the tension within the small cavity aids in its decompression. A small indentation can be felt at the site after successful aspiration, but it is not palpable within 2 or 3 days because the surrounding tissue fills the void. The recurrence rate for aspirated cysts is reported at less than 5 percent.[7]

If fluid is not returned, the lesion is solid and must be biopsied. Bloody fluid could be from the center of a necrotic tumor, a papilloma, or an intracystic carcinoma. If the mass does not disappear after aspiration, or if it refills promptly within 3 or 4 days, it is suggestive of carcinoma, and a biopsy should be scheduled. After aspiration of cysts, other previously hidden suspicious lesions may be felt, and a biopsy is again indicated.

Follow-up after the successful aspiration of breast cysts includes a return visit in 2 to 4 weeks for reexamination. If the cyst recurs it may be aspirated again, particularly if the initial cyst yielded over 15 cc. fluid and the second one appears much smaller. However, reaspiration should not be persisted in, and surgical removal is indicated. If there is no recurrence on the follow-up visit, the woman is then seen every 6 months for a routine breast examination.

It is impossible and unnecessary to excise all simple breast cysts, and an appropriately done needle aspiration is a safe and effective way to manage this problem. There is no evidence that malignant cells are spread into the needle track if the mass does turn out to be carcinoma, or that survival rates are adversely affected by a few weeks' delay between an attempted aspiration and mastectomy.

CYTOLOGY. There is mixed opinion about the usefulness of cytological study of breast fluid. Aspirated fluid from cystic lesions rarely reveals malignant cells on cytological examination and is generally not recommended unless there is reason to be suspicious of the lesion. Occasionally needle biopsies of solid lesions are done, and the specimen obtained is sent for cytological study. However, there is a high incidence of false negatives with this approach, and masses suspicious enough to warrant obtaining a specimen for cytology are generally better managed by surgical biopsy with the excision of the entire mass for study. Cytological smears of nipple discharge may be helpful when there is no palpable tumor, as one study found these positive in 6 out of 16 patients with breast cancer.[8] If physical examination and mammography do not reveal suspicious lesions in patients with abnormal nipple discharge, cytological smears of nipple secretions can be of diagnostic value. Such smears can be prepared and fixed as for a Pap smear.

BENIGN BREAST DISEASE
Fibrocystic Disease

This most common disease of women between ages 30 and 55 is also called mammary dysplasia, cystic adenosis, chronic cystic disease, and cystic mastitis. Although its etiology is unknown, the disease is thought to be estrogen-dependent because it is almost always limited to women in the reproductive years and it regresses after menopause. The cysts are often multiple, frequently bilateral, and may be either asymptomatic or painful. Rapid fluctuation in the size of the mass, and increased pain during the premenstrual phase of the cycle are common. There may be a discharge from the nipple.

A diagnosis may be established by the aspiration of the cysts or by a biopsy. Once fibrocystic disease has been diagnosed, new cysts may be aspirated as they appear if there are no signs suggestive of malignancy. Hormonal therapy has met with mixed results and is not generally recommended. Widespread fibrocystic disease presents difficulty in its management because it can easily mask early cancer. Although fibrosis and cystic change alone is not significant in relation to cancer, a biopsy with proven atypical ductal epithelial hyperplasia causes a fivefold increase in the risk of subsequent development of cancer. Women in high risk groups who present with changes in one area of the breast need to be biopsied even on mildly suspicious findings. Mammograms are also indicated more frequently for women with widespread fibrocystic disease. The breast pain associated with fibrocystic disease is best treated by avoiding trauma and wearing a good supportive brassiere both day and night.

For some women with persistent and painful fibrocystic disease, proven atypical ductal epithelial hyperplasia, or a strong family history of breast cancer, a bilateral subcutaneous mastectomy with augmentation may be the treatment of choice. The nipple, areola and a small amount of breast tissue are left and a prosthetic insert put in place in a one-step procedure. This is a major surgical procedure and the woman must weigh the risks versus the benefits of this alternative according to her own values. Women with a strong family history of early-onset breast cancer have a lifetime risk of almost 50 percent.[9]

Fibroadenoma

These benign neoplasms account for the vast majority of breast tumors in young women in their teens and early 20s. The mass is typically round, firm, discrete, movable, nontender, 1 to 5 cm. diameter, and is usually solitary but it may be multiple and bilateral. Fibroadenomas are generally asymptomatic and may enlarge rapidly and attain a great size. These masses must be removed for a definitive diagnosis, for although the likelihood of cancer is very small, it cannot be excluded. Excision is also the treatment for fibroadenomas.

Mammary Duct Ectasia

The subareolar ducts become palpable as rubbery lesions filled with a pastelike material in mammary duct ectasia. The ducts become dilated with desquamating secretory epithelium, necrotic debris, and chronic inflammatory cells. This problem occurs most commonly in perimenopausal and menopausal women, and the symptoms include pain, nipple retraction, nipple discharge, and occasionally enlarged regional lymph nodes. There is no known association with malignancy, and the treatment consists of the excision of the involved ducts and the area from which nipple discharge can be expressed.

Intraductal Papilloma and Papillomatosis

Papillomas of the ducts are a common cause of serous or bloody nipple discharge. These tiny tumors (2 to 3 mm. diameter) have a central fibrovascular stalk with delicate papilli, and are often too small to palpate. They are commonly located in a major collection duct in the subareolar area, and may be single or, less often, multiple (often called diffuse). Localizing the duct aids in finding the tumor, using gentle pressure with the fingertip at successive points around the circumference of the areola. A point often can be found where pressure produces a discharge, and a dilated duct or a small lump may be palpable here. The involved area must be excised and the tissue examined microscopically for cancer. If no mass is palpable and an involved duct cannot be localized, the patient should be reexamined weekly for one month. Mammography should be done and the nipple discharge should be examined cytologically for exfoliated cancer cells. Should the discharge persist, referral to a physician for exploration of the ducts is indicated.

Multiple papillomas (papillomatosis) are difficult to manage and may be associated with apocrine duct carcinoma. Repeated excisions may be necessary, and women with papillomatosis are considered at increased risk for cancer.

Infections

Infections of the breast can produce masses or suspicious signs, but can usually be differentiated from tumors because of the associated heat, erythema, induration, and tenderness. Inflammatory carcinoma is the exception because it closely resembles mastitis, but it usually involves more than one-third of the skin of the breast. Subareolar abscess and fistula formation is a chronic recurring infection not related to pregnancy and found in young women, with abscess formation, drainage, and often nipple inversion. Sebaceous cysts in the skin overlying the breast occasionally become infected and are readily distinguished by their superficial location. Incision and drainage or local excision are the treatments for abscesses and sebaceous cysts.

MALIGNANT TUMORS

Breast cancer is one of the major health problems affecting women. The incidence of this disease has been steadily creeping upward while the death rates have been unchanging for many years. About 88,000 new cases were diagnosed in 1976, comprising nearly 26 percent

Table 13-2
Incidence and Mortality of Breast Cancer and Other Types of Cancer in the United States

| | Estimated 1976 | | | | | | | | Actual 1973* Deaths | |
| | Incidence | | | | Deaths | | | | | |
	Male Percentage	Number	Female Percentage	Number	Male Percentage	Number	Female Percentage	Number	Male Number	Female Number
Lung	22	73,000	6	20,000	33	65,200	11	18,600	59,187	15,746
Colon and rectum	14	48,000	15	51,000	12	23,700	15	25,500	22,709	24,857
Stomach and other digest.	12	16,800	9	12,200	15	9,600	14	7,100	9,178	-
Breast	-	700	26	88,000	-	300	20	32,800	-	31,850
Uterus	-	-	14	47,000	-	-	7	11,000	-	11,774
Ovary	-	-	5	17,000	-	-	6	10,800	-	10,002
Prostate	17	56,000	-	-	10	19,300	-	-	18,830	-
Urinary	9	31,200	4	13,500	5	11,100	3	5,500	-	-
Leukemia and lymphomas	8	28,000	7	22,800	9	18,500	9	15,500	-	-

*Numbers available only for the five leading causes of cancer death by sex in 1973.
Data taken from American Cancer Society, "Cancer Facts & Figures '76" and "Cancer Statistics, 1976" in *Ca-A Cancer Journal for Clinicians*, American Cancer Society, 26, 1 (January/February, 1976).

of all new cases of cancer found in women. The death rate remains at 25 per 100,000 total population, having edged up almost 4 percent over the last decade and a half. Breast cancer is moving toward the position of the leading type of cancer in the United States in incidence, although cancer of the lung and bronchus still have the greatest mortality[10] (Table 13-2). When it is taken into account that breast cancer affects only half the population, with 99 percent of the cases being found in women, the impact is seen to be enormous.

One out of every 15 women in the United States will develop breast cancer in her lifetime. About half of these will eventually die of the disease. Incidence rates are higher in the higher socioeconomic groups, and breast cancer affects white women more often than black women, but the gap is closing rapidly. There has been a 25.7 percent increase in the incidence of breast cancer in black women from 1947 to 1969, and for 1976 it is estimated that breast cancer will comprise 22.6 percent of all new cases of cancer in nonwhite females,[11] while the annual incidence of breast cancer among all women is above 70 per 100,000.

Characteristics of Breast Cancer

The peak incidence of malignant breast lesions is between ages 40 and 60, but the disease does occur in women in their 20s and 30s, and individual risk continues to increase steadily with age. About 80 percent of the patients with breast cancer present with a usually painless lump in the breast. Less frequently, breast pain, or else nipple erosion, retraction, discharge, and itching, or redness, hardness, enlargement or shrinkage of the breast are the presenting sets of symptoms. In rare cases, an axillary mass or swelling of the arm may be the first symptom.

The early discovery of breast cancer is the most important factor in successful treatment and survival. For this reason, regular self-examination of the breasts has received considerable publicity and continues to be stressed as the best method of early detection (see page 330). There are, however, several different types of breast cancer, and the biological behavior of the disease is highly variable. Although the mean duration of life in untreated breast cancer is about 3 years, some patients die within 3 months while others survive for 5 to 30 years.[12] In some patients who have very small primary lesions and are treated promptly and appropriately, widespread metastasis and early death nevertheless occur. Generally, the course of breast cancer is related to its histologic type and grade, with well-differentiated tumors progressing more slowly. Certain types

Table 13-3
Histologic Types and Characteristics of Breast Cancers

Histologic Type	Total Percentage	Characteristics	Five-Year Survival Percentage
I. Ductal carcinoma	90	Arise from ductal epithelium	
1. Scirrhus	75	Irregular, firm, fixed; strands of atypical cells with fibrosis	54
2. Papillary	-	Soft, extensive intraductal involvement	80
3. Comedocarcinoma	-	Soft, extensive intraductal involvement	
4. Colloid	-	Mucinous epithelium, intraductal mucin	73
5. Medullary	-	Bulky, globular; hemorrhage and necrosis common	63
6. Paget's disease	3	Nipple discharge, burning and pruritis, eczema with crusting and ulceration of nipple; large pale anaplastic cells; 60% of cases have regional node metastasis	50
II. Lobular carcinoma	8	Terminal ductules and acini distended by small round malignant cells; marked tendency toward multicentricity; bilateral in 30% of cases	54
III. Sarcoma	1	Large, sharply circumscribed, similar to fibroadenomas but with more cellular, hyperplastic stroma; metastasis generally hematogenous rather than lymphatic	60
IV. Inflammatory carcinoma	3	Rapidly growing, often painful mass which enlarges the breast; skin erythematous, edematous, and warm over more than 1/3 of the breast; cancer invades subdermal lymphatics; metastases occur early and widely	Poor

are known to be particularly virulent, such as inflammatory carcinoma. It is generally believed that small, noninvasive primary tumors with no metastasis to regional lymph nodes offer the best possibilities for curative treatment (Table 13-3).

MULTICENTRICITY. Breast cancer is often multicentric, with more than one focus of malignancy within the breast. Often these "centricles" are microscopic in size and cannot be palpated but are identified on pathological examination of a breast removed for a single malignant lesion. As many as 54 percent of breast specimens from mastectomy for carcinoma were found to have more than one focus of apparent primary malignancy.[13] This spatial multicentricity is one reason why removal of the entire breast is advocated for treatment of breast cancer. Also, there is a temporal multicentricity which characterizes breast cancer. The breasts tend to respond as a single organ

to carcinogenic stimuli, accounting for the increased incidence of cancer in the remaining breast after mastectomy, which is 7 times greater than that expected for the general population. Malignancy in the remaining breast is more likely a new primary focus than a recurrence.

SIZE, GROWTH RATE, AND DOUBLING TIME. Breast cancer has a long preclinical phase, perhaps as long as 30 years, before the cell mass has increased to palpable size. Assuming that a lump can be felt when it weighs 1 Gm., or measures 1 cm. in diameter, it has gone through at least thirty doublings in size by the time it is palpable. Depending upon the type of cancer, this might take several weeks to many years. Doubling is a steady exponential growth in which the number of cells is compounded each generation, enabling a single cancer cell to become one million cells in twenty generations. If a 1-Gm. cancer is not detected and removed at this stage, after one more doubling it will weigh 2 Gm., and after two more doublings it will be 4 Gm. The length of the G-1, or resting phase of the life cycle of the tumor cell determines how rapid the doubling time is, as the other three phases have the same length of time for all types of cells (Figure 13-4). If a cancer cell divides once per month, having a 1-month doubling time, it will take 2½ years for it to attain palpable size; if another cancer cell divides once every 100 days, with a 100-day doubling time, it will not be palpable for 9 years (Figure 13-5).

The size of a breast cancer when diagnosed is one measure used to decide upon the method of treatment. Generally the larger the tumor, the greater the likelihood of advanced disease; however, this does not always hold true, as very small tumors can be associated with widespread metastasis. There is undoubtedly a period during which the tumor is confined to local growth and thus more amenable to treatment, but in many cases this may be the preclinical phase in which the mass is not palpable. This concept supports efforts to find acceptable mass screening methods more sensitive than palpation.

LOCAL EXTENSION AND METASTASIS. Fingerlike extensions from the central tumor mass into surrounding breast tissue is a common growth pattern in breast cancer. Such extensions may be in ducts, lymphatics, fascia or, less often, in blood vessels. Occasionally the skin may be involved, with satellite nodules around the primary tumor. The growth pattern is irregular, and tumor extensions are often not palpable. These fingerlike extensions account for the stellate pattern seen on mammography.

Metastasis occurs via the lymphatics and bloodstream. Since 45 percent of breast cancers occur in the upper outer quadrant, the most common site of lymphatic metastasis is the axillary chain of nodes. Axillary metastases are found in 50 to 60 percent of women undergoing radical mastectomy. The internal mammary lymph nodes are the next most commonly involved group, associated with a primary tumor located in the medial aspect of the breast or in the nipple. A 47 percent involvement of internal mammary nodes in nipple lesions and a 31 percent involvement in medial lesions have been found. The supraclavicular group of nodes are the third most commonly involved, but the

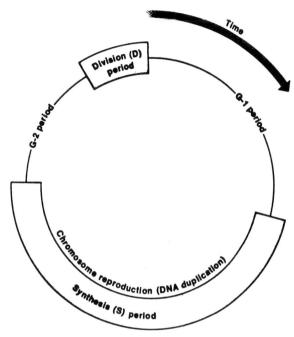

• **Figure 13-4.**   Life cycle of a cell.

involvement almost never occurs in the absence of axillary node involvement (Figure 13-6).

Distant metastasis occurs by hematogenous spread and most often involves, in order of frequency, the lungs, bones, liver, adrenals, brain, and ovaries. The bones of the pelvis, spine, femur, ribs, skull, and humerus are the most common sites of bony metastasis. Usually, dis-

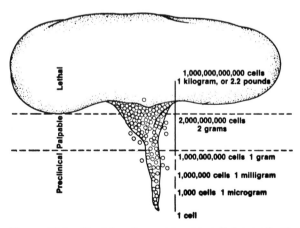

Figure 13-5.   Doubling time and exponential growth of cancer cells. R. Kushner, *Breast Cancer: A Personal History & Investigative Report* (New York: Harcourt, Brace Jovanovich, 1975), p. 44.

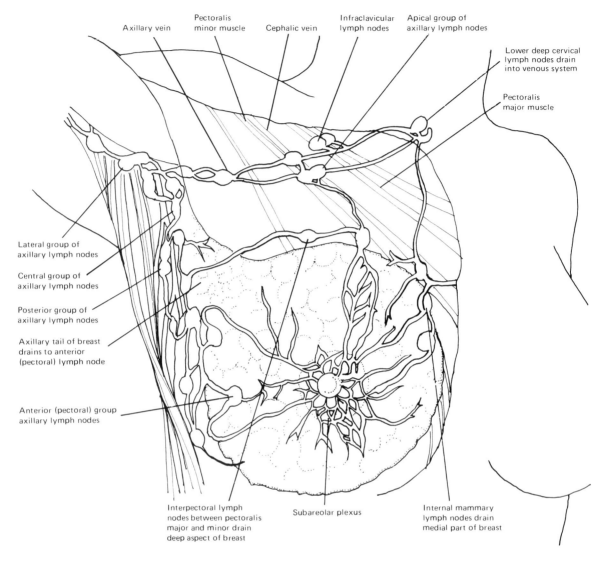

Axillary vein

Pectoralis
minor muscle

Cephalic vein

Infraclavicular
lymph nodes

Apical group of
axillary lymph nodes

Lower deep cervical
lymph nodes drain
into venous system

Pectoralis
major muscle

Lateral group of
axillary lymph nodes

Central group of
axillary lymph nodes

Posterior group of
axillary lymph nodes

Axillary tail of breast
drains to anterior
(pectoral) lymph node

Anterior (pectoral) group
axillary lymph nodes

Interpectoral lymph
nodes between pectoralis
major and minor drain
deep aspect of breast

Subareolar plexus

Internal mammary
lymph nodes drain
medial part of breast

Figure 13-6. Lymphatic drainage of the breast.

tant metastasis is preceded by regional lymphatic involvement, but not always.

Clinical Staging

The choice of treatment of breast cancer is determined mainly by the stage of the disease at the time of the initial diagnosis. The criteria used to determine the stage include the characteristics of the primary tumor (T), regional lymph nodes (N), and distant metastases (M). A subscript numeral is assigned to the T according to size of the tumor, N for the number of regional nodes involved, and M for amount

of distant metastasis. Physical examination, x-ray studies, scans, blood studies, and biopsies are utilized in determining the stage, called staging. The stages of breast cancer are generally defined as:

Stage I: The tumor is confined to the breast. There may be early signs of skin involvement such as dimpling or nipple retraction, but there are no signs of axillary or distant metastases.

Stage II: The primary tumor is as in Stage I, but there are movable, suspicious nodes in the axilla.

Stage III: The primary tumor is infiltrating the skin or chest wall, or the axillary nodes are matted or fixed.

Stage IV: Distant metastases are present.

Preoperative x-ray studies and scans are particularly useful for the detection of metastasis because the purpose of performing a mastectomy is to stop the spread of cancer beyond the breast. If metastases are present, then a mastectomy will probably be of little benefit and may delay the initiation of radiotherapy or chemotherapy. Posteroanterior and lateral chest films, and anteroposterior and lateral views of the lumbar spine and pelvis as well as a lateral skull x-ray series should be taken preoperatively in all except very early lesions. Mammography of the unaffected breast is advisable to identify any occult carcinoma.

Laboratory tests are normal in breast cancers localized to the breast and axillary nodes, but certain tests have abnormal values in the advanced disease. Disseminated cancer may cause a consistently elevated sedimentation rate. Liver metastases may be associated with an elevated alkaline phosphatase. Hypercalcemia occasionally occurs with advanced malignancy of the breast. Radionuclide scanning of the liver, bone, or brain can identify metastatic foci.

The unchanging survival rate for women with breast cancer, regardless of treatment techniques, is probably due to the existence of distant metastases at the time of primary treatment. A new era in breast cancer treatment is beginning in which chemotherapy and immunology will be more important and radical surgery less important. Careful staging and preoperative work-ups, with the selection of the most appropriate type of treatment, including other modalities than surgery, may improve survival rates. Presently, the 5-year survival rates after radical mastectomy, according to the stage of the cancer is Stage I, 75 to 80 percent; Stage II, 65 to 70 percent; Stage III, 45 to 50 percent; and Stage IV, 0.

Treatment Modalities

There is considerable controversy about the best therapy for early breast cancer. The approach is primarily surgical, with the Halsted radical mastectomy being the standard type of procedure done in the United States since its institution around 1900. There have been many approaches which use less extensive surgery—in particular, mastectomies that do not require the disfiguring and disabling excision of the pectoral muscles which is included in the Halsted radical mastectomy (see Table 13-4). Supporters of standard radical procedures argue that axillary node dissection and removal of the pectoral muscles are necessary because of early regional metastases and will result in longer survival rates.[14] Advocates of modified radicals or lesser procedures contend that survival rates are not significantly different, that there is less interference with the woman's immune system when extensive lymph node dissection is avoided, and there is less morbidity and interference with the woman's normal functioning.[15]

With minimal breast cancer—that is, in situ noninvasive tumors less than 0.5 cm. in diameter—the evidence suggests that either a modified radical (with the preservation of both pectorals) or a simple extended mastectomy (the dissection of nodes only to the lateral boundary of the pectoralis minor muscle) is sufficient treatment. With larger tumors—that is, less than 5 cm., and few low axillary nodes involved—a modified radical mastectomy, with postoperative irradiation as indicated can be used. For more extensive cancer, surgery may not be indicated or may be palliative, with irradiation or chemotherapy assuming the major therapeutic role.[16]

The modified radical mastectomy with the dissection of the lower axillary nodes seems to be the preferred procedure at present for early breast cancer. The removal of the entire breast is recommended because of the multicentric tendency of breast cancer. The removal of several axillary nodes is included because they are often the first site of metastasis, and the number of nodes involved provides information about the possibility of other metastases and suggests the need for additional therapy. Information useful in both prognosis and treatment can be obtained from the condition of axillary nodes. The removal of the pectoralis muscles and the dissection of the internal mammary nodes does not add to the effectiveness of the treatment and causes great trauma and continuing impairment of functioning in the woman.

Not all health providers agree that the removal of axillary nodes is important, however. Perhaps 50 percent of early breast cancers could be treated with a simple mastectomy, provided that there was no clinical evidence of node involvement. If metastasis did later occur in axillary nodes, they could be removed then. A small number of carefully selected patients

Table 13-4
Types of Surgery for Breast Lesions

Radical mastectomy. (Classical, Halsted) Through a vertical incision the entire breast is removed with a significant margin of skin around nipple and areola and tumor. The pectoralis major and minor muscles are removed, the axillary vein dissected, and the axillary lymph nodes dissected. A skin-thin surgical flap is left but depending upon the amount of skin removed, skin grafting may be necessary.

Extended radical mastectomy. Includes the above procedure plus excision of the internal mammary lymph nodes. Some sections of the ribs must be removed to reach the internal mammary nodes. The supraclavicular nodes may also be removed. This operation is rarely done today.

Modified radical mastectomy. The entire breast and most of the axillary lymph nodes are removed, but the pectoralis muscles are preserved. Some surgeons dissect the entire axillary chain while others leave the upper third intact. The axillary vein is stripped.

Simple (or total) mastectomy. The entire breast is removed, but the axillary nodes and pectoralis muscles are not. Some surgeons biopsy the last lymph node in the tail of the breast. If it has been invaded, either the axilla is irradiated or a radical mastectomy is done.

Partial mastectomy (segmental resection, wedge resection). The tumor and a wide segment of surrounding breast tissue, underlying fascia and overlying skin are removed; usually about one-third of the breast. Some surgeons also dissect the axillary nodes.

Lumpectomy, tylectomy, or local excision. The tumor and 3 to 5 cm. of tissue on either side are removed, retaining other breast tissue and skin.

Subcutaneous mastectomy. Breast tissue, including the axillary tail is removed through an incision beneath the breast. All breast skin including the nipple and areola and a small button of tissue under the nipple remains. A silicone implant is inserted, either during the initial surgery or several months later.

---

may do well with lumpectomy or segmental resection, providing the biological aggressiveness of the tumor is known. For some women, when the retention of the breast is an overriding concern, this approach, with regular follow-up, might be the treatment of choice. Partial mastectomies are advised only for small peripheral and localized lesions which do not involve the nipple and areola.[17]

The skill of the surgeon and the care with which the operation is done are crucial to the physical aftermath for the women. One of the major problems after axillary node dissection is lymphedema or "milk arm." The body also loses this lymphatic line of defense against infections of the hand or arm. Precise axillary dissection, with realignment of lymphatic vessels and minimal node removal, helps to prevent these problems. When the pectoralis muscles are removed and there is extensive axillary dissection, as with the Halsted radical mastectomy, limited motion of the shoulder and arm can result, as well as an extremely unsightly scar with a deep axillary cavity. Lymphedema

and continuing pain around the incision are also significant problems with the standard radical mastectomy.

THE WOMAN'S RIGHTS AS PATIENT. Breast cancer has become a major public concern that is now discussed openly and candidly. There is a strong voice of discontent with the medical community's management of this problem, as can be seen in consumer literature.[18] The traditional approach of a one-stage procedure, in which diagnostic biopsy and surgical therapy are done at the same time, has received major criticism as being a procedure that deprives the woman of any opportunity to contribute to the decision-making related to her own body. Radical versus conservative surgery is another area of contention, with women excluded from consultations on the decisions for many years. Since the medical community is undecided about the best approach, this area offers grounds for conflict between the patient and provider. Most women simply want to be included in the decision-making and to be informed about the nature of their breast lump before the final decision to remove the breast is made. They need to understand what options are possible and the future implications of these choices. Although a woman with a breast lump may initially demand lumpectomy, it is a rare patient who will not agree to follow the physician's advice once she fully understands the reasons why a more extensive procedure is indicated. Although the issue here is basically that of consumer versus professional power, consumers are only asking for a voice in decisions which affect them, not for total power over professional judgment.

The management of the initial therapy for breast cancer is not the province of the nurse practitioner, although involvement at each phase of treatment is appropriate. Education and counseling about an approaching biopsy and surgery, helping the patient and her family to understand treatment rationales and to deal with their feelings about the disease, constitutes the nurse practitioner's realm. It may be necessary, however, to act as a patient advocate in instances when there is conflict or miscommunications between physician and patient. Follow-up care, both physical and emotional, and continuing health surveillance of the cancer patient, can be done collaboratively by the nurse practitioner and the physician.

RADIOTHERAPY. There are different opinions regarding the proper use of radiotherapy in breast cancer management. Most breast cancers are slow in growing and thus relatively radioresistant, and chemotherapy seems to be more effective in controlling metastases. There is evidence, particularly from European countries and early trials in the United States, that simple mastectomy, segmentectomy, or lumpectomy, followed by radiotherapy to the lymph nodes, gives survival rates comparable to those for radical surgery.[19] With complete axillary dissection, radiotherapy seems contraindicated to this area and may increase any problems associated with lymphedema. Chest-wall irradiation postoperatively to the internal mammary and supraclavicular nodes is often used when the primary tumor is larger than 5 cm., more than 20 percent of axillary nodes are positive, and the classical grave signs are present, or if the tumor is centrally or medially placed. Preoperative irradiation to reduce a large tumor, or when there is skin involvement and multiple clinically positive axillary nodes, may improve the outcome of the surgery. Inoperable tumors such as an inflammatory carcinoma may be treated primarily by irradiation, or it can serve as palliative therapy for disseminated disease. The quality of radiotherapy is highly variable, and only supervoltage irradiation to the proper fields, done by a knowledgeable clinician, is advised. For Stage I tumors, radiotherapy is not indicated, contrary to the common practice of administering a few "prophylactic shots" postoperatively.

CHEMOTHERAPY. The use of anticancer drugs is gaining more prominence in the early management of breast cancer. Even with a small primary lesion, if more than five nodes are involved it indicates that the cancer has probably spread throughout the body, and chemotherapy is quite effective with distant metastases. Most of the anticancer drugs either prevent the reproduction of cancer cells or kill the cells during replication by binding them with receptors. These drugs affect cancer cells more than normal cells because of cancer's more rapid cell division, but normal cells undergoing replication are also vulnerable. Anticancer drugs are extremely toxic and deadly, requiring carefully controlled administration and monitoring of the patient's condition. The toxicity and subsequent side effects of all anticancer drugs are major problems, the most common being leukopenia and thrombocytopenia, hair loss, nausea and vomiting, and febrile reactions. Despite the attendant risks with chemotherapy, some oncologists think that it should be used for younger patients (age 25 to 30), even without nodal involvement, because of the long span of years in which recurrence or metastases can occur.[20] Some chemotherapeutic agents are used alone, while others are more effective in combination. Table 13-5 describes the characteristics of various chemotherapeutic agents used in the treatment of breast cancer.

ENDOCRINE THERAPY. It has long been known that some breast cancers grow more rapidly under the influence of estrogen and may regress with removal of the ovaries. Hormonal manipulation helps only about one-third of the cases, however, and an oophorectomy does not guarantee the absence of estro-

Table 13-5
Characteristics of Chemotherapeutic Agents Used in the Treatment of Breast Cancer

Drug	Class of Agent	Cell-cycle Phase	Biochemical Site of Action	Side Effects and Toxicity (Most common)
Cyclophospha-mide (Cy-toxan)	Alkylator	Nonspecific	Alkylation of DNA, RNA and/ or protein	Anorexia, nausea, vomiting, alo-pecia, leukopenia, thrombocy-topenia, hemorrhagic cystitis, fever
Doxorubicin HCL (Adriamycin)	Antibiotic	Nonspecific	—	Thrombocytopenia, leukopenia, alopecia, mucositis resembling moniliasis, myocardial damage
Cytarabine (Cy-tosar)	Pyrimidine antimeta-bolite	S-phase specific agent	Pyrimidine syn-thesis and/or incorporation into DNA	Leukopenia, thrombocytopenia, anemia, megaloblastosis, nau-sea, vomiting, diarrhea, hepatic dysfunction, stomatitis
5-fluorouracil (5-FU)	Pyrimidine antimeta-bolite	S-phase specific agent	Pyrimidine syn-thesis	Leukopenia, aphthous stomatitis, nausea, vomiting, diarrhea, weakness and lassitude, rash, alopecia, hyperpigmentation, cerebellar ataxia
Melphalan (Alk-eran)	Alkylator	Nonspecific	Alkylation of DNA, RNA and/ or protein	Anemia, neutropenia, thrombocy-topenia, nausea, vomiting, hy-peremia, GI hemorrhage, aphthous stomatitis
Methotrexate	Folic acid an-timetabolite	S-phase specific agent	Folic acid reduc-tase	Bone marrow depression, aphthous stomatitis, nausea, vomiting, diarrhea (particularly toxic in patients with liver or renal damage)
Vincristine sul-fate (Oncovin)	Alkaloid of periwinkel	M (metaphase arrest)	Assembly of mi-totic spindle protein sub-units	Neurotoxicity, alopecia, leuko-penia and thrombocytopenia at high doses

Note: Most cytotoxic agents are teratogenic and should not be used in early pregnancy.

gen, which can also be produced by the adrenals, pituitary, and possibly even by extraglandular cells. Recent technology permits a hormonal assay of breast tumors if they are available for study immediately after removal, so the hormone dependency of the particular type of breast cancer can be determined. By this technique, oophorectomy or endocrine ablation can selectively be used only for those women who might benefit from it, thus avoiding useless surgical menopause in those who will not. Some postmenopausal women have tumors which undergo remission when estrogen is given, supporting the idea that postmenopausal breast cancer is a separate entity. The use of steroid hormones such as cortisone or prednisone, and androgens may also cause tumor remission for periods of time. Hormone therapy must be individualized and is usually appropriate for widespread disease. There is evidence that all cancers eventually become hormone-independent and thus may be controlled by hormones only for limited periods of time.

POSTMASTECTOMY CARE

After their discharge from the hospital, mastectomy patients are put on a regular follow-up appointment schedule. Initially, monthly visits are indicated, then every 2 to 4 months for the next 2 years. After 2 years, visits should be every 6 months, with instructions for a monthly self-examination of the remaining breast. During return visits, the condition of the operative area is assessed and the other breast examined, problems with the affected arm explored, and the family's emotional adjustment discussed. Annual x-ray examinations of the chest and mammography of the remaining breast are done. Symptoms which might indicate metastasis are explored and appropriate laboratory and organ scans ordered.

Exercises to restore function to the affected arm are begun early. The immediate postoperative exercises consist of rotary motion of the elbow, hand, and wrist on the affected side. The arm should be elevated with a pillow when the woman is lying down. Usually functions and positions of the arm are allowed up to 60 degrees shoulder abduction. Arm abduction to 90 degrees too soon after surgery may interfere with early skin flap adherence and prolong serum formation. Full arm exercises should begin about 2 weeks postoperatively (Figure 13-7). Instructions for activities to avoid and special precautions to prevent trauma and infections must be provided at the time of the patient's discharge and must be periodically reemphasized (Table 13-6).

The American Cancer Society's Reach to Recovery program is an excellent resource for postmastectomy patients. This group of volunteers, themselves all mastectomees, visit the woman in the hospital to give her encouragement and assistance with a temporary breast prosthesis. They reinforce the instructions about arm exercises and protection. Several weeks after the patient's discharge, the volunteers make another visit to the woman at home, when additional problems can be discussed and a permanent prosthesis planned for. Most women find the Reach to Recovery program exceptionally helpful in giving them support and in assisting them to deal with anxieties and practical postmastectomy problems. Usually these volunteers will not become involved if the physician objects, although this practice may vary in different communities.

Physical Aftereffects

Women who have undergone a mastectomy report considerable differences in the amount and intensity of their pain and in the length of time before their strength and functioning return. A tight, squeezing sensation in the chest is common, with intermittent sharp, electric shocks. Pain may involve not only the area around the incision, but also the armpit, shoulder, part of the back, and inside of the arm. Numbness of the affected side of the chest is common because of the interruption of nerve pathways. Shaving under the affected arm is a strange experience because of the lack of sensation, and must be visually guided.

After a Halsted radical mastectomy, other muscles must be reeducated to take over the functions of the pectorals. Many women find this a difficult process, requiring lengthy exercise regimens before the satisfactory use of the affected arm can be regained. Skin grafts are often necessary, causing sloughing and infections, and itching is frequently a postoperative problem. Fatigue often persists for months, with a slow return to previous energy levels. Temporary or permanent lymphedema of the affected arm can be a problem, particularly with Halsted radical mastectomies and extensive axillary dissection. Mild edema cannot be seen and is felt as a tightness in the upper arm; more severe edema may require occasional elastic bandages and elevation or the continual use of an elastic sleeve. Severe lymphedema can be treated with a Jobst extremity pump to decrease the edema as much as possible before fitting the arm with an elastic sleeve. Some women notice increased lymphedema premenstrually, during hot weather, and with heavy salt intake. Exquisite tenderness and sensitivity to touch of the chest, upper arm, and shoulder may persist for several months postoperatively.

Depending on the type of surgery, the patient's scar may preclude her wearing sleeveless and low-neckline clothing. A transverse incision with modified radical or simple mastectomy greatly reduces this problem. Breast prostheses are available in various sizes and shapes to approximate the remaining breast. Although expensive, the latex-covered silicone-gel ones are weighted and feel natural to the touch and adhere to the skin so that they do not shift in position.

Emotional Impact and Adjustment

In the aftermath of the loss of a breast due to cancer, the most widespread concern seems to be the threat to life involved in having a potentially fatal disease. After surgery women want to know of their surgeon "Did you get it all?" The impact of having a chronic, life-threatening illness causes a reordering of prior-

General instructions

Often following surgery there is a tendency to drop the shoulder on the operated side, causing your other shoulder to ache. Good posture will make you feel and look better.

≫ Check your posture frequently in front of a mirror.

≫ Square your shoulders by pressing them back at every opportunity.

≫ Stand with your back against a wall with your head and both shoulders touching to get the correct feeling for good posture, then walk away from the wall keeping that position. Keep your knees relaxed and flexible, your head erect.

When you begin your exercise program, measure your progress before and after exercise each day. To do this, stand with your forehead touching the wall and toes touching the baseboard. Reach up as high as possible with your good arm and make a mark with a pencil (right arm in drawing). A family member can also help in the marking. Reach as high as possible with the arm on the operated side (left arm in drawing), while leaving your other arm resting at its maximum height on the wall. Do this slowly by moving your hand up the wall a little at a time. When you have reached as high as you can with the hand on the operated side, mark this spot on the wall. If you feel pain or tightness, rest the hand against the wall at that level you've achieved, take several deep breaths, and then continue to move the hand upward a little at a time.

Repeat this routine after the following exercises, and you will be able to easily see your progress.

Do all the following exercises as often as your doctor prescribes. Don't skip one or do it less frequently if it is difficult or hurts a little. Some pain is to be expected. Deep breathing will help you relax and will usually relieve the pain.

If you have trouble doing this exercise, have someone support the weight of your arms as they are raised. Let your elbows rest in the other person's palms.

The rising elevator exercise

Sit with your spine against the back of a straight-backed chair. Keep your head level. Rest the hand on your operated side on top of your other hand in your lap.

≫ Slowly raise your arms, keeping the elbows outward, until you feel pain or tightness (A). Breathe deeply several times until the pain or tightness eases.

≫ Continue to raise your arms. Imagine that your arms are an elevator and the signal to stop for several moments is pain or tightness.

≫ Eventually, you will be able to rest your hands on your head (B). While you are doing this breathe deeply, relax, and press your elbows outward until they are at a 90-degree angle to your head. Relax in this position.

≫ Clasp your hands and slowly slide them from the top of your head downward until they are at the back of your neck (C). Breathe deeply.

≫ When you feel relaxed and comfortable, slowly return your clasped hands to the top of your head and slowly lower your arms to your lap. Dropping your arms may cause pain.

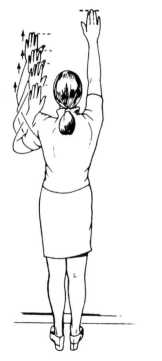

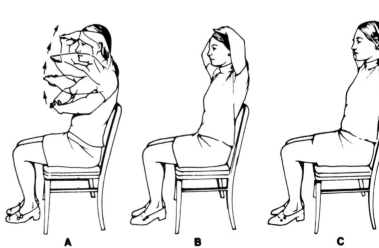

Figure 13-7. Exercises for postmastectomy patients.

The cockeyed pendulum

Imagine your arm as a pendulum that has gone cockeyed and swings in circles rather than back and forth. To get the right feeling of totally relaxing your arm and hand during this exercise, try it with the arm and hand on your unoperated side.

≫ Stand with your arm and hand on the unoperated side across the back of a straight-backed chair. Bend over from the waist and let the hand and arm on your operated side totally relax.

≫ Let the arm swing gently in small circles. Be sure that this swinging is relaxed.

≫ Periodically breathe deeply to relax even more. Continue swinging the arm in small circles until you feel tired.

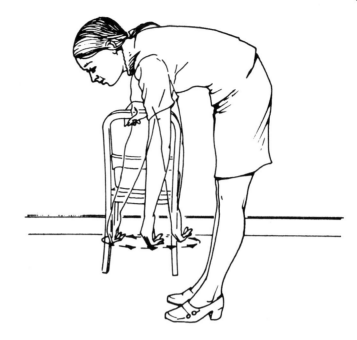

The tug rope exercise

Obtain 6–8 feet of rope and make a loop in each end. (Long strips of 3-inch gauze bandage or even an old bed sheet will do). Put the rope over a clothes hook that is well secured to a door or wall.

≫ Sit erect in a straight-backed chair—feet on floor, spine against the chair back—so that the back chair legs touch the baseboard. Look straight ahead; looking upward may cause you to feel dizzy or nauseated.

≫ Stretch your hand on the unoperated side over your head (right arm in drawing D) and grip the loop.

≫ Grasp the other loop with the hand on the operated side (E).

≫ Slowly pull down the hand on your unoperated side (right arm in drawing F), raising the arm on the operated side (left arm).

≫ When you have pain or tightness, stop, relax, breathe deeply, and then continue pulling downward with your stronger arm.

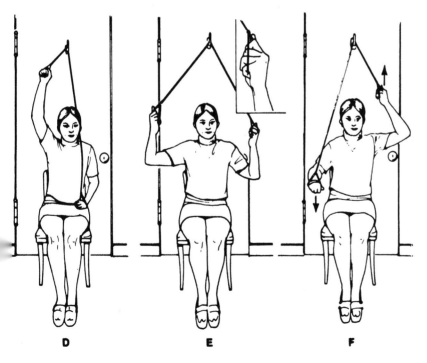

D   E   F

Table 13-6
Special Precautions for Postmastectomy Patients

After radical breast surgery, your arm is susceptible to infection and swelling because lymph nodes and lymph vessels have been removed. When infection does set in, your arm will become red, warm, and unusually hard or swollen. See your doctor immediately if this occurs. To prevent possible swelling and infection, follow these suggestions:

- Pamper your affected arm by carrying your handbag or any heavy articles with your other arm.
- Wear your wristwatch or other jewelry on the unaffected arm.
- Apply a lanolin hand cream several times daily to the hand and arm.
- Push your cuticles back with a towel after bathing. Never pick or cut cuticles or hangnails on your affected hand.
- Wear loose-fitting rubber gloves when washing dishes. Don't let the affected hand remain in water for long periods, especially when you are using a detergent.
- Use your unaffected arm when reaching into a hot oven.
- Use a thimble to avoid pinpricks when sewing.
- Get someone else to move furniture, to carry heavy objects, or to do other tasks that require excessive activity.
- Wear heavy gloves when doing light gardening; let others handle thorny plants and do the digging.
- Apply a protective insect repellent when going to areas where there may be biting insects.
- Protect your arm from sunburn. Throw a towel or other covering across the shoulder and arm while sunbathing.
- Don't permit injections, vaccinations, or blood samples to be done on your affected arm unless specifically recommended by a doctor who knows that you have had breast surgery.
- Be sure that blood pressure is taken on your unaffected arm.
- Immediately wash cuts and scratches and apply a protective covering unless the environment is clean.

Patient Care (May 15, 1975): 57.

ities, in which values and goals in life are reassessed and often changed. The need to survive generally seems to outweigh concerns about attractiveness and sexuality. Common emotional upsets include intense bitterness about why such a thing happened to them—"Why me?"; deep jealousy of women with two healthy breasts, although this is not readily expressed; rage at the physician for subjecting them to a mutilating operation (Halsted radical) without discussing the options of other procedures or explaining in advance the implications of the one-stage procedure (the shock of going in for a small biopsy and awakening with the breast gone and the chest and axilla permanently disfigured); and fury about poor follow-up care resulting in advanced metastases before the discovery that anything was wrong.

Most men seem to think that the loss of the breast itself is the main trauma, but this is not true for the majority of women. Unless something else is occurring in their emotional lives to focus their concern on their sexual attractiveness, women usually can accept the loss of a breast without devastation to their feminine identity. Married women with stable, supportive relations find that postoperative adjustment in their sex life and marital relations present no major problems. In some cases the crisis brings the couple closer together and heightens their appreciation of each other. These women, particularly the ones with young children, are most concerned about future survival and minimize the "loss of an appendage." Women with shaky marriages, or middle-aged women who are separated or divorced, experience greater difficulty in adjustment and feel the breast loss and disfigurement of surgery are much more significant. They often feel permanently handicapped in the competition to obtain or retain a man and express great bitterness and hopelessness of ever developing a satisfying relationship. The younger women press more vigorously for limited surgery and retention of the breast if possible, particularly if they are single, though an "inherent sexuality of youth" seems to bolster their confidence that the loss of a part would not cause disintegration of their heterosexual relations. Obviously any individual woman's experience is shaped by a number of factors and may or may not be similar to that of other women. Within the American value system, the price women pay to save their lives by mastectomy—loss of a breast or disfigurement—is a substantial one, with a frequent aftermath of anxiety and depression. Feeling "untouchable," with the loss of sexual desirability, dangers to interpersonal and sexual relations, and fears of breakup of marriage grow out of this value system.

Perhaps the ideal in emotional adjustment following mastectomy, as far as the man-woman relation is concerned, is embodied in this woman's personal experience:

> My husband is now, if possible, more tender and loving than he ever was before. Our love life has a brand-new dimension that wasn't there until I had the mastectomy. It's as if he suddenly realized that I was something very precious that he almost—and could still—lose. This feeling of being "cherished" like something very valuable, a treasure, is what has been added to our love.[21]

PREDICTIVE ONCOLOGY AND EARLY DETECTION

The earlier cancer is diagnosed and treated, the greater the chances for cure and longer survival. The public has been alerted to cancer warning signs and health providers are aware of the need for early detection. Interest is now focusing on the possibility of predicting cancer by identifying people at high risk due to various factors. Although our knowledge is incomplete and much research is needed, it is apparent that 3 factors are necessary to develop cancer: susceptibility, either genetic or acquired; a cancer-producing agent such as radiation, virus, or chemical; and certain cofactors such as age, sex, skin color, weight, size, and others.[22] An estimated 65 to 85 percent of all cancers are environmentally related, and about 15 percent are caused by irradiation and viruses. Cancer is considered epidemic in the United States, causing 17 percent of all deaths. Current studies indicate that there is an actual rise in incidence of breast cancer, which has become the most common type of cancer in women. By compiling data about the characteristics of the persons who develop different types of cancer, high risk or predictive profiles have been established which draw from past medical history, genetic factors, carcinogenic exposure, immune phenomena, and systemic review.[23] For some types of cancer, it has also been possible to establish low risk profiles.

High Risk Profile for Breast Cancer

Caucasian woman of northern European background and Jewish women of European ancestry are at higher risk for breast cancer than women of other backgrounds. The countries with the highest incidence of breast cancer (as determined by age-adjusted death rates per 100,000 population) include, in descending order, Netherlands, England and Wales, New Zealand, Scotland, Denmark, Northern Ireland, and Israel. The United States is thirteenth on this scale. The countries with the lowest incidence are, in ascending order, Thailand, El Salvador, Egypt, Japan, Philippines, and Mexico. Caucasian women of Latin or Mediterranean background are at reduced risk. Black women have lower incidence and mortality rates than white women in the United States, but their rate has been rapidly gaining in the last several years. This change is believed to reflect the increasing affluence among blacks and is possibly related to changes in diet or to environmental factors. Obesity is another factor which increases breast cancer risk and may be interrelated with a high consumption of animal proteins and fats including butter, lard, cheese, and whole milk. Diets which are mainly vegetarian, low in animal proteins and fats, such as oriental and Seventh Day Adventist or Mormon diets, are correlated with a low incidence of breast cancer.

There is a definite familial factor in breast cancer susceptibility, but it is not known whether this is genetic or environmental. A sister with breast cancer increases the risk most, a mother causes somewhat less risk, and having a maternal aunt or grandmother with the disease probably also increases risk, but this increase in risk only occurs if the cancer in a woman's relative was premenopausal. A history of breast abnormalities, such as fibrocystic disease, adenomas, mastitis, abscesses and injuries, increases a woman's risk. While these conditions are not premalignant, the tendency to develop benign lesions or the effects of accidents or infections may predispose the woman to develop malignancies. Several factors involved with a woman's reproductive history increase the possibility of her developing breast cancer, including early menarche, late menopause, and first pregnancy after 35 or no pregnancy. The reasons are not clearly understood, but are probably related to hormonal abnormalities and estrogen levels.

Breast cancer rarely develops in girls under 20 and was infrequently found in women under 30 until recently. The disease appears more virulent when it occurs in young women. The highest incidence of the disease occurs between the ages 42 and 47, then a plateau of about 8 years occurs, and in the early 50s the rate again begins to climb, but less steeply, until very old age. Breast cancer in young women is thought to be a different disease from breast cancer in older women.

Other factors that have been correlated with an increased risk of breast cancer include reduced estriol excretion, reduced 17-oxysteroid excretions, blood group A, and greater total body volume (height and weight). Having cancer in one breast increases the risk most significantly for developing cancer in the other breast. Table 13-7 summarizes factors which increase or decrease the risk of breast cancer, grouping them into low, intermediate, and high risk categories.

Screening Mammography

Because it has been demonstrated that mammography can detect very small breast lesions that are not palpable, the question of whether to institute the routine, widespread screening of women on a regular basis has been raised. Many projects involving screening mammography have been instituted and have been effective in diagnosing clinically occult and early Stage I disease.[24] A new development in mammography is the ability to predict a woman's probabilities of getting breast cancer based upon certain characteristics of the parenchymal pattern of the breast. A classification system has been developed in which 4 different patterns were identified and the women in the study followed to determine the incidence of breast cancer among them. The presence of prominent duct patterns, the extent of involvement, and density of the parenchyma were the criteria on which a low to high risk grouping

was established. Once a woman is known to be in the upper 2 or 3 groups, more frequent examination and mammography can be done, and minor breast changes or symptoms viewed with more suspicion. The group with minimal risk can avoid unnecessary screening or worry.[25]

Some concern has been expressed about the exposure of large numbers of women to x-rays during many years of regular screening mammograms. As radiation is known to be carcinogenic, the possibility exists that this could cause a cancer to develop, a contradiction in its basic purpose. With proper x-ray equipment, however, the dosage of radiation is very small and probably does not significantly increase this risk. Certainly regular yearly mammography is indicated for women in high risk categories. Another problem is the cost of massive screening and how such projects would be financed. Many women cannot afford this relatively expensive procedure, and the problems of availability of resources and personnel would arise with a governmental program. Presently, screening mammography is generally used selectively as risk increases.

Breast Self-Examination

Although probably every woman has heard about the importance of regular breast self-examination (BSE), a significant portion (if not the majority) do not do this simple procedure which aids so greatly in the early detection of breast cancer. The American Cancer Society has available a free pamphlet of instructions which has been widely distributed (Figure 13-8). The examination should be done once each month, about one week after the menstrual period in premenopausal women and at the first of each month in postmenopausal women. The breast tends to be engorged and more lumpy just before and during menses and is harder to examine.

Lying on the back, with one arm under the head and the shoulder supported by a pillow, use the opposite hand to examine the breast. With the fingertips together, use the flat of 3 or 4 fingers to feel the breast tissue. Palpation should be gentle and the breast lightly massaged in a circular motion. Do not squeeze, pump, or pull the breasts, but use a gentle circular pattern as you move around the breast from the outer edges toward the nipple. Be certain to cover all the breast tissue, including the

Table 13-7
BREAST-CANCER RISKS FOR U.S. WOMEN

	Who	When	Where

HIGH	1. Family history of cancer
	   Self—breast or other cancer
	   Sister
	   Mother
	   Maternal grandmother or aunts
	   Maternal first cousins
	
	2. Prior history of benign breast disease
	
	3. Reproductive history
	   Early menstruation
	   No children
	   Late (or no) beginning of sexual
	     activity
	   First child born after age 35
	   Late menopause
	
	4. Race and ethnicity
	   Jews of European ancestry
	   Non-Jews of northern European
	     background (including Iceland)
	   Affluent blacks
	
	5. Diet
	   Obesity due to high amounts
	     of animal proteins and fats, including butter, lard, cheese, whole milk
		Age 40 and up (including women over 70)	Large industrial cities, especially in the Northeast
			
			Also:
			San Francisco-Oakland
			
			Minneapolis-St. Paul
			
			Detroit
			
			Pittsburgh
			
			Iowa
			
			Colorado

MEDIUM	1–3. Average rates in the above categories
	
	4. Race and ethnicity
	   Middle-income blacks
	   Latin Americans
	   Southern European ancestries
	
	5. Diet
	   Moderate amounts of animal
	     protein and fats (e.g., Mormons)
		Ages 25-39	Medium-sized cities
			
			Also:
			Dallas-Fort Worth
			
			Atlanta

LOW	1. No family history of cancer
	
	2. No history of prior breast disease
	
	3. Reproductive history
	   Late menstruation
	   First child born before age 20
	   Early beginning of sexual activity
	   Early menopause (natural or artificial)
	
	4. Race and ethnicity
	   Jews of North African or Asian
	     ancestries
	   Non-Jews of Finnish ancestry
	   Low-income whites
	   Low-income blacks
	   American Indians
	   Oriental ancestries
	
	5. Diet
	   Mainly nonmeat protein and vegetable
	     fats (e.g., Seventh Day Adventists)
		Under age 25	Small towns and rural areas
			
			Also:
			Birmingham, Ala.

Other possible risk factors, effect unknown or subject to debate: Breast feeding, use of oral contraceptives, number of children, height, blood pressure, role of paternal ancestry, diabetes, enlarged thyroid gland, salivary-gland cancer, emotional stress, mental depression, quantity and quality of earwax secretion.

Data compiled by Rose Kushner; copyright © 1975 by Rose Kushner

It's important to see your physician as soon as possible if you discover a lump or thickening. That discovery most often represents a perfectly harmless condition. In fact, most women are told by their physicians, "You have no need to worry. Everything is fine. But you were wise to see me as soon as you did."

HERE IS HOW YOU CAN CHECK FOR YOURSELF...

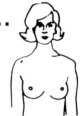

(1) In front of your mirror, arms relaxed at your sides, look for any changes in size, shape and contour . . . look for puckering or dimpling of the skin and changes on the surface of the nipples. Press each nipple gently to see if any discharge occurs.
Raise both arms over your head, and look for exactly the same things. Note differences since you last examined your breasts.

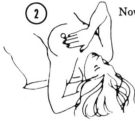

(2) Now you will be trying to find a lump or thickening. Lie down with a pillow under your left shoulder, and left hand under your head. Hold the fingers of your right hand together flat, press gently with small circular motions to feel the inner, upper portion of your left breast. Start at your breastbone and go outward toward the nipple line. Also feel the area around the nipple.

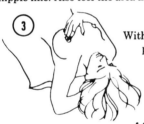

(3) With the same gentle pressure, feel the low inner part of your breast. Incidentally, in this area you will feel a ridge of firm tissue. Don't be alarmed. This is normal.

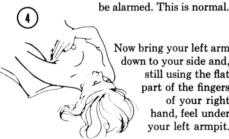

(4) Now bring your left arm down to your side and, still using the flat part of the fingers of your right hand, feel under your left armpit.

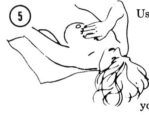

(5) Use the same gentle pressure to feel the upper, outer portion of your left breast from the nipple line to where your arm is resting.

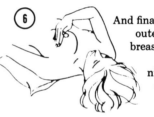

(6) And finally, feel the lower outer portion of your breast, going from the outer part of the nipple. Repeat the entire procedure, as described, on the right breast using the left hand for the examination.

YOUR OWN DOCTOR may want you to use a slightly different method of examination. Ask about this the next time you see your doctor.

A REGULAR MONTHLY SELF-CHECK CAN BE SO SIMPLE...YET SO IMPORTANT.

FOR FURTHER INFORMATION PLEASE CALL YOUR LOCAL AMERICAN CANCER SOCIETY OFFICE

6419.00/2-75

Figure 13-8. American Cancer Society technique for breast self-examination.

tail of the breast which reaches upward into the axilla. If the breast is large or pendulous, hold the side steady with one hand while examining with the other and turn slightly so the breast spreads out evenly over the chest rather than hanging off to one side. Feel deeply into the axilla and along the muscles on either side, and repeat the entire procedure for the other breast. Some women find their breasts easier to palpate when the skin is slippery from soap or oil.

A second part of the self-examination includes repeating the above procedure while standing up. Observation of the breasts in front of a mirror can help to identify minor changes in contour, symmetry, appearance of the skin, dimpling or puckers which might otherwise be missed. This is done with the arms above the head, on the hips, and leaning forward or squeezing the waist to accentuate changes. Women who become familiar with their own breasts are in the best position to discover any unusual changes or tiny lumps not there before and then to seek help early.

NOTES

1. H. Ory, et al., "Oral Contraceptives and Reduced Risk of Benign Breast Disease." *New England Journal of Medicine* 294,8 (February 9, 1976): 419-22.

2. R. Kushner, *Breast Cancer: A Personal History and an Investigative Report* (New York: Harcourt Brace Jovanovitch, 1975).

3. "Roundtable: Priorities in Managing Breast Problems." *Patient Care* 19,7 (April 1, 1975): 20-83.

4. "Roundtable: Developing Cancer Risk Factor Profiles." *Patient Care* 10,3 (February 1, 1976): 65-84.

5. G. W. Bethune, "Office Evaluation of Breast Problems." *Primary Care* 3,2 (June 1976): 263-75.

6. Kushner, *Breast Cancer*, p. 291.

7. G. P. Rosemond, W. P. Maier, and T. J. Probyn, "Needle Aspiration of Breast Cysts." *Journal of Family Practice* 1,3-4 (December 1974): 61-63.

8. G. K. Jimerson, "Breast." In S. L. Romney, et al., eds., *Gynecology and Obstetrics: The Health Care of Women* (New York: McGraw-Hill, Blakiston, 1975), pp. 919-35.

9. "Roundtable: Odds and Options in Breast Cancer Risks." *Patient Care* 19,7 (April 1, 1975): 44-55.

10. "Cancer Statistics 1976." *Ca-A Cancer Journal for Clinicians* 26,1 (January/February 1976): 14-32.

11. "Cancer Statistics 1976," pp. 2-13.

12. J. L. Wilson, "Diseases of the Breast." In M. A. Krupp and M. J. Chatton, eds., *Current Medical Diagnosis & Treatment* (Los Altos, California: Lange Medical Publishers, 1974), pp. 391-402.

13. Jimerson, "Breast," p. 930.

14. T. J. Anglem and R. E. Leber, "Operable Breast Cancer: The Case against Conservative Surgery." *Ca-A Cancer Journal for Clinicians* 23,6 (November/December 1973): 330-33.

15. G. Crile, "Operable Breast Cancer: In Defense of Conservative Surgery." *Ibid.*, pp. 334-38.

16. M. M. Romsdahl and E. D. Montague, "Managing Primary Breast Cancer." *Postgraduate Medicine* 59,2 (February 1976): 151-57.

17. "Roundtable: Sorting Out Breast Cancer Therapies." *Patient Care* 11,10 (May 15, 1975): 20-69.

18. B. Bullough, "Psychological Aspects of Breast Cancer: The Relationships Between Patients and Health Care Providers." West Coast Cancer Foundation Monograph Workshop, Carmel, California, April 5-8, 1976.

19. "Roundtable: Sorting Out Breast Cancer Therapies," pp. 33-38; and Kushner, *Breast Cancer*, pp. 277-86.

20. "Breast Problems: Managing Cancer with Chemotherapy." *Nursing Update* 6,12 (December 1975): 3-9.

21. Kushner, *Breast Cancer*, p. 252.

22. "Predictive Oncology in Family Practice." *Patient Care* 10,6 (March 15, 1976): 40-88.

23. "Assessing Problems of Cancer Prediction." *Patient Care* 10,3 (February 1, 1976): 22-85.

24. M. Moskowitz, et al., "On the Diagnosis of Minimal Breast Cancer in a Screenee Population." *Cancer* 35,5 (May 1976): 2543-52.

25. J. H. Wolfe, "Risk for Breast Cancer Development Determined by Mammographic Parenchymal Pattern." *Cancer* 35,5 (May 1976): 2486-92.

14

Abnormal Pap Smears

Cervical carcinoma is the second most frequent cancer among women, following only cancer of the breast. Half of all genital malignancies arise in the cervix, and an estimated 2 percent of American women will develop cervical cancer before the age of 80. The development and widespread use of Papanicolaou cytological smears for the detection of abnormal cervical cells in the 1940s, combined with advances in treatment, have resulted in a steady decrease in the death rate from cervical cancer. In 1930 the rate was 20 per 100,000 per year; in 1970 the number per 100,000 dropped to 8. An estimated 30,000 to 40,000 cases of cervical cancer are diagnosed yearly in the United States, about half of which are carcinoma in situ. There is considerable evidence to support the concept of cervical cancer as a progressive disease which moves in stages from atypical changes in individual epithelial cells seen in dysplasia to preinvasive (in situ), then invasive carcinoma.

The characteristics of women who have a high risk of developing cervical cancer have been identified. The key characteristic is an early age at first coitus, followed by a cluster of variables thought to be dependent upon this key factor: early marriage, low socioeconomic class, number of sexual partners, early age at first pregnancy, greater multiparity. The higher incidence of cervical cancer in blacks and Mexican-Americans is related to their lower socioeconomic status, which is associated with early marriage and childbearing. Prostitutes have a high incidence of the disease, while among celibate groups such as nuns it is very rare. Jewish women have a low risk of cervical cancer, and penile cancer is also extremely rare among Jewish men. These observations led to the idea that circumcision was protective and that the smegma of uncircumcised males had some role in carcinogenicity. Studies among Moslems and ritually circumcised males of other groups, however, compared to noncircumcised men and their sexual partners from the same locales were inconclusive in their attempts to implicate smegma. Some epidemiological features of cervical cancer suggest that its cause is a carcinogenic agent, such as a virus, which may be carried by the male. The relation between herpes simplex virus type 2 and cervical cancer is currently under investigation (see Chapter 11, Venereal Disease).

As is the case with women, certain groups of men are increasingly regarded as being at higher risk in the etiology of cervical carcinoma. The incidence of the disease in women is higher among those who have husbands with penile or prostatic cancer, a history of venereal disease, and multiple sexual partners. The increasingly liberal sexual behavior of some Jewish males is associated with an increase in cervical cancer in their wives. The occupational group of the husband has been correlated with cervical cancer or positive cytology, with a considerable increase among wives of laborers, unskilled workers, fishermen and seamen, crane and hoist operators, factory workers, miners, and lower officials in comparison to the wives of physicians, lawyers, administrators, senior officials, teachers, scientists, and clergymen. One theory concerning carcinogenic male characteristics suggests that males may have qualitative or quantitative differences in histones (basic proteins of the sperm head). These histones interact with the surface DNA of a woman's cervical cells to cause 1) an increased activation of nuclear DNA concerned with protein synthesis (and thus cell replication) and 2) an alteration of surface properties of the cell contingent on an increased content of surface DNA (thus changing cell behavior and promoting invasive properties). The basic polyamines (spermine and spermidine) found in high concentrations in human semen have a similar avidity for DNA as the basic proteins in the sperm head and are expected to show the same kind of activity vis-à-vis the metaplastic cervical cell.[1] How social class differences interact with the qualities of sperm histones or semen-polyamines is unclear.

PAP SMEAR SCREENING FOR CERVICAL CANCER

All sexually active women, regardless of age, should have regular Pap smears. It was believed that the incidence of cervical cancer in the 13- to 19-year-old age group was extremely rare; and although this is true for invasive cancer, studies have demonstrated that around 30 teenagers per 1000 screened have atypical Pap smears leading to tissue diagnosis of dysplasia or carcinoma in situ.[2] Whether sexually active or not, women ages 25 to 30 should have routine Pap smears, even though their risk for cervical cancer is low. This routine pelvic examination allows the early discovery of benign tumors, endometriosis, and ovarian cysts which are fairly common in this age group. Yearly or biennial screening is enough in women below ages 35 to 40 unless one or more high risk factors are present, such as early beginning of sexual activity, early first pregnancy, multiple sexual partners, and a history of venereal disease. For women above this age, Pap smears may be indicated every 6 months, as they are for high risk women. The incidence of cervical dysplasia increases after age 35, carcinoma in situ increases at age 40, and the peak incidence of invasive carcinoma is in the late 40s or early 50s. Semiannual Pap smears are generally not necessary for women taking oral contraceptives or with an IUD in place unless high risk factors are present.[3]

Careful endocervical specimens and scrapings from the squamocolumnar junction are most important prior to menopause. Vaginal pool specimens are often omitted in younger women because they have a false-negative rate as high as 50 percent for cervical neoplasia.[4] At menopause the incidence of cervical cancer levels off while endometrial cancer increases. Vaginal pool specimens become important therefore in the perimenopausal women, whose routine Pap smears should include endocervical, cervical, and vaginal pool samples. Suspicious endometrial cells are most likely to be found in the posterior fornix. If hormone assays are to be included, a specimen from the lateral vaginal wall is necessary. Women who have been treated for carcinoma in situ, particularly if conization was used, or who had radiation treatment for invasive carcinoma should have a Pap smear every 3 months for the first year, then every 6 months for life. Following a hysterectomy for cancer, the woman is considered at high risk for developing a vaginal neoplasm and should have a Pap smear every 6 months. After a hysterectomy for reasons other than cancer, a Pap smear is advised for women at least every 2 years to screen for vaginal cancer and because often a cuff of cervical squamous epithelium remains in the top of the vaginal vault. If the hysterectomy was performed 20 or 30 years ago or more, the cervix was often left in place and annual to biennial screening is necessary.

ANATOMY AND PHYSIOLOGY OF THE CERVIX

The cervix is the lower neck of the uterus; it is narrow and cylindrical, and enters the vagina at right angles through the anterior vaginal wall. It is 2 to 4 cm. long with an area of slight constriction, the *isthmus*, at the point of juncture with the uterine corpus. The *endocervical canal* traverses the length of the cervix opening on its superior end through the *internal os* into the uterine cavity and on its inferior end through the *external os* into the vagina. The external os has anterior and posterior lips which are usually in contact with the posterior vaginal wall, which envelops the inferior third of the cervix. The anterior vaginal wall is in contact with the upper cervix. The endocervical canal contains *crypts (plicae palmatae)*, often called glands, which have secretory cells productive of cervical mucus. The mucus undergoes cyclic changes under the influence of hormones, and the cervix also undergoes anatomic changes during the menstrual cycle. The external os progressively widens during the proliferative phase, reaching its greatest width just before ovulation. At this time cervical mucus can be seen exuding from the external os; it is usually clear white, profuse, and watery. If placed on a slide and allowed to dry, it produces the typical fern pattern characteristic of the first half of the menstrual cycle and the ovulatory period. Following ovulation the os becomes smaller in diameter and the cervical mucus becomes scant and viscid. It tends to glob, is sticky, and no longer produces a fern pattern. During menstruation the cervix is also somewhat dilated, and immediate postmenstrual cervical mucus is sparse, viscid, sticky and full of vaginal and cervical cells and leukocytes as well.

The Squamocolumnar Junction

The portion of the cervix projecting into the vagina which can be seen in a pelvic examination is called the ectocervix. It is largely covered by smooth, pink, stratified squamous epithelium which is essentially identical with vaginal epithelium. The endocervical canal is lined with columnar epithelium which appears as red, bumpy tissue resembling small clusters of grapes. This occurs because the one-layer columnar epithelium is thin enough to allow the underlying highly vascularized stroma to be seen. It was previously believed that the junction between the squamous and columnar epithelium of the normal cervix occurred at the external os and that any columnar epithelium on the ectocervix was abnormal and due to an eversion of the endocervix. Present understanding of cervical pathophysiology contradicts this belief because studies have shown that various portions of the ectocervix are covered by columnar epithelium at birth in over 70 percent of females. The presence of columnar epithelium is determined embryologically; it does not arrive there by eversion nor does it grow out of the endocervix, and it is completely normal for it to persist into adulthood for an unpredictable length of time.[5]

Under the influence of hormones and the acid vaginal secretions, this columnar epithelium on the ectocervix is transformed into squamous epithelium through a process called *metaplasia*. This normal process is particularly active during adolescence, the first pregnancy, and after the first delivery, although it occurs throughout an individual's life. There is both ingrowth from the original squamous epithelium toward the endocervical canal, and focal or patchy transformation within the ectocervical columnar epithelium itself, occurring in an orderly process. It is believed that mature columnar cells do not change into squamous cells, but that multipotent cells of the subepithelial tissue, probably stromal in origin, are the source of metaplasia.[6] The area of active metaplasia is called the *transformation zone*. Initially metaplastic squamous epithelium consists of very immature cells, which gradually develop the characteristics of mature squamous cells. These immature cells are thought to be particularly susceptible to genetic injury by environmental carcinogens; in fact, nearly all squamous neoplasia of the cervix originate in the transformation zone of the squamocolumnar junction.

Polyps and Inflammation

Cervicitis is so prevalent among women that it is difficult to find a laboratory specimen without some degree of microscopic evidence of active or chronic inflammation. The cervix is continuously exposed to trauma through coitus and childbearing, is bathed with abundant mucus secretions conducive to infection, and bacteria have ready access to the vagina and cervix due to their proximity to the body's exterior. About 90 to 95 percent of parous women have minimal, asymptomatic, and sometimes only microscopically apparent chronic cervicitis. When evident, the most common clinical manifestation is called cervical erosion, which appears as an area of granular, angry looking, inflamed tissue, with varying degrees of ulceration. There is usually a yellow mucopurulent discharge caused by the infecting organism, such as *Escherichia coli* or *Aerobacter*. Lacerations or dilatation of the external os, usually occurring during childbirth, which leaves a relatively large area of the endocervix (known as ectropion) exposed to the acid pH and bacterial flora of the vagina, predisposes women to cervicitis. The inflammatory process is countered by an attempt at repair through an upward growth of squamous epithelium which pinches off the ducts of some endocervical glands, leading to the formation of nabothian cysts. These retention cysts may be single or multiple, and they vary in size. Symptomatic acute or chronic cervicitis must be evaluated and treated (see Chapter 9, Vaginal Discharge and Itching). The most important consideration in evaluating chronic cervicitis is the exclusion of malignancy by the use of Pap smears and by a biopsy of suspicious areas.

Cervical polyps are caused by hyperplasia of the endocervical epithelium and appear as pedunculated, pear-shaped, soft, smooth, reddish growths ranging in length from a few millimeters to 3 cm. They often can be seen extruding from the cervical os, although they may occur higher in the endocervical canal and not be visible. Many women with polyps have no symptoms; if there are symptoms, however, they usually consist of menorrhagia and leukorrhea. The exact cause of cervical polyps is not known, although hormonal imbalance and changes of local response mechanisms regulating the growth of endocervical mucosa are thought to be involved. While no definite neoplastic potential has been established for polyps, occasionally a malignancy may be present in these benign-appearing structures. Polyps are removed by clamping the pedicle at its origin and gently twisting it off or by placing a ligature around the pedicle and excising the polyp. All tissue removed should be sent for pathological examination. (Figures 14-1 and 14-2 illustrate cervical anatomy and common variations.)

OBTAINING AND EVALUATING PAP SMEARS

Pap Smear Techniques

The optimal time to obtain a Pap smear is 5 to 6 days after the end of the menstrual period. The woman should not douche before coming in for the smear and should not recently have inserted vaginal medications or preparations. While smears can be obtained during menses if the flow is light, the presence of red blood cells in the specimen makes the interpretation more difficult and may obscure the presence of atypical cells. An unlubricated speculum or one lubricated only with warm water should be used, as lubricant jellies such as Lubrifax and KY jelly distort the cells and prevent accurate cytological study.

With the speculum in place and the cervix well exposed, cleanse the cervix well with a dry cotton ball to remove excess mucus. Introduce a saline-moistened cotton-tipped appli-

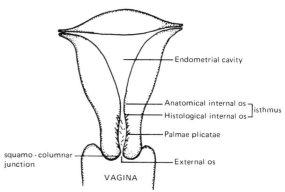

Figure 14-1. The cervix and uterus, frontal section.

cator into the endocervical canal to the level of the internal os, rotate it several times, withdraw and roll rather than smear the tip of the swab on the slide. Particularly in nulliparous and postmenopausal women, the best endocervical specimen is obtained with this technique. In women with a wide external os, some health providers prefer to use a wooden or plastic spatula to obtain endocervical specimens. Fix the slide immediately with a commercial aerosol fixative or immerse it in 95 percent ethyl alcohol solution to prevent the specimen from drying, which distorts the cells and renders the specimen useless.

After obtaining the endocervical sample, inspect the cervix to locate the squamocolumnar junction (SCJ). Using a wooden or plastic spatula, firmly scrape the SCJ and 1 cm. of tissue on each side, making two complete revolutions over the entire area. Make a thin smear on a slide and fix it promptly. If desired, both the endocervical and SCJ samples can be placed on a single slide, one on each half, but this must be done quickly to prevent their drying. It may be necessary to use a small pipette to aspirate cells from the endocervix if the SCJ cannot be seen, especially in older women who have some uterine atrophy. If a vaginal pool sample is taken, the rounded end of a wooden or plastic spatula is inserted into the posterior fornix and pressed upward against the lower portion of the cervix as it is withdrawn. A thin smear is placed on a glass slide and fixed as described above. A specimen from the midlateral vaginal wall must be included when an estrogen index is desired.

Providing the pathology laboratory with information about the woman's age, last menstrual period, use of hormones, gynecological

NORMAL NULLIPAROUS CERVIX

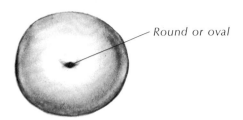

Round or oval

The nulliparous cervical os is small and either round or oval. The cervix is covered by smooth pink epithelium.

NORMAL PAROUS CERVIX

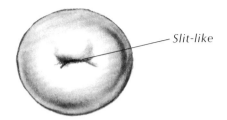

Slit-like

After childbirth, the cervical os presents a slit-like appearance.

CERVICAL POLYP

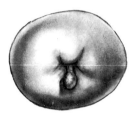

Cervical polyps usually arise from the endocervical canal, becoming visible when they protrude through the cervical os. They are bright red, soft and rather fragile. When only the tips are seen they cannot be clinically differentiated from polyps originating in the endometrium.

NABOTHIAN OR RETENTION CYSTS

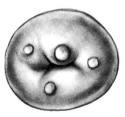

Retention or Nabothian cysts are another accompaniment of chronic cervicitis. Variable in size, single or multiple, they appear as translucent nodules on the cervical surface.

Figure 14-2. Common variations in the appearance of the cervix.

EROSION

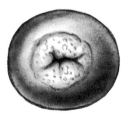

Often a manifestation of chronic cervicitis, a cervical erosion presents as a reddish area around the cervical os that bleeds easily on touch. Its name is misleading since it is not an ulcer. It represents a spread onto the cervical surface of the epithelium that normally lines the cervical canal. Differentiation from early carcinoma may require biopsy.

Table 14-1
Original Numerical Pap Smear Classifications

Class I	Normal
Class II	Normal with abnormal or "atypical benign" cells
Class III	Suspicious cells, possibly malignant
Class IV	Signs of malignancy
Class V	Definitely malignant

surgery, radiation treatment, and whether pregnant or postpartum, aids in the interpretation of specimens.

Significance of Pap Smear Reports

There is a variation in the method used by different laboratories in reporting Pap smear results. The Pap smear is intended to be used as a screening test, and further diagnostic work-up is indicated for abnormal results. The most important objective of Pap testing is to determine whether cervical cells are within normal limits or are suggestive of a malignant neoplastic process. The original numerical classifications by Dr. Papanicolaou are less often utilized by pathology labs now because they are too broad. Descriptive reports are preferred which are of more assistance in clinical decision-making.

Many laboratories no longer use numerical classifications but provide descriptive reports which allow a fuller understanding of the cellular changes seen on cytology. For example, a report could read "normal with abnormal cells, indicative of infection," or "negative with mild squamous metaplasia," or "cellular evidence of moderate dysplasia." Reports with cells indicative of malignancy may also note whether the carcinoma is in situ or invasive. Recommendations appropriate to the woman's age, menstrual history, hormone-use history, gynecological-procedure history, and so forth are often provided in the report. Specific infections due to Candida, Trichomonas, herpes vaginalis, or venereal disease may be identified, and hormonal evaluation, noting whether estrogen levels are adequate, increased, diminished or absent may be provided. Figure 14-3 shows a descriptive Pap smear report.

False negative reports of cervical lesions should not exceed 10 percent in a reliable laboratory. Invasive carcinoma is particularly likely to be involved in this false negative rate because surface inflammation and the necrosis produced by the lesion make cytological evaluation more difficult. It is most important to biopsy any suspicious lesion of the cervix or vagina at once, without awaiting the Pap smear results. The most common reason for a false negative, however, is an inadequate sample which was either improperly taken or improperly fixed. Some labs report the absence of endocervical cells on Pap smears, which alerts the provider to the possibility of inadequate samples. It is generally agreed that there is a false positive rate of 5 percent. The overall accuracy of Pap smears in detecting cervical cancer is therefore 90 to 95 percent, making it one of the most reliable screening tests in widespread use.

Cytological Findings and Disease Processes

Descriptive Pap smears identify cellular changes characteristic of physiological or pathological processes in the cervix. A report indicating metaplasia signifies that cells are undergoing the process of transformation from columnar to squamous epithelium, a normal physiologic change. Any inflammation noted on a Pap report alerts the provider to the presence of cervicitis or vaginitis, and appropriate treatment may be instituted if the patient is symptomatic. Dysplasia indicates the presence of atypical individual epithelial cells and is usually divided into the three subdivisions of mild, moderate, and severe. This is generally considered to be a precancerous condition, with less likelihood of the lesion reverting to normal epithelium as the category progresses from mild to severe. Atypical hyperplasia is an increased thickness of the epithelium, with atypical changes in the cells, similar to dysplasia. These last 2 cytological descriptions are also considered suggestive of carcinoma and indicate the need for further diagnostic work-up.

Carcinoma in situ implies that there is a lesion which has progressed from the stage of

REPORT OF PATHOLOGY DEPARTMENT

AGE 36	SEX F	DATE 9/13/77	DOCTOR Conover	IN-PATIENT	OUT-PATIENT ✓	PATH. NO. 2045

SOURCE OF SMEAR _Routine Pap Smear_   PREV. SMEAR NO.

PAPANICOLAOU SMEAR REPORT

L.M.P. **8/14/77**   PREGNANT   YES____ NO ✓

HORMONES ⊖   POST PARTUM   YES____ NO ✓

PRIOR SURGERY   RADIATION   YES____ NO ✓

DIAGNOSIS

NEGATIVE ✓   ESTROGEN

  Slightly Atypical ☐   Adequate ☐

  Atypical ☐   Increased ☐

  Suspicious ☐   Diminished ☐

REPEAT ☐   Absent ☐

NO ENDOCERVICAL CELLS ☐   TRICHOMONAS ☐

INFLAMMATION, MILD ✓   FUNGI ☐

COMMENT _mild squamous metaplasia_

0

_____ M.D.
PATHOLOGIST

PA
DATE OF BIRTH
TYPE INS.
PHYSICIAN

DATE

ADDRESSOGRAPH PLATE

LAST NAME	FIRST	MIDDLE	P.F. NO.	WARD.

Figure 14-3. Papanicolaou smear report.

hyperplasia or dysplasia to that of neoplasia but it is not invasive. The normal architecture of the epithelial cells is completely disrupted, with changes typical of carcinoma, but the basement membrane is not violated and the lesion is limited to epithelial cells and glands. Carcinoma in situ remains localized with no metastasis, and, thus, is one of the most treatable cancers. It is usually asymptomatic and the lesion often is not apparent in a routine examination. At times the mucous membrane of the cervix bleeds easily on contact, or erosion may be present on the ectocervix, but these are not pathognomonic of carcinoma in situ. Friable cervical mucosa, easy bleeding on contact, and erosion are also typical in cervicitis with inflammatory changes. To establish the diagnosis of cancer, a biopsy is necessary, with confirmation by histological sections. Carcinoma in situ is believed to be a precursor of invasive disease for the following reasons:

1. The highest incidence of carcinoma in situ occurs between ages 35 and 50, and invasive carcinoma between ages 45 and 60. This distribution suggests that carcinoma in situ precedes invasive carcinoma.
2. Epidemiologically, carcinoma in situ and invasive carcinoma follow the same social patterns.
3. In several reported studies where patients with carcinoma in situ received no major treatment, invasive carcinoma later occurred in a large percentage of patients.
4. The two lesions are histologically quite similar, and carcinoma in situ is often seen on the periphery of an invasive lesion.[7]

Cervical intraepithelial neoplasia (CIN) is a term also used to describe the histologically preinvasive carcinoma in situ, emphasizing its limitation to cells within the epithelium proper. It is considered to be an intermediate step in the progression toward invasive malignancy. That intraepithelial neoplasia is in fact malignant is supported by studies of the behavior of host-immune responses, which recognize cells of both carcinoma in situ and invasive carcinoma as malignant.[8]

Invasive carcinoma encompasses a wide range of lesions and has been divided into many stages depending upon the tissues and organs involved. The earliest stage is called microinvasive or early stromal invasion; in this stage neoplastic epithelium invades the stroma in one or more places to a depth of 3 to 5 mm.

below the base of the epithelium, but there is no lymphatic or vascular involvement. This early stage cannot be diagnosed by clinical examination, and the patient is asymptomatic. It is subdivided into classifications of microinvasion and occult cancer; the latter being lesions which exceed early stromal invasion but are still not clinically evident. Only subepithelial tissues are involved in these early invasive lesions, thus the possibility of a cure by the use of an appropriate therapy is good. The earlier the cancer is detected and the more minimal the lesion, the higher the success rate for a definitive cure. Once the tumor has spread to the pelvic wall or into adjacent structures, such as the bladder and rectum, a cure is nearly impossible to achieve. (Table 14-2, International Classification of Cancer of the Cervix, lists and describes stages of lesions.)

Clinically obvious cervical cancer occurs most frequently in multiparous women aged 45 to 55 who began sexual activity early and delivered their first child before age 20. The first symptom is usually a thin, watery, blood-tinged vaginal discharge. Intermittent, painless, abnormal intermenstrual bleeding following intercourse or douching is the classic symptom. Both of these symptoms are frequently either unnoticed by the woman or are not regarded as signs of danger. Intermenstrual bleeding becomes heavier, more frequent, of longer duration, and may be spontaneous as the malignancy enlarges. The woman's menstrual flow often seems to increase in amount and duration, as cervical bleeding combines with uterine sloughing. Eventually the bleeding will become continuous if medical attention is not sought. Late symptoms of advanced disease include referred flank or leg pain as the tumor spreads to the ureters, pelvic wall, or sciatic nerve routes; dysuria, hematuria, rectal bleeding, or intractable constipation due to bladder or rectal invasion; and edema of one or both legs as a result of lymphatic and venous blockage by extensive pelvic wall disease. Distant metastasis occur most often in the liver, lungs, vertebra, large bowel, and ribs.

The main routes of spread of cervical cancer are into the vaginal mucosa or myometrium of the lower uterine segment, the parametrium, pelvic wall, bladder, and rectum by direct extension; and into the paracervical lymphatics and from there into the obturator, hypogastric, and external iliac nodes. The prevalence of

Table 14-2
International Classification of Cancer of the Cervix

Stage	Description
Stage 0	Carcinoma in situ
Stage I	Carcinoma confined to the cervix
Stage IA1	Early stromal invasion
Stage IA2	Occult cancer
Stage IB	All other cancers limited to the uterus
Stage II	Cancer involves the vagina, but not the lower third, or infiltrates the parametrium, but not out to the sidewall
Stage IIA	Cancer involves the vagina, but there is no evidence of parametrial involvement
Stage IIB	Infiltration of the parametria, but not out to the sidewall
Stage III	Cancer involves the lower third of the vagina or extends to the pelvic sidewall
Stage IIIA	Cancer involves the lower third of the vagina, but is not out to the pelvic sidewall if the parametria are involved
Stage IIIB	Involvement of one or both parametria out to the sidewall
Stage III (urinary)	Obstruction of one or both ureters on intravenous pyelogram without other criteria for Stage III disease
Stage IV	Cancer extends outside the reproductive tract
Stage IVA	Involvement of the bladder or rectum
Stage IVB	Distant metastasis or disease outside the true pelvis

lymph node disease is closely related to the stage of the malignancy, with 15 to 20 percent having lymph node involvement in Stage I, 25 to 40 percent in Stage II, and at least 50 percent in Stage III. The choice of treatment for invasive cancer is between surgery and radiotherapy, and decisions are based upon the extent of the cancer, the patient's age and general health, and the presence and nature of complicating abnormalities. Referral to a gynecological oncologist is indicated in invasive cervical carcinoma. Five-year survival figures are closely related to the stage of disease, with comparable results obtained by both treatment techniques. Generally, all stages past Stage IIA are treated with radiotherapy. Results from two large series, one treated with radiotherapy alone and the other with surgery, are shown in percentage of disease-free survivors after 5 years as follows:[9]

In a pelvic examination, the appearance of clinically obvious carcinoma of the cervix varies widely. There are basically 3 categories of gross lesions. Exophytic lesions arise on the ectocervix and can grow to form large, friable, polypoid masses which involve varying amounts of the cervix. This type of lesion also arises within the endocervical canal and causes an enlargement of the cervix, called a "barrel-shaped lesion." Another manifestation of this type of lesion is an infiltrating tumor, which shows little visible ulceration and presents as a stony-hard cervix. The third type of lesion is ulcerative, causing erosion, and it is often associated with infection and discharge. A portion or the entire cervix may be involved, as well as the upper vaginal vault. The vast majority of cervical cancers are squamous-cell, with the remainder primarily adenocarcinomas.

Table 14-3
Five-Year Survival Rates

552 Patients With Radical Operations		2000 Patients with Radiotherapy	
Stage I	86.3%	Stage I	9.5%
Stage IIA	75.0%	Stage IIA	83.5%
Stage IIB	58.9%	Stage IIB	66.5%
Other Stages	34.1%	Stage IIIA	45.0%
		Stage IIIB	36.0%
		Stage IV	14.0%

MEANINGS FOR WOMEN

Receiving abnormal results on a Pap smear may set in motion the process of fear and panic associated with the diagnosis of cancer (see Chapter 13, Breast Masses). Certainly this fear and the denial which may be used to cope with it underlie a woman's ignoring her symptoms, such as blood-tinged, watery vaginal discharge or intermenstrual bleeding, which could serve to bring her to early treatment. The knowledge of advances in cure rates for cervical cancer is quite widespread, however, and no doubt reduces the dread associated with this disease. Public education campaigns promoting regular Pap smears have underscored the advantages of early detection, and most women know that minimal cervical cancer is curable. Despite publicity and the widespread availability of Pap smear screening, only about 35 percent of American women are regularly screened.

The internal and thus hidden aspect of the cervix and uterus, as compared to the external and very apparent aspects of the breasts, probably accounts for some difference in women's attitudes toward a hysterectomy versus a mastectomy. A hysterectomy is a very accepted operation in this culture, perhaps even fashionable, except for women who have strong identity bases in retaining their childbearing capability. Feelings about hysterectomy might range from those of the woman who has completed her family and is glad to be done with the nuisance of menstruating and its associated discomforts, to those of the woman who still desires children and perceives fertility as a major component of her personal worth, for whom the loss of her uterus is a devastating tragedy. All shades of variation exist, of course, and many women for whom fertility is not central still report a sense of loss. Menstrual function and cyclicity are so basic to the feminine self-concept that grief over the cessation of this periodic reaffirmation of their femininity, whether surgically interrupted or due to menopause, is only natural. The cavalier attitude of some physicians and other health providers toward a hysterectomy ("What does she need it for anyway?" or "The only thing the uterus is good for after childbearing is over is to get cancer.") has caused considerable resentment and hostility among women. Such attitudes are sexist in nature; certainly there is no part of the male anatomy whose loss is viewed with such casualness.

The associated meanings of cancer and hysterectomy should be discussed with patients as part of the treatment plan. Involving the husband or partner in these discussions helps him to understand and respond better to the woman's need for support. Specific treatment plans, their rationale, and the process of decision-making from diagnostic work-up to follow-up should involve the woman and her partner.

Abnormal Pap smears which are not malignant require explanations and follow-up; the premalignant results of dysplasia can be managed by several options, and the woman's individual needs and goals play a key role in therapy decisions.

MANAGEMENT OF ABNORMAL PAP SMEARS

The nature of the involvement of the nurse practitioner in the management of cases of abnormal Pap smears depends upon the type of abnormality, the nurse practitioner's preparation and expertise, and the protocols for management worked out among the health providers at the institution or organization. In cases involving more severe dysplasia and suspicious cells, a close collaboration between the nurse practitioner and the physician is necessary in the various steps toward a definitive diagnosis.

Benign Abnormal, Inflammatory

When the Pap smear report describes cells indicative of infection, clinical judgment is used regarding the treatment. Often the specific agent will be identified on the Pap report (Figure 14-3), such as Candida, Trichomonas, or Hemophilus. Many providers do not treat asymptomatic infections, but prefer simply to repeat the Pap smear in 2 or 3 months to ascertain by cytology if the inflammatory changes have resolved. If treatment for a specific infection is carried out, the Pap smear is repeated 2 to 4 weeks after the completion of the treatment. Trichomonads or yeast are occasionally reported with a normal cervical cytology; in these cases the organisms are part of the usual vaginal flora for that woman and are not causing any infection. No treatment is indicated in such cases.

Mild Dysplasia

This earliest category of cervical intraepithelial neoplasia presents a challenge to clinical decision-making. Since the potential for the dysplastic cells to revert to normal epithelium is good, some practitioners prefer to defer definitive work-up and follow the woman closely with repeat Pap smears every 4 to 6 months. Theoretically, even if the Pap smear continued to reveal a mild dysplasia, the woman could simply be followed with regularly repeated Pap smears, as long as the lesion was not progressing. Practically, however, most women cannot tolerate the anxiety of knowing that they have an abnormal Pap smear that is considered premalignant. For both the woman's and the practitioner's peace of mind, repeated mild dysplasia eventually leads to the work-up for more advanced dysplasia described next.

Moderate or Severe Dysplasia, Suspicious

The evaluation of women with Pap smear reports of dysplasia or of cells suggestive of carcinoma includes a second cytology, gross examination of the cervix, Schiller's test, cervical biopsies, and colposcopy, if it is available. The first step is to obtain a careful second Pap smear in the manner previously discussed. After the Pap smear, the cervix is cleansed with 3 percent acetic acid and carefully inspected with a good light for any grossly suspicious areas, which are biopsied with a punch biopsy forceps. Schiller's test is used, applying a 2 percent iodine solution (Lugol's) to the cervix, which stains the normal glycogen-containing squamous epithelium deep brown. Neoplastic squamous tissue remains pale, either yellow or the same color that it was before staining. Schiller's test is, however, nonspecific for neoplasia, and immature metaplastic epithelium will remain pale as will areas of preinvasive and invasive carcinoma. Normal columnar epithelium also does not take up Lugol's stain because these cells do not contain sufficient glycogen. Areas that are Schiller's pale should be described in the patient's record for future reference, and biopsies should be taken from all areas that do not take up stain. Biopsies are done after an endocervical canal curettage.

An endocervical canal curettage is carried out using the Kevorkian curette. With short, firm motions in a circumferential pattern, the endocervical canal is scraped from the internal os to the external os. It is best to first curette the upper half of the canal and then the lower half. Patients experience some discomfort and cramping but usually can tolerate curettage without sedation. After the entire canal has been curetted, all blood, mucus, and tissue debris are collected and placed on a small paper towel, molded into a small mound and placed along with the paper into a fixative. An endocervical canal curettage provides essential information needed for a thorough evaluation of abnormal Pap smears of this type. Even if the cervix shows no lesions and stains evenly with Lugol's solution, the source of abnormal cells can be within the endocervical canal and cannot be evaluated without curettage. After curettage, obtain biopsies from suspicious areas on the ectocervix. Cervical neoplasia is found predominantly on the anterior and posterior lips of the cervix, so, in the absence of abnormal appearing tissue, four-quadrant random biopsies are taken at the 2, 4, 8, and 10 o'clock positions. If colposcopy is used, biopsies are directed, and samples are taken from typical abnormal tissue.

Decision-Making Matrix

If the repeated cytology, cervical biopsies, and endocervical canal curettage show no neoplastic epithelium (negative results), the woman can be reassured that hers was a false positive test originally and that cervical carcinoma has been excluded. Another evaluation by Pap smear is done in 3 months. When the endocervical canal curettage (ECC) is negative and preinvasive cervical neoplasia (dysplasia, carcinoma in situ) is found from the biopsy, the treatment plan is based upon the patient's age, desire for more children, reliability for follow-up, and the histological appearance and extent of the lesion. Cryosurgery can be performed on patients who are good follow-up risks or who wish to preserve their fertility. Shallow conization of the cervix (a ring biopsy) can accomplish the same results. For patients who do not desire more children, a simple vaginal or abdominal hysterectomy is recommended.

If the endocervical curettage is positive for dysplasia or preinvasive neoplasia, it is necessary to exclude invasive disease. If colposcopy is not available, conization of the entire canal is carried out. If the limits of the lesion are included in the cone, and no invasive disease is found, the conization can be considered therapeutic if the reproductive function of the patient was to be preserved. The performance of high conization is associated with a significant complication rate. The immediate complications include hemorrhage, perforation, anesthetic risk, and infection; late complications include hemorrhage, cervical stenosis, infertility, and an incompetent cervix. The referral of patients to a gynecologist for colposcopy is preferred. With the use of the colposcope, if the upper limits of the disease can be seen (up to 1½ cm. of the endocervical canal is visible), the patient can be treated with cryosurgery, conization, or simple hysterectomy. If the upper limits cannot be visualized, diagnostic high conization is necessary. If invasive cancer is demonstrated by the cone biopsy, the treatment consists of either irradiation or a radical hysterectomy. Noninvasive cancer discovered by a cone biopsy is treated by a hysterectomy 24 hours after conization (Figure 14-4). If the cervical biopsy or ECC affirms the presence of invasive cancer, conization is contraindicated, and these patients should be referred to a gynecological oncologist. The stage of the disease is determined according to the extent of its spread and possible metastasis, and the treatment is based upon this evaluation.

Abnormal Smears in Pregnancy

The increased vascularity of pelvic tissues during pregnancy makes standard evaluation techniques such as biopsy, conization, and ECC extremely hazardous to both mother and fetus. Colposcopic examination is essential for an adequate evaluation because ECC is absolutely contraindicated and conization is relatively contraindicated. In 95 percent of the women examined the entire lesion can be seen colposcopically and the presence of invasion can usually be determined without biopsy. A biopsy of suspicious lesions can be done if there is doubt, provided that the means for hemostasis is available. Conization need only be done when biopsies fail to confirm the colposcopic impression of invasion. In all women who do not have invasive cancer, a vaginal delivery is allowed.[10]

Follow-up

For all women treated for cervical intraepithelial neoplasia, regardless of the method of therapy, close follow-up is mandatory. Pap smears are done every 3 months for 1 year, and then every 6 months for life. Even women treated by hysterectomy are followed according to this schedule because they are at high risk for vaginal and vulvar squamous neoplasia.

COLPOSCOPY

The use of the colposcope was introduced in 1925 in Germany to permit a more minute and comprehensive examination of the cervix. Although efforts were made to bring colposcopy to the United States in the early 1930s, interest was never sparked, and attention focused upon cytology, with the development of the Pap smear in the 1940s. Recently, interest in colposcopy as an adjunctive technique to cytology in the evaluation of cervical lesions has been renewed. The colposcope is a stereoscopic viewing instrument, actually a type of microscope, with low magnification and binocular viewing. Although various levels of magnification are available, the most widely used are between 8 and 18X. To perform a colposcopy, the cervix is cleansed with 3 percent acetic acid, which enhances the visibility of the cellular patterns of the cervical epithelium. The colposcope is focused on the transformation zone and squamocolumnar junction, and the area is inspected in a clockwise fashion. Abnormal patterns include 1) white epithelium, appearing as sharply demarcated, slightly raised, white tissue near the external os, 2) mosaic structure, due to abnormal vascular patterns, 3) punctation, also due to abnormal vascular patterns but finer than mosaic, and 4) leukoplakia, a heavy, thick, raised white lesion, often visible to the naked eye.

White epithelium, mosaic structure, and punctation are atypical epithelium and are the sites which should be biopsied. The greatest advantage of the colposcope is that it locates these atypical patterns so that a biopsy can be specifically directed rather than relying on random punch biopsies which may or may not sample abnormal areas. Leukoplakia are lesions which result from keratinization and often accompany uterine prolapse. They are often loosely attached at the base, and vigorous scraping catches part or all of the white material. Leukoplakia is not generally considered precancerous, but coexistent carcinoma does occur in some cases.

When cervical intraepithelial neoplasia has been diagnosed, the colposcope is an aid in determining further evaluation and treatment. If the upper limits of the lesions can clearly be

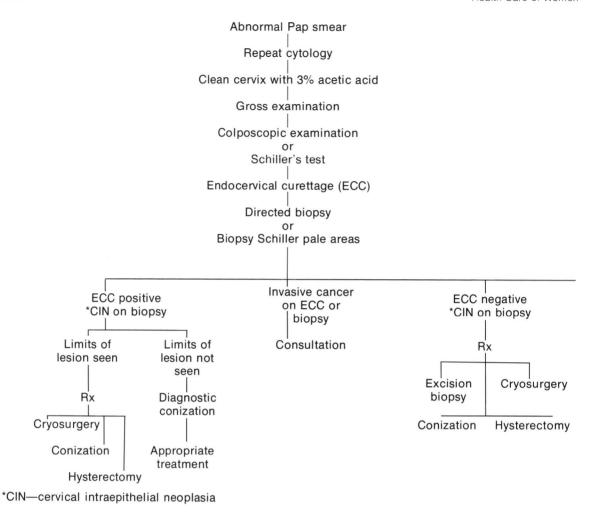

Abnormal Pap smear
|
Repeat cytology
|
Clean cervix with 3% acetic acid
|
Gross examination
|
Colposcopic examination
or
Schiller's test
|
Endocervical curettage (ECC)
|
Directed biopsy
or
Biopsy Schiller pale areas

ECC positive *CIN on biopsy

Limits of lesion seen — Limits of lesion not seen

Rx — Diagnostic conization

Cryosurgery — Conization — Hysterectomy

Appropriate treatment

Invasive cancer on ECC or biopsy

Consultation

ECC negative *CIN on biopsy

Rx

Excision biopsy — Cryosurgery

Conization — Hysterectomy

*CIN—cervical intraepithelial neoplasia

FIGURE 14-4 Decision-making matrix for the evaluation and management of abnormal pap smears

seen and the endocervical canal curettage is negative, then the disease is confined to the ectocervix and may be treated by cryosurgery or ring biopsy. If the lesion extends up into the canal beyond the vision of the colposcopist, then diagnostic conization is necessary to define the disease. With the use of an endocervical speculum, the colposcopist can visualize up to 1½ cm. of the endocervical canal. In more than 90 percent of the women examined, however, the entire lesion is confined to the ectocervix and can be identified and localized colposcopically. With directed biopsy of the worst areas, the lesion can be adequately assessed by colposcopy without conization in all but 10 percent of cases.[11]

CRYOSURGERY

Cryosurgery is the technique of freezing abnormal cervical tissue which leads to sloughing and then regeneration of normal cervical mucosa and endocervical glands. Th extent of the disease to be treated must be previously determined, and the area to be treated must be outlined. The procedure is best performed within 1 week after the cessation of menses, permitting the most active phase of regeneration to occur before the onset of the next menses and avoiding the possibility of interfering with a pregnancy. No anesthetic or analgesic is usually required, and nitrous oxide is the refrigerant most often used. Using a large speculum to provide maximum exposure, all mucus and cellular debris is removed, and the cervix then is cleansed with 3 percent acetic acid. The tissue to be frozen is moistened with saline for proper heat transfer, and the probe of the unit, at room temperature, is firmly positioned so that the largest part of the lesion is covered. The probe approximates the anatomical configuration of the cervix. If the lesion is very large, the probe may have to be repositioned for subsequent additional freezings. A tenaculum is not used to stabilize the cervix, to avoid causing bleeding.

With the cervical probe in place, the refrigerant is circulated. Ice crystalization forms first on the back of the probe tip, then spreads laterally from the edge of the probe, usually within 10 to 15 seconds. An ice ball is formed that should extend 4 to 5 cm. past the limits of the lesion onto normal appearing epithelium. This usually takes about 2 to 3 minutes, but the extent of the ice ball, not the length of time, is the important factor. Once the area to be treated has been adequately frozen, the probe is defrosted and removed. The cervix is carefully inspected to be sure that the ice ball has extended the necessary 4 to 5 cm. onto normal epithelium.

After this treatment, there are few side effects, the most common being a profuse watery discharge. Occasionally there may be spotting or cervical stenosis. By the sixth week after therapy, the cervical epithelium and endocervical glands completely regenerate leaving, in most instances, a normal cervix and endocervical canal. The difference between pretreatment cervical erosion, which appears red, angry, granular and ulcerated, and the smooth, pink, squamous epithelium posttreatment is striking.

NOTES

1. A. Singer, B. L. Reid, and M. Coppleson, "A Hypothesis: The Role of a High-Risk Male in the Etiology of Cervical Carcinoma." *American Journal of Obstetrics and Gynecology* 126, 1 (September 1, 1976): 110-15.
2. M.J. Feldman, et al., "Abnormal Cervical Cytology in the Teenager: A Continuing Problem." *American Journal of Obstetrics and Gynecology* 126, 4 (October 15, 1976): 418-21.
3. "Do Your Pap Smears Tell You Enough?" *Patient Care* 9, 11 (June 1, 1975): 112-19.
4. M. Roy, et al., "New Concepts in the Evaluation of the Abnormal Papanicolaou Smear." *Journal of Family Practice* 1, 3/4 (December 1974): 10-13.
5. *Ibid.*; and C. G. Lacey, et al., "The Abnormal Pap Test." *Continuing Education for the Family Physician* (August 1976): 21-27.
6. P. J. DiSaia, "The Cervix." In S. L. Romney, et al., eds., *Gynecology and Obstetrics: The Health Care of Women* (New York: McGraw-Hill, Blakiston, 1975), pp. 970-1002.
7. *Ibid.*, p. 988.
8. W. T. Chiang, P. Y. Wei, and E. R. Alexander, "Circulatory and Cellular Immune Responses to Squamous Cell Carcinoma of the Uterine Cervix." *American Journal of Obstetrics and Gynecology* 126, 1 (September 1, 1976): 116-21.
9. DiSaia, "The Cervix," pp. 993-94.
10. Lacey, "Abnormal Pap Test," p. 27.
11. *Ibid.*, p. 23.

15

Nervousness and Fatigue

Stress is an ever-present accompaniment of living. The human organism throughout its lifetime responds to innumerable physical and psychic events calling forth mechanisms for coping with them and adapting to them. The physiological responses to stressors follow neuroendocrine pathways, but this complex process includes a wide variety of specific reactions and the full range of intensity from so mild as to be hardly noticeable to a profound degree that is all-consuming. The observable outcomes of stress, which may be seen in the person's behavior or in manifestations of disease, are quite individual. In the broadest sense, disease can be thought of as the result of interaction between the organism and its environment, mediated by the unique characteristics of genetic inheritance and shaped by particular circumstances occurring at a given time. Many factors affect this interaction, such as the virulence of the stressor, host susceptibility, immunocompetence, environmental hazards, and attempts at treatment.

In many diseases, a specific relation between an inducing agent and a series of pathological changes in body tissues cannot be clearly identified. Such diseases are generally called "essential" or "degenerative" or "idiopathic." The changes in the target organ that produce signs and symptoms are clearly apparent, and although some of the underlying pathophysiological processes may be recognized, the actual cause of the disease process is unknown. No doubt there are many steps along the way to the frank evidence of disease, with nonspecific changes presenting a "pre-clinical syndrome." The usual response of the health provider in these cases is "you'll have to get sicker before we can find out what it is," for if a particular known disease can be diagnosed, then a specific known treatment can be given. Some of the predisease illnesses resolve spontaneously, with no identifiable residual effects; some probably progress to clinical disease entities. It has been the tradition in health care to separate disease into physical and mental spheres, and different frameworks have been developed to approach each sphere. For the human organism, however, there is no separation; stress, however experienced, affects the total organism's functions. Disease, "dis-ease," needs to be considered holistically, with the human viewed as a functioning whole.

The provider must begin with the patient's symptoms and the reasons presented for seeking care, and work through a complex maze with many blind alleys and false fronts toward a conclusion about what is wrong. The beliefs and expectations of the patient, the definitions of society about illness and its expression, and the provider's professional and personal attitudes all have their influences. The provider's approach is shaped by knowledge, understanding, and beliefs arising from these influences; one cannot see what one does not know, and one must believe something is possible before one can see it.

NERVOUSNESS AND FATIGUE AS CLUSTER SYNDROMES

Nervousness and fatigue are two common symptoms which women (and men) present as reasons for seeking care. More often than naming these feeling states, however, patients describe body sensations that are part of these syndromes. The cluster of physical sensations and the feeling state of nervousness is characterized by apprehension and tenseness; and of fatigue by tiredness and lack of energy.

"I need something for my nerves." The woman presenting with nervousness often associates a state of tension with the body sensations and feelings that she is experiencing. She reports that she feels nervous, tense, "up tight," tied up in knots, or as if she is coming apart. Or, she may describe physical symptoms which include any combination of rapid heartbeat, palpitations, chest pains, shakiness, sweating, flushing, abdominal upset, diarrhea or gas, dizziness, faintness, weakness, loss of appetite, sleeplessness, urinary frequency, headache, neck or back aches, painful feet, and numbness or tingling of her hands or feet. Blood pressure and pulse rate are often elevated, there may be a fine tremor of the hands, and hypertonicity or spasm of skeletal muscles may be felt. The skin may be flushed or pale, and excessive perspiration may be present. These signs and symptoms are the person's response to anxiety, the apprehensive tension which stems from anticipation of a danger whose source is largely unknown or unrecognized.[1]

"I just don't have any energy, I'm always tired." The woman presenting with fatigue often experiences changes in mood as well as physical sensations which cluster around a sense of feeling dragged down and low. She may report sadness, gloominess, feeling blue, miserable, hopeless, dejected, discouraged, not caring what happens, feeling empty, not interested in anything, worried, unhappy, mixed up, or other negative feelings. Changes in her body or its functioning may include the loss of energy, exhaustion, loss of weight or appetite, inability to sleep or sleeping too much, constipation, headaches, stomach upsets, heaviness in her head or chest, and vague malaise. There may be minimal body movement, melancholic facial expression, hunched posture, slow speech, decreased verbal output, or deep sighing respirations. Thoughts may get mixed up and the woman may have trouble concentrating. These signs and symptoms are some of the manifestations of depression, a problem of mood or affect which has a wide range of expression and for which there is considerable disagreement about its cause and treatment.[2]

MEANINGS FOR WOMEN

Whenever an unpleasant body sensation persists for more than a short time, it is natural to become concerned that it may signal disease. Persistent and recurrent headaches raise fears of impending strokes or brain tumors. Abdominal cramping, pain, bloating, diarrhea, or constipation eventually cause concern that something is amiss in the digestive tract—perhaps infection or cancer or some other dimly conceptualized malady of the bowels. Chest pain, palpitations, and heart consciousness create fears of heart attack. Faintness, dizziness, tremors, or numbness or tingling of the extremities lead to speculation about neurological disorders—something being wrong in the brain or nervous system. Tiredness and fatigue make women wonder if they are anemic or have a "low thyroid." Flushing, sweating, weakness, or shakiness are commonly believed to be signs of hypoglycemia, and women worry about low blood sugar or the possibility of diabetes.

These sensations in body parts, whether aches, pains, pressure, pulling, pounding, twitching, numbness, or whatever, may frighten the woman and lead to a concern that they signal disease. Just as frequently, she fears that feeling tired and dragged out are early indications of some illness. So accustomed are we to believe that any unpleasant body sensation means an abnormality for which medical aid should be sought, that it is inconceivable to some persons that such sensations can be just a normal part of the body's functioning. It is also hard for many to believe that a stress of emotional origin can create bodily symptoms seemingly unconnected with the feelings of tension or depression—thus the frequent conviction on the part of patients that their symptoms must have a physical, organic cause.

Some women may see their symptoms as an indication of aging or inadequacy. For women in a culture that glorifies youth and particularly values physical beauty in women, feelings and sensations which imply that they are aging present significant threats. Tiredness, aching muscles, a dysfunctional body for various reasons can be taken as indicators of growing older, further contributing to decreased self-esteem and feelings of depression. In young women, with the threat of growing old still far in the future, these symptoms may serve to reinforce a sense of inadequacy. Even the woman's own body cannot be depended upon; rather than being strong and healthy and serving as a solid foundation for facing life's demands, it is weak and vulnerable, subject to pains and discomforts which cannot be understood; it is unpredictable and unreliable.

The symptoms of anxiety or depression may become accepted as a personality characteristic. A woman may say, "I'm a very nervous person," or "I get depressed a lot; I'm just that way." The feelings and sensations are seen as inevitable, as inherent in her personality structure, and she does not question why or wonder if her experience could be different. This is part of low self-esteem, of not thinking one deserves anything better. These attitudes have deep cultural roots, as women have long been devalued and considered inferior to men in most societies. Women are placed in a double bind by cultural values; their affectionate and nurturant qualities are cultivated and hypocritically praised, while they soon learn that men's aggressive and dominant qualities are what society actually values, and where the real power lies. But if women move toward initiative and self-reliance (a more dominant position), their anxiety is triggered in two ways: many men and other women oppose their stepping out of woman's sanctioned role, and a conflict develops between internalized societal values and the drive for self-realization.

Or, the woman may be aware of the relation between her emotional state and her physical symptoms but feel powerless to do anything to change the situation. Such women will admit that they have a "nervous stomach" or "tension headaches," or that their nerves "cause them to break out," or that they "always have trouble sleeping." Often these are longstanding patterns for which they have been given drugs, commonly minor tranquilizers and other mood altering drugs, which have now become part of the pattern. The drugs serve as a crutch, give a false sense that something is being done, or permit enough attenuation of the symptoms that there is no motivation to get at the basis of the problem.

PSYCHOPHYSIOLOGY OF STRESS

The human is a marvelously complex creature, continuously evolving and adapting, but still inextricably connected to primal behaviors. Evolutionally, the 4 to 5 million years from the appearance of the first hominids to the present modern human is but a tiny span of time—certainly not long enough for major structural or functional changes to occur. Thus we are still heir to response patterns which had survival value in a much earlier external reality:

> Prehistoric man survived in a dangerous world because, along with an elaborate brain, he possessed the mechanisms for instant physical response when threatened. Picture such a man, many thousands of years ago, resting in the sun in front of his cave after the hunt. Suddenly he feels the shadow of a predatory animal, stalking. Without thinking he reacts with a mighty rush of automatic resources. His heartbeat quickens. His blood pressure rises. Into his blood pour hormones that send sugar to his muscles and brain, mobilizing full energy. His digestive processes turn off at once so that this energy, undiverted, can be directed toward meeting the threat. Red cells flow into the arteries to help the body take in oxygen and cast off carbon dioxide. He clubs the intruder—or flees into his cave.[3]

This reaction to danger is called the "fight or flight" response and is frequently activated in modern men and women by a wide variety of stimuli. Numerous constraints of 20th-century civilization, however, prevent people from giving full expression to such instinctive impulses. Cowboy and detective movies notwithstanding, people cannot pull a gun and shoot their adversaries when thwarted in some goal, nor punch an opponent in an argument, nor run away to some safe place whenever they feel frightened. Physical action is usually inappropriate in most instances when people now feel threatened, but this is just what their psychophysiological response has equipped them to do.

Over a period of time, the accumulated effects of these frustrated physical responses, in a complicated interplay with personality characteristics and life events, and in the absence of effective methods of adaptation, can produce stress diseases. When a stressor continues to be applied, the reaction proceeds from the initial alarm stage through a characteristic sequence which is called the General Adaptation Syndrome. Humans are subject to a wide variety of stressors, ranging from accidents, such as fractured bones, to illnesses from bacterial invasion to any type of upsetting event in life. Stressors are not always negative; such positive happenings as getting kissed, getting married, having a baby, giving a speech, and receiving a promotion also excite psychophysiological responses that create the state of stress.

Stress and the General Adaptation Syndrome

Hans Selye was prompted to explore the concept of systemic stress when as a medical student he noticed that although different diseases have unique symptoms and characteristics, they also have common attributes such as loss of weight, energy, and appetite. Certain specific changes can be identified, forming a common residual response. The cause of this response is nonspecific and can be elicited by such diverse agents as cold, heat, x-rays, poisons, infections, wounds, adrenalin, insulin, or muscular exercise. This generalized response of the body to the demands made upon it was defined by Selye as stress: "Stress is the state manifested by a specific syndrome which consists of all the nonspecifically induced changes within a biologic system."[4]

Stress causes certain changes in the structure and chemical composition of the body; some of the changes are signs of damage, some are manifestations of the body's adaptive reactions (mechanisms of defense against stress), and some are caused by physiologic functioning. While the material and energy of the body are in a constant state of flux, there is also a drive to return to an original or typical condition, to achieve balance or homeostasis. This process of regulation involves the continuous readjustment of the organism to changes in its internal and external conditions. Thus, although it is essential that a threat be reacted to, there must also be no overreaction. Many safeguards are present, both emotionally and physically, to prevent overreaction when the organism is functioning properly (Figure 15-1).

THE ALARM REACTION.   The first stage of the General Adaptation Syndrome is the alarm reaction, characterized by autonomic excitement and adrenalin discharge. There is first an initial *shock phase*, in which resistance is lowered, then a *counter-shock phase* in which defensive mechanisms become active. The neuroendocrine system is set in motion, whether the threat is first perceived by the cerebral cortex (the boss refuses you a raise, your friend has caught you in a lie) or the hypothalamus (your foot has been cut, the car in front of you is stopping suddenly). The cerebral cortex signals the hypothalamus which signals the pituitary to release adrenocorticotropic hormone (ACTH) and thyrotropic hormone (TTH). There is, however, selectivity in the release of these two hormones; for instance, TTH secretion is stimulated by the stress produced by cold, while ACTH is not part of the response to cold but is stimulated by a large group of other stressors. Also, the hypothalamus activates the splanchnic nerve which stimulates the adrenal medulla to release adrenalin and noradrenalin.

The adrenalin zap is a feeling everyone is familiar with and is the basis of the fight or flight response. There is a sudden burst of excitation, of body exhilaration that leaves the person tingly and super-alert. It would be a most pleasant experience if it were not so closely associated with fear and danger. Adrenalin is thought to be the fear hormone, and noradrenalin the anger hormone, but there is almost always a mixture of fear and anger in varying proportions. Adrenalin and noradrenalin equip the person for emergency action to meet the perceived threat. They act upon the cardiovascular system to constrict peripheral and visceral arteries and to increase the heart rate in order to rush more blood to the muscles and brain. With less blood supplied to the skin and with quickened clotting time, the person will bleed less if injured. The white blood cell count is also increased to fight a possible infection. Metabolism is speeded up, as the liver and muscles release glucose to increase the fuel supply, the spleen contracts and pushes out increased numbers of red blood cells to deliver more oxygen so that the fuel can be burned faster, and the pancreas pours out more insulin to enable the increased sugar supply to enter the cells and be utilized. The respirations become deeper and more frequent to increase the oxygen available to the red blood cells. Additionally, the thyroid cooperates by secreting thyroxine, which makes body tissues apparently more sensitive to insulin. This is a more long-term measure for dealing with stress, while adrenalin is short-term, but both are needed together and repeatedly in dealing with most stress situations. Other effects of these changes are gastrointestinal ulceration and slowed digestive processes.

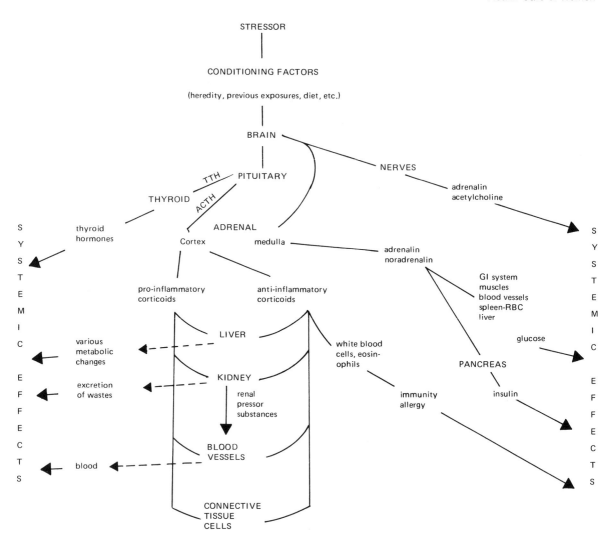

Figure 15-1. The stress response. This diagrammatic illustration of the body's stress mechanism is, of course, incomplete. Interactions between the main regulators are indicated; exact pathways of the complex secondary reactions are often not known. Selectivity at various points is individually determined by inherited and acquired characteristics.

Adrenocorticotropic hormone activates the adrenal cortex, where over 30 corticoids are produced. These are generally broken down into 2 groups, the mineralocorticoids which promote inflammation (proinflammatory) and the glucocorticoids which are antiinflammatory in action. The glucocorticoids increase the blood sugar in a slower and more persistent manner by stimulating the pancreatic glands to produce glucagon, an antagonist to insulin. Whether the proinflammatory or the antiinflammatory corticoids are most useful in responding to the threat depends upon the type and extensiveness of the problem and its progress over time. Proinflammatory corticoids are useful to contain and wall off local invaders such as the bacteria in a wound, thus preventing their spread into the bloodstream. Antiinflammatory corticoids inhibit the inflammation process when it is no longer useful, as in septicemia, balance the inflammatory reaction so it will not be excessive, and are helpful in minimizing allergic reactions such as asthma and poison oak dermatitis.

As the person mobilizes his or her defenses against the stressor, the acute alarm response decreases and the body achieves a relative homeostasis appropriate to its state of arousal. The adrenals become enlarged during the countershock phase because of their great activity. There may also be a loss of body weight.

THE STAGE OF RESISTANCE.   After this initial alarm reaction which calls forth body defenses, there follows a stage of resistance during which maximal adaptation occurs. In many instances the manifestations of this stage are the opposite of those characterizing the alarm reaction. The person achieves a state of balance, while defenses continue to fight the stressor. Depending upon the person's condition at the time of the exposure, the nature and intensity of the stressor, and other factors including medical treatment, the stage of resistance may be short and cause only mild symptoms. If, however, stress continues, lymphatic atrophy occurs with a decrease in lymphocytes and in eosinophils. This process no doubt plays a significant role in the decreased resistance to infection of people under stress.

If the stress continues, or the neuroendocrine system fails to respond properly, or the stressor itself is overwhelming, or a specific response is overused or misdirected, then the person may gradually develop a stress disease. These diseases of adaptation result from imperfections in the general adaptation syndrome and are not actually the result of some external agent but the consequences of the person's inability to meet these agents with adequate adaptive reactions. It is believed that the maladaptation of the body's response to stress plays a major role in diseases of the cardiovascular system, such as heart attacks, hypertension, angina, arrhythmias, and migraine; of the digestive system, such as ulcers, colitis, constipation and diarrhea; of the immunological system, such as infections, allergies, autoimmunity, rheumatoid arthritis, and cancer; of the musculoskeletal system, such as backache, tension headache, arthritis, and accidents; and in psychological problems, such as depression and sexual inadequacies[5] (Table 15-1).

THE STAGE OF EXHAUSTION.   If stress continues at a significant enough level, acquired adaptation is eventually lost and the person enters the stage of exhaustion. The symptoms of this stage are strikingly similar in many respects to those of the initial alarm reaction. At the end of a life under stress, there seems to be a type of premature aging due to wear and tear. Exhaustion of resources sets in, as the defense system has been gradually worn down. Selye believes that each person has a certain fixed reserve of *adaptation energy*, which is drawn upon during periods of stress and is gradually depleted over a lifetime.

People can get used to many stressors, such as cold, heavy muscular work, and worries, which at first had a very alarming effect. Yet, on prolonged exposure, eventually their resistance breaks down, and exhaustion sets in—as though something were used up during the work of adaptation. Every stress, therefore, exacts its toll, and although the person may apparently recover and resume life as usual, some portion of the adaptation energy has been taken and can never be restored. This is different from regaining vigor after resting, which occurs throughout life in healthy persons. Perhaps loss of adaptation energy is integral to the process of aging, and when all of our adaptability is used up, the failure of our most vulnerable organ occurs, and irreversible general exhaustion and death will follow.[6]

APPROACH TO MANAGEMENT

The langue of medicine is symptoms, and people have learned this well. Cultural conceptions of the sick role hold the physically ill blameless for their affliction; people "can't help it" if they are sick. It is acceptable to be absent from work due to the flu, or to cut back on responsibilities because of a strained back, or to lie down alone in a dark room for relief from a headache. In a similar vein, people can more readily identify the body sensations accompanying stress states than they can recognize the complicated underlying mechanisms. Because of culturally supported, longstanding habits of suppressing conflicts, the first level of awareness that many people experience includes one or more specific physical symptoms.

The presenting symptom or symptoms need a thorough and systematic exploration. Frequently the health provider may not suspect anxiety or depression as the basis for the patient's symptoms, for many patients show no typical signs of these conditions. Only after several visits, an appropriate work-up, and treatment has been tried will it begin to unfold

Table 15-1
Life Crisis and Health Changes

Rank	Life Event	Mean Value	Rank	Life Event	Mean Value
1	Death of spouse	100	23	Son or daughter leaving home	29
2	Divorce	73	24	Trouble with in-laws	29
3	Marital separation	65	25	Outstanding personal achievement	28
4	Jail term	63			
5	Death of a close family member	63	26	Wife begins or stops work	26
6	Personal injury or illness	53	27	Begin or end school	26
7	Marriage	50	28	Change in living conditions	25
8	Fired at work	47	29	Revision of personal habits	24
9	Marital reconciliation	45	30	Trouble with boss	23
10	Retirement	45	31	Change in work hours or conditions	20
11	Change in health of family member	44	32	Change in residence	20
12	Pregnancy	40	33	Change in schools	20
13	Sex difficulties	39	34	Change in recreation	19
14	Gain of new family member	39	35	Change in church activities	19
15	Business readjustment	39	36	Change in social activities	18
16	Change in financial state	38	37	Mortgage or loan less than $10,000	17
17	Death of a close friend	37			
18	Change in line of work	36	38	Change in sleeping habits	16
19	Change in number of arguments with spouse	35	39	Change in number of family get-togethers	15
20	Mortgage over $10,000	31	40	Change in eating habits	15
21	Foreclosure of mortgage or loan	30	41	Vacation	13
22	Change in responsibilities at work	29	42	Christmas	12
			43	Minor violations of the law	11

Life change events, by evoking adaptive efforts that are faulty in kind and duration, can lower body resistance and enhance the probability of disease occurrence. The greater the magnitude of change (mean value), the greater the probability that disease will occur and that it will be serious. The mean values of these life events are expressed in life change units (LCU) and have a high cross-cultural and cross-class consensus. By adding up the mean values of the LCUs, a total is obtained which is predictive of health change, which includes a broad spectrum of medical, surgical and psychological disorders. On the average, health changes follow life crisis by about one year.

Mild crisis	(150–199 LCU)	37 percent experienced health changes
Moderate crisis	(200–299 LCU)	51 percent experienced health changes
Major crisis	(300+ LCU)	79 percent experienced health changes

T. H. Holmes and M. Masuda: "Life Changes and Illness Susceptibility." In *Stressful Life Events: Their Nature and Effects,* B.S. Dohrenwend and B.P. Dohrenwend, eds. (New York: John Wiley & Sons, 1974), pp. 45-73. Originally published in the *Journal of Psychosomatic Research,* Vol. 11, pp 213-18, Pergamon Press, 1967.

that family or interpersonal conflicts are intimately tied to the symptomatology. In other cases, anxiety or depression may be suspected at once, and clinical judgment exercised regarding the extent of diagnostic work-up for organic problems. An atmosphere in which problems can be freely discussed and the sincere interest of the provider in identifying the problem allow the patient to bring up emotional or social material about conflicts and concerns.

The History

The usual characteristics of the presenting symptom are explored as follows:

When did it begin? How often does it occur? How long does it last? Is it constant, intermittent, or cyclic? What brings it on, makes it worse, makes it better? Is it associated with anything? Does it interfere with usual functioning? What treatment has been used, if any?

Somatic symptoms typical of anxiety include:

DIARRHEA. Slightly loose but not explosive watery stools are common. There may be some cramping, but it is not severe, and there is no tenesmus. Mucus and blood are usually absent.

URINARY FREQUENCY. Small volumes are voided, and there are no other symptoms of urinary tract infection such as dysuria, hematuria, or pyuria.

SWEATING. Usually occurs intermittently, and patients commonly complain of cold, clammy, moist hands. Only the palms or soles may be involved in some cases. Sweating with normal vital signs implies anxiety. While patients with thyrotoxicosis also sweat excessively, they report warm moist hands.

PALPITATIONS AND CHEST PAIN. The heart "skips a beat" or pounds against the chest wall, and the pain described often is not typical for cardiac pain. Frequently, patients are more aware of palpitations at night. Blood pressure is normal, and pulse rate elevated. The electrocardiogram reveals a normal tracing with sinus tachycardia.

ABDOMINAL PAIN. The pain described does not fit an organic disease, is often vague and diffuse. Nausea, usually without vomiting, and loss of appetite are common (see Chapter 12, Lower Abdominal Pain).

HEADACHE OR BACKACHE. Bilateral frontal or occipital headaches gradually increasing in intensity during the day are characteristic. These usually do not interfere with sleep but may be present upon arising. Muscle tension may also cause low back pain, which is constant and aching in quality, and may radiate to the buttocks and thighs.

Somatic symptoms typical of depression include:

CONSTIPATION. Decreased bowel activity and food intake contribute to hard and infrequent bowel movements. Gas and some cramping may be present.

HEADACHE. The most common pattern is a headache which is most severe in the morning but remains throughout the day. However, this type of headache is often indistinguishable from the tension headache, and probably the same mechanism is responsible because depression is commonly mixed with anxiety.

WEIGHT LOSS. Anorexia precedes weight loss, often with nausea but no vomiting. Usually about 10 to 15 pounds are lost. A few patients may have weight gain, particularly if they have a problem with obesity.

DRY MOUTH OR BAD TASTE. Decreased salivary secretion is the cause of these symptoms, in keeping with the general gastrointestinal hypoactivity which accompanies depression.

HEAVINESS IN HEAD OR CHEST. The depressed woman feels dragged down, as though her body has a great weight on it. This may be felt as a sense of pressure or heaviness in the head or chest. While not actually painful, this symptom does cause discomfort.

Do you feel tired even when you have enough sleep? Fatigue is the most telling sign of depression, especially when it is constant over time and not improved with adequate rest. However, fatigue is also characteristic of many illnesses such as anemia, tuberculosis, cancer, endocrine disorders, and most chronic diseases. With organic disease, the person feels most energetic in the mornings after a night's rest, gradually becoming more tired as the day progresses. People with depression often have sleep disturbances, either insomnia, difficulty in falling asleep, early awakening, or hypersomnia. They awaken feeling tired, find it hard to get going in the morning, and remain with low energy levels all day. Along with fatigue, there is a general inertia, for depressed people do not accomplish much in their daily activities, putting things off and finding reasons not to go places or become involved in projects or activities. Particularly if it is accompanied by constipation, the complaint "I'm always tired" is an almost certain clue to depression.[7]

Have you lost interest in food, family, work, friends, sex, or other activities? Loss of interest in any of these areas is a good clue to depression. Women may state that they do not feel anything any more or feel dead on the inside. Often they try to keep going and to act normally, but it is only a performance. Nothing seems to interest or stimulate them, or they cannot maintain their interest for a period of time.

Do you find it hard to make decisions? Depressed women often cannot make the smallest decision, even about what to have for dinner. They wish someone else would take over and make their decisions for them. Underlying this inability to make decisions may be the woman's need always to satisfy other people, never to make mistakes, not to commit herself to a definite opinion or course of action, or conflicts between impossible choices.

Do you often feel that something terrible is going to happen? Feelings of dread, that some disaster is impending, with elements of acute panic such as pounding heart and sweating, are signs of anxiety. These vague fears cannot be related to anything in reality. They may be accompanied by several other physical sensations of anxiety.

Are you generally tense and nervous? This overt feeling of anxiety is a common experience among women. Rarely will they be able to say just why they feel so anxious, although mention may be made of "a lot of problems" or "having many worries" or being "under a lot of pressure."

Do you find yourself continually angry, resentful, or complaining? Depressed women frequently experience conflicts with their family, friends, and co-workers. They feel constantly irritated, and often tense and anxious (anxiety often accompanies depression, although one purpose of depression is to drive the painful anxiety underground).[8] They become critical parents, nagging wives, or complaining workers and always find something to be upset about.

Are you self-critical, often feeling inferior or inadequate? Women who have set impossibly high standards for themselves will always end up falling short of their ideal self. Thus, nothing they ever do will be good enough. When these frustrations mount to an unbearable level, the woman may become depressed as a way to blot out her feelings of self-hatred. Feeling dead emotionally can be preferable to feeling a raging self-disdain.

Do you daydream a lot? Fantasizing often allows the woman to avoid facing conflicts and the feelings of anxiety which accompany them. The fantasies can become compelling, however, and make it difficult for the woman to face real life. The contrast between her wonderful imaginings and her desolate reality lead to increasing dissatisfactions and depression.

Do you alternate between periods of feeling "up" and "down"? Many women accept emotional lability and moodiness as a part of their character. Their continual emotional seesaw causes problems, however, in relations with others and in their own sense of contentment. Alternating between times of driven activity and inertia is very trying. In its more pronounced form it is called a manic-depressive condition.

Do you cry easily and frequently? Bursting into tears for no reason or at the slightest provocation can indicate depression. Women are culturally permitted to cry more freely than men, and tears accompany both joy and sorrow. Crying is appropriate, helpful, and therapeutic under the right circumstances, but when unpredictable outbursts of crying occur often and inappropriately, they are most likely the tears of impotent rage in a depressed person. There is a sense of helplessness, that nothing will ever change, a feeling of hopelessness with depression. Tears also can be mourning for a loss—in the case of a depressed woman, loss of some dream or goal or ideal.

Do you feel "in a fog" or "unreal"? This strange disjointed dreamlike feeling of being separate from reality, is part of depression. Women may report that their head feels full or heavy, that something has snapped inside, that they feel dazed. This fogginess is a defense reaction to suppress powerful feelings which the woman cannot face, usually including rage, deprivation, and anxiety. To prevent these feelings from erupting into consciousness, depression serves as an anesthetic, but it suppresses positive as well as negative feelings.

Do you have trouble concentrating or do you keep going over certain thoughts? Difficulty in concentrating and maintaining attention, as well as ruminative thought processes, are typical of depression. Often women focus upon the things that upset them most or that they hate most about themselves or their situations.

Have you considered committing suicide? Suicidal thoughts should always be taken seriously, and an appropriate referral must be made. This is often a last resort to escape or avoid painful feelings that can no longer be tolerated when no other options are perceived. The woman may say she just wants to die, wants her misery to end, her family would be better off without her, she doesn't deserve to go on living, or other expressions of hopelessness and despair. Asking the depressed person about suicidal thoughts is usually appreciated as an expression of the provider's concern and does not cause the nonsuicidal person to move in that direction.[9]

Do you have any current health problem? Are you under care? Do you take any medications? Chronic illness can precipitate depression as part of the disease process or as a response to the impact of the illness. Withdrawal from drugs such as amphetamines, barbiturates, and narcotics can trigger depression. The use of alcohol or tranquilizers often masks depression. Antihypertensive medications, especially reserpine, and cortisone or ACTH can cause depression. Recent surgery involving the loss of some part of her body, particularly the removal of her uterus or breast, or a tubal ligation often provokes serious conflicts in women, which may be translated into depression or anxiety. A long-term illness associated with nausea, such as hepatitis, often has depression as an accompaniment.

Have there been any recent changes, problems, or stresses in your life? Emotional losses are a common cause of depression, including the loss of employment, the loss of a loved one, retirement, or menopause. Changes in work, marital relations, children leaving home or having problems, and a myriad of life happenings may be enough to tip a precarious balance in a marginally adjusted woman, leading to anxiety or depression which reaches symptomatic levels.

Physical Examination

The physical examination depends largely upon the presenting symptoms and the systems implicated by them. Whether the symptom is headache, abdominal pain, diarrhea, palpitations, back pain, or whatever, the appropriate systems should be carefully examined. If the woman presents many symptoms (a positive review of systems), it may be necessary to schedule a complete physical examination and laboratory testing. It is difficult to assess whether her complex of symptoms may indicate organic disease without a thorough and systematic work-up.

FATIGUE. When the patient's symptoms are characterized by or cluster around fatigue, yet there is no history of chronic disease, the diagnoses to be ruled out include anemia, hypothyroidism and, possibly, diabetes. The physi-

cal signs of these diseases should be carefully searched for. In *anemia*, there may be no signs, or if they are present they can include pallor of the skin and conjunctiva, fissure of the lips, brittle nails, and warm pinkish palms. A history of heavy menses may be elicited. In *hypothyroidism*, signs could include dry hair, falling or thinning hair, loss of lateral eyebrows, dry rough skin, hoarseness, periorbital edema, dull expression, and slow return phase of the Achilles tendon reflex.[10] *Diabetes* produces few signs in the early stages, so a history of polyuria with increased thirst and appetite, loss of weight, and slow-healing infections are more useful indicators. *Neurological dysfunction* may be manifest by paresthesias, and vascular insufficiency by faint peripheral pulses, bruits, and ulcerations. Changes in the ocular fundi occur later in the disease.

NERVOUSNESS. With symptoms that cluster around nervousness, depending upon the specific symptoms, the diagnoses to be ruled out include hyperthyroidism (thyrotoxicosis), hypoglycemia, pulmonary emboli or, possibly, carditis. *Hyperthyroidism* produces sweating and warm, moist skin, tachycardia, arrhythmia, fine tremor of the fingers and tongue, and lid lag. There may or may not be an enlargement of the thyroid and prominent eyes (early expothalmos). *Hypoglycemia* is probably better thought of as hyperinsulinemia, when a relative carbohydrate intolerance or excessive carbohydrate intake triggers the oversecretion of insulin, causing a precipitous drop in blood sugar to abnormally low levels. Although blood sugar usually reaches normal levels within a short time, during the time that levels are quite low the patient experiences typical shakiness, tremor, sweating, weakness, dizziness, and nervousness. *Pulmonary emboli* might occasionally present as nervousness and chest pain, with tachycardia, arrythmia, dyspnea, and hemoptysis. A key element in the history would be the absence of previous similar episodes. Anxiety reactions tend to be recurrent. *Carditis* is manifested in chest pain and is exaggerated by breathing or coughing, and there may be tachycardia, hypotension, pericardial friction rub and dyspnea.[11]

If nervousness is associated with gastrointestinal symptoms, a different set of diagnostic possibilities arises. *Diarrhea* could be associated with diverticulitis, colitis, gastroenteritis, or parasitic infections. Anorexia and abdominal pain could be early signs of appendicitis (see Chapter 12, Lower Abdominal Pain).

Diagnostic Tests

The most useful diagnostic tests for women presenting with fatigue or nervousness, without significant medical history and with a low index of suspicion for organic pathology, are the *complete blood count (CBC)* and *urinalysis*. The complete blood count will generally rule out anemia, infection, and blood dyscrasias. The urinalysis will provide information about diabetes, urinary infections, and renal diseases. If the patient is concerned about diabetes or hypoglycemia, and desires further testing, the 2 or 3 hour *glucose tolerance test* can generally verify these conditions if they are present. When thyroid abnormalities are suspected, or if the patient feels strongly that she has "low thyroid," then a *thyroid panel* can be done, including T-4 (bound), T-3 uptake, and the T-7 calculation. It is important to do these tests together to create a check and balance system, especially if the woman is on oral contraceptives, which can cause an increased T-3 and T-4.

Immediate consultation with a physician is in order if pulmonary emboli or carditis is suspected. For gastrointestinal symptoms, diagnostic tests in addition to the complete blood count and urinalysis are usually delayed; if the symptoms such as diarrhea persist for several weeks, stool tests for blood, ova and parasites, and bacteria, and possibly a barium enema and sigmoidoscopy may be ordered later.

Treatment of Anxiety

When anxiety presents as a cluster of physical symptoms, the process of the diagnostic work-up is often itself therapeutic. Such patients not infrequently bring in a list on which they have carefully chronicled their many body sensations and unusual feelings. They want to be sure no data are omitted and that the practitioner is fully aware of all the ills that plague them. It is best to take each one of the patient's symptoms and explore it, both through her history and a physical examination. Appropriate lab tests are ordered, but it is wise to keep these simple and not to engage in an extensive work-up unless positive signs of organic disease are present.

Simple anatomic and physiological explanations for each symptom help the patient to understand how emotions can cause, for example, a spasm of the paraspinous muscles or gastrointestinal hypermotility, which in turn cause real and painful symptoms. Repeated explanations may be necessary because anxiety interferes with cognitive functioning and misunderstandings are common. Recognizing that the "mind can do so much to the body" is a significant step in accepting the fact that a state of anxiety can underlie the patient's symptoms. The next question then becomes obvious: Why is the patient so anxious?

If the patient can come to ask this question of herself, reasoning with the practitioner through the signs and symptoms and lab results, a foundation is established for beginning to consider other aspects of the patient's life as sources of anxiety. Some patients are "overaware" of body processes, overconcerned with their health, and worried that the slightest symptoms may mean disease. Because attention is focused so often on body sensations, this person is more aware of those normally below the threshold of perception. Minor aches, pains, and strange body sensations are usually unnoticed or overlooked by the less sensitive person. But the "overaware" person translates whatever insecurity she feels unconsciously into a concern over her physical well-being.[12] If the woman is able to carry on a busy, generally satisfying life and can think of no major problems which might be the sources of her anxiety, this explanation of being "overaware" of body processes may give her a way to deal with her benign but bothersome symptoms. The practitioner can even give some positive compliments to the patient for being aware of her body, thus more likely to seek care early and note significant danger signs. Encouraging an acceptance of some minor discomforts as part of the normal functioning of the body, with intermittent exaggerations due to tensions and stresses, will, it is hoped, give the patient more latitude before she becomes concerned about symptoms.

If the patient is willing to move toward exploring family, interpersonal, work, or other conflicts as a source of her anxiety, pointing out some of the dynamics involved can be useful. A preoccupation with somatic symptoms serves to keep the woman's attention from unpleasant and anxiety-provoking feelings—usually anger, hostility, aggressive feelings, impotent rage, sexual feelings, guilt, or shame. There may also be an element of assuaging guilt through suffering, and a number of secondary gains from "being ill," such as excuses for failure, avoiding responsibilities, postponing decisions, evoking love and attention from others, or escaping painful and intolerable life situations. If specific problems in the patient's life are brought up, they can be discussed and possible alternatives for dealing with them may be examined.

The process of resolving the conflicts underlying the patient's anxiety can take varying amounts of time, depending upon how conscious and near the surface they are and how ready to deal with them the woman is. Family therapy, counseling, or psychotherapy may be indicated, with the nurse practitioner participating to the extent of her personal expertise, or the nurse practitioner may refer the patient to community resources for such therapy.

DRUG THERAPY. The use of antianxiety drugs must be approached carefully because it is easy to fall back upon this chemical method of symptom relief while largely avoiding the underlying cause of the disturbance. The short-term use of antianxiety agents, however, is justifiable in many instances. Some diminution of the level of anxiety may be necessary before the patient can focus on an exploration of its emotional causes. Or, the woman may be aware of underlying conflicts and attempting to find her solutions to them, but the toll of anxiety in loss of sleep and agitation make it difficult for her to cope with her problems on a day-to-day basis.

The most commonly used antianxiety agents are the minor tranquilizers diazepam (Valium) and chlordiazepoxide HCL (Librium) (Table 15-2). These drugs have the effect of relieving anxiety and tension but are not useful for major psychotic symptoms such as delusions and hallucinations. Valium has been found to be more effective in anxious patients with painful musculoskeletal problems because of its muscle relaxing effects. Patients with gastrointestinal symptoms often do better on Librium. Both drugs can produce a degree of sedation, but it is quite variable. Librium has less sedative effect than Valium. The beginning doses are Valium 5 mg. three or four times a day, and Librium 10 mg. four times a day.[13] The patient must be advised to take the first dose at home

or to avoid driving until the degree of sedation the drug causes has been established. A small number of patients become mildly confused or giddy on these drugs and are told to call if they experience unusual affects.

A follow-up visit in a week, then regularly while the patient is on drug therapy is recommended. Other types of treatment should be undertaken, and the patient should be informed that the tranquilizer is meant for short-term use, not as a solution to the problem (see pages 364 to 365 for a discussion of issues surrounding the use of mood-altering drugs).

Another minor tranquilizer commonly used for anxiety is meprobamate (Miltown or Equanil) 400 mg. three or four times a day. As with the other tranquilizers, the patient must be cautioned that alcohol can potentiate the drug's effects and vice versa, and people often become intoxicated more easily.

Treatment of Depression

Depression is often a hard diagnosis for the patient to face because the very purpose of this emotional wet blanket is to suppress from consciousness painful or frightening feelings. When the woman is presenting depression through body symptoms (masked depression), the symptoms permit her to express her distress without confronting the conflicts which underlie the process. Patients at first may reject the idea that they are depressed, insisting that they are "run down" or have chronic back problems or headaches and that they would feel fine if only these conditions could be cleared up. It is incumbent upon the practitioner to move the patient along skillfully in the diagnostic reasoning process so that when all the data are put together from her history, examination, and lab tests, the inevitable conclusion points away from organic and toward emotional problems. The diagnosis of depression rests not only on the elimination of organic disease as the cause of a woman's symptoms, but also on the presence of several characteristic factors: dysphoric mood, fatigue, weight or appetite loss, loss of general or sexual interest, insomnia or hypersomnia, trouble in concentrating, self-reproach or guilt, retardation of movement or speech, or thoughts of death or suicide.[14]

Accepting the diagnosis of depression implies for the patient that she must make some changes in her life or else be willing to con-

Table 15-2
Drugs in the Treatment of Anxiety and Depression

ANTIANXIETY DRUGS

	Dosage Range (mg.) per day	Sedative Action	Other Factors
Benzodiazepines			
Chlordiazepoxide HCL (Librium)	15–40	+	High safety factor
Diazepam (Valium)	4–40	+ +	
Oxazepam (Serax)	30–60	+	
Chlorazapate Dipotassium (Tranxene)	15–60	+	
Propanedioles			
Meprobamate (Miltown, Equanil)	400–1600	+ + + +	High toxicity, relatively low therapeutic value
Tybamate (Tybatran, Solacen)	750–2000	+ + +	

TRICYCLIC ANTIDEPRESSANTS

Sedating			
Amitriptyline HCL (Elavil)	100–300	+ + + +	Autonomic side effects predominate
Nortriptyline HCL (Aventyl)	20–100	+ +	"
Doxepin HCL (Adapin, Sinequan)	75–300	+ + + + +	Extrapyramidal side effects predominate
Energizing			
Imipramine HCL (Tofranil)	100–300	+ +	Autonomic side effects predominate
Desipramine HCL (Norpramine, Pertofrane)	100–300	+ +	"
Protriptyline HCL (Vivactil)	20–50	+	"

tinue with her present symptoms and mood. If the woman is ready to explore the sources of her dissatisfaction and conflict, a discussion of family relations, marital or partner relations, work, goals, and other problems may help in determining the causes of her depression. Depending upon the type of conflicts in the woman's life, a number of different therapeutic approaches can be utilized. Marriage counseling, family therapy, individual counseling or psychotherapy, or group therapy are some of the options. Women's groups, which provide for the sharing of experiences and the support of personal growth, are often very helpful in coping with depression and in finding ways for a woman to make the changes which are necessary for her to eliminate the causes of the conflicts in her life.

Conflict is always one of the cornerstones of depression and may arise from several basic dynamics. An ideal of the perfect self is developed through a set of internalized "shoulds," the do's and don'ts which people come to believe about themselves in the process of growing up. This causes the person to restrict her life; it limits acceptable choices, and sets her up for failure. Inevitably the perfect self cannot be realized, and these failures to live up to her shoulds make the woman despise herself. This may cause unbearable anxiety which is suppressed through depression. Or, feeling so worthless, the woman desperately seeks affirmation from others, doing anything needed to gain approval. Such self-effacement leads to anger, a hopeless rage which also is suppressed through depression. The woman may become detached and uninvolved to escape conflicts with her shoulds, but human needs for closeness and intimacy are continually at odds with detachment, producing another conflict.[15]

There is a growing school of thought that biochemical alterations are the basis of depression. The "catecholamine hypothesis" identifies neurotransmitter chemicals as the agents for affective disorders; in the central nervous system decreases in norepinephrine and serotonin levels cause depression, while increases result in mania. Reserpine depletes these catecholamines, with depression the result. Monamine oxidase (MAO) is critical in the metabolic breakdown of these amines, and any blockage of MAO will increase the amines and lift the depression. An increase of MAO will hasten the degradation of amines and promote depression. With aging there is an increase of MAO activity in the brain, corresponding to increased depression in older persons. Estrogen inhibits MAO, and with menopause as estrogen activity drops, MAO activity increases, leading to more frequent depression in menopausal and postmenopausal women. There also appears some genetic predisposition to depression.[16]

There is, no doubt, a biochemical pathway for depression, just as there must be a particular chemical or electrical activity in the brain associated with all emotions and cognitive functions. The question is one of cause and effect: do these biochemical changes initiate the chain of events which leads to depression or are they produced after stressors and conflicts have activated certain glands or cells to trigger the biochemical response? Loss is also associated with depression, whether loss of a loved one, loss of some life goal, loss of some mode of expression such as one's work, or loss of a body part. The grief reaction or mourning which accompanies loss is normal and must be differentiated from depression. Mourning is related to a specific event and, although intense, usually does not prevent people from functioning. There is a fairly rapid decline in the intense signs of mourning, with a gradual lessening of the feelings of sadness and loss. Although depression is characterized by sadness, a specific event often cannot be identified, functioning is impaired, and the feelings of loss persist at significant levels for an undue time.

DRUG THERAPY. Antidepressive drugs are quite effective in relieving depression, and some practitioners believe that they should be used in preference to insight therapy. The rum-inative thoughts typical of depression, the circular reasoning and immobilization, often make it very difficult for the depressed person to benefit from a discussion of feelings and conflicts. Interrupting these mental processes and forcing a biochemical change in the brain with drugs brings about changes in mood more rapidly. As in treating anxiety, drugs have a legitimate place in the treatment of depression as long as they are not seen as the sole solution to the problem. Antidepressives permit a relative balance to be attained by the patient, relieve much inertia and fatigue, and improve her other symptoms, such as insomnia. With this help, patients may be capable of exploring emotional factors and benefitting from other types of therapy.

The antidepressant drugs include two pharmacological classes, the imipraminelike drugs (Tofranil, Elavil, Sinequan, Vivactil) which are also called tricyclics, and the MAO inhibitors (Parnate, Nardil). Tricyclics are selected according to the degree of sedation likely to optimize function during drug therapy. The more sedative tricyclics are Sinequan and Elavil; the less sedative are Vivactil and Tofranil. The beginning doses for all but Vivactil are 25 mg. four times a day; for Vivactil 5 mg. four times a day. Some patients require larger doses, which can later be adjusted. The sedative effect of these drugs appears about 1 hour after taking the pill, which could cause waves of sedation during the day. Orthostatic hypotension and dizziness, though not common, may occur at about the same time. One way to avoid this symptom is by giving the tricyclic in one dose at night, rather than splitting it during the day. For instance, Elavil 25 mg. three tablets at bedtime achieves its highest sedative action during the night, thus relieving insomnia, but continues to have its antidepressive effect all day.

The MAO inhibitors are less commonly used because they are less effective than the tricyclics and may cause a hypertensive crisis if the patient eats foods high in tyramine content. In the few patients who do not respond to tricyclics, however, MAO inhibitors may produce a good response and are particularly useful for women who are sensitive to emotional rejection.[17] The nurse practitioner should consult with a psychiatrist when considering the use of an MAO inhibitor.

Both classes of antidepressant drugs act in a slow manner, and clinical improvement may not occur until after 1 to 3 weeks of therapy. Patients must be informed of this, and the importance of taking the medications daily in order to build up to therapeutic effects must be carefully explained. Regular follow-up visits as long as the patient is on drug therapy are advised, with the institution of additional forms of treatment (counseling, family therapy) provided either by referral or by experienced nurse practitioner-physician teams.

The more acutely depressed women can be reassured that their present state of feeling will eventually improve in a matter of weeks or a few months, for this is common in women who have been previously reasonably adjusted and functioning well. A chronic low-grade depression may persist, however, indicating the need for dealing with the underlying conflicts. Some women remain more or less depressed throughout their lives unless their motivation to confront conflicts is somehow spurred and they find the courage to make the changes necessary for them to lead more satisfying and fulfilling lives (Figure 15-2).

PHILOSOPHICAL CONSIDERATIONS

Women's Status, Anxiety and Depression

Women are particularly prone to depression and its predecessor, anxiety. Men, of course, can be anxious or depressed but generally manifest their conflicts in other ways: falling prey to the stress diseases of heart attacks, hypertension, ulcers, and disabling musculoskeletal back problems. Although both sexes are subject to a lifetime of stresses, their different status, social roles, and consequent personality organization make them prone to different ways of becoming ill. Empirical knowledge indicates that women utilize the health care system more, take more over-the-counter and prescription drugs, have more apparently psychosomatic illness, use more mood-altering drugs, and are more often depressed than men. These reactions to stress are attributed to women's subordinate status and the destructive effects of male domination. The female-inferior male-superior social dichotomy is, however, a two-edged sword which exacts a heavy toll on both sexes and prevents the full expression of human potential for men as well as for women.

Some observers have noted that when

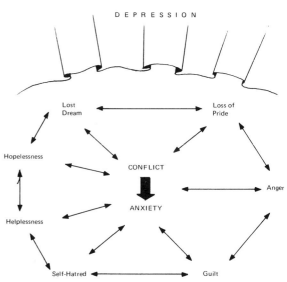

Figure 15-2. Components of anxiety/depression.

women attain power, they are as destructive as men to those in subordinate positions, leading to a hypothesis that human nature is intrinsically egotistical and exploitative. From this view, domination is the "stuff of life," and we are locked into never-ending competition and struggle for power, their most extreme expression being war. There are, however, certain nonaggressive societies characterized by cooperation rather than competition, demonstrating that other social organizations are possible. One explanation of this apparent contradiction in human nature is that all humans are basically affectionate, as manifest by the early nurturant mother-child bond, and that exploitative social institutions are necessary to disrupt affectional bonds and to push persons of either sex into dominating others.

An exploitative power group existing within a society forms an extremely potent force, both for the assumption of real power and for the promotion of attitudes which value aggressive personalities as "powerful" and gentle personalities as "weak." Such cultural distortions push men more easily into dominant positions, perhaps because men are not childbearers or because women are slightly more gentle and affectionate by genetic and hormonal endowment. For centuries of civilization, there have been exploiters and the exploited, with women having inferior positions to men of their own class, and the family serving as a "transmission belt for power-based authoritarian values, personified by the father." Even in such exploitative societies, it is hard to suppress childhood experiences of warmth, gentleness, and affection, to mold men into "expendable warriors" and women into "inferior childbearers." The inherent contradictions between affectionate experiences during childhood and the later dehumanized, exploitative relations of adulthood create serious conflicts in both sexes. Because men are required to suppress affectionateness more severely and to follow a more confusing path to gender identity (their initial identification is with a nurturant, loving mother), there is a greater need for men to be powerful and to devalue women. Their real power in male-dominated societies, reinforced by laws and customs, forces the living-out of this culture-myth that men are superior in all ways to women.

The price paid for the molding of men and women into these roles, in addition to the human suffering of the exploited and the devastation of war, is a different cognitive and emotive style, with typical patterns of mental illness for the two sexes. An exploitative society trains men in aggression, distorting their affectionate natures and going against their earliest experiences. Men suffer guilt and "go crazy" through developing strange, radical transformations of their selves and the world; compulsions and obsessions such as sexual deviations (transvestism, fetishism, sadomasochism, exhibitionism, voyeurism, child-molesting, and rape), obsessional neurosis, schizophrenia, alcoholism, and drug addiction. Women are trained to be loving and affectionate, in keeping with their early experiences, and have a more direct path to gender identity. But society devalues affection and scorns gentleness, placing women in subjugated, inferior positions in the external world and in relation to men. Women "go crazy" by collapsing into an abysmal state of fear, helplessness, sadness, and self-hatred which produces anxiety, depression, and hysteria. A chronic state of shame characterizes these conditions, because women are ashamed of their loving feelings which have no reward in society's marketplace, yet are their only way to any degree of value and acceptance.[18]

In nonexploitative societies, the status of women is higher and there is more equality between the sexes. There also tends to be less illness and anomie when cooperation is the social mode and when all members have a valued and recognized place in the social structure, including children, women, and the elderly.

THE ROOTS OF CHANGE. Perhaps the era of human inequality and exploitative societies is slowly waning, though it is by no means close to an end. The mid-20th century has seen an uprising of consciousness of human rights and a massive reaction against exploitation, as exemplified in the Civil Rights Movement, the Women's Movement, the protest against the Vietnam war and the compulsory draft, the "third world" people's fights for self-determination, and "La Raza" and the Chicano Movement. Indeed, a strong current of change permeates American society, upheaving old traditions and sacrosanct cultural institutions. But there is resistance every step of the way, both from those in power and from their effectively socialized subordinates. The struggle for equality, for the right to pursue personal fulfillment in individual ways, with no channels artificially closed because of characteristics one is born with, must continue on a personal, community, and societal level for a long time to come.

But women do have choices, and many of the roots for change lie within themselves. Women can understand the bases for anxiety and chronic low-grade depression and can take action to improve their situations. In an excellent and perceptive book, Helen DeRosis and Victoria Pellegrino present theories and practical exercises for self-help for women with depression: *The Book of Hope: How Women Can Overcome Depression.* Women are encouraged to use physical activity, to keep a notebook detailing their lost dream, lost pride, anger, guilt, self-hatred, hopelessness, helplessness, and conflicts related to these problems. There are specific questions and exercises to analyze them, with explanations of how stereotyped expectations and scripts from childhood set women up for conflicts and lead to compulsive beliefs and behaviors. Support is given to the questioning of traditional social values and childhood teachings in order to arrive at a new belief-system compatible with women's growth and full maturation. Concepts of femininity, women's role, and man-woman relations may all have to be changed if women are to overcome depression and feel truly alive.

... if dependency is seen to be a natural state for women, then depression will always be a natural state, too. ... You will have to keep trying to find your lost self through your own efforts, your own strengths. These are the wellsprings of your own hopefulness. To recover, to be well is a *possible dream*. Be persistent; be tenacious, be courageous. And most of all, be hopeful.[19]

Many paths to self-realization are available today in professional or lay groups and organizations which promote personal awareness and growth. There are encounter groups, Gestalt group therapy, Rogerian groups, EST, existential therapy, Esalon, women's groups, Transcendental Meditation, other Eastern approaches such as Sufism and Yoga, Arica, Rolfing, and many other paths. Although there are dangers of faddism and evangelism, reputable groups have much to offer in helping people find pathways for constructive change. Some sort of shock, whethr directly to the body or through the cerebral cortex, is basic to all the therapies: challenge the organism, force a change of pace, shake it up, free it from old patterns, get it moving, functioning, flowing.

Use of Mood-Altering Drugs

Drug use is a widespread problem, met with conflicting viewpoints, and here only the prescription antianxiety and antidepressant drugs will be considered. The nurse practitioner will be faced repeatedly with the decision of beginning or renewing these drugs for women. A well-thought-out philosophy of drug use will be invaluable in managing cases of anxiety and depression. There has unquestionably been an abuse of mood-altering drugs through medical routes, particularly of Valium, to the point where some providers simply will not prescribe it. Mood pills do not really solve problems; they only obscure them and make them less painful. This palliation reduces the likelihood that action will be taken to correct the situation or that the person will listen to danger signals from physical and emotional sensations. Although mood pills are not physically addictive, patients do develop a psychic dependency on them with their long-term use. Patients come to believe that they cannot do without their pills and perceive the rebound of anxiousness or fatigue which they experience when stopping the pills as withdrawal. These

unpleasant feelings drive the person to seek the pills again, and the cycle repeats itself.

Physicians have been accused, not altogether without basis, of using mood-altering drugs in treating women to avoid dealing with the conflicts and anxieties which are at the basis of the presenting problems. Many women are labeled "crocks" because of their persistent physical symptoms with negative objective findings, and they are dismissed with drugs which dampen their anxieties and alleviate their depressions. In one study it was found that women constituted 76 percent of antidepressant drug users, 72 percent of users of minor tranquilizers, and 80 percent of diet pill users (uppers, amphetamines).[20] The drug industry makes considerable profits from the sale of psychoactive drugs. At community pharmacies in the U.S., these account for more than 200 million prescriptions per year at a retail cost of almost one billion dollars. About 17 to 20 percent of all prescriptions, or one in five, are written for psychoactive drugs. The use of minor tranquilizers alone has increased nearly 78 percent since the mid-1960s.[21,22] Approximately 11 percent of the annual expenditures on health care in the U.S. goes to the drug industry. Although drug treatment is appropriate and indicated in many cases, there is an obvious economic benefit derived in part from the miseries of women (the majority consumers of health care) which has caused cynicism and bitterness toward providers and toward the health system as a whole.

A decision must be made in each individual case; is the use of a mood-altering drug appropriate or is it contributing to perpetuating the problem? Generally, short-term use with fairly identifiable sources of conflict is well supported, especially if the woman is aware of and taking some action to deal with her situation. Or, in conjunction with another method of therapy, short-term mood alterers can aid progress. But what of the long-term user, the woman who already has been on Valium or Miltown for years, the woman who can't do without her pills, and undoubtedly will go elsewhere if denied here; or the woman whose cultural, family, economic, and social situation impose impossible restrictions on insight, change or growth, and whose pills are helping her to "get by" day by day? These cases pose much harder problems in deciding for or against the use of mood-altering drugs. The individual practitioner's clinical judgment must enter, as well as standards for practice in the setting.

The human organism is genetically programmed for growth, mental and emotional as well as physical, both male and female. The unfolding and flowering of the magnificent human potential is within each of us, as is the drive to be all that we can be, to realize our abilities to their fullest extent. People must be hurt and damaged to suppress their growth, and the stresses produced will come out in some way. Women in particular must struggle to grow, fighting emotional and cultural barriers.

NOTES

1. C. H. H. Branch, *Aspects of Anxiety* (Philadelphia: J. B. Lippincott Company, 1968), pp. 9-11.
2. A. T. Beck, *The Diagnosis and Management of Depression* (Philadelphia: University of Pennsylvania Press, 1973), pp. 3-40.
3. W. McQuade and A. Aikman, *Stress* (New York: E. P. Dutton, 1974), p. 5.
4. H. Selye, *The Stress of Life* (New York: McGraw-Hill, 1956), p. 54.
5. McQuade, *Stress*, pp. 21-90; and M. H. Appley and R. Trumbull, "On the Concept of Psychological Stress." In Appley and Trumbull, eds., *Psychological Stress: Issues in Research* (New York: Appleton-Century-Crofts, 1967), pp. 3-4.
6. Selye, *Stress of Life*, p. 66.
7. "Tip-Offs that You're Dealing with Depression." *Patient Care* 8,6 (March 15, 1974): 178-207.
8. H. DeRosis and V. Y. Pellegrino, *The Book of Hope: How Women Can Overcome Depression* (New York: Macmillan, 1976), p. 7.
9. S. Soreff, "Depression and the Middle Aged Woman." *Primary Care* 2,4 (December 1975): 609-14.
10. A. J. Hoole, R. A. Greenberg, and C. G. Pickard, *Patient Care Guidelines for Family Nurse Practitioners* (Boston: Little, Brown, 1976), pp. 276-78 and 286-88.
11. O. Horowitz and J. H. Magee, *Index of Suspicion in Treatable Disease* (Philadelphia: Lea & Febiger, 1975), pp. 494, 525.
12. Branch, *Aspects of Anxiety*, pp. 106-10.
13. "Office Therapy for Anxiety/Depression." *Patient Care* 7,14 (August 1, 1973): 27-52.
14. J. G. Williams, "Common Errors in the Treatment of Depression." *American Family Physician* 14,2 (August 1976): 61-64.
15. DeRosis and Pellegrino, *Book of Hope*, pp. 3-59.
16. Soreff, "Depression," p. 611.
17. "Office Therapy for Anxiety/Depression," pp. 27-52.
18. H. B. Lewis, *Psychic War in Men and Women* (New York: New York University Press, 1976), pp. xv-xix, 59, 86, 198-99, 233-34, and 266-67.
19. DeRosis and Pellegrino, *Book of Hope*, pp. 289-99.
20. E. Frankfort, *Vaginal Politics* (New York: Quadrangle Books, 1972), pp. 107-8.
21. M. E. Jarvick, ed., *Psychopharmacology in the Practice of Medicine* (New York: Appleton-Century-Crofts, 1977), p. xv.
22. M. Silverman and P. R. Lee, *Pills, Profits & Politics* (Berkeley and Los Angeles: University of California Press, 1975), pp. 274, 293.

16

Socialization of Women

In providing sensitive and sympathetic health care for women, it is necessary to understand the many forces shaping women's behavior. Women's heritage, including their history through the progress of civilization, their current socialization, and the milieu in which they live are all components of which the health provider should be aware. While it is invalid to assume that an individual woman possesses a certain general characteristic, knowledge of the broad factors which affect contemporary women adds an important dimension to women's health care. Each woman encountered by the nurse practitioner needs an individualized approach. The truths in one woman's life may be inapplicable to another, and the sources of problems and conflicts are quite varied. With this in mind, a framework can be established to examine the socialization of women and the significance of women's roles and identity to the provision of health care.

Two factors which have widespread influence upon many women, cutting across subgroup values and cultural norms, are the human drive toward growth and the changing roles of women in society. Because of women's history of restricted roles, their opportunities for personal growth and expression of their abilities have often been limited. Women's part in reproduction seems to have indelibly stamped their options, and the functions of their bodies to have shaped their abilities and possibilities. Men's part in reproduction, however, is not considered so pivotal in the expression of their capabilities. Why women's role and status have so thoroughly derived from bi-

ological function, and why these have been assigned lower value and a secondary position in society are the enigmas.

> The overwhelming evidence so far is that virtually no society in the world provides women equal status with men. Although anthropologists have found that women are given considerable social recognition and power in some societies, there exists no society in which their publicly recognized power exceeds that of men.[1]

> Though the status of women in society varied in the past, sometimes higher, sometimes lower, there has been a practical universal unanimity of the male to ascribe a relative inferiority to the female.[2]

So pervasive is this differentiation between social status and role based on sex that it is easy to conclude this is the natural order, biologically or constitutionally ordained. Diverse cultures assign different functions to males and females, but there is great variation in what is contained in culturally approved functions. In some cultures, women plow fields and tend flocks, while in others they are considered too delicate for strenuous work. Women may be artisans who innovate basketry, weaving and pottery, or the culture may define them as having no creative talents. Their counsel may be valued as wise and humane, or their minds thought to be incapable of comprehending worldly affairs. They may offer wit and intellectual stimulation in conversation, or appear dulled by the details of simple domesticity. In some instances, women are cast as the guardians of society's moral standards, while at other times they seduce men from virtue and higher purpose. They may barter and trade deftly, or not be able to manage any economic interface. The stalwart, courageous molder of family life contrasts with the perennial adolescent incapable of serious purpose. Women can forge a life on a dangerous frontier, or they must be protected from the strain of public life in carefully buttressed homes.

What is considered the normal, natural function of women in one culture may be viewed with repugnance and astonishment in another. A given task may be believed contrary to woman's nature in one place and integral to her nature in another. Among social groups, the only functions completely monopolized by women are childbearing and suckling, and those almost always performed by men are war-making and hunting. Society is responsible for shaping the roles carried out by men and women:

> This variety and diversity in the roles and status of women testify to the influence of culture and structure in fashioning the social order and argue against a simple biological determinism. Biological capacity merely limits the part each person can play in human reproduction. Society, through its interpretation of what it means to be female or male, and through its establishment of patterns of appropriate behavior for women and men, transforms biological potential into social actuality.[3]

Women now appear to be on the threshold of an era of great opportunity. They are largely able to control reproductive function. Before this, any fertile sexually active woman could expect to be pregnant the majority of her adult years. Laws have been changed gradually over the last quarter century to allow women to own and control property, make contracts and agreements, vote in national and local elections, serve in the judicial and legislative processes, and recently to bar discrimination in education and employment. The ground swell for human rights, particularly civil rights for minority and ethnic groups, has created a climate in which relationships between people can be reexamined and old values and practices questioned. The women's movement has focused awareness on the deep-seated discontent of large numbers of·women with their restricted roles.

Although many barriers have been removed, the most pervasive and profound factors affecting equality between the sexes continue to support a subordinate status for women. These factors involve the shaping of identity, the psychological and structural determination of social status and role, and the values, traditions and beliefs which prevail in the culture. This chapter examines the many factors contributing to the socialization of women, the resultant feminine behaviors and characteristics, and some of the problems socialization poses for both women and men.

The stresses of living which grow out of contradictory values cause considerable morbidity among women. The changes now occurring in women's roles are unsettling and a source of conflict for many women and men. In a complex variety of personal expressions, life stresses and role changes often produce symptoms which motivate people to seek care from the health system. Whether manifest as depression or anxiety, or converted physically to such symptoms as abdominal pain or headaches, the expressions of stress and conflict can be more effectively treated when the psychosocial sources of this behavior are understood.

DEVELOPMENT OF GENDER IDENTITY AND SEX ROLES

The basis of the differences in appearance and behavior between women and men rests in a complex interaction of genetic and environmental factors. There is no dichotomy between "nature and nurture," but rather a genetic code requiring certain species-specific environmental boundaries for its proper expression. The genetic information contained in chromosomes interacts with the environment on many different levels, however, and among humans it is inordinately difficult to trace the effects of biological factors through the maze of other determinants, particularly cultural and social forces, which govern behavior. The effects of sex chromosomes on reproductive organs and body configurations are indirect and are mediated through hormones. The impact of sexual dimorphism on other than reproductive behavior is even less clear, and is subject to considerable controversy.

That there are probably some genetically determined differences in behavioral potentials is a cause of concern for women who are fighting their subjugation. From Freud's contention that "biology is destiny" to the male chauvinist's notions that "genetics justifies sexism," women have had to struggle against the use of their "feminine characteristics" to relegate an inferior social status and limit life choices. Very little is actually known about hereditary psychological differences, but there is beginning evidence that the sexes vary on some important characteristics: sociability (also called person-orientation), spatial ability, field independence, and aggression.[4] When there is widespread agreement that certain qualities are superior, for instance aggression is better than sociability, the groundwork is laid for discrimination. While the tendency to ignore sex differences has the advantage of stressing the common humanity of both sexes, it does not promote understanding of the subtle influences of genetic components. It is possible that women's greater sociability provides a basis for their subjugation: "To put it bluntly, they are easier to exploit."[5]

Genetic and Hormonal Sex

The beginning of sexual development is initiated by the X or Y chromosome supplied by the male parent, which pairs with the X chromosome from the female parent. The XX or XY combination then passes the sexual program to the primordial gonad. The primitive genital ducts of the embryo are identical until about six weeks after conception, when under chromosomal influence the gonads of the XX embryo become ovaries and the XY embryo, testes. Androgenic hormones secreted by the testes then stimulate the Wolffian ducts, which give rise to most of the male reproductive system, and probably suppress the Mullerian ducts, from which the female genital structures develop. If the fetal gonads do not secrete hormones, however, the fetus always continues to differentiate the reproductive anatomy of a female. Thus, the presence of androgens produces a male differentiation, while their absence leads to female differentiation.[6]

This situation of "adding something" to make a male implies that nature's basic propensity is to produce a female. In an XX embryo, if the gonads are removed before the seventh week so they do not produce estrogen, the embryo still develops normal female anatomy. Circulating maternal estrogens are not necessary for female differentiation; when embry-

onic reproductive tracts (minus gonads) are removed and kept alive *in vitro* for sufficient time, the growth pattern in all (both XX and XY) remains female. Mammalian embryos are innately female, and no ovarian inductor substance is needed for female differentiation, as all have genetically determined basic female morphology. The morphogenesis of primordial sexual organs is a result of hormonal exaggeration or suppression of inherent growth tendencies. This organization pattern is initially given in the female, and it must be acquired in the male through androgenic induction.

Of the entire primordial reproductive tract, it appears that the Mullerian and Wolffian ducts are the only basically dimorphic structures. They have separate origins, the latter from the embryonic kidneys and the former probably from peritoneal evaginations. Fetal androgens must suppress the Mullerian ducts, but the Wolffian ducts degenerate in females without suppression by fetal or maternal estrogens. The remainder of the genital tract is basically female, as shown by the large genital tubercle (glans and corpora cavernosi), the labioscrotal folds, the urethral-labial folds, and the vestibule of a seven-week embryo which are well-defined and clearly female in form and general configuration (Figure 16-1). The innate femaleness of mammalian embryos was known to biologists as early as 1957 (with 15 years of prior research), but has received little attention. Most texts still refer to the "undifferentiated" embryonic phase, rather than acknowledge the primacy of female morphology. This forces a reversal of long-held concepts about the nature of sexual differentiation; rather than the clitoris being a "vestigial penis," it is embryologically correct to say that the penis is an exaggerated clitoris, the scrotum is derived from the labia majora, and the original libido is female (Figures 16-2 and 16-3).[7]

Certain patterns of organization in the brain are also responsive to the presence or absence of androgens during a critical time of brain development. Neural pathways that will subsequently influence certain aspects of sexual behavior, probably involving the hypothalamus, are established. The endocrine system and the peripheral and intracranial nervous systems which serve the genital organs are part of this brain dimorphism. This neural sexual differentiation mediates reproductive behavior and

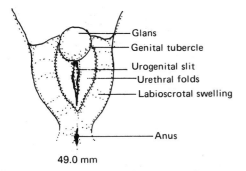

Figure 16-1. External genitalia of a 7-week embryo. The 7-week embryo is just entering the differentiation stage. Although this embryo is female, its sex could be determined only by the Barr body chromosome test. The 7-week male embryo appears exactly the same.

cyclicity of gonadal function. What other types of behavior it influences are slowly being unraveled.

Early Physical and Behavioral Differences

Certain differences are observable between the sexes during the prenatal period. The female fetus develops more quickly, has a faster heartbeat, and is more hardy as seen in lower rates of spontaneous abortion, perinatal and infant mortality. Geneticists speculate that the female's survival advantage from conception

Figure 16-2. External genital differentiation in the human fetus.

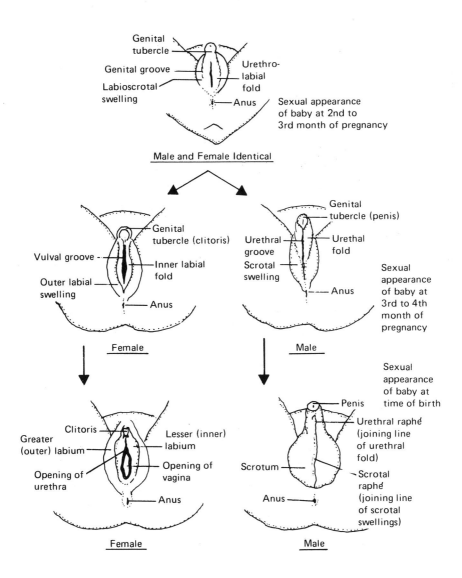

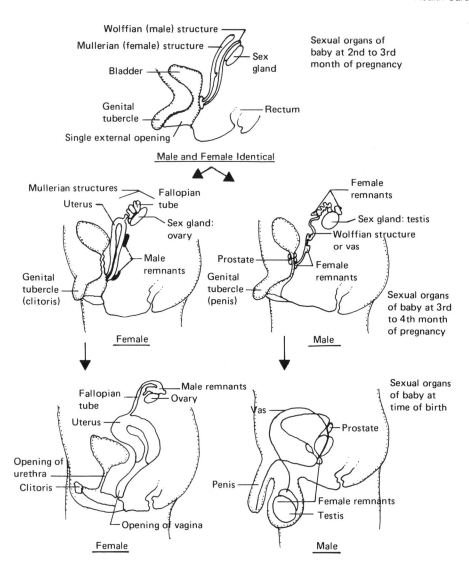

Figure 16-3. Differentiation of internal sex organs in the human fetus.

onward is because she has two X chromosomes, so a defective gene on one X chromosome can be suppressed by the second X. The male's Y chromosome does not carry any genes to act as a mediating force for his X chromosome.[8]

At birth, female infants are smaller in length and weight, have less muscle mass, are less active, but are more advanced developmentally. They have greater sensitivity to touch, taste and pain, and this may include sound and light as well. Females retain their sensitivity into adulthood. Infant girls show greater attentiveness to human faces than do boys, and are able to discriminate between photos of faces and line drawings at 3 months, which boys fail to do. Six-month-old girls show more interest in human faces than in geometrical forms, while the opposite is true of boys. Girls babble more at this age also, and prefer more novel auditory patterns than boys. Differences in perceptual discrimination in favor of girls are still present at 10 months.

Factors are thus present at birth and during infancy which enable girls to be more attentive to the human face and more reactive to complex and varied stimuli. These could permit women to become more sensitive to other humans and more perceptive of many types of input. Such characteristics are assets to women's care-taking functions, but can also be used by society to increase their susceptibility to social approval. Boys, on the other hand, can be pushed by cultural expectations to place greater interest in things than people, capitalizing upon their somewhat lesser human orientation and sensitivity in infancy.

Infants of both sexes are affectionate and social by biological nature, though it appears females have a slight edge over males. Infant girls attach earlier to their mothers and are more distressed by separation, showing stranger anxiety about 2½ months sooner than boys, and crying more for their mothers when separated. Newborn girls do more sympathetic crying in response to another infant's crying. Boys startle more both in sleeping and waking states, have periods of penile erection and are generally more irritable. Mothers handle babies differently according to sex. Boys are held farther away, more often in a standing or sitting position, are stimulated and aroused more, and attended more frequently during their first 3 weeks because they cry and fuss more. Girls are held closer and more gently, sleep more and cry less, and are imitated more by their mothers who feel more at ease and have a sense of sameness with female babies. As boys are harder to pacify, by 3 months mothers attend them less when they cry, while girls receive more attention when crying at this age. Girls respond better to mother's intervention and boys are less consolable, attesting to smoother interaction between mothers and their infant girls.

Infants are aggressive when physically uncomfortable or in need of attention. Aggression is initiated to restore mother's lost ministrations. Toddlers become angry over habit training and fight over possessions. Older children become angry over insults, and their aggression becomes more person-oriented and retaliatory. Rather than simply instrumental, their aggression is hostile as they try to retrieve their dignity. The immediate stimuli for aggression, whether instrumental or hostile, are the same in both girls and boys; thus their "aggressive equipment" is the same. However, numerous studies have shown that boys are much more aggressive and hostile, and that girls have more positive attitudes toward other people; these

same findings hold true for adults. It appears that boys and men are more aggressive because there are more cultural pressures operating against their affectionateness.[9]

Girls bring qualities to the interaction with their mothers that produce responses leading to a smoother relationship. This feeds back into the girl's sociability, creating close ties. Boys also bring certain qualities, but these create a sense of differentness in the mother and a more uncomfortable relationship. Sociability is not reinforced as much, and the maternal tie is not as close. This differential treatment of infants is setting the groundwork for personality and behavioral differences typical of women and men.

Socialization into Sex Roles

As soon as a baby is born and the shape of the genitals perceived, a chain of communication is set into motion based upon "Its a girl!" or "Its a boy!" This communication is passed from person to person and encompasses all people the baby ever encounters; day to day, year to year, from birth to death. Communication based on sexual differences is so universal and habitual that most people are unaware that they are shaping the child's gender identity, that there could be options in their response to the child's signals, and that there is no preordained eternal verity dictating the expressions of sexual dimorphism.

Parents treat girls and boys differently. This begins with pink and blue color coding at birth, subtle differences in tone of voice, use of sex-appropriate pronouns, more frequent verbal interaction with girls, rougher handling for boys, touching boys less often and in fewer places, comforting and cuddling girls more, and distinctly different types of dress.As children grow, girls are expected to be neater and cleaner, to sit with thighs together, to adopt feminine posture and body movements, and to wear more adornments. Girls' hair is kept longer, brushed and curled, decorated with ribbons and clips, and their interest in clothes and appearance encouraged. The child's core gender identity has taken form by 18 months of age.[10]

Toys and Play. At 13 months babies do not show clear-cut preferences for sex-appropriate toys, but by 3 years they are aware that boys should not play with dolls. When given male and female dolls and asked to match these to their own sex, children were inconsistent in their choice at age 3, but were usually accurate by age 4. By age 5 to 6 both sexes correctly match the sex of dolls, themselves, and their future role as parent, though boys do this earlier than girls. Children prefer same-sex playmates by age 2. By age 6 to 7 gender-appropriate play preferences are strongly established, although boys are more uniformly masculine in preferences than girls are uniformly feminine. These differences are expanded in games of later childhood, which may contribute to developing different skills. Girls are encouraged to play quietly and reconstruct domestic roles, while boys play active and rough games. Because boys intercept a moving ball more often in their games, they build experience in visual-motor coordination, and judgment of distance, speed, and trajectory. This probably contributes to later superiority in mathematical and spatial ability.[11]

DISTINGUISHING FEMALE AND MALE ROLES.   Observation of women and men around them, subtle reinforcement, and explicit instruction enable children to distinguish female from male roles. Books and pictures provide role models for childhood and adult behavior. The overwhelming majority of children's books portray women in a stereotyped and limited way, identifying them as wives and mothers who receive praise for attractiveness, and have status by virtue of their relationship with important men. Men are shown in a wide variety of occupations, admired for their achievements, intelligence, and daring. Girls are taught to have low aspirations because so few opportunities are open to them. The family and home is to be their focus, or their work world consists of glamour and service. Television and films reinforce these traditional concepts of women.[12]

SEX ROLE PREFERENCE.   At age 3, both girls and boys decidedly prefer the mother role. Small children like best the parent who caters to their material needs, expresses affection for them, plays with them most, and punishes them least. By age 5, however, most boys and a significant number of girls prefer the masculine role. Girls desire to be boys more often

than boys wish to be girls, and boys show a much stronger preference for the masculine role than girls do the feminine one. As each year passes, more girls want to identify with the masculine role, and fewer boys with the feminine role. There is a social class difference in this, with upper- and middle-class boys preferring the male role strikingly more often than lower-class boys.

Children clearly perceive the superior status and privileges of the masculine role, except in lower classes where it is not so prestigious. They learn it is better to be a man than a woman, because men exhibit the traits which our society rewards with privilege and prestige. As children grow into their teens, they increasingly ascribe desirable traits to boys and undesirable ones to girls. Boys express a progressively better opinion of themselves, while girls' self-concepts progressively decrease.

TAKING ON SEX ROLES.   Although the male adult role is preferable, boys experience difficulty learning appropriate sex-role behavior due to lack of continuous male role models, the rigidity and harshness of masculine sex-role requirements, and the negative nature of the learning process. By age 2, boys have become aware they are different from their mothers. The boy must work harder to get her affection, but soon renounces this or finds himself in conflict with his father's rights to mother. To become like the powerful owner of mother, the source of supply, the valued role, boys must give up much affectionateness as well as other "feminine" qualities. As boys have less exposure to male role models, they often pattern themselves after a male stereotype and show exaggerated masculine behavior, encouraged by male peer groups. Demands that boys exhibit masculine behavior come much earlier and are enforced more vigorously than with girls, with a strong emphasis on *not* engaging in feminine (sissy) behavior. The boy's anxiety is provoked; he is asked to do something not clearly defined for reasons he cannot appreciate, and enforced with threats, punishments, and anger by those closest to him. He strains to be masculine, in virtual panic at being caught doing something feminine, and is often hostile toward anything hinting at femininity, even women themselves.[13] With his basically affectionate nature in conflict with demands for dehumanization, the boy has more trouble with gender identity, and men may find their fury and longing fusing into sadism, violence, sexual abberations, or dissociative thought disorders.

Girls have a consistent role model, the same-sex parent with whom they can readily identify. They are allowed a wider range of behaviors and are punished less severely for deviation (being a tomboy). Due to heightened perceptiveness and sensitivity to people, girls are better able to assess and anticipate parental wishes. This, combined with greater verbal ability, enables girls to minimize discord. They are less pressured to give up infantile behaviors such as dependency. Because parents want their daughters to be passive and nurturing, they discourage assertion and independence. The self-concept of the girl remains linked to the evaluation of others, she has a higher need for approval and acceptance, and her self-esteem rests largely on how she is valued and responded to in relationships. An internal frame of reference is frequently not developed, nor is an independent sense of self.

The girl's socialization is also anxiety-provoking, however, because children understand the relative worth of the two sexes early. Girls also find many "boy's activities" intrinsically more enjoyable and exciting. The role the girl is being pushed into is clearly not the more desirable one. Being encouraged to adopt and perform a set of behaviors held in low esteem causes anxiety and considerable internal conflict, for the girl realizes that her loved model (mother) receives neither recognition nor satisfaction from these activities.[14] Mother, whom the girl is like and with whom her identity is so intertwined, is to be scorned as weak and powerless, the devalued sex. And yet, the girl must follow suit. With affectionateness encouraged yet exploited in the service of others, and the very role she is forced to adopt the source of her low status, the woman is prone to collapse into depression and self-hatred.

The well-socialized girl is a conforming person, very susceptible to cultural values and social expectations. She is forced to be dependent upon people, to seek continual feedback so she can assess whether she is attractive, nurturing, and passive. She must court the acceptance of others in order to obtain those experiences which can establish her appropriate sex-typed behavior. In keeping with the expectation that they will devote their lives to others, women are trained to understand and respond to people.

The well-socialized boy is self-reliant, using his internal scale of values as a measure of self-worth. His system of self-esteem is relatively independent of the evaluation of others, and he is admired when he pursues individual principles despite opposition, or selects behaviors he believes appropriate. In keeping with the expectation that they will venture into the world and make a place for themselves, men are trained to understand the workings of things. They may also be trained to accept the idea that people may be treated as if they were things.

SCHOOL EXPERIENCES. The educational system generally reinforces sex-role stereotypes. Girls are subjected to a series of pressures to conform to traditional feminine roles, beginning with the message that they are not as important as boys. The people that students study are predominately men—more stories are written about men, men are portrayed as the bearers of knowledge and wisdom, and rarely are women mentioned as important in history, government, or science. Girls are steered toward subjects which reinforce traditional roles, and away from masculine classes such as physics, advanced algebra, and shop. There are several well-established differences in intellectual functioning between the sexes, reflecting the social prescription that men's assignment is to master things and women's to understand people.

Verbal ability. Girls exceed boys in most aspects of verbal performance throughout the preschool and early school years. Girls say their first word earlier, speak more clearly and at a younger age, use longer sentences, and are more fluent. Boys catch up on vocabulary by the time they enter school, but girls learn to read sooner, and more boys are in remedial programs. Through all the school years, girls do better in grammar, spelling and word fluency. (Language also reflects social ability.) Girls' earlier verbalization and consistent linguistic superiority may be due to earlier and stronger development of left cerebral dominance; this may be a genetic effect amplified by culturally encouraged people-orientation.

Number ability. Girls learn to count at an earlier age than boys, a fact that is probably related to their verbal ability. There are no consistent differences in arithmetic skill until high school, when boys show clear superiority. Girls tend to drop out of this area as it is thought unnecessary to their roles and even a handicap to femininity. There is an obvious connection between mastery of mathematics and performing well in the world of things and the marketplace.

Spatial ability. Very young children do not differ in spatial tasks, but by the early school years boys do consistently better, and this difference continues into adulthood. Spatial ability involves the capacity to organize information about objects in space, such as aiming at a target, arranging objects in a two-dimensional pattern, or having a good sense of direction. This ability is necessary in dealing with things and inanimate objects, and the male organization of self with clear boundaries fosters this.

Field independence. The ability to keep an object separate in perception from the context in which it is embedded is called field independence, since it requires separating the object out of its field. Men are better at this, partly because of their capacity to visualize space. There seems a brief period, around age 5, when girls are superior in this disembedding skill. However, by late adolescence boys are clearly superior. An overlapping concept involved with field independence is the capacity to group different objects according to common elements. Boys generally use analytic groupings more often, but the age at which this occurs is not clearly established.[15]

Field independence and analytic grouping are used as a measure of analytic ability, and thus intelligence. As sex differences are not apparent generally until high school, these abilities are probably acquired as a differential result of socialization. The superior linguistic ability of girls is apparent before age 2, however, suggesting an innate factor. Even the definition of intelligence thus has a sex bias.

Gaps in the Socialization Process

It is obvious that not all women take on the culturally prescribed feminine role. This results because pressures on women to conform are not unidimensional, and women do not internalize the feminine role completely. During school girls learn the value society places on achievement, success, competition, leadership, and productivity. Often girls are socialized in an ambivalent fashion, being rewarded both for typically feminine behavior and also for some typically masculine behavior. Parents are proud when their daughter excels at school, is elected to class office, is outstanding in sports, or achieves in other ways. Double messages frequently are delivered, such as "do well" but "don't do too well."

Women are motivated to achieve, as part of an unflowering of their inherent potential, the same as men. George Bernard Shaw expressed this concept nicely:

> People sometimes wonder what is the secret of the extraordinary knowledge of women which I show in my plays. They very often accuse me of having acquired it by living a most abandoned life. But I never acquired it. I have always assumed that a woman is a person exactly like myself, and that is how the trick is done.[16]

However, there is often great anxiety when women attempt to achieve outside traditional feminine roles. Women fear success because it often implies a loss of femininity in cultural terms. Pursuing a successful career is associated with strong fears of social rejection and doubts about normality. The bright woman worries about both failure and success; if she fails she is not living up to her own standards; if she succeeds she is not living up to social expectations. Men do not experience such ambivalence, for they are actively encouraged to do well. Women's ambition is thus thwarted by the motive to avoid success, as competition will lead to negative consequences: social disapproval, loss of popularity, loss of femininity, suggestion of abnormality, distrust or outright prejudice from men.[17]

A different type of socialization often occurs for the black girl who, instead of being discouraged from aspiring to college or a career, is often actively supported by her family. As black girls grow, they believe few men can fit the model of protector and supporter, and may be discouraged from reliance on men and marriage for future security. Black mothers who headed their families had higher educational aspirations for their daughters than their sons. But, in intact black families, there was still equal aspiration for girls and for boys, in contrast to white families.[18]

PATHS AND OBSTACLES TO EQUALITY

The status of women within any particular society may be assessed by an examination of these common activities:

1. Political expression. Do women have rights (to join in community decisions, to vote, hold property, or public office) that are now enjoyed by men? Do important segments of the female population show clear signs of dissatisfaction or a sense of injustice compared with men? Is a social movement for women's rights in progress?
2. Work and mobility. Are women's movements deliberately more restricted than men's? Are they active in the labor force? Do the jobs they hold enjoy equal rank with those held by men? Is their pay roughly equivalent and do they enjoy the same amount of leisure?
3. Family formation, duration and size. Are women subject to greater control and limitations in their choice of a marriage partner than men? Do they have the same right to divorce? What are the consequences if they are single or widowed? What are the restrictions on their movements beyond the family?
4. Education. Do females have the same access to educational opportunities as boys? Is their curriculum the same? Do they reach the same levels of educational attainment?
5. Health and sexual control. Are females subject to higher mortality or more serious physical or mental illnesses than males? Are they prevented from limiting conceptions and birth?
6. Cultural expression. Do women make identifiable contributions to religious culture, the arts, or practical artifacts and inventions? Are they symbolically portrayed to be as valuable and worthy of respect as are men?[19]

In the United States, with its diversity of regional styles, multicultural heritage and socioeconomic disparities, the positions individual women or subgroups may occupy range from conceptually free and equal to clearly secondary and dependent. However, social structures are not fully supportive of equality between the sexes and the powerful process of female socialization still works to limit women's options. The repercussions of several changes in the late 20th century are now being felt in all major institutions of our society. Urbanization and job specialization, invention of machines to do most heavy work, and the change in family ecology as women have fewer children and these children spend larger portions of their time in schools, are having significant effects. It is increasingly possible for women and men to do each other's jobs, with a marked shift from the two-sphere theory of sex roles (men as providers, women as caretakers) to a shared role pattern. Efforts are underway to establish rules in social institutions that are fair to both sexes, and more recognition given to qualities of women's experience which have previously been devalued or overlooked.

Given these changes, there is often a question of why more women do not take advantage of their new opportunities and attain high levels of achievement or recognition. Again, the effects of attitudes and values often outweigh the potential of the spirit:

> We overlook the fact that the society has spent twenty years carefully marking the woman's ballot for her, and has nothing to lose in that twenty-first year by pretending to let her cast it for the alternative of her choice. Society has controlled not her alternatives but her motivation to choose any but one of those alternatives.[20]

Marriage and the Family

Significant changes are happening in the American family as unprecedented numbers of women enter the work force, the childbearing period is compressed, women have a longer middle age, and the percentage of divorces is greater. These changes are reflected in the efforts of many couples to work out a different division of labor, the emergence of different marriage forms, and governmental measures to assume support for certain family functions as women are less often full-time housewives. Husbands are sharing more in housekeeping activities and child care, wives assuming more responsibility for family income. In many families there is strain around changing the traditional division of labor, however, often resulting in the working wife being burdened with the domestic demands as well as her duties at work, creating an integrative crisis for women.

Pressures exist to redraft marriage, divorce, custody and tax laws to treat women and men in a more egalitarian way. Marriage is commonly considered a contract freely entered into by partners on an equal footing, but in fact there are many inequities for women. The husband can legally force his wife to have intercourse against her will, for by definition of law he cannot be guilty of raping his own wife. The compulsory nature of sex in marriage extends to the wife's rights to intercourse also, but she has a harder time insisting on her husband's performance of conjugal duties. The household services a wife performs are part of her marital duties, and are such an essential part of what the law considers a husband entitled to, that it does not recognize any agreement between spouses that the wife be paid for these services.

The legal responsibilities of a wife are to live in the home established by her husband, perform domestic chores, and care for husband and children. The husband is obligated to provide her with basic maintenance and necessities according to his income. She has no right to any part of his cash income, nor legal voice in spending it. Domicile laws hold that a wife is obliged to accompany her husband wherever he establishes a household, or she can be charged with desertion. In community property states, husbands generally have rights to manage and control property, with superior rights and interest in it.[21]

Though reasons for granting divorce vary, there is a trend toward no-fault laws. Current estimates are that nearly 40 percent of all first marriages during the 1970s will end in divorce, making divorce almost half as prevalent as marriage. Throughout the country divorce settlements are changing the traditional practice of awarding child custody to the woman and requiring support payments from the man, reflecting less sex stereotyping.

Perhaps nothing better symbolizes women's secondary status than the practice of name change after marriage. By assuming her husband's surname, a woman loses her identity and becomes submerged, both psychologically and civilly, into the man's. The woman who lived for some 20 years as a certain person no longer exists; yet men undergo no such drastic identity change upon marrying. The custom of taking a husband's name is a remnant of when wives were the legal property of husbands, and is typical of patriarchal systems. Patrilineal descent also emphasizes the importance of the man over the woman. Increasingly women are retaining their birth names after marriage, or hyphenating surnames. Petty harassment and

some legal penalties may result from this, though states vary in their laws and legal opinions. Under the common law codes, any person has the right to use any name chosen as long as this is not done to defraud someone else. Under the civil law codes, a woman does not lose her patronymic name through marriage, as her legal name never varies and she never acquires her husband's name by law.

Women generally use their husband's name because of social custom, and not because the law requires it, although most are not aware of this. Only one state, Hawaii, has a statute (passed in 1860) requiring wives to adopt their husband's names. This came about because of the strong tradition for native Hawaiian women to use their own names. The Hawaiian law was changed in 1976 to allow each partner to declare the surname each may use upon marriage. Many states require people to file name change petitions, reregister to vote, and notify officials to retain a valid driver's license, motor vehicle registration, or certificate of title when their name changes "by marriage or otherwise." Some states have no laws regulating name change, and any person may lawfully change her or his name merely by using it exclusively and consistently.[22]

The use of titles in address also discriminates against women. Assigning the title Miss or Mrs. immediately designates a woman's marital status; not so the ambiguous Mr. The sexual double standard is involved, as sexual respectability and availability are announced to the world for women but not for men. The rapid spread of women's using Ms. testifies to their frustration with this daily reminder of sex-linked inequities.

Income tax and social security legislation discriminate against women by assuming that most married women are occupied as wives/mothers and are supported by a wage-earning husband. Income-splitting and joint return tax provisions benefit couples when the wife has no paid work, and the deduction system often penalizes the double-income family. Social security benefits are calculated on the assumption that wives are dependent on their husbands, and often retired female workers find that benefits based on their own earnings are less than their benefits as dependent wives. The unpaid contribution of the wife/mother is not well recognized. However, before 1978 if a woman divorced before 20 years of marriage (even if she maintained the home for 19 years), she could not claim any social security benefits.[23] The time limit for these social security benefits is now 10 years. This unpaid labor of women in the home is not included in the Gross National Product, nor do women derive retirement benefits or labor law protections regarding minimum wage, vacation, hours, environmental safety, overtime compensation, and so forth.

Education

The education system presently encourages males and hampers females, as it is primarily geared to train men for their careers, and generally rewards the male rather than female role. Implicit and explicit discrimination against women is apparent in male-oriented educational goals and values, sex stereotyping in the curriculum, small numbers of women in upper faculty ranks, calendars and admissions policies which provide barriers to women, and differences in family support mechanisms.

Title IX of the Higher Education Act of 1972 prohibits discrimination on the basis of sex in educational programs or activities receiving federal financial assistance. This provides a legal basis for protest against unequal treatment of women, and prevents a sex-tracking system where girls are required to take home economics and are limited in sports, while boys must take shop and more extensive sports, and opens all classes to both sexes. The Women's Educational Equity Act of 1974 calls for development of new curricula, programs for women on all levels, improved counseling, women's resource centers, and community education about opportunities for women. Hopefully these will change the statistics on women's achieving degrees and college positions.

Although women's grades in high school and college are almost uniformly higher than men's, their attrition rates are also much higher. Women cluster in fine arts, education, and the humanities in college (50 percent of the student body) and are decreasingly found in social sciences (33 percent) and biological and physical sciences (20 percent). Reasons for these disparities reside in the differential socialization of girls and boys, the institutional encouragement of boys and discouragement of girls to cultivate spatial, analytic and mathematic skills, the unequal impact of family responsibilities, and the discriminatory structures and attitudes within the educational system itself.

Because 65 percent of public school teachers are women but only 15 percent of these are principals, young girls are denied leadership models. Texts and curricula communicate a narrow range of roles for women and reinforce the importance of men. Counselors discourage girls from certain fields and careers. Family responsibilities weigh more heavily on women and delay and obstruct their progress through college and graduate school. A wife is an asset to the male student, however, who receives more financial assistance for "dependents," and who is freed from personal maintenance services to pursue his studies. Women in graduate school rely more on outside financial support from family while men obtain loans or employment; thus working and lower-class women may be unable to pursue higher education due to lack of family financial resources.

The full-time teaching or full-time student model, with minimal effort to accommodate absences due to childbearing or care of small children, serves to handicap women in professional pursuits. Continuing education now offers an opportunity for many women to resume their education, but still graduate degrees require intensive and concentrated study.

Occupation

During the 1970s the proportion of women in the work force has grown to 44 percent. However, women are clustered in a few fields with one-fourth of all women workers employed as secretaries, domestics, school teachers, and waitresses. Women generally stay at the lower rungs of the career ladder, receive lower salaries than men, and are underrepresented in the higher ranks in every occupation. Very few are in the most prestigious professions (9 percent of physicians, 5 percent of lawyers, and 28 percent of college professors and administrators are women.)[25]

There is no single dominant profile of the working woman. A woman is more likely to work if she has a good education, her children are older, or her husband's income is not high. It is suggested that women remain on the lower end of the occupational scale because they must invest more of their time and efforts in their families, and because of sex labels on certain kinds of work. Women and minority workers are offered marginal, seasonal and parttime jobs more often because they are less well trained and perceived as more likely to quit. Employers are less willing to invest fringe

Table 16-1
Women and Men in Higher Education 1972-1974[24]

	% of High School Degrees	% of Baccalaureate Degrees	% of Masters Degrees	% of Doctoral Degrees	% College Instructors	% Asst. Professors	% Associate Prof.	% Full Professors
Women	50	43.7	40.6	15.8	47.6	25	6	3
Men	50	56.3	59.4	84.2	52.4	75	94	97

benefits, security, on-the-job training and pensions to these fringe workers. Therefore, women are at a disadvantage in promotions, pay and security.

The earnings of fulltime women workers were 66 percent those of males in the early 1970s. This represents little change from the 50 to 60 percent of men's wages that women were paid in 1910.[26] Women in the professions are less likely to achieve at the same level as men because they more often interrupt their careers, either by taking several years off to raise small children, or by leaving positions because of their husband's change of job, often having to settle for what they can find around their new home.

It is evident that long-term structural conditions and attitudes in industrial society perpetuate women as second-class workers. There are several legal remedies for sex discrimination in employment now in effect, but the problem is inadequate enforcement. The Equal Pay Act prohibits paying a woman at a lower rate than a man for doing substantially the same work, if the jobs require equal skill. Title VII of the Civil Rights Act of 1964 prohibits discrimination on the basis of race, color, religion, sex, or national origin in all aspects of employment. Executive Order 11246 (1965) prohibits discrimination in employment under federal contracts, and Executive Order 11478 (1969) prohibits discrimination in employment by the federal government itself. Litigation arising from these laws has removed restrictions on hours or conditions of work applying to women only, because the effects of these were to deprive women of access to higher paid jobs which might require, for instance, overtime work, nighttime work, or lifting certain weights. Also overridden was the practice of employers not to hire women with preschool age children.[27]

Enforcement of antidiscrimination laws is not enough, in itself, to remedy the barriers to women's full participation in the occupational sphere. Work schedules and production techniques will have to be restructured, provisions made for institutional supports to women's family roles (such as child care or home help services), and retraining and counseling services made widely available. Maternity benefits and leaves are important to facilitate equal opportunities for women, but the recent U.S. Supreme Court ruling that employers need not include maternity among health benefits (yet often include many types of elective surgery for men) is a serious setback.[28]

Politics and Law

In 1963 the Commission on the Status of Women reported that many states treated women inequitably through laws on jury service, child custody, guardianship, property rights, inheritance, and protective work legislation and discriminated against women in employment and education. Although the due process clauses of the 5th and 14th Amendments refer to "any person," the courts previously had refused to consider women fully "persons" and generally supported the constitutionality of laws treating women as an inferior class. The U.S. Supreme Court elucidated this view in a decision made a century ago upholding the refusal of the State of Illinois to allow women to practice law:

> The natural and proper timidity and delicacy which belongs to the female sex evidently unfits it for many of the occupations of civil life. The constitution of the family organization, which is founded in the divine ordinance, as well as in the nature of things, indicates the domestic sphere as that which properly belongs to the domain and functions of womanhood.... The paramount destiny and mission of women are to fulfill the noble and benign offices of wife and mother. This is the law of the Creator.[29]

In a country guaranteeing freedom of religion, separation of church and state, and equality under the Constitution, such a judgment is a travesty on justice. However, court rulings up until the early 1970s continued to reflect the prevailing social attitudes that women belonged in the home, were rightly treated as "a class by herself," were the reproductive instruments of the state, and needed protection and guidance of men. As recently as 1961 the U.S. Supreme Court upheld a Florida law treating men and women differently in selection for jury duty, noting that the "woman is still regarded as the center of home and family life."[30] This use of women's functions in the home as a basis for treating women and men differently under the law has relegated the woman to a service class, in which her status under the Constitution is that of a servant to man and the State.

In 1973 the U.S. Supreme Court made a landmark decision in *Frontiero v. Richardson* when it ruled against armed services regulations that denied dependents of female members the same benefits as dependents of male members. A more enlightened view of the status of women under the Constitution was expressed:

> ... in part because of the high visibility of the sex characteristic, women still face pervasive, although at times more subtle, discrimination in our educational institutions, on the job market and perhaps most conspicuously, in the political arena ... statutory distinctions between the sexes often have the effect of invidiously relegating the entire class of females to inferior legal status without regard to the actual capabilities of its individual members. ... With these considerations in mind, we can only conclude that classifications based upon sex, like classifications based upon race, alienage, or national original, are inherently suspect. ... [31]

The most powerful force in changing the legal and political status of women was the rise of the new feminist movement in the 1950s and 1960s. The efforts of the National Organization of Women (NOW), the Women's Equity Action League, and the National Women's Political Caucas promoted enforcement of the new antidiscrimination laws, supported court cases representing feminist positions, and monitored new legislation affecting women's status. Consciousness-raising groups were an outgrowth of women's activities in the civil

rights movement, in which they were excluded from leadership and often relegated to traditional feminine functions. Feminist sentiment has had an effect on the larger U.S. population; a 1971 Harris poll showed that 42 percent of women favored the aims of the women's movement and 41 percent opposed them, while in a 1975 poll 59 percent favored and 28 percent opposed them.[32]

Other legal breakthroughs occurred in the U.S. Supreme Court's decisions in *Griswold v. Connecticut*, which in 1965 struck down state laws against dissemination and use of contraceptives, and *Roe v. Wade* and *Doe v. Bolton* which in 1973 upheld women's Constitutional rights to abortion. These decisions provided women the right to physical self-determination and control of the uses of their body.

The Equal Rights Amendment (ERA) was finally passed by Congress in 1972, after being introduced every year since 1923. It states simply that "Equality of rights under the law shall not be denied or abridged by the United States or any State on account of sex." Proponents argue this is needed to provide a certain and consistent remedy to the hodgepodge of state laws, regulations, and informal practices which treat women unfairly. It would provide a uniform basis for designing alternatives as laws are changed. Primarily, though, it would be a national statement that women are full and equal citizens and that the democratic principle does apply to all. Opponents declare the ERA is not necessary because of the several laws, orders and court opinions which prohibit discrimination on the basis of sex. They fear that the implications of a broad Constitutional amendment would, for instance, mandate women and men to use the same toilet facilities and dormitories, and do battle side-by-side in armed services. Such separation would be legally permissible if done to protect rights of privacy and did not operate to deny any individual of rights. The underlying goal of opponents, of course, is to maintain separate (and inferior) status for women. The backlash to women's rights is apparent in the failure of the ERA to achieve ratification by 38 states to date, and the attempt of some states to rescind their prior ratification.

Women have become more visible in the political arena, but still are poorly represented in leadership positions. In 1975 a total of 51 women were serving in high offices such as governor, lieutenant governor, and secretary of state. There were 599 women in state legislatures in 1974.[33] In 1976, a total of 18 women (and 417 men) serviced in the U.S. House of Representatives.[34] The U.S. Senate in 1977 had no female members, and a woman has never been elected to the Senate completely in her own right. Only 11 women have ever been Senators, all either appointed to fill vacancies or elected after being appointed to complete a dead husband's term. Muriel Humphrey's appointment in 1978 to complete her deceased husband Hubert's term continues this pattern.

Images and Interpersonal Behavior

Cultural expression of female images is changing and contradictory. While many forces in media, religion, and the arts have recently shown remarkable willingness to question old symbols and role models, counterforces continue to support traditional images. Polarization regarding the appropriate images for women is readily apparent. On one hand, women have penetrated the male bastion of television newscasters, launched successful feminist publications, and established scholarly women's studies programs. Wearing pants has been popularized, and changes are occurring in language use with such terms as "chairperson" and growing awareness that calling adult women "girls" is inappropriate. Political images provide more respect for women as the public is exposed to such competent Congresspeople as Barbara Jordan of Texas and Elizabeth Holtzman of New York. Agitation of women for ordination has questioned the legitimacy of an all-male priesthood. There has been a revival of women writers and artists, and a challenge of the male definition of what constitutes great art. Women historians are exploring their sex's contributions to building society and promoting a focus on other channels of power and influence than those illuminated by the chronicles of war, battle and succession of kings.

On the other hand, media portrayals of women are still heavily weighted toward their household maintenance and personal nurturant roles. Female scholarship is often suspect and subject to sex bias in critique. Daily, women receive nonverbal reminders of their inferior status through print and electronic images showing females serving, tending to, and admiring males. Women as sex objects are still used to sell a wide variety of products.

In interpersonal relations, there are many indicators of female deference and submission. Symmetrical familiarity occurs in interactions between equals, but commonly men will touch women more often, use women's first names while they are addressed more formally, and will initiate familiar interactions, such as joking with the opposite sex, more often than women. Men have greater latitude than women in assuming body positions and in swearing, and they interrupt, challenge and question more often in discussions. It is well-ingrained that men are the initiators of intimacy, as they call women for dates and propose marriage. Clothes also communicate status, and women's styles tend to restrict action and reveal body contours, instead of being comfortable and functional as are men's clothes.

Self-disclosure generally has an inverse relationship with power, and women are expected to reveal not only more of their bodies but more of themselves. Greater access by one person to information about another person provides a resource the other person does not have. Although this may be more apparent than real power, it still conveys a status difference. Women have been noticed to have a smaller "personal space," being approached more closely than men with a shorter initial speaking distance. Gestures of submission are more frequent in women, including gazing at men to obtain cues of social approval, tilting the head when looking directly at men, and hesitating or apologizing. Staring directly, pointing and touching can be subtle nonverbal threats, and the corresponding gestures of submission are lowering the eyes, falling silent when interrupted or pointed at, and cuddling to the touch. Such gestures of submission are considered socially desirable secondary characteristics of the female role.[35]

Health and Sexual Control

Women have lower mortality rates than men until very old age, past 85 years of age. The life expectancy of a woman who was 60 years old in the early 1970s is nearly 80 years, while that of a man in the same situation is slightly over 75. The health problems of women increasingly include the chronic diseases of middle age and illnesses resulting from stress and tension. Emotional or mental illnesses take a heavy toll among women. In the control of reproduction, the U.S. birth rate is at a record low of 14.9 births per thousand people, and the fertility rate is 1.9 children per woman. Contraception and abortion information and services are widely utilized by women of diverse backgrounds. However, many women are concerned about dangers and side effects of current contraceptives, and urge research on male methods and safer female methods. There is a strong antiabortion movement promoting a Constitutional amendment prohibiting abortion and laws restricting access. The recent U.S. Supreme Court ruling that it is constitutional to deny federal medical aid assistance for elective abortions reinstitutes a double standard of care for the poor woman.[36]

As part of women's activities to improve health care, there is greater emphasis on self-help, preventive care, and consumer knowledge. The health professions are feeling the impact of women's changing roles, as the overwhelming numbers of women in health (primarily nurses) become aware of their low status and relative powerlessness. The consciousness-raising of nurses is spurred by books such as Marlene Grissum and Carol Spengler's *Womanpower and Health Care*[37] and Jo Ann Ashley's *Hospitals, Paternalism & the Role of the Nurse.*[38] The repetition of society's attitudes and expectations of women in the microcosm of health care delivery led to the traditional role of the nurse: a woman who was compassionate, intuitive, cooperative, and subordinate. The physician's role reflected that of men in society: intelligent, decisive, objective, and dominant. Sexism has been described as the most fundamental problem in nursing,[39] and the last several years have seen a tremendous upsurge among nurses to improve their image, attain positions of greater power and influence, increase their earnings, and achieve a more colleagial relationship with medicine. The nurse practitioner movement reflects one such approach to changing nursing's role, as nurses seek greater voice in health care policy and decision-making and greater impact on the health delivery system.

The medical profession often fosters an ideology of sex differences which perpetuates the inferiority of women. The usual stereotypes are present regarding women's biological and emotional makeup, with assumptions made about women's capabilities and drives which reflect a male sex bias. Misinformation about female sexuality is still prevalent among physicians. The social status quo is maintained when physicians define women who are dis-tressed or unhappy with their present lives as ill or maladjusted,[40] and avoid dealing with difficult problems of change and conflict by overprescribing antidepressants or tranquilizers.

The Women's Movement

American women began a revival of the movement for women's rights in the 1960s when Betty Friedan described the "problem that has no name" in her pivotal book, *The Feminine Mystique.*[41] With prosperity and material comforts beyond any previously known, women yet felt a sense of dissatisfaction, a yearning for something more than their domestic existence. Although this seemed a new phenomenon, it actually was a continuation of a long struggle which had laid dormant for 50 years. American feminism has its roots in conditions of the colonial period when women sought greater freedom in the religious realm, and continued through the early industrial period of the late 1800s as they pushed for rights to control their earnings, retain their property, vote, and receive an education. The movement constricted its goals to winning the vote in the early 1900s, although there were always fringe groups desiring greater rights and more equality for women. The economic crisis of the 1930s and World War II preoccupied national efforts, and a striving for return to normality and recovery of lost or delayed goals led to an exaggeration of traditional female and male characteristics in the decades after the war. By the 1960s, however, women's desire for something more than the wife/mother domestic role gained momentum that led to challenge of the old order of sex roles, and by 1970 women's liberation was a household phrase. Feminism has emerged as a strong national force, with well-known leaders and an ideology which is bringing about many changes in economic, educational, social, and political fields.

Among the goals in the National Organization of Women's "Bill of Rights" are an equal rights Constitutional amendment, enforcement of laws banning sex discrimination in employment, maternity leave rights in employment and social security benefits, tax deductions for home and child care expenses for working parents, child care day centers, equal job training and allowance opportunities for women in poverty, and the right of women to control their reproductive lives.[42]

As sex role differences are felt to be a result of common expectations for behavior growing out of society's fundamental beliefs, values and myths, feminists believe that changes must be brought about in both cultural orientations and institutional structures so a blurring and overlapping can occur between the roles of women and men. Rigid role expectations are felt to be equally dehumanizing for both sexes, and in a society affirming human freedom there should be wide possibilities for individual expression. Some of the components of such a society would include an economic system based on merit, definitions of manhood freed from dependence on violence and aggression, shared family maintenance and support functions, honest sexual relations, and the elimination of sexism in education, law, religion, literature, manners and fashion.[43]

PROVIDING HEALTH CARE TO WOMEN

When the health care provider meets the woman patient, any number of the factors discussed in this chapter may have affected the individual woman's life. Ranging from the radical feminist to the woman content with her traditional role, women will possess a wide variety of personal values and ascribe to many different life styles. It is the art of nursing which enables a response appropriate to individual needs, open to multiple definitions of worth and nonjudgmental in the professional sphere. A new candidness in health care, and a growing orientation toward partnership with the patient in management of health problems and illnesses, will enhance the process of providing truly individualized care.

Whenever problems with health occur, the repercussions are felt by the people with whom the patient has attachments, and in a more remote way, by the community. Even a minor illness, such as a bladder infection or vaginitis, raises questions such as why did it occur now and how can future occurrences be prevented. The answers involve the woman's entire ecology—her relations, her work, her identity and sense of self, nutritional and physiological status, environmental exposures, and the habits and practices of daily living. Part of the health provider's response to women patients can often be founded in an understanding of the effects of women's socialization, following assessment of individual applicability. Another dimension may be added to the treatment rep-

ertoire, through utilizing community resources which assist women in personal growth and development of self-awareness. Women's groups and counselors with expertise in the impact of changing roles are increasingly available, and may be a key component in helping women patients deal with both physical and emotional problems.

NOTES

1. J. Z. Giele and A. C. Smock (eds.), *Women: Roles and Status in Eight Countries* (New York: John Wiley & Sons, 1977), p. 3.
2. V. L. Bullough, *The Subordinate Sex—A History of Attitudes Toward Women* (Baltimore: Penguin Books Inc., 1974), p. 17.
3. Giele and Smock, *Women*, p. 385.
4. H. B. Lewis, *Psychic War in Men and Women* (New York: New York University Press, 1976), p. 30.
5. E. Maccoby and C. Jacklin, *The Psychology of Sex Differences* (Stanford: Stanford University Press, 1974), p. 215.
6. J. Money and A. A. Ehrhardt, *Man & Woman, Boy & Girl* (Baltimore: The Johns Hopkins University Press, 1972), p. 2.
7. M. J. Sherfey, *The Nature & Evolution of Female Sexuality* (New York: Random House, 1972), pp. 37-48.
8. Lewis, *Psychic War*, p. 31.
9. *Ibid.*, pp. 61-86.
10. Money and Ehrhardt, *Man & Woman*, p. 176.
11. *Ibid.*, pp. 180-182.
12. J. Freeman (ed.), *Women: A Feminist Perspective* (Palo Alto, Calif.: Mayfield Publishing Co., 1973), pp. 110-112.
13. *Ibid.*, pp. 113-114.
14. *Ibid.*, pp. 115-117.
15. Lewis, *Psychic War*, pp. 95-100.
16. A. Adams and M. L. Briscoe, *Up Against the Wall, Mother . . .* (Beverly Hills, Calif.: Glencoe Press, A Division of the Macmillan Co., 1971), p. 199.
17. *Ibid.*, pp. 379-386.
18. D. B. Kandel, "Race, Maternal Authority and Adolescent Aspirations." *American Journal of Sociology*, 76, 6 (May 1971): 999-1020.
19. Giele and Smock, *Women*, pp. 4-5.
20. Freeman, *A Feminist Perspective*, p. 133.
21. *Ibid.*, p. 73.
22. S. D. Ross, *The Rights of Women: A Basic ACLU Guide to Women's Rights* (New York: Discus Books/Published by Avon Books, 1973), pp. 239-247.
23. Giele and Smock, *Women*, p. 327.
24. *Ibid.*, pp. 328-331.
25. *Ibid.*, pp. 319-320.
26. *Ibid.*, pp. 322.
27. Freeman, *A Feminist Perspective*, pp. 329-330.
28. "Pregnancy Sick Pay—Another Ruling With Widespread Impact." *U.S. News & World Report*, December 20, 1976, p. 31.
29. *Bradwell v. Illinois*, 83 U.S. (16 Wall.) 130 (1872).
30. *Hoyt v. Florida*, 386 U.S. 57, 62.
31. *Frontiero v. Richardson*, 93 Sup. Ct. 1764.

32. *Women Today*, 1975, p. 72.

33. Giele and Smock, *Women*, p. 317.

34. A. Golenpaul (ed.), *Information Please Almanac* (New York: Simon & Schuster, 1977), p. 31.

35. Freeman, *A Feminist Perspective*, p. 398.

36. M. Denes, "The Abortion Decision: A Case of Moral Myopia." *New Times*, August 5, 1977, p. 17.

37. M. Grissum and C. Spengler, *Womanpower and Health Care* (Boston: Little, Brown & Co., 1976).

38. J. A. Ashley, *Hospitals, Paternalism, & the Role of the Nurse* (New York: Teachers College Press, 1976).

39. V. Cleland, "Sex Discrimination: Nursing's Most Pervasive Problem." *American Journal of Nursing* 71, 8 (August 1971): 1542-1547.

40. R. Levinson, "Sexism in Medicine." *American Journal of Nursing* 76, 3 (March 1976): 426-531.

41. B. Friedan, *The Feminine Mystique* (New York: W.W. Norton, 1963).

42. G. G. Yates, *What Women Want* (Cambridge, Mass.: Harvard University Press, 1975), pp. 45-46.

43. G. Steinem, "What It Would Be Like If Women Win." In M. E. Adelstein and J. G. Pival (eds.), *Women's Liberation* (New York: St. Martin's Press, 1972), pp. 85-88.

Index